Handbook of
Stress, Coping, and Health
Second Edition

Handbook of
Stress, Coping, and Health
Second Edition

Implications for Nursing Research, Theory, and Practice

Edited by
Virginia Hill Rice, PhD, RN, CNS, FAAN
Wayne State University

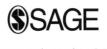

Los Angeles | London | New Delhi
Singapore | Washington DC

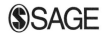

Los Angeles | London | New Delhi
Singapore | Washington DC

FOR INFORMATION:

SAGE Publications, Inc.
2455 Teller Road
Thousand Oaks, California 91320
E-mail: order@sagepub.com

SAGE Publications Ltd.
1 Oliver's Yard
55 City Road
London EC1Y 1SP
United Kingdom

SAGE Publications India Pvt. Ltd.
B 1/I 1 Mohan Cooperative Industrial Area
Mathura Road, New Delhi 110 044
India

SAGE Publications Asia-Pacific Pte. Ltd.
33 Pekin Street #02-01
Far East Square
Singapore 048763

Acquisitions Editor: Christine Cardone
Editorial Assistant: Sarita Sarak
Production Editor: Karen Wiley
Copy Editor: Terri Lee Paulsen
Typesetter: C&M Digitals (P) Ltd.
Proofreader: Allyson Rudolph
Indexer: Joan Shapiro
Cover Designer: Candice Harman
Marketing Manager: Liz Thornton
Permissions Editor: Karen Ehrmann

Printed in the United States of America

Library of Congress Cataloging-in-Publication Data

Handbook of stress, coping, and health : implications for nursing research, theory, and practice / editor, Virginia Hill Rice. — 2nd ed.
p. cm.

Includes bibliographical references and index.

ISBN 978-1-4129-9929-8 (cloth : acid-free paper)

1. Stress (Physiology)—Handbooks, manuals, etc.
2. Stress (Psychology)—Handbooks, manuals, etc.
3. Stress management—Handbooks, manuals, etc.
4. Stress (Psychology)—Research—Methodology—Handbooks, manuals, etc.
5. Nursing—Research—Methodology—Handbooks, manuals, etc.
I. Rice, Virginia Hill.

QP82.2.S8H357 2012
616.9'8—dc23
2011030163

This book is printed on acid-free paper.

11 12 13 14 15 10 9 8 7 6 5 4 3 2 1

CONTENTS

PART V. STRESS, COPING, AND HEALTH: MEDIATING AND MODERATING FACTORS

DETAILED CONTENTS

PART III. STIMULUS-ORIENTED STRESS

PART V. STRESS, COPING, AND HEALTH: MEDIATING AND MODERATING FACTORS

PREFACE

Interest in the phenomena of stress and coping and their relationship to health has reached an all-time high not only in psychology and the behavioral sciences but also in nursing. Stress, coping, and health content has become an integral part of nursing curricula, theory, research, and practice at all educational and practice levels. There are undergraduate programs whose structural underpinnings are built on the relationships among these constructs; most, if not all, undergraduate textbooks include content in this area (e.g., Carrieri, Lindsey, & West, 2003; Lewis, Dirksen, Heitkemper, & Bucher, 2010; Porth, 2010).

At the master's level, stress, coping, and health are core content in most graduate programs and are essential knowledge for certification at the advanced practice level. (See American Nurses Credentialing Center Commission on Certification.) At the doctoral level, there are many schools and colleges that offer a minor in this area of study (e.g., University of Michigan, Wayne State University). Over the last 10 years (2000–2010) 265 stress, coping, and health nursing research studies have been listed in the Cumulative Index for Nursing and Allied Health Literature (CINAHL); 92 are for dissertation research with an eye to the future. The extensive attention given to these phenomena individually is reflected in the periodical literature for nursing. CINAHL cites more than 2,800 stress and coping articles published under these keywords since 1982, more than 1,900 in the last decade. When stress and coping topical areas are specified, such as life events, sense of coherence, or type A personality pattern (see Chapters 6, 8, and 13 in this text), the number of citations increases exponentially. For the above reasons it is necessary to update the content of selected chapters in the first edition (Rice, 2000) and to add new chapters that all address the current state of nursing science.

The stress, coping, and health field is a broad one, developing across many disciplines, including nursing, psychology, medicine, sociology, and biology. This has resulted in an unevenness and lack of systematic development. Nonetheless, the contributing authors and I believe there is much to be gained through exploring a cross-section of developments in the field. An attempt has been made to synthesize the stress, coping, and health findings of the past 50-plus years in this 2nd edition. The book's content reflects the evolution and testing of various theoretical models of stress, coping, and health from other disciplines including the general adaptation syndrome (Selye, 1936), Transaction Model of Stress and Coping (Lazarus & Folkman, 1984), and Allostasis & Allostatic Load Theory (McEwen, 2007; McEwen & Wingfield, 2003) and their particular relevance for the profession and the discipline of nursing and to examine nursing theory models that have evolved from these constructs including those of King (1981), Levine (1973), and Roy's Adaptation Model (Roy, 1984; Roy & Andrews, 1991). (See Chapters 1, 2, and 9.) Ryan-Wenger (1992) used three perspectives—growth and development theory (Piaget, 1971), transactional model of stress and coping (Lazarus, 2000), and ecological theory (Bronfenbrenner, 1979)—to derive a theory of stress, coping, and health in children. (See Chapter 10 of this text.)

Of necessity, choices of content have been made throughout because of the extraordinary breadth, depth, and longevity of the field. Selected for inclusion in this book was content considered to be the most thoroughly developed and studied by the discipline and profession of nursing. Every attempt has been made to present a balance between theoretical development, research, measurement, and implications for nursing science and practice and to critique the content within those contexts.

Part I, Chapter 1 is the introduction and overview. The author discusses the diverse conceptualizations of stress, coping, and health and the importance of these for nursing and other disciplines. It also addresses some of the major problems and issues surrounding the various conceptualizations. Part II, Chapter 2 presents the response-oriented theories of stress, beginning with the hallmark works of Cannon (1932) and Selye (1936). In these models, stress is considered to be within the person as a result of some internal or external stressor and is viewed as a nonspecific response to any demand on the organism. Recent nursing investigations that have used this perspective include adults experiencing surgery (Karlsson, Mattsson, Johansson, & Lidell, 2010; Slater, 2010), heart disease (Robley, Ballard, Holtzman, & Cooper, 2010), chronic hypertension (Chummun, 2009; Doshi, Zuckerman, Picot, Wright, & Hill-Westmoreland, 2003), music therapy (Nilsson, 2009), and caregiver stress (Thompson et al., 2004). Studied also were children with cancer (Hinds et al., 2003) and pain (Ramelet, Abu-Saad, Rees, & McDonald, 2004) and adolescents with immune reactivity (Kang, Kim, & Suh, 2004).

Chapters 3, 4, and 5 address the issues of stress, coping, and immunity; epigenetics; and the physiological measures of the stress response. It is this area of research that is critical for the growth of nursing science and for documenting the biological effects of stress and coping on health at the cellular infrastructure, metabolic organization, and system levels.

Part III, Chapter 6 presents the stimulus-oriented theories of stress, in which stress is viewed as the spark or catalyst. It is considered to come from without, and the human organism responds both psychologically and physiologically. The assumption is that change in itself is stressful (regardless of individual differences) and that there is inherent stress in events such as death, pain, divorce, and loss, no matter who is experiencing them. The body of knowledge regarding stressful life events and their effects on health and illness has been well developed and is important to many disciplines, including nursing. The reason for its widespread interest stems from the large body of evidence supporting the premise that stressful life events and environmental

conditions do have an impact on physical and psychological reactions, and, in some cases, on health and illness.

The major life events work of psychologists Holmes and Rahe (1967) is key in this area. Over the past three decades, stressful life event or stress-as-stimulus theoretical underpinnings have changed very little. Measurements, however, have taken on diverse characteristics. In Table 6.1 are a variety of life-change measures developed for children, adolescents, adults, older adults, families, the ill, and the healthy.

In contrast to major life events, relatively minor day-to-day irritating and joyous experiences called *hassles* and *uplifts* are proposed to have a greater effect on psychological well-being and health (Lazarus, 1984; Kanner, Coyne, Schaefer, & Lazarus, 1981). Recent nursing studies of health outcomes in terms of hassles or uplifts or both include depression (Ravindran, Matheson, Griffiths, Merali, & Anisman, 2002), quality of sleep in older adults with Alzheimer's disease (Song, Dowling, Wallhagen, Lee, & Strawbridge, 2010), perinatal mood disturbances (Monk, Leight, & Fang, 2008), and alcohol dependency (Boyd, Baliko, Cox, & Tavakoli, 2007). Chapter 6 examines the life event and hassles and uplifts perspectives.

Chapter 7 addresses how computer information technology (CIT) and computer-mediated communications (CMC), including information systems (IS), computerized behavioral programs (CBPs), social networks (SN), and e-health applications help individuals to improve or alter lifestyle behaviors that have the potential to play an important role in stress, coping, and health outcomes. Research has documented the use of the Internet and e-mail for health care information (Baker, Todd, Wagner, & Bundorf, 2003), health care professionals' decisions to accept telemedicine technology (Chau & Hu, 2002), and using the technology acceptance model to explore public health nurses' intentions toward web-based learning (Chen, Yang, Tang, Huang, & Yu, 2007).

Part IV examines interactional and transactional theories useful for nursing science including salutogenesis (the origins of health) and sense of coherence (Antonovsky, 1979) and the evolution of Lazarus's (1966) and Lazarus and Folkman's (1984) stress and coping models. Researchers using these theoretical perspectives in studies of nursing phenomena include Langeland, Wahl, Kristoffersen, and Hanestad

(2007), who examined *salutogenesis* among adults with mental health problems; Fok, Chair, and Lopez (2005), who documented sense of coherence, coping, and quality of life following critical illness; and Forbes (2001), who tested the effects of enhancing mastery and sense of coherence on health in older adults. Using Lazarus's theories, clinical nursing studies documented coping with chronic heart failure (Yu, Lee, Kwong, Thompson, & Woo, 2008), asthma (Vinson, 2002), chronic illness among HIV-infected women (Bova, 2001), chronic pain (Dysvik, Natvig, Eikeland, & Lindstrøm, 2005; Knussen & McParland, 2009) and the intensive care unit experience (Cronqvist, Theorell, Burns, & Lutzen, 2001). Other theoretical positions are proposed for stress, coping, and health in children (Chapter 10), adolescents (Chapter 11), and the workplace (Chapter 12).

Part V examines mediating and moderating factors found to affect the relationships among stress, coping, and health. These include antecedent variables such as temperament (Carless, Douglas, Fox, & McKenna, 2006), family relationships (McCubbin & McCubbin, 1993), and culture (Giger & Davidhizar, 2002). Other factors include social support (Abualrub, Omari, & Abu Al Rub, 2009; Cadzow & Servoss, 2009), hardiness (Smith & Gray, 2009), resilience (Zautra, Hall, & Murray, 2010), sense of mastery (Pudrovsa, Schieman, Pearlin, & Nguyen, 2005) and personal control (Jacelon, 2007). (See Chapters 13 and 14.) In Chapter 15 the authors note additional psychosocial stressors (e.g., personality patterns, moods, and environmental factors) that have been linked to behavioral risk factors, atherogenesis, development and progression of cardiovascular disease (CVD), poorer health outcomes following acute CVD events, and activation of neuroendocrine and immunologic dynamics (G. E. Miller, Chen, & Cole, 2009). Chapter 16 provides a framework for understanding acute myocardial infarction (AMI) care-seeking behavior. The Acute Myocardial Infarction Coping Model was developed by Alonzo and Reynolds (1997, 1998) and is now being tested.

Chapters 17 through 21 provide in-depth knowledge on factors known to affect the stress, coping, and health dynamic. These include quality of life (QOL) (Halvorsrud, Kirkevold, Diseth, & Kalfoss, 2010), hope and hopelessness (Farran, Herth, & Popovich, 1995; J. F. Miller, 2007), self-regulation and illness representation (Reynolds, 2003), self-efficacy (Champion, Skinner, & Menon, 2005; Majer, Jason, Olson, & North; Siela, 2003), and uncertainty (Mishel, 1991; Mishel, Germino, Lin, Pruthi, & Wallen, 2009).

Chapter 22 proposes a theoretical model that includes most of the concepts discussed in the book. Its purpose is to provide some direction for a more holistic view of stress, coping, and health and to point the way for future research and model building in nursing science. It is clear that our understanding of how stress-related variables affect coping and health is evolving, and much of it stems from models developed in other disciplines. For example, Toth's (1988) cardiovascular recovery model was derived from Selye's (1936) general adaptation syndrome, Pollock's (1989) work was "borrowed" from Kobasa's (1979) hardiness model, and Norbeck's (1981) social support model was founded on the work of Cobb (1976). Scott, Oberst, and Dropkin's stress-coping model (1980) and Mishel's (1991) uncertainty models were both derived from the work of Lazarus and Folkman (1984). Descriptions of the respective model, theory, or constructs follow with a discussion of the level of theory development within nursing science and a schematic representation. A critical examination of the empirical adequacy of the model, theory, or construct in nursing and related disciplines is followed by a detailed description of measures of the phenomenon. Intervention tables are included in some, but not all, of the chapters. Lastly, implications of the construct, concept, or theory for practice, theory development, and future research are discussed.

This book is intended as a primary source for graduate students in nursing and for other health care disciplines and may serve as a secondary source for undergraduate students. The book has considerable utility as a reference work for researchers and scholars in nursing and a variety of other health sciences. For the clinician, it can be a guide to the most pertinent findings for the understanding, prevention, intervention, and treatment of stress-related disorders. It has significant importance for those in stress, coping, and health theory development and testing who wish to have foundational knowledge. This book is very important because no other comprehensive handbook was found that addresses specifically the state of the knowledge of stress, coping, and health in and for nursing.

REFERENCES

Abualrub, R. F., Omari, F. H., & Abu Al Rub, A. F. (2009). The moderating effect of social support on the stress-satisfaction relationship among Jordanian hospital nurses. *Journal of Nursing Management, 17,* 870–878.

Alonzo, A., & Reynolds, N. (1997). Responding to symptoms and signs of acute myocardial infarction: How do you educate the public? *Heart & Lung, 26,* 263–272.

Alonzo, A. A., & Reynolds, N. R. (1998). The structure of emotions during acute myocardial infarction: A model of coping. *Social Science and Medicine, 46*(9), 1099–1110.

Antonovsky, A. (1979). *Health, stress and coping.* San Francisco, CA: Jossey-Bass.

Baker, L., Todd, H., Wagner, S., & Bundorf, M. K. (2003, May). Use of the internet and e-mail for health care information: Results from a national survey. *Journal of the American Medical Association, 289,* 2400–2406.

Bova, C. (2001). Adjustment to chronic illness among HIV-infected women. *Journal of Nursing Scholarship, 33*(3), 217–223.

Boyd, M. R., Baliko, B., Cox, M. F., & Tavakoli, A. (2007). Stress, coping, and alcohol expectancies in rural African-American women. *Archives of Psychiatric Nursing, 21*(2), 70–79.

Bronfenbrenner, U. (1979). *The ecology of human development.* Cambridge, MA: Harvard University Press.

Cadzow, R. B., & Servoss, T. J. (2009). The association between perceived social support and health among patients at a free urban clinic. *Journal of the National Medical Association, 101*(3), 243–250.

Cannon, W. B. (1932). *The wisdom of the body.* New York, NY: Norton.

Carless, D., Douglas, K., Fox, K., & McKenna, J. (2006). An alternative view of psychological well-being in cardiac rehabilitation: Considering temperament and character. *European Journal of Cardiovascular Nursing, 5,* 237–243.

Carrieri, V., Lindsey, A., & West, C. (2003). *Pathophysiological phenomena in nursing: Human responses to illness* (3rd ed.). Philadelphia, PA: W. B. Saunders.

Champion, V., Skinner C., & Menon, U. (2005). Development of a self-efficacy scale for mammography. *Research in Nursing & Health, 28*(4), 329–336.

Chau, P. Y. K., & Hu, P. J. (2002). Investigating healthcare professionals' decisions to accept telemedicine technology: An empirical test of competing theories. *Information and Management, 39,* 297–311.

Chen, J., Yang, K. F., Tang, F. I., Huang, C. H., & Yu, S. (2007). Applying the technology acceptance model to explore public health nurses' intentions towards web-based learning: A cross-sectional questionnaire survey. *International Journal of Nursing Studies, 45*(6), 869–878.

Chummun, H. (2009). Hypertension: A contemporary approach to nursing care. *British Journal of Nursing, 18*(13), 784–789.

Cobb, S. (1976). Social support as a moderator of life stress. *Psychosomatic Medicine, 38,* 300–314.

Cronqvist, A., Theorell, T., Burns, T., & Lutzen, K. (2001). Dissonant imperatives in nursing: A conceptualization of stress in intensive care in Sweden. *Intensive and Critical Care Nursing, 17*(4), 228–236.

Doshi, J. A., Zuckerman, I. H., Picot, S. J., Wright, J. T., & Hill-Westmoreland, E. E. (2003). Antihypertensive use and adherence among African American caregivers and noncaregivers. *Applied Nursing Research, 16*(4), 266–277.

Dysvik, E., Natvig, G. K., Eikeland, O. J., & Lindstrøm, T. C. (2005). Coping with chronic pain. *International Journal of Nursing Studies 42,* 297–305.

Farran, C., Herth, K., & Popovich, J. (1995). *Hope and hopelessness: Critical clinical constructs.* Thousand Oaks, CA: Sage.

Fok, S. K., Chair, S. Y., & Lopez, V. (2005). Sense of coherence, coping and quality of life following critical illness. *Journal of Advanced Nursing, 49*(2), 173–181.

Forbes, D. A. (2001). Enhancing mastery and sense of coherence: Important determinants of health in older adults. *Geriatric Nursing, 22*(1), 29–32.

Giger, J. N., & Davidhizar, R. (2002). The Giger and Davidhizar transcultural assessment model. *Journal of Transcultural Nursing, 13,* 185–188.

Halvorsrud, L., Kirkevold, M., Diseth, A., & Kalfoss, M. (2010). Quality of life model: Predictors of quality of life among sick older adults. *Research and Theory for Nursing Practice: An International Journal, 24*(4), 241–259.

Hinds, P. S., Srivastava, D. K., Randall, E. A., Green, A., Stanford, D., Pinlac, R., & Taylor, K. (2003). Testing the revised stress-response sequence model in pediatric oncology nurses. *Journal of Pediatric Oncology Nursing, 20*(5), 213–232.

Holmes, T. H., & Rahe, R. (1967). The social readjustment rating scale. *Journal of Psychosomatic Research, 12,* 213–218.

Jacelon, C. S. (2007). Theoretical perspectives of perceived control in older adults: A selective review of the literature. *Journal of Advanced Nursing, 59*(1), 1–10.

Kang, D. H., Kim, C. J., & Suh, Y. (2004). Sex differences in immune responses and immune reactivity to stress in adolescents. *Biological Research for Nursing, 5*(4), 243–254.

Kanner, A. D., Coyne, J. C., Schaefer, C., & Lazarus, R. S. (1981). Comparison of two modes of stress measurement: Daily hassles and uplifts versus major life events. *Journal of Behavioral Medicine, 4*, 1–39.

Karlsson, A., Mattsson, B., Johansson, M., & Lidell, E. (2010). Well-being in patients and relatives after open-heart surgery from the perspective of health care professionals. *Journal of Clinical Nursing, 19*(5-6), 840–846.

King, I. (1981). *A theory for nursing: Systems, concepts, process.* New York, NY: John Wiley.

Kobasa, S. C. (1979). Stressful life events, personality, and health: An inquiry into hardiness. *Journal of Personality and Social Psychology, 37*, 1–11.

Knussen, C., & McParland, J. (2009). Catastrophizing, ways of coping and pain beliefs in relation to pain intensity and pain-related disability. *Journal of Pain Management. 2*(2), 203–215.

Langeland, E., Wahl, A. K., Kristoffersen, K., & Hanestad, B. R. (2007). Promoting coping: Salutogenesis among people with mental health problems. *Issues in Mental Health Nursing, 28*, 275–295.

Lazarus, R. S. (1966). *Psychological stress and the coping process.* New York, NY: McGraw-Hill.

Lazarus, R. S. (1984). Puzzles in the study of daily hassles. *Journal of Behavioral Medicine, 7*, 375–389.

Lazarus, R. S. (2000). Toward better research on stress and coping. *American Psychologist, 55*(6), 665–673.

Lazarus, R. S., & Folkman, S. (1984). *Stress, appraisal, and coping.* New York, NY: Springer.

Levine, M. (1973). *Introduction to clinical nursing* (2nd ed.). Philadelphia, PA: F. A. Davis.

Lewis, S. L., Dirksen, S. R., Heitkemper, M. M., & Bucher, L. (2010). *Medical-surgical nursing: Assessment and management of clinical problems.* Maryland Heights, MO: Elsevier, Health Sciences Division.

Majer, J. M., Jason, L. A., Ferrari, J. R., Olson, B. D., & North, C. S. (2003). Is self-mastery always a helpful resource? Coping with paradoxical findings in relation to optimism and abstinence self-efficacy. *The American Journal of Drug and Alcohol Abuse, 29*(2), 385–399.

McCubbin, M. A., & McCubbin, H. I. (1993). Family coping with health crises: The Resiliency Model of Family Stress and Adaptation. In C. Danielson, B. Hamel-Bissel, & P. Winstead-Fry (Eds.). *Families, health, and illness.* New York, NY: Mosby.

McEwen, B. S. (2007). Physiology and neurobiology of stress and adaptation: Central role of the brain. *Physiological Reviews 87*, 873–904.

McEwen, B. S., & Wingfield, J. C. (2003). The concept of allostasis in biology and biomedicine. *Hormone Behavior, 43*(1), 2–15.

Miller, J. F. (2007). Hope: A construct central to nursing. *Nursing Forum, 42*(1), 12–19.

Miller, G. E., Chen, E., & Cole, S. (2009). Health psychology: Developing biologically plausible models linking the social world and physical health. *Annual Review of Psychology, 60*, 501–524.

Mishel, M. H. (1991). The measurement of uncertainty. *Nursing Research, 30*, 258–263.

Mishel, M. H., Germino, B. B., Lin, L., Pruthi, R. S., & Wallen, E. M. (2009). Efficacy of a decision making uncertainty management intervention in early stage prostate cancer. *Patient Education and Counseling*, 349–359.

Monk, C., Leight, K. L., & Fang, Y. (2008). The relationship between women's attachment style and perinatal mood disturbance: Implications for screening and treatment. *Archives of Women's Mental Health, 11*(2), 117–129.

Nilsson, U. (2009). Soothing music can increase oxytocin levels during bed rest after open-heart surgery: A randomised control trial. *Journal of Clinical Nursing, 18*(15), 2153–2161.

Norbeck, J. (1981). Social support: A model for clinical research and application. *Advances in Nursing Science, 3*, 43–59.

Piaget, J. (1971). *Biology and knowledge.* Chicago, IL: University of Chicago Press.

Pollock, S. E. (1989). The hardiness characteristic: A motivating factor in adaptation. *Advances in Nursing Science, 11*, 53–62.

Porth, C. (2010). *Essentials of pathophysiology: Concepts of altered health states* (5th edition). Philadelphia, PA: J. B. Lippincott.

Pudrovsa, T., Schieman, S., Pearlin, L. I., & Nguyen, K. (2005). The sense of mastery as a mediator and moderator in the association between economic hardship and health in late life. *Journal of Aging and Health, 17*, 634–660.

Ramelet, A., Abu-Saad, H. H., Rees, N., & McDonald, S. (2004). The challenges of pain measurement in critically ill young children: A comprehensive review. *Australian Critical Care, 17*(1), 33–34.

Ravindran, A. V., Matheson, K., Griffiths, J., Merali, Z., & Anisman, H. (2002). Stress, coping, uplifts, and quality of life in subtypes of depression: A conceptual model and emerging data, *Journal of Affective Disorders, 71*, 121–130.

Reynolds, N. R. (2003). The problem of antiretroviral adherence: A self-regulatory model for intervention. *AIDS Care, 15*(1), 117–124.

Rice, V. H. (2000). *Handbook of stress, coping, and health: Implications for nursing theory, research, and practice* (1st ed.). Thousand Oaks, CA: Sage.

Robley, L., Ballard, N., Holtzman, D., & Cooper, W. (2010). The experience of stress for open heart surgery patients and their caregivers. *Western Journal of Nursing Research, 32*(6), 794–813.

Roy, C. (1984). *Introduction to nursing: An adaptation model* (2nd ed.). Englewood Cliffs, NJ: Prentice Hall.

Roy, C., & Andrews, H. (1991). *The Roy Adaptation Model: The definitive statement.* Norwalk, CT: Appleton & Lange.

Ryan-Wenger, N. M. (1992). A taxonomy of children's coping strategies: A step toward theory development. *American Journal of Orthopsychiatry, 62*(2), 256–263.

Scott, D. W., Oberst, M., & Dropkin, M. (1980). A stress coping model. *Advances in Nursing Science, 3*(1), 9–23.

Selye, H. (1936). A syndrome produced by diverse nocuous agents. *Nature, 138,* 132–135.

Siela, D. (2003). Use of self-efficacy and dypsnea perceptions to predict functional performance in people with COPD. *Rehabilitation Nursing, 28*(6), 197–204.

Slater, R. (2010). Impact of an enhanced recovery program in colorectal surgery. *British Journal of Nursing, 23,* 19–21.

Smith, M. S., & Gray, S. W. (2009). The courage to challenge: A new measure of hardiness in LGBT adults. *Journal of Gay & Lesbian Social Services, 21*(1), 73–89.

Song, Y., Dowling, G. A., Wallhagen, M. I., Lee, K. A., & Strawbridge, W. J. (2010). Sleep in older adults with Alzheimer's disease. *Journal of Neuroscience Nursing, 42*(4), 190–198.

Thompson, R. L., Lewis, S. L., Murphy, M. R., Hale, J. M., Blackwell, P. H., Acton, G. J., & Bonner, P. N. (2004). Are there sex differences in emotional and biological responses in spousal caregivers of patients with Alzheimer's disease? *Biological Research for Nursing, 5*(4), 319–330.

Toth, J. (1988). Measuring the stressful experience of hospital discharge following acute myocardial infarction. In C. Waltz & O. Strickland (Eds.), *Measurement of nursing outcomes* (pp. 3–23). New York, NY: Springer.

Vinson, J. A. (2002). Children with asthma: Initial development of the Child Resilience Model. *Journal of Pediatric Nursing, 28*(2), 149–158.

Yu, D. S., Lee, D. T., Kwong, A. N., Thompson, D. R., & Woo, J. (2008). Living with chronic heart failure: A review of qualitative studies of older people. *Journal of Advanced Nursing, 61*(5), 474–483.

Zautra, A. J., Hall, J. S., & Murrary, K. E. (2010). Resilience: A new definition of health for people and communities. In J. W. Reich, A. J. Zautra, & J. S. Hall (Eds.), *Handbook of Adult Resilience* (pp. 3–29). New York, NY: Guilford.

ABOUT THE EDITOR

Virginia Hill Rice, PhD, RN, CNS, FAAN, is Professor of Nursing at the Wayne State University College of Nursing and the Karmanos Cancer Institute. She holds a doctorate in social psychology and a master's degree as a clinical nurse specialist in medical–surgical nursing. She has an extensive history of funded research and numerous publications and presentations in the field of stress, coping, and health; patient teaching; and tobacco use. Dr. Rice received the Nightingale Award for Excellence in Nursing Research, the Midwest Nursing Research Society's (MNRS) Stress and Coping Research Section's Advancement of Science Award, the MNRS Distinguished Contributor to Nursing Research in the Midwest Award, and a 2010 Leadership Award for Community Research Collaboration. She is a fellow in the American Academy of Nursing and received the 2010 Wayne State University College of Nursing's Lifeline and Distinguished Alumni Award. Dr. Rice was the editor of the 1st edition of this text, in 2000.

ABOUT THE CONTRIBUTORS

Angelo A. Alonzo, PhD, is currently a Research Scientist at the Yale School of Nursing and professor emeritus in Sociology at The Ohio State University. His research and scholarly activities have focused on examining behaviors surrounding seeking health care for a cardiac problem. He is also involved in curriculum development and evaluation in India for the Indian Ministry of Health, Yale University, and the William J. Clinton Foundation. Prior appointments have been with the National Heart, Lung and Blood Institute of the National Institutes of Health as a Research Sociologist and as a Consultant to the National Heart Attack Alert Program.

Neveen Farag Awad, PhD, is a Management Consultant. Her doctorate was in Information Systems and Manufacturing from the Wayne State University School of Business. Her research interests include online word of mouth, online trust, and information personalization and privacy. Dr. Awad received the Marcy Maguire Fellowship, awarded to a female PhD student whose research carries the greatest potential business impact. Her research has appeared in several journals including *Management Information Systems Quarterly, Journal of Management Information Systems, International Journal of E-Business Research,* and *Communications of the ACM,* among others.

Cecilia R. Barron, PhD, RN, CNS, is an Associate Professor Emeritus at the University of Nebraska Medical Center College of Nursing. She holds a doctorate in developmental psychology and served as coordinator of the graduate psychiatric mental health nursing area at the University of Nebraska for many years. Her research, publications, and presentations are in the field of stress, coping, and health, especially as personality influences perceptions of stress and use of coping strategies.

She is an active member of the American Psychological Association in the divisions of Health Psychology and Psychology of Religion.

Alexandra G. Broussard, BS, is a graduate student in the pediatric nurse practitioner program at The Ohio State University. She received a bachelor's degree in psychology from Xavier University in New Orleans, Louisiana. She was a research assistant in the Ryan-Wenger Research Lab at the Research Institute at Nationwide Children's Hospital and participated in several research studies related to the quality of care and safety of hospitalized children.

Judith A. Cohen, PhD, RN, is a Professor of nursing at the University of Vermont. She obtained her PhD in nursing from Wayne State University. She is past president of the Vermont State Nurses Association and a Captain in the U.S. Naval Reserve (retired) Nurse Corps. Dr. Cohen's expertise, research interests, and publications are focused in the areas of cardiovascular nursing, reflective practice, nursing theory, caring science, qualitative research methods, health policy, and stress and coping. Dr. Cohen is Vice President of the Vermont Ethics Network Board. She has received the University of Vermont's Kroepsch-Maurice Award for Teaching Excellence, Vermont State Nurses Association Service Award for Leadership, Jackie Gribbons Leadership Award for Vermont Women in Higher Education, and Sigma Theta Tau International Honor Society (Kappa Tau Chapter) Outstanding Nurse Award for Excellence in Education and Excellence in Research Award.

Dina Tell Cooper, PhD, is a National Cancer Institute Postdoctoral Fellow at the Loyola University Chicago Niehoff School of Nursing. She holds a doctorate in developmental psychology and is completing her postdoctoral training in the field of psychoneuroimmunology. As part of the training, Dr. Tell Cooper directs a National Cancer Institute–funded study that examines the effectiveness of mindfulness-based stress reduction (MBSR) on reducing stress reactivity, improving psychological well-being and immune function in women with breast cancer. She has presented this work at professional conferences in the field of stress. Since the start of her postdoctoral training, Dr. Tell Cooper has further developed her interest in behavioral epigenetics, including investigating how early-life experiences contribute to the changes in epigenetic mechanism of gene regulation and influence behavior and health.

Holli A. DeVon, PhD, RN, is an Associate Professor in the Betty Irene Moore School of Nursing at the University of California, Davis. Her current research examines the influence of gender on symptom characteristics during acute coronary syndromes and psychosocial and biological stressors in women with cardiovascular disease. Dr. DeVon has had numerous research articles published in multidisciplinary journals. She has presented her research findings at national and international meetings. Dr. DeVon received the new investigator award from the American Heart Association, Cardiovascular Nursing Council in 2002 and the Sage/MNRS best paper award in 2007.

Alana L. Ferguson, BA (Hon), MA, is a Health Research Facilitator and Innovation Analyst for the Office of the Associate Vice-President Research-Health (University of Saskatchewan)/Vice-President Research and Innovation (Saskatoon Health Region). She holds a master's degree in sociology from the University of Saskatchewan (2009). Her thesis explored women's experiences of stress and coping with arm problems after breast cancer. Over the past five years she has published and presented in the area of qualitative health research, with specific interests in phenomenology, ethno-drama, and participatory action research.

Alissa L. Firmage, MSN, NP-C, is currently a family nurse practitioner practicing in Salt Lake City, Utah. She graduated from Yale School of Nursing, where her master's praxis research incorporated the Acute Myocardial Infarction Coping Model and focused on the post-traumatic stress effects of an AMI . There, she was also a Health & Wellness fellow at the Yale McDougal Center for Graduate Student Life, where she coordinated health and wellness programs, services, and resources, including stress management and mindful meditation workshops. She holds a BA in human biology, with a concentration in disease prevention and health promotion from Stanford University. She has worked at Yale, Stanford University Medical Center, and the Navajo Area Indian Health Service. As a member of the Navajo Tribal Nation, she was awarded a Navajo Nation Graduate Fellowship. She is a member of the AANP, Sigma Theta Tau International Honor Society of Nursing, and the Utah Nurse Practitioner Association.

Marlene Hanson Frost, PhD, RN, AOCN, is a Professional Associate in research and Assistant Professor of Oncology at Mayo Clinic, Rochester, Minnesota. Dr. Frost received her undergraduate nursing degrees from Rochester Community College, Rochester, Minnesota, and Mankato State University, Mankato, Minnesota. Her master's degree with a major in nursing is from the University of Minnesota, and her doctorate with a major in nursing is from the University of Texas at Austin. Dr. Frost's research is in the areas of women's cancers, benign breast disease, individuals at increased risk for cancer, and those at increased risk for poor psychosocial adjustment. Specific foci include quality of life; patient-reported outcomes; satisfaction and psychosocial function following prophylactic mastectomy; issues surrounding stress and coping in women with benign breast disease, breast and gynecologic cancers; and interventions to promote adjustment to a diagnosis of cancer.

Carolyn Marie García, PhD, MPH, RN, is an Assistant Professor in the School of Nursing at the University of Minnesota and holds an adjunct faculty appointment in the School of Public Health. Her program of research is focused on adolescent mental health promotion and employs community-based participatory methods to develop, implement, and evaluate school-based, family-centric interventions for youths and their families. She has worked as a public health nurse for more than 15 years in teen clinics and adult detention centers from rural Rwanda to post-9/11 Red Cross disaster relief centers in Washington, D.C. As a sexual assault nurse clinician, she provides care for women immediately after an assault. She teaches courses on public health nursing and qualitative research methods and advises undergraduate and graduate students' programs in nursing and public health. She currently serves as co-chair of the Stress and Coping Research Section of the Midwest Nursing Research Society.

Barbara Harris, PhD, RN, is a visiting Assistant Professor at DePaul University, Department of Nursing. She directs the psychiatric–mental health component of the Master's Entry to Nursing Program at DePaul and has over 25 years of experience in psychiatric–mental health nursing, including several years working on a stress disorders unit.

Martha E. (Beth) Horsburgh, PhD, RN, is a Professor in the School of Public Health at the University of Saskatchewan, Saskatoon, Saskatchewan, Canada. She presently holds a joint appointment as the Associate Vice President, Research-Health at the University, and as Vice President of Research & Innovation, for the Saskatoon Health Region. Dr. Horsburgh plays an important role leading the development of health research and innovation initiatives across the university and the health region, while addressing the needs of patients, researchers, and other stakeholders. She holds a doctorate in nursing and has a long history of funded research and numerous publications and presentations in the field of self-care and care-giving for adults within the context of living with chronic illness.

Linda Witek Janusek, PhD, RN, FAAN, is a Professor and holder of the Niehoff Endowed Chair for Research at the Marcella Niehoff School of Nursing, Loyola University. She holds a doctorate in physiology from the University of Illinois–Chicago. She has a consistent record of NIH-funded research focused on understanding the influence of emotions and behavior on neuroendocrine stress reactivity and immune responses in vulnerable populations experiencing psychosocial stress. Scientific contributions include documenting the dynamics of stress-induced immune dysregulation in women across the breast cancer trajectory and demonstrating the effectiveness of mindfulness-based stress reduction on improving quality of life, enhancing coping effectiveness, and facilitating restoration of immune function in women after breast cancer treatment. Her recent program of research is directed toward investigating the contribution of life adversity and psychosocial stress on epigenetic regulation of immune function and inflammatory processes. She is a fellow in the American Academy of Nursing.

Richard S. Lazarus, PhD, a distinguished scholar, researcher, and Professor Emeritus of Psychology at the University of California, Berkeley, passed away in 2002. His research interests included projective methods, individual differences in perception, and perceptual defense. Mainly he focused on psychological stress, emotions, and coping, moving the field of psychology away from behaviorism. Professor Lazarus was awarded a Guggenheim Fellowship in 1969–1970. In 1984, the California Psychological Association gave him special recognition for his outstanding contributions, and in 1989, the American Psychological Association gave him one of its highest awards for Distinguished Scientific Contribution. He was the author or co-author of more than 200 scientific articles and 20 books, including *Psychological Stress and the Coping Process* (1966), which is considered a classic; *Stress, Appraisal, and Coping* (with S. Folkman) (1984); *Emotion and Adaptation* (1991); *Passion and Reason* (with B. Lazarus) (1994); and *Stress and Emotion: A New Synthesis* (1999). We thank him for his most valuable contributions to this text and to nursing science.

Gail Low, PhD, RN, is an Assistant Professor, Faculty of Nursing at the University of Alberta in Edmonton, Alberta, Canada. Her teaching background is in care of the frail elder in community settings, chronic illness management, theory and research on aging, and community health. She has practiced extensively in general surgical and respiratory nursing, and geriatric outreach in acute care, and home care nursing. She also was a clinical nurse specialist in extended care and transitional care settings. Her program of research focuses on quality of life among older adults. Specialized interests in this area include determinants of COPD-specific and nondisease-specific quality of life. She is currently embarking on research projects pertaining to active aging and its relationship to quality of life, happiness, and life satisfaction, and attitudes to aging. She has also examined the psychometrics of quality of life and related instruments for use with older people.

Brenda L. Lyon, PhD, RN, CNS, FAAN, is a Professor Emeritus of the Indiana University

School of Nursing. Currently, Dr. Lyon is President of Health Potentials Unlimited, LLC, founded in 1975, which is her private practice for counseling individuals suffering from stress-related physical illness and offering workshops nationally on how to conquer stress. She is also Vice President of Aircom Manufacturing, Inc. and Medivative Technologies, LLC, where she evaluates new medical devices to be used in patient care or to assist individuals in self-care. At Indiana University she taught stress counseling in the MSN program for 38 years and stress and coping research in the PhD program for 15 years. She is a co-founder of the Midwest Nursing Research Society's Stress & Coping Section and is a recipient of the section's Advancement in Science Award. She has numerous publications and is a Fellow in the American Academy of Nursing.

Carol L. Macnee, PhD, RN (1949–2008), was the Research Director and a Professor at the University of Wyoming, Fay W. Whitney School of Nursing. Her research interests included examining the process of smoking cessation and other health behavior changes from a stress and coping perspective and examining outcomes of nursing care with homeless and indigent clients. She received numerous honors including the Excellence in Nursing Award in Research from Sigma Theta Tau, Nurse of the Year in Research from East Tennessee State University, and the Rackham Non-Traditional Student Award from the University of Michigan. Dr. Macnee was noted for her keen ability to make difficult information understandable for students and for patients. She co-authored a textbook with Dr. Susan McCabe titled *Understanding Nursing Research*. Dr. Macnee died in an automobile accident in December 2008. We are most grateful for her valuable contribution to the 1st edition of this text.

Faith Martin, PhD, is a Research Fellow in the Applied Research Centre for Health and Lifestyle Interventions at Coventry University, United Kingdom. She holds a doctorate in psychology, awarded by the University of Bath, and her PhD work addressed perceived quality of life of people living in poverty in northeast Thailand. Her postdoctoral research focuses on the design and evaluation of self-management interventions for people living with chronic illnesses, to facilitate coping and well-being. She is a member of the British Psychological Society.

Herbert L. Mathews, PhD, is Professor of Microbiology and Immunology, Stritch School of Medicine, Loyola University of Chicago. His research has evaluated the effects of psychosocial and physiological distress on immune function in a number of different clinical paradigms. The focus of that work has been on immune effector genes, immune effector function, and physiological and psychological constructs. Special emphasis is placed upon an understanding of the epigenetic basis for psychosocial distress mediated immune dysregulation.

Susan McCabe, EdD, RN, CS (1949–2008), was an Assistant Professor of Nursing at the University of Wyoming, Fay W. Whitney School of Nursing. Her specialty was treatment of psychiatric disorders and the process of care for homeless and indigent clients. Susan had been a faculty member at East Tennessee State University, College of Micronesia in the Marshall Islands, and Crouse Irving School of Nursing in Syracuse, New York. She received numerous professional awards and honors including the Hendricks Lectureship Award from the International Society of Psychiatric Mental Health Nurses, Excellence in Leadership Award from the American Psychiatric Nurses Association, and Psychiatric Nurse of the Year from the Tennessee State Nurses Association. She co-authored the textbook, *Understanding Nursing Research*, with Dr. Carol Macnee. Dr. McCabe died in an automobile accident in December 2008. We are most grateful for her valuable contribution to the 1st edition of this text.

Merle H. Mishel, PhD, RN, FAAN, is the Kenan Professor of Nursing at the School of Nursing, University of North Carolina at Chapel Hill and director of the doctoral and postdoctoral program. She directs a T32 pre- and postdoctoral training grant in Interventions to Prevent and Manage Chronic Illness. She has a PhD in social psychology and is recognized as one of the major theorists in nursing. She is the developer of the Uncertainty in Illness Theory and the Re-conceptualized Uncertainty Theory. She has also produced Uncertainty Scales. Her theory work and measures, available in 15 languages, are used in countries around the world in both graduate and clinical programs. Dr. Mishel has been funded by NINR and NCI for seven intervention studies with breast and prostate cancer patients. Her Theory of Uncertainty is built around the original work in psychology on stress and coping and she has extended that work.

Anita E. Molzahn, PhD, RN, FCAHS, is a Professor and Dean in the Faculty of Nursing at the University of Alberta, Edmonton, Alberta, Canada. She holds a master's degree in nursing and a PhD in sociology from the University of Alberta. Dr. Molzahn's clinical practice is in nephrology nursing and transplantation. Her research focuses on quality of life in relation to chronic illness. Her interest in quality of life has led to studies relating to organ donation and studies that include quality of life measurement as an outcome. Dr. Molzahn is the Canadian principal investigator in the WHOQOL Group, an international research group working with the World Health Organization (WHO) on the development and testing of a series of instruments to measure quality of life, including the WHOQOL-100, WHOQOL-BREF, and WHOQOL-OLD. She is currently using narrative inquiry with people with life-threatening illness, transitions from pediatric to adult dialysis settings, and photographic methods to enhance safety culture in dialysis units.

Rose C. Nanyonga, MSN, RN, FNP-C, graduated from Baylor University School of Nursing with a Family Nurse Practitioner specialty. From 2005 to 2008 she worked as the Director of Nursing at the International Hospital Kampala (IHK), in Uganda, then as Director of the teaching arm of IHK to help establish an International Hospital School of Nursing, and finally as the Director of Clinical Services for International Medical Group in Uganda. In 2009 she enrolled in the PhD program at Yale University. Her research focuses on HIV, health policy, and workforce development. In particular, she hopes to examine the mechanisms necessary to enhance and expand the role of nurses in developing countries as a strategy for improving access and distribution of health services. She has worked with her PhD advisor to develop a Master's HIV Specialty curriculum for the Indian Institute of Advanced Nursing (IIAN) practice. She is a recipient of the Jonas Nurse Leaders Scholar Award.

Jessie Kemmick Pintor, MPH, is a Doctoral Student in Health Services Research, Policy, & Administration at the University of Minnesota School of Public Health, where she received her MPH in Maternal and Child Health in 2009. During her master's program, she assisted in the development and facilitation of a school-based stress and coping intervention study of Latina adolescents through the University of Minnesota School of Nursing. The program consisted of sharing circles, body/mind exercises, and skill-building activities intended to increase use of healthy coping. Participation in this study led to her master's thesis exploring acculturation, stress, and coping in Latina adolescents. Prior to pursuing graduate studies, she worked for six years at a social service agency serving Latino immigrant families focusing primarily on healthy youth development. Her current research addresses immigration and health care policy, particularly the barriers that exist for immigrant communities in accessing quality care.

Marilyn Plummer, MSN, RN, PhD-C, is a doctoral student at the School of Nursing, University of Victoria, Victoria, B.C., Canada. Her dissertation relates to health inequities, housing, and women. Also she is teaching in the undergraduate nursing program at Camosun College in Victoria. Marilyn is a public health nurse with an unconventional practice background. She has worked with First Nations and Inuit families in the Northwest Territories and Nunavut for approximately 10 years. She also worked for Doctors Without Borders in Rwanda in 1994–1995. Prior to teaching, she worked in public health nursing with Vancouver Island Health Authority. Her research interests include public health nursing, health inequality/inequity, women's health, quality of life, stress and coping, nursing education, and curriculum development.

Edith D. Hunt Raleigh, PhD, RN, is Dean of the Graduate School and Research and Professor of Nursing at Madonna University in Livonia, Michigan. Her research and teaching interests focus on coping and hopefulness in chronic physical conditions and hospice. As a postdoctoral fellow at the University of Michigan, she developed the Multidimensional Hope Scale. She has published in a number of journals and book chapters. She has extensive experience with evidence-based practice, having served as nurse researcher for Harper-Grace Hospitals in Detroit during the 1980s. She has served on the editorial board of the *Journal of Nursing Measurement* and is currently on the editorial board of *Research in Nursing & Health*. She was named Michigan Top Nurse in 1996 by *Metropolitan Women* magazine and is a member of the Advisory Board (formerly Board of Directors) for the Moody Theological Seminary–Michigan.

Betty A. Rambur, PhD, RN, is a Professor of Nursing and Health Policy and Director of the Holly and Robert Miller Caring for Nurses Initiatives at the University of Vermont. From 2000 to 2009 she served as Dean of the College of Nursing and Health Sciences at The University of Vermont. Dr. Rambur received her MS and PhD in nursing from Rush University in Chicago, Illinois, and maintains an active program of research primarily focused on health services, the nursing workforce, and organizational dynamics including moral stress. In 2007, Dr. Rambur's research was honored by Sigma Theta Tau International. In 2007 to 2008, she was selected from a national pool as an American Council on Education (ACE) Fellow. This is a leadership development program preparing select individuals for senior leadership in university administration. Dr. Rambur currently directs the Holly and Robert Miller Caring for Nurses Initiative at the University of Vermont.

Nancy R. Reynolds, PhD, RN, C-ANP, FAAN, is a Professor of Nursing at Yale University. She has been conducting research examining illness behavior in the context of HIV/AIDS for more than 20 years. Her work is guided by self-regulation theory and focused on the psychological and social aspects of an HIV diagnosis as related to illness perceptions and self-management strategies (especially antiretroviral adherence behavior). She has a long history of funding from the National Institutes of Health as a principal investigator and co-investigator of several large, interdisciplinary, domestic and international, multisite studies. She has developed and established the effectiveness of a self-regulation guided adherence counseling intervention delivered by telephone. The self-regulation model is currently being applied to a variety of illness populations and settings. Dr. Reynolds is also actively engaged in HIV-related global health initiatives in India, China, Ghana, and Russia.

Virginia Hill Rice, PhD, RN, CNS, FAAN, is Professor of Nursing at the Wayne State University College of Nursing and the Karmanos Cancer Institute. She holds a doctorate in social psychology and a master's degree as a clinical nurse specialist in medical–surgical nursing. She

has an extensive history of funded research and numerous publications and presentations in the field of stress, coping, and health; patient teaching; and tobacco use. Dr. Rice received the Nightingale Award for Excellence in Nursing Research, the Midwest Nursing Research Society's (MNRS) Stress and Coping Research Section's Advancement of Science Award, and the MNRS Distinguished Contributor to Nursing Research in the Midwest Award. She is a fellow in the American Academy of Nursing and received the 2010 Wayne State University College of Nursing's Lifeline and Distinguished Alumni Award. Dr. Rice was the editor of the 1st edition of this text in 2000.

Elizabeth Roe, PhD, RN, is Associate Professor of Nursing at Saginaw Valley State University in University Center, Michigan. She holds a PhD in nursing from Wayne State University and a Master of Science in medical–surgical nursing from University of Michigan, Ann Arbor. She has completed research on treatment seeking in women with myocardial infarction using the Acute Myocardial Infarction Coping Model. She has made numerous presentations and publications on evidence-based practice.

Nancy A. Ryan-Wenger, PhD, RN, CPNP, FAAN, is Director of Nursing Research at Nationwide Children's Hospital in Columbus, Ohio, and a Principal Investigator for the Center for Innovation in Pediatric Practice at the Research Institute at Nationwide Children's Hospital. She was awarded Professor Emeritus from The Ohio State University after 28 years of teaching in the College of Nursing. She holds a PhD in nursing from Case Western Reserve University and is a certified pediatric nurse practitioner. Dr. Ryan-Wenger has numerous publications and research grants related to stress, coping, and stress-related symptoms in children. Her widely used instrument, the School-agers' Coping Strategies Inventory, is translated into six languages. She received the Advancement of Science Award from the Stress and Coping Research Section of the Midwest Nursing Research Society. She is a fellow in the American Academy of Nursing.

Karen L. Saban, PhD, RN, APRN, CNRN, is an Assistant Professor in the Marcella Niehoff School of Nursing at Loyola University Chicago and is a Research Health Scientist in the Center for Management of Complex Chronic Care at the Edward Hines, Jr., VA Hospital. Dr. Saban's research focuses on the psychological and physiological stress response of persons who are suffering from brain injury and their families, including ischemic stroke and traumatic brain injury. She is particularly interested in how the social environment influences the stress response and its role in health disparities.

Debra Siela, PhD, RN, CCNS, ACNS-BC, CCRN, CNE, RRT, is an Assistant Professor of Nursing at Ball State University School of Nursing in Muncie, Indiana. She has a doctorate from Rush University College of Nursing and is certified as a Clinical Nurse Specialist in both adult health and acute/critical care nursing. She is also certified as a Nurse Educator. She conducts research about the effects of self-efficacy on people with COPD, ventilator weaning, and patient falls. She speaks at national conferences regarding pulmonary topics and issues. She publishes articles on clinical topics and research findings. She also works in the role of a Clinical Nurse Specialist consultant with Siela Nurse Consultants.

Matthew R. Sorenson, PhD, RN, is an Assistant Professor of Nursing at DePaul University and a Clinical Scholar in the Department of Physical Medicine and Rehabilitation at Northwestern University's Feinberg School of Medicine. He obtained his doctorate from Loyola University, Chicago and completed a 3-year postdoctoral program in research and neurology at Edward Hines Jr. VA Hospital. His clinical practice includes work in psychiatric and physical rehabilitation settings. He has received awards for community work and is featured in the book *Ordinary People, Extraordinary Lives: The Stories of Nurses.* He previously served as chair of the Stress and Coping Research section of the Midwest Nursing Research Society. His program of research examines stress and coping in those with multiple sclerosis.

Jill Mattuck Tarule, EdD, is a Professor of Educational Leadership and Policy at the University of Vermont. She has served as an Associate Provost, a Dean, and in other academic leadership roles in three institutions. She holds a doctoral degree from the Harvard Graduate School of Education, and an honorary doctorate from the University of New Hampshire School for Lifelong Learning. She is co-author of *Women's Ways of Knowing: The Development of Self, Voice*

and Mind and co-editor of *Knowledge, Difference and Power: Essays Inspired by Women's Ways of Knowing* and *The Minority Voice in Educational Reform: An Analysis by Minority and Women College of Education Deans,* as well as articles and chapters on leadership, adult learners, and moral development and stress. She received the Pomeroy Award for Outstanding Contributions to Teacher Education and the Gender Equity Architect Award, both from the American Association of Colleges for Teacher Education.

Patricia W. Underwood, PhD, RN, FAAN, is an Executive Associate Dean for academic programs and an Associate Professor at the Frances Payne Bolton School of Nursing, Case Western Reserve University. She has conducted several studies examining stress, coping, and social support within the context of childbirth from quantitative and qualitative perspectives. The latter included a national study examining how women make decisions regarding infant feeding and how these decisions are maintained in the face of significant challenge and/or the absence of support. She has developed a model for measuring perceived satisfaction with five forms of social support that can be adapted to accommodate situation salient sources.

Carol Vallett, EdD, is a Research Associate Professor in the College of Education and Social Services at the University of Vermont. She holds an educational doctorate from the University of Vermont, where she was also the Dean of Continuing Education from 2002 to 2009. Dr. Vallett's research interests are in positive organizational behavior, organizational virtuousness, and organizational culture, particularly in educational institutions.

Linda S. Weglicki, PhD, MSN, RN, earned her PhD in Nursing from the University of Michigan in health promotion and risk reduction. She earned a master's degree in community health nursing from Wayne State University in Michigan. Dr. Weglicki's research has focused on health promotion in ethnically diverse urban populations. She has published in a variety of interdisciplinary journals in the areas of stress, coping, and health. Her publications and presentations have specifically included studies of tobacco prevention/cessation including water-pipe and cigarette smoking by youth, adolescent pregnancy and parenting, e-health applications to promote health behaviors by older adults, and environmental risks associated with air pollution. Dr. Weglicki is an advocate of interdisciplinary research collaboration and partnerships in order to promote translational research. Currently, Dr. Weglicki is the Chief, Officer of Extramural Programs, Division of Extramural Activities, National Institute of Nursing Research, National Institutes of Health. Dr. Weglicki's contributions to this book chapter and the contents herein do not reflect the views of the National Institutes of Health or the U.S. Government.

Joan Stehle Werner, DNS, RN, is Professor Emeritus of Nursing at the University of Wisconsin–Eau Claire (UW–EC). During her 27 years of tenure at UW–EC, her research focused on occupational stress and health in various populations and on stress and quality of care in long-term care. Her program of research included preventive and protective factors in stress and health, including spirituality and quality of life, in diverse populations including various patient groups, people receiving dialysis, and adults with chronic mental illness. She has authored or co-authored several chapters and articles on stress, coping, spirituality, and related topics. Her educational research and writings were in the area of clinical reasoning. Dr. Werner's areas of teaching expertise were nursing practice in adult health, human responses, research, psychiatric nursing, and nursing adults with chronic mental illness. During her retirement, Dr. Werner has continued to provide consultation on scholarly works of colleagues.

Ann W. Wieseke, PhD, APRN-BC, QBHP, is an Associate Professor of Nursing at the Ball State University School of Nursing in Muncie, Indiana. She has a doctorate from Indiana University College of Nursing and is a certified Adult Nurse Practitioner. She conducts research about self-efficacy and exercise, ethical–economic issues, and health care economics. She has published articles and presented on topics such as maternal depression and ethical–economics issues. She currently practices in a community mental health setting, primarily seeing patients with endocrine disorders.

Vicki L. (Sharrer) Wilson, MSN, RN, CNP, is Professor of Nursing at Ohio University, Zanesville. She is certified and has practiced as a pediatric nurse practitioner in a pediatric practice for 16 years. She has a 20-year history of research and publications on stress, coping, and stress symptoms in school-age children.

Jill M. Winters, PhD, RN, is Dean, Professor, and CEO of the Columbia College of Nursing. She holds a doctorate in nursing. She has a long history of funded research and numerous publications and presentations in the field of anxiety, stress, coping, health, and disease. She received awards for her research from such organizations as the Canadian Society of Telemedicine, the American Telemedicine Association, Midwest Nursing Research Society, the American Association of Critical Care Nurses, and the Wisconsin Nurses Association. She was named the American Nurses Foundation Virginia Stone Scholar.

PART I

INTRODUCTION

1

STRESS, COPING, AND HEALTH

A Conceptual Overview

BRENDA L. LYON

lthough the term *stress* as it relates to the human condition has been in the scientific literature since the 1930s and in the nursing literature since the late 1950s, the word did not become popular vernacular until the late 1970s and early 1980s. Today, the term is used in everyday vocabulary to capture a variety of human experiences that are disturbing or disruptive in some manner: "You wouldn't believe how much stress I had today!" "I was really stressed out."

Subjective sensations commonly experienced in conjunction with "feeling stressed" are headache, shortness of breath, light-headedness or dizziness, nausea, muscle tension, fatigue, gnawing in the gut, palpitations, loss of appetite or hunger, and problems with sleep. Behavioral manifestations of stress commonly reported are crying, smoking, excessive eating, drinking alcohol, fast talking, and trembling. It is also commonplace for people to complain that stress negatively affects their functioning. It impairs their mental concentration, problem solving, decision making, and the ability to get work done in an efficient and effective manner (Barling, Kelloway, & Frone, 2004; Goleman & Gurin, 1993; Ornstein & Sobel, 1988; Pelletier, 1992, 1995; Thompson, 2010).

The word *stress* began appearing in nursing journals in the 1950s. Stress, as a construct, was not widely recognized by nurse researchers until the 1970s (Lyon & Werner, 1987). It gained recognition as a phenomenon of interest for nursing because anecdotal data from patients and empirical evidence from researchers suggested that stress and health were inextricably related concepts. Nursing, as a discipline, was not alone in recognizing the importance that stress played in health. Other health-related disciplines had already begun to contribute to both theory development and empirical testing of the phenomenon of stress and its connection with health.

Many different disciplines (e.g., psychology, social psychology, nursing, and medicine) have identified stress and coping as important variables affecting health. It has been linked to the onset of diseases, such as cardiovascular conditions (Benschop et al., 1998; Dimsdale, Ruberman, & Carleton, 1987; Ornish, 2007; Ornish, Scherwitz, & Doody, 1983; Pashkow, 1999), cancer (Cohen & Rabin, 1998; Siegel, 1986), breast cancer (Antonova & Mueller, 2008), and colds (Cohen et al., 1998; Cohen, Tyrrell, & Smith, 1991), as well as the exacerbation of symptoms such as asthma (Fitzgerald, 2009; Wright, Rodriquez, & Cohen, 1998), irritable bowel syndrome (Bennett, Tennant, Piesse, Badcock, & Kellow, 1998; Dancey, Taghavi, & Fox, 1998), ulcerative colitis (Whitehead & Schuster, 1985), arthritis (Crofford, Jacobson, & Young, 1999; Straub, Dhabhar, Bijlsma, & Cutolo, 2005), respiratory diseases (Nielson, Kristensen, Schnohr, & Gronbaeck, 2008), skin disorders (Lebwohl &

Tan, 1998), and diabetes (Fitzgerald, 2009; Inui et al., 1998; Surwit, Schneider, & Feinglos, 1992).

In addition, stress has been linked to symptomatic experiences such as headaches (Davis, Holm, Myers, & Suda, 1998; Fanciullacci, Allessandri, & Fanciullacci, 1998; Armstrong, Wittrock, Robinson, 2006; Bjorling, 2009), musculoskeletal pain (Dyrehag et al., 1998; Finestone, Alfeeli, and Fisher, 2008), gastrointestinal upset (Whitehead & Schuster, 1985), hyperventilation (Ringsberg & Akerlind, 1999), insomnia (Vgontzas et al., 1998), and fatigue (Maes, 2009). Also, coping behaviors have been identified as mediating the effect of stress on blood sugar (Cox & Gonder-Frederick, 1992; Fukunishi, Akimoto, Horikawa, Shirasaka, & Yamazaki, 1998; Sultan, Jebrane, & Heurtier-Hartemann, 2002), heart rate (Fontana & McLaughlin, 1998; Suarez & Williams, 1989), and blood pressure (Rozanski & Kubzansky, 2005; Schnall, Schwartz, Landsbergis, Warren, & Pickering, 1998).

The experience of stress, particularly chronic stress, takes a significant toll on the well-being of individuals in terms of emotional and physical discomforts as well as functional ability. Health care utilization research has repeatedly demonstrated that from 30% to 80% of all physician office visits are for illness experiences that are nondisease based with stress as the common contributor (Cummings & Vandenbos, 1981; Sobel, 1995). As early as 1982, the United States Clearing House for Mental Health Information reported that industry had lost $17 billion in production capacity due primarily to stress-related problems. In addition, it was estimated in the late 1980s that $60 billion was lost annually by businesses because of stress-related physical illness (Matteson & Ivancevich, 1987). It has been estimated by the National Institute for Occupational Safety and Health that businesses lose up to $300 billion per year due to stress-related absenteeism, lost productivity, retraining, and stress-related health care costs (National Institute for Occupational Safety and Health, 2010).

Although it is commonly accepted that stress affects health, all of the psychobiological connections are not understood. For example, why does a person who has had an unpleasant interaction with his or her supervisor develop a tension headache? Or why does a woman who is struggling to balance the demands of work and home develop stomach pains every Monday morning? Theoretical developments in the areas of stress, coping, and health have been hampered by confusion regarding each of these concepts.

The purpose of this chapter is to present an overview of the theoretical approaches to explaining the concepts of stress, coping, and health and their interrelationships with some historical perspectives. Problems and issues regarding the conceptualizations will be identified. Attention will be paid to reconciling some of the diverse views of stress, coping, and health for nursing.

THEORETICAL APPROACHES TO DEFINING STRESS, COPING, AND HEALTH

In this section, I present an overview of the conceptualizations of the stress and health connection. The content regarding coping will appear, as appropriate, in the presentation of each of the major theoretical orientations to stress. Discussion of each construct includes identification of conceptual and theoretical problems and measurement challenges. The theoretical orientations to explaining stress have been categorized into three types: response based, stimulus based, and transactional based.

Stress as a Response

The response-based orientation was initially developed and examined by Hans Selye and summarized in *The Stress of Life* (1956). He was a pioneer in the development and testing of theory pertinent to stress from a physiological and medical perspective. As a physician, he was intrigued by the common inflammatory responses he observed in patients regardless of their particular disease or exposure to medical problems and procedures. Many of Selye's main concepts stemmed historically from Cannon's (1932) notion that sympatho-adrenal changes are "emergency functions."

Selye viewed stress as a response to noxious stimuli or environmental stressors and defined it as the *"nonspecific response of the body to noxious stimuli"* (Selye, 1956, p. 12). Thus, he defined stress as a response, and it became the dependent variable in stress research. His work focused on describing and explaining a physiological response pattern known as the general adaptation syndrome (GAS) that was focused on retaining or attaining *homeostasis,* which refers to the stability of physiological systems that maintain life (e.g., body temperature, heart rate, glucose levels). The following are the basic premises of his theory: (a) The stress response (GAS) is a defensive response that does not depend upon the nature of the stressor; (b) the GAS, as a defense reaction, progressed in three well-defined stages (alarm, resistance, and exhaustion); and (c) if the GAS is severe enough and/or prolonged, disease states could result in death or the so-called diseases of adaptation.

In his early work, Selye (1956) proposed that cognitive variables such as *perception* played no role in contributing to the initiation or moderation of the GAS. In his 1983 edition of *The Stress Concept: Past, Present, and Future,* he extended his thinking to include both negatively and positively toned (eustress) experiences that could be contributed to and moderated by cognitive factors. It is important to note, however, that Selye's basic theoretical premise that stress was a physiological phenomenon was not altered. In the absence of a modification of his theory, it was not possible to explain *psychological stress.* This could not be done in the context of a theory that was strictly limited to physiology and neglected cognitive-perceptual factors. In fact, problems inherent in a normative or generalized response theory were demonstrated when Mason (1971, 1975a, 1975b) disconfirmed the *non-specificity* of physiological responses to noxious stimuli in rats and monkeys.

Although Selye did not specifically address the concept of coping in his work, his notions of *defense* and *adaptation* are conceptually similar to that of coping. The alarm reaction phase of the GAS is triggered when there is a noxious stimulus. This reaction is characterized by sympathetic nervous system stimulation. In the second phase, or stage of resistance, physiologic forces are mobilized to resist damage from the noxious stimulus. Often, the stage of resistance leads to adaptation or homeostasis or the disappearance of symptoms and does not progress to the third stage of exhaustion. The stage of resistance can also lead to diseases of adaptation, such as hypertension, arthritis, and cancer. Exhaustion can occur when the stressor is prolonged or sufficiently severe to use up all of the adaptive energy. It is important to note that Selye conceptualized adaptive energy as being limited by an individual's genetics. That is, each

individual is proposed to have a certain amount of adaptive energy, similar to a bank account, from which he or she can withdraw, but cannot deposit. When adaptive energy is depleted, death ensues (Selye, 1983).

Much of the early stress response–based research tested Selye's theoretical propositions using animal models with the intent of extrapolating the results to humans. Since the late 1970s, there have been many attempts to measure the stress response in humans using such indices as heart rate, blood pressure, plasma and urinary cortisols, and antibody production. As Lindsey (1993) correctly noted, however, it is not possible to capture the proposed *stress response* and the magnitude of the response by such variables alone.

There are several theoretical, measurement, and practice-related problems with defining stress as a *nonspecific response to noxious stimuli* or, as Selye (1983) stated, to any stress-inducing demand or stressor. First, the generality of the definition as the sum of all nonspecific reactions of the body obscures the more specific response patterns of psycho-physiological responses. As early as 1957, Schachter demonstrated differential autonomic responses for anger and anxiety.

In 1967, Arnold summarized the empirical evidence of how the physiological correlates of anger and fear differed. Fear demonstrates primarily an adrenergic effect, whereas anger demonstrates primarily a cholinergic effect. By the mid-1970s, there was evidence that a single emotion such as anxiety could trigger different physiological responses depending on how a person coped with it (Schalling, 1976).

Second, Selye uses the term *stressor* to refer to the *noxious* condition that triggers the response and the term *stress* to refer to both the initial impact of the stressor (alarm reaction) on tissues and the adaptive mechanisms that are a reaction to the stressor. In addition, conceptual confusion about the meaning of the term *stress* was heightened because Selye sometimes defined stress as the wear and tear, damage, or disease consequences of prolonged GAS responses. Third, the absence of cognitive factors such as appraisal and meaning shortchanged what occurs in psychological stress and fourth, the normative nature of the nonspecific physiological response pattern or GAS does not allow for individual differences in perception of a stimulus situation or how a person uniquely copes with a threatening situation.

In a classic study, Ursin, Baade, and Levine (1978) demonstrated that effective coping behavior produced a significant reduction in physiological activation. Their study of parachutist trainees found that general ability level, defense mechanisms, motivation, and role identification explained "considerable portions" of the variance in the stress response. Increased activation of the hypothalamic-pituitary-adrenocortical (HPA) axis was positively correlated only with defense mechanisms and low performance, whereas cortisol levels returned to baseline as coping processes were established. In general, the Ursin et al. study supported the idea that an individual's perception of a threatening situation and his or her coping behavior are the primary determinants of the neuroendocrine response pattern.

The Allocastic Load framework developed by McEwen and Steller (1993) is a more holistic view of the factors affecting the physiological correlates of stress and coping responses. Fifth, the measurement of stress as a dependent variable must be operationalized by physiological variables. It has long been known that there is a disassociation between subjective experiences and objective signs of both the central and the autonomic nervous systems (Lacey, 1967). Sixth, in terms of adoption of the theory to guide nursing practice, the assumptions underlying the theory are not compatible with nursing's philosophical presuppositions, rendering its application to nursing practice awkward at best. Specifically, the presupposition that each individual is unique and that perception or meaning is central to one's personal experiences is not compatible with Selye's tenants.

In their critical review of nursing research on stress, Lyon and Werner (1987) noted that from 1974 to 1984 approximately 24% of the studies used a response framework to study stress. As noted earlier, the use of the response framework necessitated that stress be the dependent variable, that is, the disruption caused by a noxious stimulus or stressor. Commonly, stress has been defined in nursing research by both psychological and physiological measures. Physiological measures were typically vital signs (Guzzetta & Forsyth, 1979), urinary Na:K ratio and 17-ketosteroids (Far, Keene, Samson, & Michael, 1984), cardiovascular complaints (Schwartz & Brenner, 1979), anxiety (Guzzetta & Forsyth, 1979), or all these.

Most of the research studies critically reviewed by Lyon and Werner used independent variables such as relaxation (Tamez, Moore, & Brown, 1978) or information (Toth, 1980) that were purported to mediate between the stressor (commonly assumed to be hospitalization, a threatening medical procedure, or a unit transfer) and the stress response. Use of such mediating variables is inconsistent with Selye's theoretical propositions.

A recent OVID Nursing Data Base search of the funded research literature from 2000 to 2010 using the key words "stress response and physiological stress" generated two articles. Neither of the studies was grounded in Selye's theory. Additionally, none of the literature searches using the key words "stress and Selye," "coping and Selye," and "stress physiology and Selye" generated funded-research studies during the 2000–2010 decade.

Contrary to Selye's GAS theory, studies of stress using the response-based orientation to stress in humans indicate that stress is stimulus- or situation-specific and subject to individual response. Although there is limited empirical support for the "nonspecific and uniform response" to noxious stimuli in humans, there is abundant evidence that a person's perception of an event and his or her coping behaviors do vary as physiological correlates (Eriksen & Ursin, 2006).

Stress as a Stimulus

In the 1960s, psychologists became interested in applying the concept of stress to psychological experiences. Masuda and Holmes (1967) and Holmes and Rahe (1967), stimulated by their interest in what happens when a person experiences *changes* in life circumstances, proposed a stimulus-based theory of stress. This approach treated life changes or *life events* as the stressor to which a person responds. Therefore, unlike the response-based model, stress is the independent variable in this formulation.

The work of the aforementioned researchers resulted in the development of tools known as the Social Readjustment Rating Scale (SRRS) and Schedule of Recent Experiences (Holmes & Rahe, 1967), both of which were purported to measure *stress* defined and measured *as the adjustment or adaptation required by selected major life changes or events*. The central proposition of this model is that too many life changes in a relatively short period of time increase one's vulnerability to illness. The SRRS consisted of 42 life events (e.g., marriage, loss of a loved one, pregnancy, vacation, divorce, retirement, and change in residence) that were assigned *a priori* weights derived from the estimated amount of adjustment the events would require (Holmes & Rahe, 1967). In their early research with Navy recruits, the researchers demonstrated a small but significant relationship between the adaptation scores (assigned to different events) and illness experiences during the subsequent year.

The stimulus-based model was built on assumptions that are inherently problematic in explaining human phenomena. The primary theoretical proposition was based on the premise that (a) life changes are normative and that each life change results in the same readjustment demands for all persons, (b) change is stressful regardless of the desirability of the event to the person, and (c) there is a common threshold of readjustment or adaptation demands beyond which illness will result. During their early work, Holmes and Rahe viewed the person as a passive recipient of stress. Furthermore, stress was conceptualized as an additive phenomenon that was measurable by researcher-selected life events that had pre-assigned normative weights. Later in their work, however, the researchers incorporated consideration of a person's interpretation of the life event as a negative or positive experience (Rahe, 1978).

During the 1970s, hundreds of studies were conducted on the ability of life event scores to predict illness. Illness was typically assessed as morbidity or disease states. Collectively, these studies have consistently accounted for not more than 4% to 6% of the incidence of illness with low correlations of .20 to .30 (Johnson & Sarason, 1979a). One important explanation for why the low correlations reached statistical significance is that sample sizes in these studies were typically very large. The low correlations may also simply reflect the fact that people commonly experience stress that is not necessarily related to major life changes.

Sarason, Johnson, and Siegel (1979) developed a different measure, the Life Experiences Survey (LES), that not only incorporated the person's view of whether the life event was desirable or undesirable, but also incorporated the degree of impact the event had on the individual's life. This 57-item self-report measure has been widely used in life stress studies. Despite the fact that development of the LES represented a theoretically useful step forward in the assessment of life stress, researcher-selected events do not have a uniform effect on individuals and many other factors influencing the stress-health outcome relationship were found (Johnson & Sarason, 1979b; Lazarus & Folkman, 1984). Despite the fact that LES correlations with illness (operationalized as disease) were higher than those achieved by the SRRS, they were still very low. It is plausible that these low correlations were contributed to by researchers neglecting to assess other factors such as social support, hardiness, and perceived control.

An important study, disconfirming the central postulate of the stimulus-based approach, was conducted by Kobasa in 1979. She introduced the notion of *hardiness* as an important moderator variable. Initially, hardiness was described as (a) a strong commitment to self, (b) a vigorous attitude toward the environment, (c) a sense of meaningfulness, and (d) an internal locus of control. Kobasa assessed these elements by using several different extant surveys, including the Internal-External Locus of Control Scale, the Alienation Test, and the Achievement Scale of the Personality Research Form. In a study of 837 middle- and upper-level executives, the findings showed that those with higher levels of hardiness had lower illness scores despite scoring higher on significant life events (SRRS). Executives who had higher SRRS scores and low hardiness scores, however, had significantly more illness. Kobasa demonstrated that hardiness was a powerful moderator of stress as measured by SRRS and illness.

Although Kobasa (1979) found a mediating effect for hardiness on the relationship between life events and health outcomes, there have been inconsistent findings in other studies. Manning, Williams, and Wolfe (1988) found hardiness, rather than acting as a mediator between stress and health outcomes, to have direct effects on emotional and psychological factors thought to be related to well-being and work performance. These included a higher quality of life, more positive effect, and fewer somatic complaints.

A construct closely related to hardiness but different enough to be a more powerful mediator between life event stress and illness is *sense of coherence* (Antonovsky, 1987). Sense of coherence (SOC) is characterized by (a) comprehensibility—the degree to which a situation is predictable and explicable, (b) manageability—the availability of sufficient resources (internal and external) to meet the demands of the situation, and (c) meaningfulness—the degree to which life's demands are worthy of the investment of energy. Persons with a high SOC have a tendency to view the world as ordered, predictable, and manageable. Importantly, Antonovsky (1987) argued that we often ask the wrong question—that is, "Why do some people become ill?"—when, perhaps we should be asking, "Why do people stay healthy despite life stress?"

Notwithstanding the dominance of the stimulus approach to studying the relationship between life event stress and illness (disease) in the 1970s and early 1980s, the value of this paradigm in explaining the relationship between stress and illness was not confirmed. In an attempt to come to grips with the issues regarding the *a priori* weighted measures of major life events, Kanner, Coyne, Schaefer, and Lazarus (1981) proposed a measure of chronic daily hassles and uplifts—the Hassles Scale consisting of 117 items and the Uplifts Scale containing 135 items. Hassles were defined as "relatively minor" daily experiences and demands that are appraised as threatening or harmful, and uplifts are favorable experiences and events. On the Hassles Scale, respondents indicated whether or not an occurrence of any of the experiences "hassled or bothered" them within the past week or month and, if so, whether the hassle was "somewhat," "moderately," or "extremely" severe. Similarly, on the Uplifts Scale, respondents indicated if they experienced an event as an uplift, a positive event, and, if so, to what extent was it positive ("somewhat," "moderate," or "extremely"). Using the Hassles Scale and a life events questionnaire, Delongis, Coyne, Dakof, Folkman, and Lazarus (1982) were able to demonstrate, through a multiple regression analysis, that the hassle scores were more strongly associated with somatic health than were life event scores. Interestingly, the uplift scores made very little contribution to health that was independent of hassles. Despite the stronger performance of hassles in predicting illness, the authors concluded that the experiences of daily hassles or uplifts were insufficient in predicting health outcomes.

In 1987, Lyon and Werner noted that approximately 30% of the nursing research on stress

from 1974 to 1984 used a stimulus-based or life event approach. In fact, Volicer and Bohannon (1975) adapted the SRRS to stressful events of hospitalization and developed the Hospital Stress Rating Scale (HSRS). Consistent with findings from other disciplines, the correlations between life event as HSRS scores and physical and mental disruptions were small in magnitude ($r = .20$–$.28$). By the late 1980s, the stimulus-based approach to defining and measuring stress without appraisal had fallen out of favor in nursing.

A recent search of the OVID Nursing Data Base for research literature from 2000 to 2010 using the key words "stress and life events," "coping and life events," and "stress, illness, and life events" generated 628 funded research reports. In all of these studies the focus was on discrete life events such as divorce, environmental disasters, or traumatic experiences such as rape, incest, and unexpected hospitalization in an intensive care unit. None of the studies used tools developed to measure life events consistent with the assumptions underlying the "stress as a stimulus" conceptualization posed by Holmes and Rahe (1967).

In 1993, Werner significantly modified and extended the notion that stress and health-related responses were triggered from events. She proposed a framework to examine trigger events or stimuli that resulted in the experience of stress or significant physical or psychosocial reaction. Werner labeled the trigger event a *stressor* and proposed that there are four types of stressors: event, situation, conditions, and cues. An *event* is something noteworthy that happens. A *situation* is composed of a combination of circumstances at any given moment. A *condition* is a state of being, and a *cue* is a feature indicating the nature of something perceived (see Table 1.1).

In addition to identifying types of stressors, Werner identified ways to categorize them with respect to locus (internal or external), duration, and temporality (acute, time limited; chronic, intermittent; and chronic), forecasting (predictable or unpredictable), tone (positive or negative), and impact (normative or catastrophic). Integrating these elements, she proposed an organizing schema for stressor research in nursing. Although it is unlikely that specific responses to stressors in any of the categories proposed by Werner would be the same across individuals, it might be possible to identify common themes within specified categories in similar cultures.

Table 1.1   Organizing Schema for Stressor Research in Nursing

Stressor category	Working definition
Life-Related Normative (L-RN)	Events, situations, conditions, or cues which are usually expected, which most experience, and which require adjustment or adaptation
Health/Illness-Related Normative (HI-RN)	Events, situations, conditions, or cues which are related to health or to illness, and/or treatment for these, and which are usually expected, which most experience, and which require adjustment or adaptation
Life-Related Catastrophic (L-RC)	Events, situations, conditions, or cues which are generally unpredictable, usually infrequent, and commonly result in dire consequences in addition to requiring adjustment or adaptation
Health/Illness-Related Catastrophic (HI-RC)	Events, situations, conditions, or cues which are related to health or to illness, and/or treatment for these, and which are generally unpredictable, usually infrequent, and commonly result in dire consequences in addition to requiring adjustment or adaptation

SOURCE: From Werner (1993, pp. 17–18). Copyright © 1993 by Sigma Theta Tau International.

Stress as a Transaction

As a social-personality psychologist, Richard Lazarus became interested in explaining the dynamics of troublesome experiences. He developed and tested a transactional theory of stress and coping (TTSC) (Lazarus, 1966; Lazarus & Folkman, 1984). He believed that stress as a concept had heuristic value, but in and of itself was not measurable as a single factor. Lazarus (1966) contended that stress did not exist in the *event* but rather is a result of a transaction between a person and his or her environment. As such, stress encompasses a set of cognitive, affective, and coping factors.

Precursor models to Lazarus's TTSC theory included those proposed by Basowitz, Persky, Korchin, and Grinker (1955); Mechanic (1962); and Janis (1954). Each of these models, although different in many ways, shared some commonalities. Basowitz et al. defined stress as feelings that typically occur when an organism is threatened. In Mechanic's (1962) model of stress, it is defined as "discomforting responses of persons in particular situations" (p. 7). The factors proposed to influence whether or not a situation is experienced as discomforting include the abilities or capacities of the person, skills and constraints produced by group practices and traditions, resources available to the person in the environment, and norms that

define where and how the individual could be comfortable in using the means available. Behavior that a person uses to respond to demands is termed *coping behavior*. Janis (1954) proposed a model of disaster that included three major phases of stress: (a) the threat phase, in which persons perceive objective signs of danger; (b) the danger impact phase, in which the danger is proximal and the chance of the person escaping injury is dependent on the speed and efficiency of their protective actions; and (c) the danger-of-victimization phase, which occurs immediately after the impact of the danger has terminated or subsided. In addition to these early models of stress that introduced the importance of *assigned meaning* and *coping options* to understanding the origin of discomforts, there were psychosomatic stress models that incorporated personal perception as a determinant of organic processes (Alexander, 1950; Dunbar, 1947; Grinker & Speigel, 1945; H. G. Wolf, 1950; C. T. Wolf, Friedman, Hofer, & Mason, 1964).

Due in part to the early works of all the aforementioned researchers, by the 1960s stress had become a popular construct in psychological, psychosomatic, and nursing research. Including his own research findings, Lazarus's 1966 book, *Psychological Stress and the Coping Process,* represents an elegant theoretical integration of all the research findings on stress and its interrelationship with health through the early 1960s. The theoretical framework that Lazarus posed to explain the complex phenomenon of stress was a major impetus for the field of cognitive psychology because his framework consistently emphasized the important role that *appraisal* or self-evaluation plays in how a person reacts, feels, and behaves.

Lazarus (1966) and Lazarus and Folkman (1984) asserted that the primary mediator of person–environment transactions was appraisal. Three types of appraisal were identified: primary, secondary, and reappraisal. *Primary appraisal* is a judgment about what the person perceives a situation holds in store for him or her. Specifically, a person assesses the possible effects of demands and resources on well-being. If the demands of a situation outweigh available resources, then the individual may determine that the situation represents (a) a potential for harm or loss (threat) or that (b) actual harm has already occurred (harm) or (c) the situation has potential for some type of gain or benefit (challenge). It is important to note, however, that the perception of challenge in the absence of perceived potential for harm was not considered a stress appraisal.

The perception of threat triggers *secondary appraisal,* which is the process of determining what coping options or behaviors are available to deal with a threat and how effective they might be. Often, primary and secondary appraisals occur simultaneously and interact with one another, which makes measurement very difficult (Lazarus & Folkman, 1984).

Reappraisal is the process of continually evaluating, changing, or relabeling earlier primary or secondary appraisals as the situation evolves. What was initially perceived as threatening may now be viewed as a challenge or as benign or irrelevant. Often, reappraisal results in the cognitive elimination of perceived threat.

There are many situational factors that influence appraisals of threat, including their number and complexity; person's values, commitments, and goals; availability of resources; novelty of the situation; self-esteem; social support; coping skills; situational constraints; degree of uncertainty and ambiguity; proximity (time and space), intensity, and duration of the threat; and the controllability of the threat. What occurs during appraisal processes determines emotions and coping behaviors (Lazarus, 1966; Lazarus & Folkman, 1984).

Other important concepts in Lazarus's transactional framework for stress include coping and stress emotions. Unlike the response-based or stimulus-based orientation to stress discussed earlier, the transactional model explicitly includes coping efforts. Coping is defined as *"constantly changing cognitive and behavioral efforts to manage specific external and/or internal demands that are appraised as taxing or exceeding the resources of the person"* (Lazarus & Folkman, 1984, p. 141). This definition clearly deems coping as a process-oriented phenomenon, not a trait or an outcome, and makes it clear that such effort is different from automatic adaptive behavior that has been learned. Furthermore, coping involves *managing* the stressful situation; therefore, it does not necessarily mean *mastery*. Managing may include efforts to minimize, avoid, tolerate, change, or accept a stressful situation as a person attempts to master or handle his or her environment.

Lazarus and Folkman (1984) warned against "stage"-type models of coping because they tend to create situations in which a person's behavior is judged to be inside or outside the norm by the way they deal with a stressful situation over time. A common example of a stage model is that proposed by Kubler-Ross (1969) for death and dying. It is not uncommon for health care providers to inappropriately judge a person's grief response because of the expectation that a person must experience all the predicted stages of grief and only cycle through them one time. Although there may be commonalties or patterns in certain situations that are similar in terms of both the nature of the situation and the cultural ways of responding, there is probably not a dominant pattern of coping.

In 1966, Lazarus identified two forms of coping: direct action and palliative. In 1984, Lazarus and Folkman changed the names of these two forms to problem-focused and emotion-focused, respectively. *Problem-focused coping* strategies are similar to problem-solving tactics. These strategies encompass efforts to define the problem, generate alternative solutions, weigh the costs and benefits of various actions, take actions to change what is changeable, and, if necessary, learn new skills. Problem-focused efforts can be directed outward to alter some aspect of the environment or inward to alter some aspect of self. Many of the efforts directed at self fall into the category of reappraisals—for example, changing the meaning of the situation or event, reducing ego involvement, or recognizing the existence of personal resources or strengths.

Emotion-focused coping strategies are directed toward decreasing emotional distress. These tactics include such efforts as distancing, avoiding, selective attention, blaming, minimizing, wishful thinking, venting emotions, seeking social support, exercising, and meditating. Similar to the cognitive strategies identified in problem-focused coping efforts, changing how an encounter is construed without changing the objective situation is equivalent to reappraisal. The following are common examples: "I decided that something a lot worse could have happened" or "I just decided there are more important things in life." Unlike problem-focused strategies, emotion-focused strategies do not change the meaning of a situation directly. For example, doing vigorous exercise or meditating may help an individual reappraise the meaning of a situation, but the activity does not directly change the meaning. Emotion-focused coping is the more common form of coping used when events are not changeable (Lazarus & Folkman, 1984).

Lazarus (1966) and Lazarus and Folkman (1984) summarize a large body of empirical evidence supporting the distinction between emotion (palliative) and problem-focused (direct-action) coping. In addition, the evidence indicates that everyone uses both types of strategies to deal with stressful encounters or troublesome external or internal demands. Folkman (1997), based on her work in studying AIDS-related caregiving, proposed an extension of the model regarding the theoretical understanding of coping. Her study involved measurement of multiple variables of psychological state (depressive symptomatology, positive states, and positive and negative affect), coping, and religious or spiritual beliefs and activities. Each caregiver participant was interviewed twice. Although participants reported a high level of negative psychological states as expected, they also reported high levels of positive affect. Interestingly, the interview data, when examined along with quantitative analyses, revealed that the coping strategies associated with positive psychological states had a common theme, "...searching for and finding positive meaning. Positive reappraisal,

problem-focused coping, spiritual beliefs and practices, and infusing ordinary events with positive meaning all involve the activation of beliefs, values, or goals that help define the positive significance of events" (p. 1215). Folkman cites many studies that support her conclusion that finding positive meaning in a stressful situation is linked to the experience of well-being.

Another important construct in Lazarus's (1966, 1991) transactional model is emotion—specifically emotions that are considered to be stress emotions. These include, but are not limited to, anxiety, fear, anger, guilt, and sadness (Lazarus, 1966, 1991; Lazarus & Folkman, 1984). Lazarus (2000) presents cogent arguments for the explanatory power of the cognitive theory of emotion. Although thoughts precede emotions, (that is, emotions are shaped by thought processes) emotions can in turn affect thoughts. The primary appraisal of threat and the specific meaning of the situation to the person triggers a particular stress emotion consistent with its meaning. He presents his evolution of a model of stress, coping, and discrete emotions in the earlier edition of this text (pp. 195–222). It is reproduced as Chapter 9 here.

Lazarus (1966) and Lazarus and Folkman (1984) link stress-related variables to health-related outcomes. All of the constructs in their transactional model, when taken together, affect adaptational outcomes. The theorists propose three types of adaptational outcomes: (a) functioning in work and social living, (b) morale or life satisfaction, and (c) somatic health. They view the concept of health broadly to encompass physical (somatic conditions, including illness and physical functioning), psychological (cognitive functional ability and morale—including positive and negative effects regarding how people feel about themselves and their life, including life satisfaction), and social (social functioning). Table 1.2 presents a comparison of the response-based, stimulus-based, and transactional-based conceptualizations of stress, coping, and health outcomes. (See Table 1.2.)

A recent search of the OVID Nursing Data Base for funded research reports from 2000–2010 using the key words "stress and Lazarus" and "coping and Lazarus" generated 48 articles and 34 articles, respectively, totaling 82 studies. It is clear that the transactional or TTSC theory orientation to stress continues to inform nursing research.

Table 1.2   Stress, Coping, and Health Outcomes as Defined in Stress Theories

Scientific view	Conceptualization of stress	Conceptualization of coping	Health outcomes
Response based (Selye, 1956, 1983)	Stress is the nonspecific response to any noxious stimulus. The physiological response is always the same regardless of stimulus—the general adaptation syndrome (GAS).	There is no conceptualization of coping per se. Instead, Selye used the concept of "resistance stage," the purpose of which is to resist damage (this concept is part of the GAS).	On the basis of the assumption that each person is born with a finite amount of energy and that each stress encounter depletes energy stores that cannot be rejuvenated, it was proposed that stress causes "wear and tear on the body" that can result in various diseases based on the person's genetic propensity.
Stimulus based (Holmes & Rahe, 1967)	The term *stress* is synonymous with "life event." Life events are "stress" that require adaptation efforts.	Coping is not defined.	A summative accumulation of adaptation efforts over a threshold level makes a person vulnerable to developing a physical or mental illness (operationalized as disease) within 1 year.
Transaction based (Lazarus, 1966; Lazarus & Folkman, 1984)	The term *stress* is a "rubric" for a complex series of subjective phenomena, including cognitive appraisals (threat, harm, and challenge), stress emotions, coping responses, and reappraisals. Stress is experienced when the demands of a situation tax or exceed a person's resources and some type of harm or loss is anticipated.	Coping is conceptualized as efforts to ameliorate the perceived threat or to manage stress emotions (emotion-focused coping and problem-focused coping).	Adaptational health outcomes are conceptualized as short term and long term. Short-term outcomes include social functioning in a specific encounter, morale in the positive and negative affect during and after an encounter, and somatic health in symptoms generated by the stressful encounter. Long-term outcomes include social functioning, morale, and somatic health. Both short-term and long-term health outcomes encompass effective, affective, and physiological components.

The Concept of Health

Each of the three theoretical perspectives described above incorporates proposed links between stress and health. It is clear that both the stimulus-based and the response-based models were developed based on a biomedical orientation to health in which illness is operationalized as disease and health is viewed as the absence of disease. The transaction model, however, views health as a subjective phenomenon that encompasses somatic sense of self and functional ability.

Health is an elusive term. It is a term that many people think they understand until they are asked to define or describe it and then asked how they would measure it. It has been described as a value judgment, as an objective state, as a subjective state, as a continuum from illness to wellness, and as a utopian state (rarely achievable). Contributing to the confusion about health are the related concepts of wellness, well-being, and quality of life.

Despite the common origin of the word health from *hoelth*, an Old English word meaning safe or sound and whole of body (Dolfman, 1973), there is no one contemporary meaning for the construct. During the twentieth century, many attempts have been made by the lay community to define health in a manner that has broad applicability. These global definitions, however, are confusing and make it difficult, if not impossible, to clearly operationalize. This confusion has particularly important ramifications when one considers that health is a target goal shared by many professions and the federal government.

Health-related professions offer definitions of health that give rise to discipline-specific foci for diagnosis and treatment. Such definitions are not necessarily problematic. In fact, these differences have probably contributed to targeted and efficient efforts to generate knowledge about different aspects of the human condition. However, there are three important problems with discipline-specific definitions for which we must use caution.

The first is that discipline-specific health perspectives partition the holistic phenomenon of health in such a manner that the whole picture of the human condition and how persons feel and are doing is lost. The second is that too often the discipline's perspective on health is adopted by other disciplines when there is not a good match in terms of the disciplines' philosophical presuppositions and social mandate. An excellent example is the nursing field adopting the medical model definition of health as the absence of disease. A third problem is that the acceptance of a discipline-specific view of health by policy-making groups necessarily leads to health policy decisions that may not be in the best interest of the population as a whole.

The Biomedical View of Health

The most popular and widely held view of health is the biomedical one. Medicine has traditionally viewed health from an objective stance and defines it as the absence of disease or discernible pathology and defines illness as the presence of same (Engel, 1992; Kleinman, 1981; Millstein & Irwin, 1987). On the basis of this perspective, medicine's social mandate has been the diagnosis and treatment of disease. Public health professionals and government agencies commonly adopt the biomedical model and use morbidity and mortality statistics as an index of the population's health.

The biomedical model, as noted by Antonovsky (1979), is a dichotomous model. Consistent with this perspective, a person who has a chronic disease cannot have health or be considered well. Furthermore, a logical extension of the dichotomous model is that a person cannot be healthy in the presence of disease.

Nursing's View of Health

Nursing has been critical of the narrow confines of the biomedical model as a perspective for nursing and its adoption by government agencies (Hall & Allan, 1987; Leininger, 1994; Lyon, 1990). Many nurses in practice and nurse educators, however, commonly adopt the biomedical view and equate illness and disease using the terms interchangeably. Likewise, concepts of health and wellness are used interchangeably, logically resulting in the conclusion that persons who have chronic diseases are not and cannot be described as well. Because health and wellness are targeted outcomes, it is imperative that nursing be clear on how it defines these concepts. This is particularly important in developing theoretical models linking stress, coping, and health that can serve as a framework for nursing research and practice. Nursing must define health in a manner that (a) is consistent with its philosophical presuppositions, (b) is measurable, (c) is empirically based, and (d) captures outcomes that are sensitive to nursing interventions or therapeutics.

Currently, there is little unity regarding a definition of health as a central concept for nursing. Considered an essential ingredient of nursing's theoretical meta-paradigm (i.e., person, environment, health, and nursing), nurse theorists have elected to define health in the context of their proposed models. Florence Nightingale (1860/1969) wrote that health is *"not only to be well, but to be able to use well every power we have to use"* (p. 26). Although one cannot be sure what Nightingale actually meant by the word *well*, Selanders (1995) argues she meant *"being the best you can be at any given point in time"* (p. 26). This allows for an individual to be healthy even if not *medically* well. Some additional light is shed on the meaning of wellness because it is clear that Nightingale viewed disease and illness as distinctly different phenomena. It is interesting to speculate that if Florence Nightingale were writing her *Notes on Nursing* today, she most certainly would have included stress as one of the many nondisease-based causes of symptoms experienced by patients.

Tripp-Reimer (1984) proposed a two-dimensional health state with an *etic* perspective (disease–nondisease) that reflects an objective interpretation of health data and an *emic* perspective (wellness–illness) that represent the subjective experience. Four health states are possible within her model. Tripp-Reimer proposes that this approach is particularly useful cross-culturally when perceptions of heath differ between scientifically educated providers and the client. Newman (1986) views health as the totality of life processes that are evolving toward expanded consciousness. Man represents only one stage of this evolution. Orem (1995) distinguishes between health and wellness. She defines health as a state characterized by soundness or wholeness of human structure and bodily and mental functions. Wellness, she notes, is a state characterized by experiences of contentment, pleasure, and movement toward maturation and achievement of the human potential (personalization). Engagement in self-care facilitates this process of personalization. Other nurses offering conceptualizations of health include Henderson (1966), King (1981), Lyon (1990), Newman (1986), Parse (1992), Paterson and Zderad (1976), Peplau (1952, 1988), and Rogers (1970). Health is defined in many ways within the discipline of nursing (See Table 1.3). Commonly shared attributes of health inherent in all of these definitions, however, is that it is a subjective experience that encompasses how a person is feeling and doing. These commonly shared attributes are apparent in Keller's (1981) analysis of definitions of health. A subjective orientation to defining health is quite different from the medical definition of health as an objective phenomenon manifested by the absence of disease or pathology.

Regarding the possibility of a single definition of health for nursing, Meleis (1990) points out that, "although diversity should be accepted and reinforced, there is a need for unity in perspective that represents the territory of investigation, the territory for theoretical development" (p. 109).

Table 1.3   Nursing-Focused Conceptualizations of Health

Author	*Definition of Health*
Henderson (1966)	Health is viewed in terms of a person's ability to perform 14 self-care tasks and a quality of life basic to human functioning.
Peplau (1952, 1988)	Health is defined as forward movement of the personality that is promoted through interpersonal processes in the direction of creative, productive, and constructive living.
Rogers (1970, 1989)	Health is defined as a value term for which meaning is determined by culture or the individual. Positive health symbolizes wellness.
Orem (1971, 1980, 1995)	Health is defined as a *state* that is characterized by soundness or wholeness of bodily and mental functioning. It includes physical, psychological, interpersonal, and social aspects. Well-being is the individual's perceived condition of existence.
King (1971, 1981)	Health is defined as a dynamic state of the life cycle; illness is an interference in the life cycle. Health implies continuous adaptation to stress.
Neuman (1989)	Health is defined as reflected in the level of wellness.
Parse (1981, 1989)	Health is defined as a lived experience—a rhythmic process of being and becoming.
Tripp-Reimer (1984)	Health is defined as encompassing two dimensions, the etic (objective) and the emic (subjective), which include both disease/nondisease and illness/wellness.
Lyon (1990)	Health is defined as a person's subjective expression of the composite evaluation of somatic sense of self (how one is feeling) and functional ability (how one is doing). The resulting judgment is manifested in the subjective experience of some degree of illness or wellness.

This unity in perspective would also help to shape the target goals of nursing's unique contributions to society and could serve as a practical guideline for assessment, diagnosis, and intervention. The importance of using a definition of health that can be operationalized and used to guide nursing practice and research cannot be overemphasized.

A nursing-oriented definition of health consistent with the theme that health is a subjective phenomenon that is operationalizable has been proposed by Lyon (1990). Lyon defined *health as a subjective representation of a person's composite evaluation of somatic sense of self (how one is feeling) and functional ability (how one is doing)*. As such, health is manifested in the subjective judgment that one is experiencing wellness or illness. These subjective experiences are dynamic and are an outgrowth of person and environmental interactions. As long as a person is capable of evaluating how he or she is feeling and doing at some level, the person has health. For example, an infant, although unable to utter words, is capable of evaluating somatic sensations and functional ability. Likewise, a fundamental assumption underlying nursing practice is that all persons who have brain waves have the capability of sensing their environment and the capability of experiencing discomfort or comfort. Therefore, even persons who are unconscious should be treated in a manner that assumes that they can sense discomfort and comfort. Defined in this manner, both illness and wellness are health outcomes. The target goals for nursing care are to promote and maintain wellness (comfortable somatic sensations and functional ability at capability level) and to prevent or alleviate illness (somatic discomfort and a decline in functional ability below capability level). Illness and wellness are conceptualized as different phenomena, not as opposite or polar ends of the same phenomenon.

Illness as defined by Lyon (1990) is the subjective experience of somatic discomfort (emotional or physical or both) that is accompanied by some degree of functional decline below the person's perceived capability level. Illness occurs on a continuum from low ("I'm not feeling well") to high ("I'm very ill or sick"). The experience of somatic discomfort and a decline in functional ability can be the consequence of both disease and, importantly for nursing, factors other than disease (nondisease-based factors) that are amenable to nursing interventions (Lyon, 2010) (see Figure 1.1).

Nursing's unique health-related contribution to society is the prevention of and diagnosis and treatment of factors other than disease contributing to or causing illness (Lyon, 1990). No other discipline focuses on the prevention or alleviation of nondisease-based etiologies of illness. In fact, it is interesting to note that the concept of *cure* is applicable to illness experiences. That is, in addition to preventing somatic discomforts and functional disability caused by nondisease-based factors, nursing therapeutics also can cure *illness* by eliminating or altering nondisease-based factors that are causing symptoms (Loomis & Wood, 1983). Symptoms such as pain, fatigue, nausea, and a decline in functional ability, such as skin breakdown, falling, and inability to swallow, need to be addressed.

Wellness is characterized by Lyon (1990) as the experience of somatic comfort (emotional and physical) and a functional ability level at or near the person's perceived capability level. There is an abundance of research to demonstrate that people commonly judge themselves to feel well even in the presence of chronic, debilitating, or life-threatening diseases when they are somatically comfortable and can function at their highest capability level (Dasback, Klein, Klein, & Moss, 1994; Long & Weinert, 1992; Okun, Zautra, & Robinson, 1988; Stuifbergen, Becker, Ingalsbe, & Sands, 1990). Evaluation of somatic sense of self and functional ability is ongoing and can change from moment to moment. The important distinction in Lyon's (1990) definition of functional ability is that a person's subjective evaluation of functional ability is a comparison between what the individual believes his or her capability level is and what he or she is actually able to do. This view allows for adjustments of perceived capability downward or upward. Therefore, during the early phases after diagnosis of rheumatoid arthritis, a person may not only be experiencing physical discomfort but also be viewing their self as not being able to measure up to previously held standards and expectations of functional ability. As a consequence, the person judges himself or herself to be experiencing some degree of illness. After a diminished level of functioning has become the person's norm (along with learning to live with some degree of discomfort), however, the individual with rheumatoid arthritis actually might judge himself or herself as quite well.

Some in nursing may, at first glance, be concerned about using a subjective definition

Figure 1.1   Disease-Based and Nondisease-Based Etiologies of Illness With Medical and Nursing Interventions

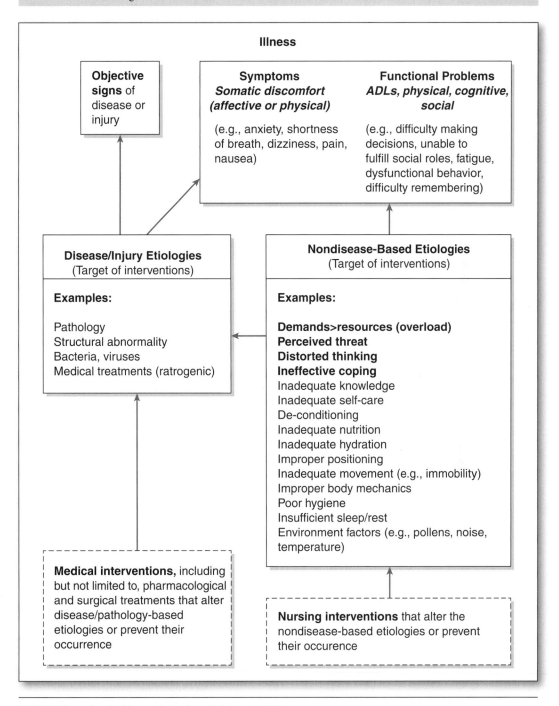

of health as a framework to guide nursing practice. That is, what do you do with the person who has had a stroke yet perceives himself or herself as well? Nothing? Of course not, it is important to note, however, that the individual with a stroke may not do anything unless he or she deems his actions (e.g., taking medications and changing lifestyle) as both salient and important. Helping patients to elevate and to maximize their awareness of slight somatic discomforts (e.g., extremity weakness) or slight problems with functional ability (e.g., decreased mobility) is important in stimulating therapeutic self-care actions (Lyon, 2002). Figure 1.2 presents of graphic of this perspective.

The understanding that both illness and wellness can be experienced in the presence or absence of disease and that nursing's unique contribution is focusing on the diagnosis and treatment of factors other than disease (nondisease based) contributing to illness is a fundamental cornerstone of nursing. Grasping this idea is what makes it possible for nurses to see possibilities for patients to experience wellness in the presence of a chronic and/or life-threatening disease. Knowledge about nondisease-based factors, such as stress, that can contribute to somatic (physical or emotional) discomfort and declines in functional ability increases a nurse's repertoire of intervention possibilities to help patients. It is imperative that nursing develop and/or adopt measurements of health outcomes that demonstrate the efficacy of stress- and coping-focused nursing interventions. In Chapter 22, Lyon and

Figure 1.2   Linking Nursing Interventions to Health Outcomes

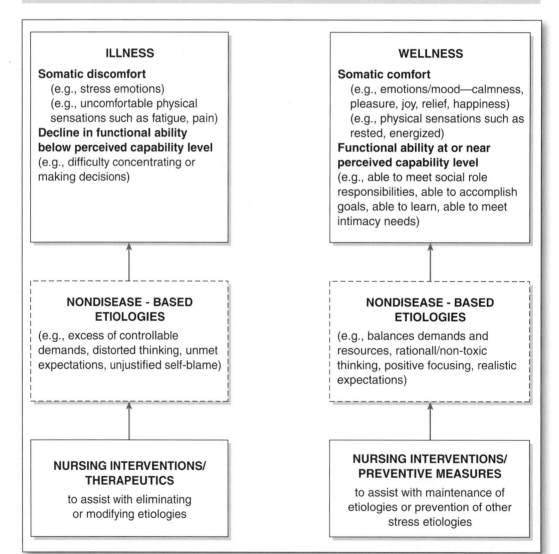

ILLNESS

Somatic discomfort
(e.g., stress emotions)
(e.g., uncomfortable physical sensations such as fatigue, pain)
Decline in functional ability below perceived capability level
(e.g., difficulty concentrating or making decisions)

WELLNESS

Somatic comfort
(e.g., emotions/mood—calmness, pleasure, joy, relief, happiness)
(e.g., physical sensations such as rested, energized)
Functional ability at or near perceived capability level
(e.g., able to meet social role responsibilities, able to accomplish goals, able to learn, able to meet intimacy needs)

NONDISEASE - BASED ETIOLOGIES
(e.g., excess of controllable demands, distorted thinking, unmet expectations, unjustified self-blame)

NONDISEASE - BASED ETIOLOGIES
(e.g., balances demands and resources, rationall/non-toxic thinking, positive focusing, realistic expectations)

NURSING INTERVENTIONS/ THERAPEUTICS
to assist with eliminating or modifying etiologies

NURSING INTERVENTIONS/ PREVENTIVE MEASURES
to assist with maintenance of etiologies or prevention of other stress etiologies

Rice present a conceptual model for nursing that links stress, coping, and health. This chapter has provided a historical overview of stress, coping, and health and its importance for the profession and discipline of nursing.

REFERENCES

Alexander, F. (1950). *Psychosomatic medicine: Its practices and application*. New York, NY: Norton.

Antonova, L., & Mueller, C. R. (2008). Hydrocortisone down-regulates the tumor suppressor gene BRAC1 in mammary cells: A possible molecular link between stress and breast cancer. *Genes, Chromosomes & Cancer, 47*(4), 341–352.

Antonovsky, A. (1979). *Health, stress, and coping*. San Francisco, CA: Jossey-Bass.

Antonovsky, A. A. (1987). *Unraveling the mystery of health: How people manage stress and stay well*. San Francisco, CA: Jossey-Bass.

Armstrong, J. F., Wittrock, D. A., & Robinson, M. D. (2006). Implicit associations in tension-type headaches: A cognitive analysis based on stress reactivity processes. *Headaches, 46*(8), 1281–1290.

Arnold, M. B. (1967). Stress and emotion. In M. H. Appley & R. Trumbull (Eds.), *Psychological stress: Issues in research* (pp. 123–150). New York, NY: Appleton-Century-Crofts.

Barling, J., Kelloway, E. K., & Frone, M. R. (2005). *Handbook of work stress*. Thousand Oaks, CA: Sage.

Basowitz, H., Persky, H., Korchin, S. J., & Grinker, R. R. (1955). *Anxiety and stress*. New York, NY: McGraw-Hill.

Bennett, E. J., Tennant, D. C., Piesse, C., Badcock, C. A., & Kellow, J. E. (1998). Level of chronic life stress predicts clinical outcome in irritable bowel syndrome. *Gut, 43*(2), 256–261.

Benschop, R. J., Greenen, R., Mills, P. J., Naliboff, B. D., Kiecolt-Glaser, J. K., Herbert, T. B., . . . Cacioppo, J. T. (1998). Cardiovascular and immune responses to acute psychological stress in young and old women: A meta-analysis. *Psychosomatic Medicine, 60*(3), 290–296.

Bjorling, E. A. (2009). The momentary relationship between stress and headaches in adolescent girls. *Headache, 49*(8), 1186–1197.

Cannon, W. B. (1932). *The wisdom of the body* (2nd ed.). New York, NY: Norton.

Cohen, S., Frank, E., Doyle, W. J., Skoner, D. P., Rabin, B. S., & Gwaltney, J. M. (1998). Types of stressors that increase susceptibility to the common cold in healthy adults. *Health Psychology, 17*(3), 214–223.

Cohen, S., & Rabin, B. S. (1998). Psychologic stress, immunity, and cancer. *Journal of the National Cancer Institute, 90*, 30–36.

Cohen, S., Tyrrell, D. A. J., & Smith, A. P. (1991). Psychological stress and susceptibility to the common cold. *New England Journal of Medicine, 325*, 606–612.

Cox, D. M., & Gonder-Frederick, L. (1992). Major developments in behavioral diabetes research. *Journal of Consulting and Clinical Psychology, 60*, 628–638.

Crofford, L. J., Jacobson, J., & Young, E. (1999). Modeling the involvement of the hypothalamic-pituitary-adrenal and hypothalamic-pituitary-gonadal axes in autoimmune and stress-related rheumatic syndromes in women. *Journal of Women's Health, 8*(2), 203–215.

Cummings, N. A., & Vandenbos, G. R. (1981). The twenty year Kaiser-Permanente experience with psychotherapy and medical utilization: Implications for national health policy and national health insurance. *Health Policy Quarterly, 1*, 159–175.

Dancey, J. C. P., Taghavi, M., & Fox, R. J. (1998). The relationship between daily stress and symptoms of irritable bowel: A time-series approach. *Journal of Psychosomatic Research, 44*(5), 537–545.

Dasback, E. J., Klein, R., Klein, E. K., & Moss, S. E. (1994). Self-rated health and mortality in people with diabetes. *American Journal of Public Health, 84*, 1775–1779.

Davis, P. A., Holm, J. E., Myers, T. C., & Suda, K. T. (1998). Stress, headache, and physiological disregulation: A time-series analysis of stress in the laboratory. *Headache, 38*(2), 116–121.

Delongis, A. D., Coyne, J. C., Dakof, G., Folkman, S., & Lazarus, R. S. (1982). Relationship of daily hassles, uplifts, and major life events to health status. *Health Psychology, 1*, 119–136.

Dimsdale, J. E., Ruberman, W., & Carleton, R. A. (1987). Conference on behavioral medicine and cardiovascular disease: Task force 1: Sudden cardiac death, stress and cardiac arrhythmias. *Circulation, 76*(Suppl. 1), 198–201.

Dolfman, M. L. (1973). The concept of health: An historic and analytic examination. *Journal of School Health, 43*(8), 491–497.

Dunbar, H. F. (1947). *Mind and body*. New York, NY: Random House.

Dyrehag, L. E., Widerstrom-Noga, E. G., Carlsson, S. G., Kaberger, K., Hedner, N., Mannheimer, C., & Andersson, S. A. (1998). Relations between self-rated musculoskeletal symptoms and signs and psychological distress in chronic neck and shoulder pain. *Scandinavian Journal of Rehabilitation Medicine, 30*(4), 235–242.

Engel, G. L. (1992). The need for a new medical model: A challenge for biomedicine. *Family Systems Medicine, 10*(3), 317–331.

Eriksen, H. R., & Ursin, H. (2006). Stress—It is all in the brain. In B. B. Arnetz & R. Ekman (Eds.),

Stress in health and disease (pp. 46–68). Weinheim, Germany: WILEY-VCH.

Fanciullacci, C., Allessandri, M., & Fanciullacci, M. (1998). The relationship between stress and migraine. *Functional Neurology, 13*(3), 215–223.

Farr, L., Keene, A., Samson, D., & Michael, A. (1984). Alterations in circadian excretion of urinary variables and physiological indicators of stress following surgery. *Nursing Research, 33,* 140–146.

Finestone, H. M., Alfeeli, A., & Fisher, W. A. (2008). Stress-induced physiologic changes as a basis for the biopsychosocial model of chronic musculoskeletal pain: A new theory? *Clinical Journal of Pain, 24*(9), 767–775.

Fitzgerald, P. J. (2009). Is elevated noradrenaline an aetiological factor in a number of diseases? *Autonomic & Autacoid Pharmacology, 29*(4), 143–156.

Folkman, S. (1997). Positive psychological states and coping with severe stress. *Social Science and Medicine, 45*(3), 207–221.

Fontana, A., & McLaughlin, M. (1998). Coping and appraisal of daily stressors predict heart rate and blood pressure levels in young women. *Behavioral Medicine, 24,* 5–16.

Fukunishi, I., Akimoto, M., Horikawa, N., Shirasaka, K., & Yamazaki, T. (1998). Stress, coping and social support in glucose tolerance abnormality. *Journal of Psychosomatic Research, 45*(4), 361–369.

Goleman, D., & Gurin, J. (1993). *Mind-body medicine: How to use your mind for better health.* New York, NY: Consumer Report Books.

Grinker, R. R., & Speigel, J. P. (1945). *Men under stress.* Philadelphia: Blakiston.

Guzzetta, C. E., & Forsyth, G. L. (1979). Nursing diagnostic pilot study: Psychophysiologic stress. *Advances in Nursing Science, 2,* 27–44.

Hall, B. A., & Allan, J. D. (1987, June). Sharpening nursing's focus by focusing on health. *Nursing and Health Care,* 315–320.

Henderson, V. (1966). *The nature of nursing.* New York, NY: Macmillan.

Holmes, T., & Rahe, R. (1967). The social readjustment rating scale. *Journal of Psychosomatic Research, 12,* 213–233.

Inui, J. A., Kitaoka, H., Majima, M., Takamiya, S., Uemoto, M., Yonenaga, C., . . . Taniguchi, H. (1998). Effect of the Kobe earthquake on stress and glycemic control in patients with diabetes mellitus. *Archives of Internal Medicine, 158*(3), 274–278.

Janis, I. (1954). Problems of theory in the analysis of stress behavior. *Journal of Social Issues, 10,* 12–25.

Johnson, J. H., & Sarason, I. G. (1979a). Moderator variables in life stress research. In I. G. Sarason & C. D. Spielberger (Eds.), *Stress and anxiety, Volume 6* (pp. 151–168). New York, NY: John Wiley.

Johnson, J. H., & Sarason, I. G. (1979b). Recent developments in research on life stress. In

V. Hamilton & D. Warburton (Eds.), *Human stress & cognition: An information processing approach* (pp. 205–233). New York, NY: John Wiley.

Kanner, A. D., Coyne, J. C., Schaefer, J. C., & Lazarus, R. S. (1981). Comparison of two modes of stress measurement: Daily hassles and uplifts versus major life events. *Journal of Behavioral Medicine, 4,* 1–39.

Keller, M. J. (1981, October). Toward a definition of health. *Advances in Nursing Science,* 43–52.

King, I. (1971). *Toward a theory for nursing: General concepts of human behavior.* New York, NY: John Wiley.

King, I. (1981). *A theory for nursing: Systems, concepts, process.* New York, NY: John Wiley.

Kleinman, A. (1981). The failure of Western medicine. In P. R. Lee, N. Brown, & I. Red (Eds.), *The nation's health* (pp. 18–20). San Francisco, CA: Boyd & Fraser.

Kobasa, S. C. (1979). Stressful life events, personality, and health: An inquiry into hardiness. *Journal of Personality and Social Psychology, 37,* 1–11.

Kubler-Ross, E. (1969). *On death and dying.* New York, NY: Macmillan.

Lacey, J. I. (1967). Somatic response patterning and stress: Some revisions of activation theory. In M. H. Appley & R. Trumbull (Eds.), *Psychological stress: Issues in research* (pp. 14–42). New York, NY: Appleton-Century-Crofts.

Lazarus, R. S. (1966). *Psychological stress and the coping process.* New York, NY: McGraw-Hill.

Lazarus, R. S. (1991). *Emotion and adaptation.* New York, NY: Oxford University Press.

Lazarus, R. S. (2000). Evolution of a model of stress, coping, and discrete emotions. In V. H. Rice (Ed.), *Handbook of stress, coping, and health: Implications for nursing research, theory, and practice.* Thousand Oaks, CA: Sage.

Lazarus, R. S., & Folkman, S. (1984). *Psychological stress and the coping process.* New York, NY: Springer.

Lebwohl, M., & Tan, M. H. (1998). Psoriasis and stress. *Lancet, 351*(9096), 82.

Leininger, M. (1994). Nursing's agenda of health care reform: Regressive or advanced-discipline status? *Nursing Science Quarterly, 7*(2), 93–94.

Lindsey, A. M. (1993). Stress response. In V. Carrieri, A. M. Lindsey, & C. M. West (Eds.), *Pathophysiological phenomena in nursing: Human responses to illness* (pp. 397–419). Philadelphia, PA: W. B. Saunders.

Long, K. A., & Weinert, C. (1992). Descriptions and perceptions of health among rural and urban adults with multiple sclerosis. *Research in Nursing and Health, 15,* 335–342.

Loomis, M. E., & Wood, D. J. (1983). Cure: The potential outcome of nursing care. *Image: The Journal of Nursing Scholarship, 15*(1), 4–7.

Lyon, B. (1990). Getting back on track: Nursing's autonomous scope of practice. In N. Chaska

(Ed.), *The nursing profession: Turning points* (pp. 267–274). St. Louis, MO: C. V. Mosby.

Lyon, B. (2002). Psychological stress and coping: Framework for post-stroke psychosocial care. *Topics in Stroke Rehabilitation, 9*(1), 1–15.

Lyon, B. L. (2010). Clinical reasoning model: A clinical inquiry guide for solving problems in the nursing domain. In J. S. Fulton, B. L. Lyon, & K. A. Goudreau (Eds.), *Foundation of clinical nurse specialist practice* (pp. 61–76). New York, NY: Springer.

Lyon, B., & Werner, J. S. (1987). Stress. In J. Fitzpatrick & R. L. Taunton (Eds.), *Annual review of nursing research* (Vol. 5, pp. 3–22). New York, NY: Springer.

Maes, M. (2009). Inflammatory and oxidative and nitrosative stress pathways underpinning chronic fatigue, somatization and psychosomatic symptoms. *Current Opinion in Psychiatry, 22*(1), 75–83.

Manning, M. R., Williams, R. F., & Wolfe, D. M. (1988). Hardiness and the relationship between stressors and outcomes. *Work & Stress, 2*(3), 205–216.

Mason, J. W. (1971). A re-evaluation of the concept of "non-specificity" in stress theory. *Journal of Psychiatric Research, 8,* 323–333.

Mason, J. W. (1975a). A historical view of the stress field (Part I). *Journal of Human Stress, 1,* 6–12.

Mason, J. W. (1975b). A historical view of the stress field (Part II). *Journal of Human Stress, 1,* 22–36.

Masuda, M., & Holmes, T. H. (1967). Magnitude estimations of social readjustments. *Journal of Psychosomatic Research, 11,* 219–225.

Matteson, M. T., & Ivancevich, J. M. (1987). *Controlling work stress: Effective human resource and management strategies.* San Francisco, CA: Jossey-Bass.

McEwen, B. S., & Stellar, E. (1993). Stress and the individual: Mechanisms leading to disease. *Archives of Internal Medicine, 153,* 2093–2101.

Mechanic, D. (1962). *Students under stress.* New York, NY: Free Press.

Meleis, A. I. (1990). Being and becoming healthy: The core of nursing knowledge. *Nursing Science Quarterly, 3*(3), 107–114.

Millstein, S. G., & Irwin, C. E. (1987). Concepts of health and illness: Different constructs or variations on a theme? *Health Psychology, 6,* 515–524.

National Institute for Occupational Safety and Health. (2010). *Stress at work.* Retrieved July 7, 2007, from http://www.cdc.gov/niosh/topics/stress/

Neuman, B. (1989). *The Neuman systems model* (2nd ed.). Norwalk, CT: Appleton & Lange.

Newman, M. A. (1986). *Health as expanding consciousness.* St Louis, MO: C. V. Mosby.

Nielson, N. R., Kristensen, T. S., Schnohr, P., & Gronbaek, M. (2008). Perceived stress and cause-specific mortality among men and women: Results from a prospective study. *American Journal of Epidemiology, 168*(5), 481–491.

Nightingale, F. (1969). *Notes on nursing: What it is and what it is not.* New York, NY: Dover. (Original work published 1860)

Okun, M. A., Zautra, A. J., & Robinson, S. E. (1988). Hardiness and health among women with rheumatoid arthritis. *Personality and Individual Differences, 9,* 101–107.

Orem, D. E. (1971). *Nursing: Concepts of practice.* New York, NY: McGraw-Hill.

Orem, D. E. (1980). *Nursing: Concepts of practice* (2nd ed.). New York, NY: McGraw-Hill.

Orem, D. E. (1995). *Nursing: Concepts of practice* (5th ed.). New York, NY: McGraw-Hill.

Ornish, D. (2007). Dr. Dean Ornish's program for reversing heart disease. In A. Monat, R. S. Lazarus, and G. Reevy (Eds.), *The Praegar handbook of stress and coping.* Westport, CT: Praegar.

Ornish, D. M., Scherwitz, L. W., & Doody, S., Jr. (1983). Effects of stress management training and dietary changes in treating ischemic heart disease. *Journal of the American Medical Association, 249,* 54–59.

Ornstein, R., & Sobel, D. (1988). *The healing brain.* New York, NY: Simon & Schuster.

Parse, R. R. (1981). *Man-living-health: A theory of nursing.* New York, NY: John Wiley.

Parse, R. R. (1989). Man-living-health: A theory of nursing. In J. Riehl-Sisca (Ed.), *Conceptual models for nursing practice* (3rd ed.). Norwalk, CT: Appleton & Lange.

Parse, R. R. (1992). Human becoming: Parse's theory of nursing. *Nursing Science Quarterly, 5,* 35–42.

Pashkow, F. J. (1999). Is stress linked to heart disease? *Cleveland Clinic Journal of Medicine, 66*(2), 75–77.

Paterson, J. G., & Zderad, L. T. (1976). *Humanistic nursing.* New York, NY: John Wiley.

Pelletier, K. R. (1992). Mind-body health: Research, clinical and policy implications. *American Journal of Health Promotion, 6,* 345–358.

Pelletier, K. R. (1995). Between mind and body: Stress, emotions, and health. In E. Goleman & J. Gurin (Eds.), *Mind body medicine: How to use your mind for better health* (pp. 18–38). New York, NY: Consumer Reports Books.

Peplau, H. (1952). *Interpersonal relations in nursing.* New York, NY: G. P. Putnam.

Peplau, H. (1988). The art and science of nursing: Similarities, differences and relations. *Nursing Science Quarterly, 1,* 8–15.

Rahe, R. H. (1978). Life change and illness studies: Past history and future directions. *Journal of Human Stress, 4,* 3–14.

Ringsberg, K. C., & Akerlind, I. (1999). Presence of hyperventilation in patients with asthma-like symptoms but negative asthma test responses: Provocation with voluntary hyperventilation and mental stress. *Journal of Allergy and Clinical Immunology, 103*(4), 601–608.

Rogers, M. (1970). *The theoretical basis of nursing.* Philadelphia, PA: F. A. Davis.

Rogers, M. (1989). Nursing: A science of unitary, irreducible, human beings: Update 1990. In E. A. M. Barrett (Ed.), *Vision of Rogers's science-based nursing* (Publication No. 15–2285, pp. 5–11). New York, NY: National League for Nursing.

Rozanski, A., & Kubzansky, L.D. (2005). Pscyhologic functioning and physical health: A paradigm of flexibility, *Pschosomatic Medicine, 67,* Supplement 1, S47–S53.

Sarason, I. G., Johnson, J. H., & Siegel, J. M. (1979). Development of the life experiences survey. In I. G. Sarason & C. D. Spielberger (Eds.), *Stress and anxiety, Volume 6* (pp. 131–149). New York, NY: John Wiley.

Schachter, J. (1957). Pain, fear, and anger in hypertensives and normotensives: A psycho-physiologic study. *Psychosomatic Medicine, 19,* 17–29.

Schalling, D. (1976). Anxiety, pain, and coping. In I. G. Sarason & C. D. Spielberger (Eds.), *Stress and anxiety, Volume 3* (pp. 49–71). New York, NY: Hemisphere.

Schnall, P. L., Schwartz, J. E., Landsbergis, P. A., Warren, K., & Pickering, T. G. (1998). A longitudinal study of job strain and ambulatory blood pressure: Results from a three-year follow-up. *Psychosomatic Medicine, 60*(6), 697–706.

Schwartz, L. P., & Brenner, Z. R. (1979). Critical care unit transfer: Reducing patient stress through nursing interventions. *Heart & Lung, 8,* 540–546.

Selanders, L. C. (1995). Florence Nightingale: An environmental adaptation theory. In C. M. McQuiston & A. A. Webb (Eds.), *Foundations of nursing theory: Contributions of 12 key theorists.* Thousand Oaks, CA: Sage.

Selye, H. (1956). *The stress of life.* New York, NY: McGraw-Hill.

Selye, H. (1983). The stress concept: Past, present, and future. In C. L. Cooper (Ed.), *Stress research: Issues for the eighties.* New York, NY: John Wiley.

Siegel, B. (1986). *Love, medicine, and miracles.* New York, NY: Harper & Row.

Sobel, D. S. (1995). Rethinking medicine: Improving health outcomes with cost-effective psychosocial interventions. *Psychosomatic Medicine, 52,* 234–244.

Straub, R. J., Dhabhar, F. S., Bijlsma, J. W., & Cutolo, M. (2005). How psychological stress via hormones and nerve fibers may exacerbate rheumatoid arthritis. *Arthritis & Rheumatism, 52*(1), 16–26.

Stuifbergen, A. K., Becker, H. A., Ingalsbe, K., & Sands, S. (1990). Perceptions of health among adults with disabilities. *Health Values, 14*(2), 18–26.

Suarez, E. C., & Williams, R. B. (1989). Situational determinants of cardiovascular and emotional reactivity in high and low hostile men. *Psychosomatic Medicine, 51,* 404–418.

Sultan, S., Jebrane, A., & Heurtier-Hartemann, A. (2002). Rorschach variables related to blood glucose control in insulin-dependent diabetes patients. *Journal of Personality Assessment, 79*(1), 122–141.

Surwit, R. S., Schneider, M. S., & Feinglos, M. N. (1992). Stress and diabetes. *Diabetes Care, 15,* 1413–1422.

Tamez, E., Moore, M., & Brown, P. (1978). Relaxation training as a nursing intervention versus pro re nata medication. *Nursing Research, 27,* 160–165.

Thompson, H. L. (2010). *The stress effect: Why smart leaders make dumb decisions—and what to do about it.* San Francisco, CA: Jossey-Bass.

Toth, J. C. (1980). Effect of structure preparation for transfer on patient anxiety on leaving coronary care unit. *Nursing Research, 29,* 28–34.

Tripp-Reimer, T, (1984). Reconceptualizing the construct of health: Integrating emic and etic perspectives. *Research in Nursing and Health, 7,* 101–109.

Ursin, H., Baade, E., & Levine, J. S. (Eds.). (1978). *Psychobiology of stress: A study of coping man.* New York, NY: Academic Press.

Vgontzas, A. M., Tsigos, C., Bixler, E. O., Stratakis, C. A., Sachman, K., Kales, A., . . . Chrousos, G. P. (1998). Chronic insomnia and activity of the stress system: A preliminary study. *Journal of Psychosomatic Research, 45,* 21–31.

Volicer, B. J., & Bohannon, M. W. (1975). A hospital stress rating scale. *Nursing Research, 24,* 352–359.

Werner, J. S. (1993). Stressors and health outcomes: Synthesis of nursing research, 1980–1990. In J. Barfather & B. Lyon (Eds.), *Stress and coping: State of the science and implications for nursing theory, research, and practice* (pp. 11–38). Indianapolis, IN: Sigma Theta Tau International.

Whitehead, W. E., & Schuster, M. M. (1985). *Gastrointestinal disorders: Behavioral and physiological basis for treatment.* San Diego, CA: Harcourt Brace Jovanovich.

Wolf, C. T., Friedman, S. B., Hofer, M. A., & Mason, J. W. (1964). Relationship between psychological defenses and mean urinary 17-hydroxycorticosteroid excretion rates: A predictive study of parents of fatally ill children. *Psychosomatic Medicine, 26,* 576–591.

Wolf, H. G. (1950). Life situations, emotions and bodily disease. In M. L. Reymert (Ed.), *Feelings and emotions* (pp. 284–335). New York, NY: McGraw-Hill.

Wright, R. J., Rodriquez, M., & Cohen, S. (1998). Review of psychosocial stress and asthma: An integrated biopsychosocial approach. *Thorax, 53*(12), 1066–1074.

PART II

RESPONSE-ORIENTED STRESS

2

Theories of Stress and Its Relationship to Health

Virginia Hill Rice

Conceptualizations of stress and the stress response have varied in form and context throughout the centuries. Florence Nightingale wrote in *Notes on Nursing* (1860/1969),

> In watching disease, both in private houses and in public hospitals, the thing which strikes the experienced observer most forcibly is this, that the symptoms or the sufferings generally considered to be inevitable and incidental to the disease are very often not symptoms of disease at all, but of something quite different—of the want of fresh air, or of light, or of warmth, or of quiet, or of cleanliness, or of punctuality and care in the administration of diet, of each or of all of these. (p. 8)

Nightingale believed that all patients were experiencing some *stress* (as it was later to be called) regardless of their illness. She wrote to nursing, "If you knew how unreasonably sick people suffer from reasonable causes of distress, you would take more pains about these things" (p. 104). Nursing's challenge is to facilitate the "reparative process" (p. 9). More than 70 years later, Hans Selye (1936), a young medical student at the University of Prague, wrote,

> Whether a man suffers from a loss of blood, an infectious disease, or advanced cancer, he loses his appetite, his muscle strength, and his

ambition to accomplish anything; usually the patient also loses weight and even his facial expression betrays that he is ill. (p. 19)

He labeled this phenomenon the "syndrome of just being sick" and pursued the catalysts and processes of this syndrome in the laboratory and in his medical practice for more than 50 years. He described it as "stress-response theory" and systematically examined its relationship with health. Other researchers of the stress-response phenomenon include Mason (1971), McEwen (1998), and McEwen and Wingfield (2003). This chapter examines, in depth, the development of stress-response theory and the wealth of research, theory development, and clinical implications that have been derived from the work.

STRESS-RESPONSE THEORY

Selye (1976a) initially proposed a triadic model as the basis for the stress-response pattern. The elements included adrenal cortex hypertrophy, thymicolymphatic (e.g., the thymus, the lymph nodes, and the spleen) atrophy, and gastrointestinal ulcers. These three, he reasoned, were closely interdependent; they seemed to accompany most illnesses and were provoked no matter what the stimulus or illness. Selye could evoke the response in laboratory rats with agents such as formalin, enzymes, hormones, heat, and cold, and he observed it in patients with such diverse health problems as infections, cancer, and heart disease. He noted that the syndrome probably represented an expression of a generalized "call to arms" of the body's defensive forces in reaction to excessive demands or provocative stimuli. Selye (1936) called this *nonspecific* response to damage of any kind *stress*. Later, he used the term *stressor* to designate the stimulus that provoked the stress response (Selye, 1976b). To derive a conceptualization of stress, Selye (1974) chose to delineate what it was not. He wrote that stress is not:

1. simply nervous tension; it can occur in organisms without nervous systems or in anesthetized or unconscious patients.

2. an emergency discharge of hormones from the adrenal medulla; although catecholamines are a part of the stress reaction, they are not the only hormones activated, and they play no role in generalized inflammatory diseases or local stress reactions.

3. everything that causes a secretion of the adrenal cortex (i.e., corticoids); adrenocorticotropic hormone (ACTH) can stimulate the release of corticoids without producing a stress response.

4. always the nonspecific result of damage; normal activities, such as tennis or a passionate kiss, can produce a stress response without conspicuous damage.

5. the same as a deviation from homeostasis (Cannon, 1932), the body's steady state: Reactions to loud noises, blinking of the eye, or contracting a muscle may cause deviations from the resting state without evidence of a generalized stress reaction.

6. anything that causes an alarm reaction: It is the stressor that is the stimulus and not the stress itself.

7. identical with the alarm reaction: These reactions are characterized by certain end-organ changes caused by stress and, hence, cannot be stress.

8. a nonspecific reaction: The pattern of the stress response is specific, although its cause and effects may vary.

9. necessarily bad: The stress of success, challenge, and creativity is positive, whereas that of failure, anxiety, and infection can be negative.

10. to be avoided: Stress cannot be avoided. It is ubiquitous; it is an essential ingredient of life.

Selye viewed stress as the common denominator of all adaptive reactions in the body and complete freedom from stress as death (Selye, 1974).

In his first publication on stress in *Nature* in 1936, Selye defined stress as *"the nonspecific response of the body to any demand made on it"* (p. 32). Following criticisms for being too vague, confusing, and ambiguous, he offered the following operational definition: Stress is *"a state manifested by a specific syndrome which consists of all the nonspecifically induced changes within the biological system"* (Selye, 1976b, p. 64). He proposed that such changes were measurable and occur at both the system and the local level. The entire stress process at the system level, including the threat and the individual's reaction to it, he called the general adaptation syndrome (GAS). (See Figure 2.1.) The regional response (e.g., localized inflammation where microbes have entered the body) he termed the local adaptation syndrome (LAS). The GAS and LAS are seen as closely coordinated, with the GAS acting as backup (Selye, 1976a). The GAS is described in detail in the following section.

General Adaptation Syndrome

Selye (1950, 1956) noted that throughout history aspects of stress and the stress phenomenon floated aimlessly like loose logs on the sea, periodically rising and falling in waves of popularity and disgrace. He attempted to bind together these loose logs of observable facts with solid cables (workable theories) and secure them with a resulting raft (GAS) by mooring it to generally accepted classical medicine in space and time. In space, the three fixed points were the triad of adrenal, thymicolymphatic, and intestinal changes. In time, three distinct phases were identified as the *alarm reaction, resistance stage,* and *exhaustion stage.* (See Figure 2.1.) Bringing together these points of space and time, he reasoned, permitted stress to be less ethereal and more amenable to scientific inquiry.

Selye (1976b) labeled this process general "because it was produced only by agents which have a general effect upon large portions of the body," adaptive "because it stimulated defense

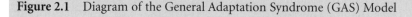

Figure 2.1 Diagram of the General Adaptation Syndrome (GAS) Model

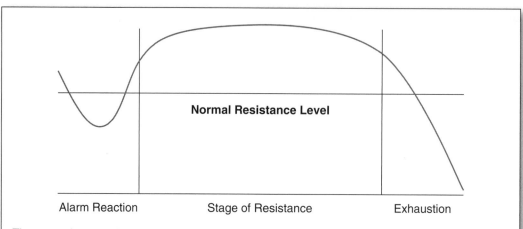

Normal Resistance Level

Alarm Reaction   Stage of Resistance   Exhaustion

The general adaptation syndrome is thought to be the main reason why stress is such an abundant source of health problems. By changing the way our body normally functions, stress disrupts the natural balance—the homeostasis—crucial for well-being. It can also subtract years from our lives by speeding up the aging process. Resistance is the name of the game when it comes to disease. Stress is one of the most significant factors in lowering resistance and triggering the various mechanisms involved in the disease process. By learning relaxation and stress management techniques, you'll improve your overall health as well as your odds of living a disease-free life.

SOURCE: Health News Network, http://www.healthnewsnet.com/gap.html

and, thereby, helped in the acquisition and maintenance of a state of inurement," and syndrome "because its individual manifestations are coordinated and, even partly, dependent upon one another" (p. 38). This response to stimuli, he noted, included (a) the direct effect of the stress on the organism, (b) internal responses that stimulated tissue defense to destroy the damaging threat, and (c) internal responses that caused tissue surrender by inhibiting unnecessary or excessive defense. He noted, "Resistance and adaptation depend on a proper balance of these three factors that occur during the general adaptation syndrome" (p. 56).

In addition to the three theoretical stages of the GAS (i.e., alarm, resistance, and exhaustion), Selye (1976b) identified level of function and normal level of resistance as other constructs in his model. In routine day-to-day situations, he wrote, the organism functions within a level of normal resistance or homeostasis. Self-regulating and balancing devices, as well as problem solving, facilitate maintenance and adaptation to routine stressors and stress. Responses are automatic or habitual adaptations. When a stressor is encountered that exceeds current adaptive resources, an alarm is initiated. The alarm reaction involves activation of the hypothalamic-pituitary-adrenalcortical (HPA) axis.

Alarm Stage

Selye wrote that, even as a demand is being appraised and possible specific responses are being tested, certain cells in the hypothalamus are being alerted to a state of emergency. There is a generalized stimulation of the autonomic nervous system during this initial shock phase of the alarm reaction. A nonspecific breakdown of resistance occurs; sympathetic nervous system activity is suppressed, accompanied by a decrease in muscle tone, hypotension, and hypothermia. Other manifestations include hemoconcentration, hypocholoremia, hypoglycemia, and acidemia. Generalized protein catabolism occurs with altered capillary and cell membrane permeability. The initial shock stage can last from a few moments to as long as 24 hours depending on the intensity of the stressor and the vulnerability of the individual.

A counter-shock phase follows if the stressor persists or the individual is weak or both. This phase is characteristic of the *fight-or-flight* reaction described by Cannon (1932). It involves stimulation of the sympathoadrenal medullary system with the release of catecholamines (epinephrine and norepinephrine). Epinephrine causes dilation of bronchi and pupils; increases in respirations, blood pressure, heart rate, blood volume, blood clotting, perspiration, alertness, blood supply to vital organs, and energy; and causes a decrease in peristalsis. Norepinephrine leads to peripheral vasoconstriction, renin secretion, and stimulation of aldosterone, which in turn causes sodium retention and potassium secretion. Simultaneously, the signal induces secretion of the corticotrophin-releasing factor (CRF) by median eminence cells in the hypothalamus. CRF is conveyed down the portal-venous system into the adenohypothysis, in which it triggers the release of the adrenocorticotropic hormone (ACTH) that is carried throughout the vascular system, acting directly on the adrenal cortex and regulating the secretions of a variety of hormones known collectively as the corticoids. Corticoids are carried to all parts of the body, inducing numerous effects, including gluconeogenesis, thymicolymphatic involution, eosinopenia, peptic ulcers, and decreased immune-inflammatory reactions.

Usually secreted in lesser amounts are proinflammatory cortocoids. They stimulate proliferative ability and the reactivity of connective tissue to build strong barricades to resist invasion, increase the platelet count, and cause protein catabolism. The corticoid hormones are known as *syntoxic* because they facilitate coexistence with the stressor pathogen either by reducing sensitivity to it or by encapsulating it within a barricade of inflammatory tissue. These are distinguishable from the *catatoxic* hormones that enhance the destruction of potential pathogens, mostly through the induction of poison-metabolizing enzymes in the liver. The effects of all these substances can be modulated or conditioned by other hormones (e.g., thyroxin), nervous reactions, diet, heredity, health state, and tissue memories of previous experiences with stress.

Symptomatically, the individual may complain of chest pain, palpitations, a racing heart, headache, dysphagia, or all these. Other manifestations include intestinal cramping, dysmobility, dysnea, feelings of lightheadedness, muscle tremors, joint pain, and bruxism. If survival of the organism is at all possible, a stage of resistance follows the alarm reaction. It is called the *stage of resistance* because opposition to a particular stressor has been established, but resistance to most other stressors tends to be less than normal. Manifestations of the second stage are the antithesis of the alarm reaction stage. In the former, for example, the adrenal cortex discharges its hormone-containing secretions into the bloodstream; consequently, the stores of the gland are depleted. In the stage of resistance, the cortex accumulates an abundant reserve of secretory granules.

Resistance Stage

The resistance stage is evidenced by a dramatic reduction in the alarm reaction as full resistance to the stressor is being established. Developmental (homotrophic) adaptation occurs in the tissues that must intensify their characteristic functional activity for the body to transcend the stressor. There is an attempt to maintain a higher level of functioning in the presence of the stressor as enlargement and multiplication of preexisting cell elements occur without qualitative change. Heterotrophic adaptation, involving tissue readjustment and transformation to perform diverse functions, also occurs at this time. The stage of resistance may be viewed as an attempt at survival through a carefully balanced use of the body's syntoxic and catatoxic defense mechanisms to facilitate coexistence of the organism and the stressor (Selye, 1976a).

Exhaustion Stage

If the organism is not able to return to a normal level of resistance (i.e., prealarm reaction homeostasis) or the initial insult is too overwhelming, a third stage, the stage of exhaustion, ensues. At this time, endocrine activity is heightened; high circulating levels of cortisol begin to have pronounced negative effects on the circulatory, digestive, immune, and other systems. The symptoms are strikingly similar to those of the initial alarm reaction, but such a high level of resistance cannot be maintained indefinitely. Human resources become depleted, and permanent damage to the system through *wear and tear* or death or both is likely to occur. In the usual course of events, the organism would experience all the GAS stages. Surprisingly little has been written about this final stage of adaptation, and few studies have been performed.

GAS Assumptions

The following assumptions are foundational to the general adaptation syndrome theory: (a) Any demand, positive or negative, can provoke the stress response; (b) the stress response is characterized by the same chain of events and pattern of physiological correlates regardless of the stressor or stimulus that provoked it; (c) what occurs systematically in the GAS is evident to a much lesser degree in the LAS; (d) the occurrence of the LAS or GAS or both defines the occurrence of stress; (e) the theory de-emphasizes differences among stimuli and organisms; and (f) the theory presumes adaptive resources are genetically determined and finite. According to Selye (1976a), every individual is endowed with a genetically predetermined quantity and quality of adaptative energy that may be spent with conservative discretion (producing a longer life) or with a reckless abandon (a shorter but more colorful existence).

Many criticisms of Selye's conceptualization of stress and the GAS have been raised by Mason (1971) and others. Mason identified the following: (a) Stress has too many ambiguous meanings (he thought that Selye should have coined a new word rather than selected one already in use); (b) stress is an abstraction—it has no real independent existence; (c) stress has been applied to both the agent and the consequence; (d) the stress response cannot be both specific and nonspecific; (e) there have been few attempts to arrive at a consensus definition and operationalization for the term stress; and (f) the stress definition and the GAS do not take into consideration cognition, perception, and interpretation of the stimulus.

Some of these concerns were addressed by Selye (1976c) in his article, "Forty Years of Stress Research: Principal Remaining Problems and Misconceptions." He argued that stress is the nonspecific response of the body to any demand, that the stressor is the agent that produces it, and that the GAS is the chronological development of the response to stressors when their action is prolonged. Selye wrote that the terms *nonspecificity* and *specificity* could be applied to both the eliciting agent and the response. By nonspecific is meant the *generalized effects or responses that are characteristic of many stimuli or agents—that is, the manifestations of the alarm reaction with secretion of ACTH, the catecholamines, thymicolymphatic involution, and so on.* These, he argued,

are elicited by innumerable agents that make intense and systemic demands on the organism. Perception of a green light, however, is a highly specific response. It can occur only when given light wavelengths reach the retina. Selye noted that the stress response was affected by conditioning factors, such as age, genetic predisposition, sex, and exogenous treatments, and that these factors can cause the same stimulus to act differently in different individuals and to act differently in the same individual at different times.

Although *perception* and *cognition* were not identified in Selye's early work, he attempted to distinguish between agreeable (healthy) and disagreeable (pathogenic) stress as qualitatively different phenomenon. The first he called *eustress* and the latter, *distress*. He wrote that the body undergoes virtually the same nonspecific response during eustress and distress. In the former, however, there is much less damage. This notion of *appraisal* was addressed further by Selye's addition of perception, interpretation, and assessment to his 1985 model (Tache & Selye, 1985). According to Selye, perception and interpretation had not been developed because they were outside the realm of expertise of physiologists (such as himself) who had proposed the original theory (Tache & Selye, 1985).

Coping With Stress

Although not specified in his earlier works, Selye introduces the notion of coping in this later model (Tache & Selye, 1985). Coping he defined as *adapting* to stress situations. This is accomplished in our society, he wrote, "*by removing stressors from our lives, by not allowing certain neutral events to become stressors, by developing a proficiency in dealing with conditions we do not want to avoid, and by seeking relaxation or diversion from the demand*" (p. 20). Tache and Selye (1985) summarized the essential points of Selye's model of stress as follows:

1. All life events cause some stress.

2. Stress is not bad per se, but excessive or unnecessary stress should be avoided whenever possible.

3. The stressor is the stimulus eliciting a need for adaptation; stress is the response.

4. The nonspecific aspects of the body's reaction to an agent may not be as obvious as the specific effects. Sometimes, only disease or

dysfunction will make an individual realize that he or she is under stress.

5. Stress should be monitored through a battery of parameters.

6. Stress should not be equated with only ACTH, corticoid, or catecholamine secretions. These seem to manifest the main pathways of nonspecific adaptation; they are but a few of the elements of a very complex scheme, however.

7. Removal of the stressor eliminates stress.

They noted that stress is the price that organisms pay to survive as animals, and humans pay that same price to accomplish what they consider to be great things.

Stress, Disease, and Illness

According to Selye (Tache & Selye, 1985), the nervous and hormonal responses to stressors, as discussed previously, aid survival. He believed the demand-induced neuro-hormonal changes are carefully balanced to enhance the organism's capacity to meet challenges and, thus, are adaptive. If, however, there is an excess of defensive or submissive bodily reactions, then diseases of adaptation can occur. Conditions in which such maladaption is a factor include high blood pressure, diseases of the heart and blood vessels, diseases of the kidney, eclampsia, rheumatic and rheumatoid arthritis, inflammatory diseases of the skin and eyes, infections, allergies and hypersensitivity diseases, nervous and mental diseases, sexual dysfunctions, digestive diseases, metabolic diseases, cancer, and diseases of a compromised immune system. Simonton, Simonton, and Creighton (1978) and Goodkin, Antoni, and Blaney (1986) all proposed a strong relationship between stress and cancer. Matthews and Glass (1981) suggested a similar relationship between stress and heart disease.

Leidy (1989) presented the physiological processes of stress as a useful framework for nursing to understand the dynamics of chronic illness, its evolution, and trajectory. She suggested that the manifestations of chronic health problems such as chronic obstructive lung disease could be interpreted as expressions of chronic stress that evolve as a consequence of environmental stressors, such as cigarette smoking or prolonged exposure to air pollutants, and the individual pulmonary system vulnerability. She also noted the association between stress and nutritional imbalances, obesity, and diabetes mellitus.

Bryla (1996), a nurse researcher, reviewed the literature that addressed the relationship between stress and the development of breast cancer and the mediator effects of the immune system. She used published articles, book chapters, books, and workbooks from nursing and the medical literature as sources. The studies showed a positive relationship existed between stress and the development of breast cancer although the exact mechanism was not clear. Most of the researchers tended to characterize women who developed breast cancer or who experienced progression of the disease or both as having certain personality traits and being over-responsive to emotional stress. These traits include emotional suppression, depression, conflict avoidance, repressive coping style, uncertainty, extroversion, and sexual inhibitions. The inability to manage anger (so-called *anger in*), masochism, aggressiveness, and hostility (masked with a facade of pleasantness) all seem to contribute to breast cancer risk (Bahnson, 1981; Cooper, Cooper, & Faragher, 1989; Fox, 1983; Grassi & Cappellari, 1988). It has been suggested that the immune system might mediate the physiologic influence of stress on breast cancer (Hulka & Moorman, 2001; Peled, Carmil, Siboni-Samocha, & Shoham-Vardi, 2008). Bryla points out the problem of isolating an individual's perception of stress from the extraneous factors that often coexist with it (e.g., fear and depression).

Other studies have noted the connection between stress and breast cancer as a "stress-related" weakening of the immune system that, in turn, allows cancer cells to proliferate (Greer & Watson, 1985; Levy et al., 1990; Park & Kang, 2008; Watson, Pettingale, & Greer, 1984). This includes the effect of heuristic thinking (Facione, 2002). Measurable physiological effects include lymphocytopenia, thymus involution, and decreases in eosinophils, monocytes, macrophages, and T cells. Other changes are decreases in antibody production, inhibition of natural killer cells, and loss of tissue mass in the spleen and peripheral lymph nodes (Vitaliano, Scanlan, Ochs, Siegler, & Snyder, 1998). To date, most studies have been correlational and retrospective in nature, involving women who have already been diagnosed with cancer. Not considered was the potential potent influence of the cancer diagnosis, itself. Other methodological concerns included the diverse *operationalization* of the stress concept. For the most part, stress has been measured as an emotion, such as anxiety, hostility, depression, or anger, or as physiological data. Linkages between manifest emotions and, for example, changes in heart rate and experienced stress have, at best, been inferred. Means to establish more direct linkages and measurements are necessary.

Bleiker and van der Ploeg (1999) reviewed 27 studies of the psychosocial factors in the etiology of breast cancer. Seven of the studies were retrospective, 12 were quasi-prospective, and 8 were prospective. The reviewers failed to find conclusive results and noted that there was a lack of specific knowledge on the relationship between breast cancer development and psychosocial factors, such as stressful life events, coping styles, depression, and the ability to express emotions. They concluded that at least three hypotheses have been described to explain a possible relationship between the psychosocial variables and cancer development. The first proposes a biological pathway in which stress through the central nervous system and the endocrine system compromises the immune system leading to cancer development. The second assumes that psychological variables are related to high-risk lifestyle behaviors—for example, personality characteristics lead to cigarette smoking, which in turn leads to increased risk for cancer. A third hypothesis suggests that an unknown factor (possibly hormonal or genetic) may be responsible for the increased risk for cancer and for the increased chance of having a given personality trait. The authors concluded that much prospective research is needed to explicitly determine the personality–cancer relationship. Butow et al. (2000) noted that the evidence for a relationship between psychosocial factors and breast cancer is weak at best. The strongest predictors seem to be emotional repression and severe life events. Future research would benefit from a stronger theoretical grounding and greater methodological rigor.

Carrieri-Kohlman, Lindsey, and West (2003), in *Pathophysiological Phenomena in Nursing: Human Response to Illness,* depict pathological consequences associated with the stress response and describes conditions antecedent to it. These physiological manifestations include lipolysis, proteolysis, gluconeogenesis, and urea-genesis. Antecedent conditions include multiple traumatic insult, ischemia, hypoxia, burns, surgery, sepsis, and loss of a loved one and other catastrophic socio-psychological losses. Fauci and others (2008), in *Harrison's Principles of Internal Medicine* (17th edition), describe clinical manifestations of many stress-related disorders, including depression, ulcers, and hypertension. The proposed relationship between stress and health and illness is explicated further in these texts.

OTHER STRESS RESPONSE THEORISTS

Although Selye was the pioneer of stress response theory, other early contributors in the field included Mason (1971), McEwen (1998), and McEwen and Mendelson (1983). Mason believed that coping processes were constantly shaping the endocrine response to stressors and that this response varied with the particular properties of the stimuli. He disagreed with Selye that there was a nonspecific response to stimuli. Mason coined the term "psycho-endocrinology," thus attributing to mental processes some of the variance in the endocrine response to stressful stimuli.

Like Selye, McEwen and Mendelson (1983) and McEwen (1998, 2000) believed that a stressor was an event that challenged *homeostasis,* with disease the consequence of failure of the normal adaptive system. These scientists proposed that psychological stress (such as fear and anxiety) involved perceived threats to homeostasis and that these were likely to evoke psychosomatic reactions, such as gastric ulcers and immunosuppression. The focus of their work was on the neuroendocrine response of the brain to stressors and the development of depressive symptoms. They found glucocorticoids to be one of the body's natural antidepressants. These researchers believed the important first mediator of the GAS was psychological. This is discussed in more detail in subsequent chapters.

Allostasis and Allostatic Load Theories

The work of McEwen (1998, 2000), Sterling and Eyer (1988), and McEwen and Wingfield (2003) laid the foundation for the allostasis and allostatic load theories. They proposed that *homeostasis* is the regulation of the body to a balance, by single-point tuning such as blood oxygen level, blood glucose, or blood pH. On the other hand, allostasis proposes maintenance of stability outside of the normal homeostatic range where an organism must vary all the parameters of its physiological systems to match them appropriately to chronic demands (i.e., reset the system parameters to a new set point). The main hormonal mediators of the stress response in this situation are cortisol and epinephrine (adrenaline). They have both protective and damaging effects on the body. (See Figure 2.2.)

Allostasis implies that many, if not all, physiological functions are mobilized or suppressed as reflected in a cascade of brain–organism interactions overriding local regulation. In the short run, they are essential for adaptation, maintenance of homeostasis, and survival *allostasis*. Yet, over longer time intervals, when called upon frequently, they exact a cost (i.e., an *allostatic load*) that can accelerate disease processes. Allostatic load can be measured in the physiological systems as chemical imbalances in the autonomic nervous system, central nervous system, and neuroendocrine and immune system activity as well as perturbations in the diurnal rhythms, and, in some cases, plasticity changes to the brain structures. McEwen (2000) identifies a number of physiological indicators for determining allostatic load. These include systolic and diastolic blood pressures, high-density lipoproteins (HDL) and total cholesterol, glycosylated hemoglobin (HbA1c) levels of glucose metabolism over time, serum dihydroepiandrosterone (DHEA-S), 17-Hydroxycorticosteroids or 24-hour urinary cortisol excretion, and overnight urinary noradrenaline and adrenalin excretions. Cortisol, noradrenalin, adrenalin, and DHEA are identified as the four primary mediators

A search of the Cumulative Index of Nursing and Allied Health Literature (CINAHL) found six research studies in the recent decade (2000–2010) that used the allostasis theoretical framework. Shannon, King, and Kennedy (2007) used the framework to understand and evaluate perinatal health outcomes. Weiss and others (2007) looked at degree of obesity, glucose allostasis, and the major effectors of glucose tolerance in youth. Carlson and Chamberlain (2005) studied allostatic load and health. Chronic stress to explain posttraumatic brain injury depression (Bay, Kirsch, & Gillespie, 2004), chronic stress and depression in community-dwelling survivors (Bay, Hagerty, Williams, Kirsch, & Gillespie, 2005), and job stress related to allostatic load (Li et al., 2007) all used allostasis theory. There is a great deal of interest in conducting nursing research using the allostasis and allostatic load models.

Stress Response Measurement

The first physiological axis to become activated during the stress response is the autonomic nervous system (ANS). Primary ANS indicators of the stress response include heart rate, respiratory rate, blood pressure, heart rate variability, cardiac output, and electro-dermal activity. In addition, a rate pressure product has been used as a reliable noninvasive indicator of myocardial oxygen demand and impedance cardiography has been employed to determine noninvasive estimates of cardiac output and peripheral vascular resistance (Sherwood, 2010). An additional measure includes the finger arterial blood pressure. The finger arterial blood pressure monitoring method (i.e., Finapres, Datex Ohmeda) facilitates continuous finger arterial pressure waveforms (Imholz, Wieling, van Montfrans, & Wesseling, 1998). The equipment is easy to use and provides a method for continuous measurement of blood pressure changes. Although there are conflicting reports (e.g., Jagomägi, Raamat, & Talts, 2001; Jagomägi, Raamat, Talts, Länsimies, & Jurvelin, 2003) regarding its utility in the clinical setting in which treatment options are determined by blood pressure measurements, it provides a noninvasive method for tracking momentary blood pressure changes in stress studies (Imholz et al., 1998). Blood pressure measurements have been used as indicators of psychological and physiological stress in many, many recent research studies (i.e., Artinian, Washington, Flack, Hockman, & Jen, 2006; Han et al., 2010; Jefferson, 2010; Mikosch et al., 2010). Heart rate measures also have been used as indicators of psychological and physiological stress in many studies (e.g., Matsubara et al., 2011; McKay, Buen, Bohan, & Maye, 2010).

Nurse researchers have also used many of the biomarkers of the stress response including cotinine for tobacco users (Boran et al., 2010), urinary Na+/K+ ratios and 17-ketosteroids (Farr, Keene, Sampson, & Michael, 1984; Jia, Hong, Pan, Jefferson, & Orndoff, 2001), and plasma cortisol levels (Page & Ben-Eliyahu, 1997; Herrington, Olomu, & Geller, 2004). Farr et al. (1984) found altered circadian excretion of urinary catecholamines in postoperative surgical patients. Lanuza and Marotta (1987) reported cortisol elevations in cardiac pacemaker implant patients, and Lanuza (1995) found elevated cortisol levels in both coronary artery bypass graft patients and patients undergoing implantation

Figure 2.2   Allostatic Load

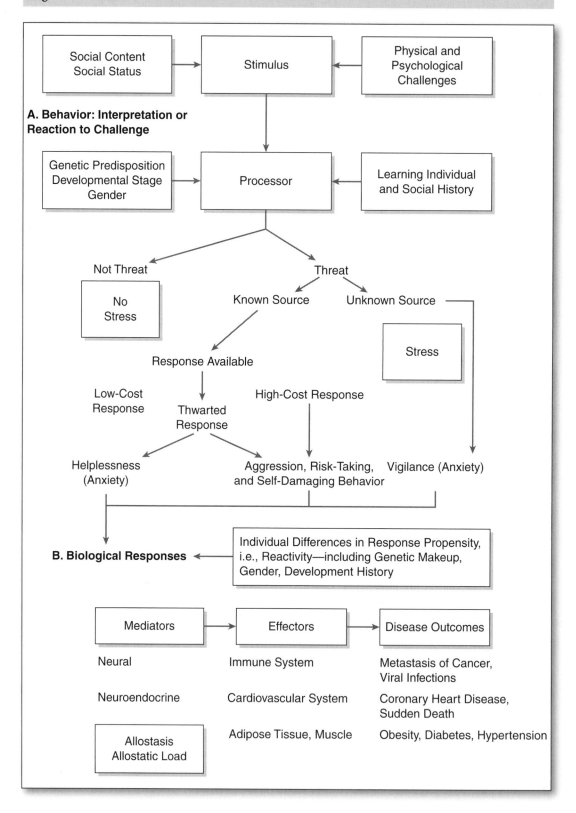

NOTE: Conceptual model of biology and behavior in which responses that are stressful result from the interpretation of, and behavioral and physiologic responses to, environmental challenges that may be stressful to some individuals and less or not stressful to others. (A) Physical and psychological challenges operate within social context that includes individual social status. The processing of this information by the nervous system is biased by factors such as genetic predisposition that are operated on by developmental history, learning, and socioeconomic status; developmental age and gender are also important factors. Interpretation of a stimulus as threatening results in behavioral responses that vary in degree and cost to the individual and that are therefore stressful to varying degrees. Nonthreatening situations and low-cost responses are not considered stressful because they do not elevate physiologic responses. Stress refers to responses that are costly in terms of arousal of physiologic systems and elicitation of behaviors that are harmful. Thwarted responses may lead to aggression or result in helplessness that is similar to a response being unavailable. High-cost responses, which may include aggression, are ones that consume energy and that further increase risk to additionally challenge. All these responses, including vigilance and helplessness, have biological counterparts, and they feed back to influence additional stimulation and processing of that stimulation. (B) Behavioral responses are accompanied by neural and neuroendocrine responses that act on effectors, such as the immune and cardiovascular systems and adipose tissue and muscle. Chronic or repeated stimulation of these effectors may be due to thwarted or high-cost responses or to anxiety associated with vigilance or helplessness and may lead to allostatic load that, over time, increases risk for pathology and disease. Acute stress more readily precipitates disease when chronic stress has laid a pathophysiologic foundation (McEwen & Stellar, 1993).

of an automatic cardioverter or defibrillator device. Strahler and others studied aging diurnal rhythms and chronic stress using salivary alpha-amylase and cortical levels (Strahler, Berndt, Kirschbaum, & Rohleder, 2010) and salivary alpha-amylase levels across different age groups (Strahler, Mueller, Rosenloecher, Kirschbaum, & Rohleder, 2010). Chapter 5 of this text presents other various stress response measures, including their source, research, reliability, validity, sensitivity, and specificity.

Stress Response Empirical Adequacy

During the past 60 to 70 years, thousands of studies have sought to explicate stress theory and the stress response. Selye (1979) wrote "30 books and about 15,000 technical articles on the subject" (p. xi) and produced *Selye's Guide to Stress Research* (1980) to present the then-current state of the knowledge of the stress concept. Included in Volume 1 are a preface and epilogue by Selye and the seminal works of Dohrenwend and Dohrenwend on life events theory, Lazarus's psychological stress and adaptation model, and Frankenhaeuser's psychoneuroendocrine approaches to the study of stressful person–environment transactions. Studies of stress as a response have been conducted in such

diverse fields as business, law, pharmacy, psychology, anthropology, education, sociology, physiology, and philosophy. A major portion of the research has been conducted in the scientific fields of medicine and nursing because of the hypothesized relationships between stress and disease and stress and illness.

A MEDLINE search of the literature (since 1966), using the key word "stress," generated more than 95,000 citations; with "Selye" as the key word, 212 references resulted. When the focus-phrase "general adaptation syndrome" was added, 100 additional studies were indicated. Sampled literature indicates that stress as a response has been examined in adults experiencing surgery (Karlsson, Mattsson, Johansson, & Lidell, 2010; Lanuza, 1995; Slater, 2010), social isolation (Nicholson, 2009), living with a spinal cord injury (Chen & Boore, 2008), heart disease (Brown, 1976; Kasl, 1996; Robley, Ballard, Holtzman, & Cooper, 2010), panic (Lopez-Ibor, 1987; Desborough, 2000), fatigue (Aldwin, 2007; Eidelman, 1980), cancer (Vitaliano et al., 1998), biofeedback (Zolten, 1989), and antibody malproduction (Herbert & Cohen, 1993). It has been used to study music therapy (Bally, Campbell, Chesnick, & Tranmer, 2003; Nilsson, Rawal, & Unosson, 2003), children with cancer (Hinds et al., 2003), pain (Ramelet, Abu-Saad,

Rees, & McDonald, 2004), caregivers (Thompson et al., 2004), and chronic hypertension (Calhoun, 1992; Chummun, 2009; Doshi, Zuckerman, Picot, Wright, & Hill-Westmoreland, 2003). In addition, stress as a response has been used for the development of a culturally sensitive stress measure (Ruiz, Fullerton, Guerrero, Garcia-Atwater, & Dolbier, 2006) and for examining workplace demands of professional nurses (McVicar, 2003; Santamaria, 2001).

In the Cumulative Index for Nursing and Allied Health Literature (CINAHL) (dating from 1982), there were more than 11,000 references in nursing journals for the key word "stress as a response." There are 143 references for "Selye" and 94 for "general adaptation syndrome". In the last decade (2000–2010) there have been 283 "stress as a response" nursing studies. As examples, researchers have evaluated nursing interventions (Han et. al., 2010), stress in neonatal intensive care unit parents (Mackley, Locke, Spear, & Joseph, 2010), adolescent coping (Garcia, 2010), open heart surgery experiences for patients and their caregivers (Robley, Ballard, Holtzman, & Cooper, 2010), irritable bowel responses to acute stress (FitzGerald, Kehie, & Sinha, 2009), recovery from colorectal surgery (Slater, 2010), violence and women's health (Symes et al., 2010), and job stress in professional nursing (Chen, Chen, Tsai, & Lo, 2007; Ulrich et al., 2010; van den Tooren & de Jonge, 2008).

STRESS RESPONSE NURSING KNOWLEDGE

Stress response nursing knowledge has been generated in theory development, nursing practice, and empirical research. Each of these content areas will be reviewed in this section.

Theory Development

Conceptualization of stress as a response has contributed to the development of many theories and models now being used in nursing science and practice. Among those detailed here is Roy's Adaptation Model (RAM).

Roy's Adaptation Model (RAM)

Sister Callista Roy developed one of the earliest nursing theories in 1964 while she was still a graduate student. The model has some of the characteristics of systems theory and some of the characteristics of stress and interaction theories. Roy borrowed and expanded on theories from others, including Selye (1936), Helson (1964), and Maslow (1970). She has continued to expand her model from its inception to the present (Galbreath, 2002). RAM focuses on the individual (person) as a bio-psychosocial adaptive system and describes nursing as a humanistic discipline that *"places emphasis on the person's own coping abilities to achieve health"* (Roy, 1984, p. 32).

This model relies heavily on stress theory, the notion of adaptation, and the ability of nursing to facilitate client adaptation or coping with stress. (See Figure 2.3.) From stress theory, Roy selected the concepts of stressor, stress, and adaptation for her model. She defines stress as *"a constantly changing point, made up of focal, contextual, and residual stimuli, which represent the person's own standard of the range of stimuli to which one can respond with ordinary adaptive responses"* (Roy, 1984, pp. 27–28). *Focal stimuli* are the internal and external demands immediately confronting the organism (e.g., a need for cancer surgery). *Contextual stimuli* are all other internal and external factors in the given situation (e.g., fear of dying). *Residual stimuli* are factors that may be affecting current emotions and behaviors but whose effects are not clearly validated (e.g., having a mother who died from cancer).

Stress, for Roy, represents the person's adaptive level. She wrote, "The human system has the capacity to adjust effectively to changes in the environment and, in turn, to affect the environment" (p. 22). She defined adaptation as "that which promotes the integrity of the person in terms of survival, growth, reproduction, and mastery" (p. 51). A person's adaptation level is determined by the combined effect of the three classes of stimuli (input). Health results when adaptation reaches the optimal level of the individual's potential to meet his or her physical, psychosocial, and self-actualization needs. The individual uses both innate and acquired biological, psychological, or social adaptive mechanisms or all three.

Roy's model postulates that there is an interchange between the adaptive system (individual) and various stimuli (input) from the environment and from the adaptive system. Responses to stimuli are processed through subsystems that

Figure 2.3   Roy's Adaptation Model (RAM)

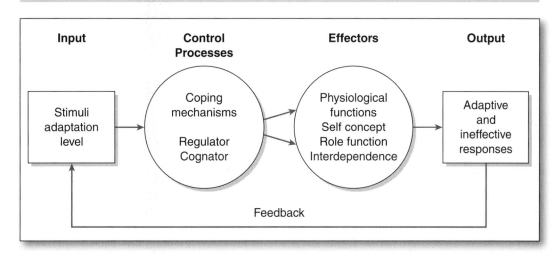

SOURCE: Sister Callista Roy (1984), *Introduction to Nursing: An Adaptation Model* (2nd ed.). Retrieved from http://currentnursing.com/nursing_theory/application_Roy%27s_adaptation_model.html

include two control mechanisms as coping processes and four adaptive modes. One control mechanism is the *regulator subsystem*. It responds automatically via neural, chemical, and endocrine processes. Stimuli from the internal and external environment (through the senses) act as inputs to the nervous, circulatory, and endocrine systems of the body. Automatic, unconscious (coping) responses are produced. The second subsystem, a *cognator*, receives input from external and internal stimuli that involve psychological responses concerned with the process of perception (the link between the regulator and cognator), learning, judgment, and emotion.

The four modes are (a) physiological functioning (biological integrity derived from basic needs), (b) self-concept (interaction with others and the psychic integrity regarding perception of self), (c) role functioning (social integrity and the performance of duties based on positions within society), and (d) interdependence (seeking of help, affection, and attention along with relationships with significant others and support systems) (Roy & Andrews, 1991). Adaptation, Roy (1984) noted, may occur predominantly in one mode or simultaneously in several.

The output of the adaptive system is either adaptation or maladaptive (ineffective) responses. Ineffective responses (coping) result in illness. Adaptive coping results in health. The

goal of nursing is to "maintain and enhance adaptive behavior and to change ineffective behavior to adaptive" (p. 59). According to Roy, each individual has finite adaptive potential that is affected by the conditions of the person or the individual's state of coping. This introduces the idea of control into stress, which goes beyond earlier theories of stress in which the individual was considered a passive recipient of stimuli. It also reflects a more optimistic view of the human capability and potential.

Roy's Adaptation Model Empirical Adequacy

Roy's Adaptation Model has served to guide the development of nursing curriculum, the sophistication of nursing practice, and nursing research (Frederickson, 2000). A search of CINAHL revealed 324 references to Roy's Adaptation Model. Since its inception, the model has been supported through research in practice and education (Bakan & Akyol, 2008; Bower & Baker, 1976; Chiou, 2000; DeSanto-Madeya, 2006; Jones, 1978; Mitchell & Pilkington, 1990; Rambo, 1983; Ryan, 1996; Zhan, 2000). Fawcett and Tulman (1990) built a program of research around RAM, and many midrange theories have been derived from the model (e.g., Calvert, 1989; Hamilton & Bowers, 2007; Ryan, 1996). The study by Sercekus and Mete (2010) provides yet another example of using RAM to guide nursing interventions. Roy has authored 7 books (e.g., Andrews & Roy, 1986; Roy, 1984; Roy & Andrews, 1991), 21 articles, and numerous book chapters. Summary reviews of Roy's work can be found in Alligood and Marriner-Tomey (2006), Marriner-Tomey and Alligood (2006), and George (2002).

Critical Analysis of RAM Theory

Evaluation of RAM in terms of its level of theory development (using criteria proposed by Walker, 1994, and Walker & Avant, 1988) has shown it to be appropriately meaningful for nursing, logically adequate with well-defined concepts, and useful for guiding nursing practice, education, and research. It has been shown to be generalizable across age groups, health conditions, cultures, and time periods (Bakan & Akyol, 2008; Chiou, 2000; Jackson, 1990; Weiland, 2010; White, Richter, & Fry, 1992; Yeh (2001, 2003). RAM is fairly complex with numerous components and proposed relationships, thus reducing its parsimony. The model has generated many hypotheses that have been subjected to empirical testing through research (Aaronson & Seaman, 1989; Innes, 1992; Inouye, Albert, Mohs, Sun, & Berkman, 1993; Zhan, 2000).

Other theories for nursing that have incorporated stress response include Levine's (1973) four conservation principles, Neuman's (1982) systems model, and King's (1971, 1981) theory of goal attainment. These models are critically examined in the text *Nursing Theorists and Their Work* (Marriner-Tomey & Alligood, 2006), and their utility and application are described in *Nursing Theory: Utilization & Application* (Alligood & Marriner-Tomey, 2006). Nursing theories as a basis for professional nursing practice includes the most recent description of the RAM (George, 2002).

A Midrange Stress Model: An Example

The Psychophysiological Stress Model (PSM), an example of a midrange theory, was created by Toth (1984) as a result of her dissertation and used to direct her program of research. She designed it to explain the interplay of multiple stressors on affective and physiologic behavior that increased the likelihood of relapse in acute myocardial infarction (AMI) patients. This model was based on the work of Selye (1956, 1980) and the physiologic consequences of stress (Guyton, 1986). Stress was theoretically defined as *"a generalized stimulation of the autonomic nervous system that alerts a person to the presence of stressors arising from an actual or perceived threat"* (Toth, 1993, p. 36). The response of AMI patients to physiologic stressors translated into the specific consequences analogous to Selye's stage of alarm. Toth proposed that her model explained both the disease process that could result in an AMI and the negative consequences of multiple stressors in the recovering AMI patient.

Key concepts in her model include stressors (physiological, psychological, environmental, and sociocultural), psychophysiological stress, and conditioning effects. Toth noted that with stressors there are increases in heart rate, blood pressure, and myocardial oxygen consumption and that turn, in turn, leads to an increase in myocardial ischemia and the possibility of fatal dysrhythmias or reinfarction. Therefore, assessing stress level at hospital discharge for AMI patients was important to determine who may be at risk for a subsequent AMI. It was also essential for practitioners planning discharge patient care.

Psychophysiological Stress Model Measurement Development

Toth (1988) used the PSM to guide the development of Stress of Discharge Assessment Tool (SDAT). It is a 60-item, norm-referenced, self-report measure that is completed by acute myocardial infarction (AMI) patients at the time of their hospital discharge. The first 46 items assess stressors common to most AMI patients; 14 additional items measure the effects of stressors that may be specific to some AMI patients (e.g., those that relate to employment). Scoring is on a 5-point, Likert-type scale that assesses the degree of consensus with the items from "strongly agree" to "strongly disagree." Summative scores range from 60 to 300 points; the higher the score, the higher the experienced stress.

Scale items were determined through a literature search and reviewed by an eight-member panel of expert clinicians for content validity. Construct validity was examined with a sample of 104 AMI patients who completed the SDAT 48 hours prior to hospital discharge. Scores ranged from 86 to 168; 72% were within one standard deviation of the mean. Internal consistency, using a Cronbach's alpha coefficient, was .85. Toth proposed that such assessment information is needed before initiation of interventions to reduce the stress response.

Six hypotheses were generated based on Toth's model. Each examined the value of factors measured by the SDAT to predict magnitude of stress following AMI prior to discharge in 104 adults. Variables included persistent symptoms, socioeconomic status (SES), age, previous AMI history, marital status, and severity of AMI. Only severity of AMI was significantly related to the stress response at hospital discharge. Toth (1987) found that older and younger AMI patients generally experienced similar stressors; younger patients, however, were less worried about having another AMI and had felt less sick during their hospitalization. Both age groups believed their partners worried about them too much and this was a source of stress. In a subsequent study, Toth (1993) found that women did not differ from men at hospital discharge in the magnitude of stress experienced as their most stressful concerns were the severity of AMI or their age. Women, however, had and reported more persistent cardiac symptoms than men. Findings from these studies serve to guide the nurse clinician in ensuring that AMI clients receive appropriate referrals for stress management or cardiac rehabilitation or both on discharge. Toth suggested that the SDAT be tested with other AMI samples and that SDAT scores be used as a dependent variable in assessing the effectiveness of different types of stress reduction and cardiac rehabilitation programs.

Critical Analysis of Psychophysiological Stress Model (PSM)

PSM, in terms of its level of theory development using criteria proposed by Walker and Avant (1988), has been shown to be appropriately meaningful in identifying persons in need of nursing care. It is useful to guide nursing practice in the planning of discharge care for AMI patients and their families. The model has logical adequacy in that all its key concepts are defined or specified by Toth. The theory has generated testable hypotheses and an instrument (SDAT) to operationalize concepts in the model. The PSM has shown generalizability across age groups and race (Toth, 1987) and

gender (Toth, 1993). The PSM is fairly complex, with numerous components and proposed relationships when the physiological elements are explicated, thus reducing its parsimony. Empirical adequacy is limited. To date much of the research has been conducted by the designer of the model.

STRESS RESPONSE AND CLINICAL PRACTICE MODELS

Many clinical practice models have evolved from the work of Selye and from response theory. Some of these are described briefly in the following sections.

An Adaptation Model for Nursing Practice

Jones (1978) designed an adaptation model for practice. She proposed that the interaction among unmet basic needs (as identified by Maslow, 1970), adaptability (as described by Selye, 1976b), and location on an illness–wellness scale (Dunn, 1959) constituted relative health. She conceptualized each of these factors on a continuum from below average to a high level. Envisioned as a linear model, a line can be plotted from any point on the basic needs continuum to its opposite apex and intersect with another line similarly plotted on the adaptability continuum. Thus, a person's position on the illness–wellness continuum is determined by finding where basic needs and adaptability lines intersect and drawing a vertical line from that point down to the illness–wellness continuum. As a person's position on either their basic needs or adaptability lines changes, so does their position on the illness–wellness continuum. For example, an older adult with hypertension who is low on adaptability but whose basic needs for normotension are being largely met may be placed at the point of average health. If the need to manage the hypertension increases, while adaptability remains the same, health will move in a direction below average.

Kidder (1989) offered a midrange framework that examined five factors (stress, coping, development, social support, and immunocompetence) from a bio-psychosocial perspective to gain a clearer understanding of why some children in intensive care recover faster than others. Her definition of physiological stress was derived from the work of Selye. She concluded that a child's recovery from a critical illness is not merely a matter of providing the correct medical treatment at the appropriate time. Knowledge and analysis of the stressors in the child's environment, the child's ability to cope, developmental age, availability of social supports, and competence of the child's immune system are needed by nursing for understanding, planning, and implementing effective care.

Stress Response and Nursing Intervention Research

In this section, a sampling of the nursing research intervention studies guided by Selye's stress response theory and conducted in the past 10 years (2000–2010) are presented. A CINAHL review revealed 230 studies over that period of time; 33 were doctoral dissertations. Examples include reducing the stress response in adults with surgery (Mertin, Sawatzky, Diehl-Jones, & Lee, 2007), and in children with cancer (Hinds, 2000); gender differences in the stress response (Motzer & Hertig, 2004); the neuroendocrine and immunological correlates of chronic stress (Van den Berghe, 2001); the role of stress neuropeptides (Papathanassoglou, 2010); and psychological stress and anxiety in middle and late childhood (Washington, 2009).

Stress Response, Nursing Research Reviews, and Meta-Analyses

Three reviews of the stress response as a perspective for nursing research were examined. Lindsey (1983) reviewed nursing research studies of physiological phenomena between 1970 and 1980. She reported 141 studies divided into 3 categories: (a) phenomena investigated were primarily individual-related ($n = 66$), (b) phenomena studied were primarily related to the environment ($n = 25$), and (c) studies focused on some aspect of nursing therapeutics ($n = 50$). Following a detailed examination of all the studies, Lindsey concluded that a wide variety of physiological phenomena have been studied with relatively small sample sizes. Most of the studies were either preliminary in nature or

pilot studies, most were single investigations without follow-up, few were replications or extensions, and most were imprecise or lacking in theoretical underpinnings.

Doswell (1988) focused her review on nursing research studies conducted between 1977 and 1987 that had examined physiological responses to stress. She found 19 studies, which she divided into four categories: life events, vocal stress, hospitalization and environmental stressors, and miscellaneous (covering single studies). The majority of the physiological response variables were studied in cardiovascular patients. All subjects were adults. The reviewer concluded that nursing studies of physiological responses to stress were only nominally linked to a conceptual framework. In addition, the number of published nursing studies was too small and too disjointed to provide any consistent support for stress-response relationships. She concluded that the research during that decade included a majority of single diverse studies measuring single cardiovascular variables using Selye's theory of stress. There was little attempt to build a systematic body of nursing knowledge in this area.

Werner (1993) conducted the third review. She examined the nursing research literature for studies on stressors and health outcomes between 1980 and 1990; she found seven studies that had a stress response theoretical orientation. Werner noted that a diminishing number of nursing researchers were using Selye's perspective of physiological stress as a response. She reasoned that this is the consequence of nursing taking a much broader view of the human condition in response to stress. It also may be related to the increasing interest in Lazarus's transactional model, with its heavy emphasis on cognition and appraisal (Lazarus & Folkman, 1984). Lyon and Werner (1987) noted that response models of stress are incompatible with nursing's view of the holistic human experience. Focusing on physiological phenomena without consideration of the person's perspective, psyche, and emotions was seen as only treating one half of the person.

In an effort to arrive at a solid evidence-based nursing practice (Melnyk & Fineout-Overholt, 2010), meta-analyses are being conducted to combine and solidify the results of intervention studies that address the same research hypotheses. Six meta-analytic studies conducted in the past decade have addressed the stress-response issue. They include (1) psychological interventions for needle-related procedural pain and distress in children and adolescents (Uman, Chambers, McGrath, & Kisely, 2006); (2) psychosocial interventions for reducing fatigue in cancer patients (Goedendorp, Gielissen, Verhagen, & Bleijenberg, 2009); (3) psychosocial and psychological interventions for preventing postpartum depression (Dennis & Creedy, 2004); (4) preventing occupational stress in health care workers (Ruotsalainen & Verbeek, 2006); (5) noninvasive interventions for improving well-being and quality of life in patients with lung cancer (Solà, Thompson, Casacuberta, & Lopez, 2004); and (6) support for mothers, fathers, and families after a perinatal death (Flenady & Wilson, 2008).

Conclusion

There is a very long history of stress-response theory and its evolution in psychology, medicine, and nursing. It has led to numerous theoretical models, thousands of research studies and publications, and the development of health care provider curricula and interventions. Selye (1936) might be considered the founding father of stress-response theory. It was one of the most significant contributions to the field of stress and coping. He designed it to describe, predict, and explain living organisms' physiological reactions to ubiquitous life stressors. He gave it prominence and detail with his general adaptation syndrome (GAS). The GAS is able to describe and explain, in part, physiological responses to stressors. Noticeably absent, however, is the connection between the body and the mind. It is this missing piece that has given the theory limited usefulness for nursing.

Some of the early research in nursing also examined the stress response physiologically; in addition, nursing has sought to assess, predict, and explain both the physiological and the psychosocial components of stress. With the need to understand the patient as a whole, nursing moved rather quickly toward using models and theories that took into consideration both components. This is reflected in the broad adoption of biopsychosocial models, measurements, and intervention arenas of research. These developments in stress, coping, and health are further explicated in this book.

References

Aaronson, L., & Seaman, L. (1989). Managing hypernatremia in fluid deficient elderly. *Journal of Gerontological Nursing, 15*, 29–36.

Aldwin, C. (2007). *Stress, coping, and development* (2nd ed.). New York, NY: Guilford.

Alligood, M. R., & Marriner-Tomey, A. (2006). *Nursing theory: Utilization & application* (3rd ed.). St. Louis, MO: Mosby.

Andrews, H., & Roy, C. (1986). *Essentials of the Roy Adaptation Model.* Norwalk, CT: Appleton-Century-Crofts.

Artinian, N. T., Washington, O. G. M., Flack, J. M., Hockman, E. M., & Jen, K. C. (2006). Depression, stress, and blood pressure in urban African-American women. *Progress in Cardiovascular Nursing, 21*(2), 68–75.

Bahnson, C. (1981). Stress and cancer: The state of the art. *Psychosomatics, 22*, 207–220.

Bakan, G., & Akyol, A. D. (2008). Theory-guided interventions for adaptation to heart failure in Turkey. *Journal of Advanced Nursing, 61*(6), 596–608.

Bally, K., Campbell, D., Chesnick, K., & Tranmer, J. E. (2003). Effects of patient-controlled music therapy during coronary angiography on procedural pain and anxiety distress syndrome. *Critical Care Nurse, 23*(2), 50–51, 53–58.

Bay, E., Hagerty, B. K., Williams, R. A., Kirsch, N., & Gillespie, B. (2005). Chronic stress, salivary cortisol response, interpersonal relatedness, and depression among community dwelling survivors of traumatic brain injury. *Journal of Neuroscience Nursing, 37*, 4–14.

Bay, E., Kirsch, N., & Gillespie, B. (2004). Chronic stress conditions do explain posttraumatic brain injury depression. *Research, Theory and Nursing Practice, 18*(2–3), 213–228.

Bleiker, E., & van der Ploeg, H. M. (1999). Psychosocial factors in the etiology of breast cancer: Review of a popular link. *Patient Education and Counseling, 37*, 201–214.

Boran, A., Shotar, A., Khatib, A., Hamza, M., Hadidi, M. S., & Rice, V. H. (2010). Patterns of cotinine excretion among diabetic, cardiac patients and healthy smokers in Jordan. *Research Journal of Biological Science, 5*, 476–483.

Bower, H., & Baker, B. (1976). The Roy Adaptation Model: Using the adaptation model in a practitioner curriculum. *Nursing Outlook, 24*, 686–689.

Brown, A. (1976). Effect of family visits on the blood pressure and heart rate of patients in CCU. *Heart & Lung, 5*, 291–296.

Bryla, C. (1996). The relationship between stress and the development of breast cancer: A literature review. *Oncology Nursing Forum, 23,* 441–448.

Butow, P. N., Hiller, J. E., Price, M. A., Thackway, S. V., Kricket, A., & Tennant, C. C. (2000). Epidemiological evidence for a relationship between life events, coping style, and personality factors in the development of breast cancer. *Journal of Psychosomatic Research, 49*(3), 169–181.

Calhoun, D. (1992). Hypertension in blacks: Socioeconomic stressors and sympathetic nervous system activity. *American Journal of Medical Sociology, 304,* 306–311.

Calvert, M. (1989). Human-pet interaction and loneliness: A test of concepts from Roy's Adaptation Model. *Nursing Science Quarterly, 2*(4), 194–202.

Cannon, W. B. (1932). *The wisdom of the body.* New York, NY: Norton.

Carrieri-Kohlman, V., Lindsey, A., & West, C. (2003). *Pathophysiological phenomena in nursing: Human responses to illness* (3rd ed.). Philadelphia, PA: W. B. Saunders.

Carlson, E., & Chamberlain, R. (2005). Allostatic load and health disparities: A theoretical orientation. *Research in Nursing & Health, 28*(4), 306–315.

Chen, H.-Y., & Boore, J. (2008). Living with a spinal cord injury: A grounded theory approach. *Journal of Nursing and Healthcare of Chronic Illness* in association with *Journal of Clinical Nursing 17,* 5a, 116–124.

Chen, Y., Chen, S., Tsai, C., & Lo, L. (2007). Role stress and job satisfaction for nurse specialists. *Journal of Advanced Nursing, 59*(5), 497–509.

Chiou, C. (2000). A meta-analysis of the interrelationships between the modes in Roy's Adaptation Model. *Nursing Science Quarterly, 13*(3), 252–258.

Chummun, H. (2009). Hypertension—a contemporary approach to nursing care. *British Journal of Nursing, 18*(13), 784–789.

Cooper, C., Cooper, R., & Faragher, E. (1989). Incidence and perception of psychosocial stress: The relationship with breast cancer. *Psychological Medicine, 19,* 415–422.

Dennis, C. L., & Creedy, D. K. (2004). Psychosocial and psychological interventions for preventing postpartum depression. *Cochrane Database of Systematic Reviews,* Issue 4.

DeSanto-Madeya, S. (2006). The meaning of living with spinal cord injury 5 to 10 years after the injury. *Western Journal of Nursing Research, 28,* 265–289.

Desborough, W. (2000). The stress response to trauma and surgery. *British Journal of Anesthesia, 85*(1), 109–117.

Doshi, J. A., Zuckerman, I. H., Picot, S. J., Wright, J. T., Jr., & Hill-Westmoreland, E. E. (2003). Antihypertensive use and adherence and blood pressure stress response among black caregivers and non-caregivers. *Applied Nursing Research, 16*(4), 266–277.

Doswell, W. (1988). Physiological responses to stress. *Annual Review of Nursing Research, 7,* 51–69.

Dunn, H. (1959). *High level wellness.* Arlington, VA: R. W. Beatty.

Eidelman, D. (1980). Fatigue toward an analysis and unified definition. *Medical Hypotheses, 6,* 517–526.

Facione, N. C. (2002). Perceived risk of breast cancer: Influence of heuristic thinking. *Cancer Practice, 10*(5), 256–262.

Farr, L., Keene, A., Sampson, D., & Michael, A. (1984). Alterations in circadian excretion of urinary variables and physiological indicators of stress following surgery. *Nursing Research, 33,* 140–146.

Fauci, A. S., Braunwald, E., Kasper, D. L., Hauser, S. L., Longo, D. L., Jameson, J. L., & Loscalzo, J. (Eds.). (2008). *Harrison's principles of internal medicine* (17th ed.). New York, NY: McGraw-Hill.

Fawcett, J., & Tulman, L. (1990). Building a programme of research from the Roy Adaptation Model of nursing. *Journal of Advanced Nursing, 15,* 720–725.

FitzGerald, L. Z., Kehoe, P., & Sinha, K. (2009). Hypothalamic-pituitary-adrenal axis dysregulation in women with irritable bowel syndrome in response to acute physical stress. *Western Journal of Nursing Research, 31*(7), 818–836.

Flenady, V., & Wilson, T. (2008). Support for mothers, fathers and families after perinatal death. *Cochrane Database of Systematic Reviews,* Issue 1.

Fox, B. (1983). Current theory of psychogenic effects on cancer incidence and prognosis. *Journal of Psychosocial Oncology, 1,* 17–31.

Frederickson, K. (2000). Nursing knowledge development through research: Using the Roy Adaptation Model. *Nursing Science Quarterly, 13*(1), 13–17.

Galbreath, J. (2002). Roy Adaptation Model: Sister Callista Roy. In J. B. George (Ed.), *Nursing theories: The base for professional nursing practice* (pp. 295–338). Upper Saddle River, NJ: Prentice Hall.

Garcia, C. (2010). Conceptualization and measurement of coping during adolescence: A review of the literature. *Journal of Nursing Scholarship, 42*(2), 166–185.

George, J. B. (2002). *Nursing theories: The base for professional nursing practice* (5th ed.). Upper Saddle River, NJ: Prentice Hall.

Goedendorp, M. M., Gielissen, M. F. M., Verhagen, C. A. H. H. V. M., & Bleijenberg, G. (2009). Psychosocial interventions for reducing fatigue during cancer treatment in adults. *Cochrane Database of Systematic Reviews,* Issue 1.

Goodkin, K., Antoni, M., & Blaney, P. (1986). Stress and hopelessness in the promotion of cervical intraepithelial neoplasia to invasive squamous cell carcinoma of the cervix. *Journal of Psychosomatic Research, 30,* 67–76.

Grassi, L., & Cappellari, L. (1988). State and trait psychological characteristics of breast cancer patients. *New Trends in Experimental and Clinical Psychiatry, 4,* 99–109.

Greer, S., & Watson, M. (1985). Towards a psychobiological model of cancer. Psychological considerations. *Social Science and Medicine, 20,* 773–777.

Guyton, A. (1986). *Textbook of medical physiology* (7th ed.). Philadelphia, PA: W. B. Saunders.

Hamilton, R. J., & Bowers, B. J. (2007). The theory of genetic vulnerability: A Roy Model exemplar. *Nursing Science Quarterly, 20*(3), 254–264.

Han, L., Li, J. P., Sit, J. W. H., Chung, L., Jiao, Z. Y., & Ma, W. G. (2010). Effects of music intervention on physiological stress response and anxiety level of mechanically ventilated patients in China: A randomised controlled trial. *Journal of Clinical Nursing, 19*(7–8), 978–987.

Helson, H. (1964). *Adaptation level theory.* New York, NY: Harper & Row.

Herbert, T., & Cohen, S. (1993). Stress and immunity in humans: A meta-analytic review. *Psychosomatic Medicine, 55,* 364–379.

Herrington, C., Olomu, I., & Geller, S. (2004). Salivary cortisol as indicators of pain in preterm infants: A pilot study. *Clinical Nursing Research, 13*(1), 53–68.

Hinds, P. S. (2000). Fostering coping by adolescents with newly diagnosed cancer. *Seminars in Oncology Nursing, 16*(4), 317–336.

Hinds, P. S., Srivastava, D. K., Randall, E. A., Green, A., Stanford, D., Pinlac, R., . . . Taylor, K. (2003). Testing the revised stress-response sequence model in pediatric oncology nurses. *Journal of Pediatric Oncology Nursing, 20*(5), 213–232.

Hulka, B. S., & Moorman, P. G. (2001). Breast cancer: Hormones and other risk factors. *Maturitas, 38,* 103–113.

Imholz, B. P., Wieling, W., van Montfrans, G. A., & Wesseling, K. H. (1998). Fifteen years experience with finger arterial pressure monitoring: Assessment of the technology. *Cardiovascular Research, 38*(3), 605–616.

Innes, M. (1992). Managing upper airway obstruction. *British Journal of Nursing, 9*(14), 732–735.

Inouye, S., Albert, M., Mohs, R., Sun, K., & Berkman, L. (1993). Cognitive performance in a high-functioning community-dwelling elderly population. *Journal of Gerontology, 48,* 146–151.

Jackson, B. (1990). Social support and life satisfaction of black climacteric women. *Western Journal of Nursing Research, 12,* 25–27.

Jagomägi, K., Raamat, R., & Talts, J. (2001). Effect of altering vasoactivity on the measurement of finger blood pressure. *Blood Pressure Monitoring, 6,* 33–40.

Jagomägi, K., Raamat, R., Talts, J., Länsimies, E., & Jurvelin, J. (2003). Effect of deep breathing test on finger blood pressure. *Blood Pressure Monitoring, 8*(5), 211–214.

Jia, Q. L., Hong, M. F., Pan, Z. X., Jefferson, & Orndoff, S. (2001). Quantification of urine 17-ketosteroid sulfates and glucuronides by high-performance liquid chromatography–ion trap mass spectroscopy. *Journal of Chromatography B: Biomedical Sciences and Applications, 750*(1), 81–91.

Jefferson, L. L. (2010). Exploring effects of therapeutic massage and patient teaching in the practice of diaphragmatic breathing on blood pressure, stress, and anxiety in hypertensive African-American women: An intervention study. *Journal of National Black Nurses Association, 21*(1), 17–24.

Jones, P. (1978). An adaptation model for nursing practice. *American Journal of Nursing, 78,* 1900–1906.

Karlsson, A., Mattsson, B., Johansson, M., & Lidell, E. (2010). Well-being in patients and relatives after open-heart surgery from the perspective of health care professionals. *Journal of Clinical Nursing, 19*(5–6), 840–846.

Kasl, S. V. (1996). The influence of the work environment on cardiovascular health: A historical, conceptual, and methodological perspective. *Journal of Occupational and Health Psychology, 1,* 42–56.

Kidder, C. (1989). Reestablishing health: Factors influencing the child's recovery in pediatric intensive care. *Journal of Pediatric Nursing, 4,* 96–103.

King, I. (1971). *Toward a theory for nursing: General concepts of human behavior.* New York, NY: John Wiley.

King, I. (1981). *A theory for nursing: Systems, concepts, process.* New York, NY: John Wiley.

Lanuza, D. (1995). Postoperative circadian rhythms and cortisol stress response to two types of cardiac surgery. *American Journal of Critical Care, 4,* 212–220.

Lanuza, D., & Marotta, S. (1987). Endocrine and psychologic responses of patients to cardiac pacemaker implantation. *Heart & Lung, 16,* 496–505.

Lazarus, R. S., & Folkman, S. (1984). *Stress, appraisal, and coping.* New York, NY: Springer.

Leidy, N. (1989). A physiological analysis of stress and chronic illness. *Journal of Advanced Nursing, 14,* 868–876.

Levine, M. (1973). *Introduction to clinical nursing* (2nd ed.). Philadelphia, PA: F. A. Davis.

Levy, S., Herberman, R., Lee, J., Whiteside, T., Kirkwood, J., & McFeeley, S. (1990). Estrogen receptor concentration and social factors as predictors of natural killer cell activity in early-stage breast cancer patients. *Natural Immune Cell Growth Regulation, 9,* 313–324.

Li, W., Zhang, J. Q., Sun, J., Ke, J. H., Dong, Z. Y., & Wang, S. (2007). Job stress related to glyco-lipid allostatic load, adiponectin and visfatin. *Stress and Health, 23,* 257–266.

Lindsey, A. (1983). Stress response. In V. Carrieri-Kohlman, A. Lindsey, & C. West (Eds.), *Pathophysiological phenomena in nursing: Human responses to illness* (2nd ed.). Philadelphia, PA: W. B. Saunders.

Lopez-Ibor, J. (1987). The meaning of stress, anxiety, and collective panic in clinical settings. *Psychotherapy and Psychosomatics, 47,* 168–174.

Lyon, B., & Werner, J. (1987). Stress. In J. Fitzpatrick & R. Taunton (Eds.), *Annual review of nursing research.* New York, NY: Springer.

Mackley, A. B., Locke, R. G., Spear, M. L., & Joseph, R. (2010). Forgotten parent: NICU paternal emotional response. *Advanced Neonatal Care, 10*(4), 200–203.

Marriner-Tomey, A., & Alligood, M. R. (2006). *Nursing theorists and their work* (6th ed.). St. Louis, MO: Mosby.

Maslow, A. H. (1970). *Motivation and personality* (2nd ed.). New York, NY: Harper & Row.

Mason, J. W. (1971). A re-evaluation of the concept of "non-specificity" in stress theory. *Journal of Psychiatric Research, 8,* 323–333.

Matsubara, T., Arai, Y. C., Shimo, K., Nishihara, M., Sato, J., & Ushida, T. (2011). Comparative effects of acupressure at local and distal acupuncture points on pain conditions and autonomic function in females with chronic neck pain. *Evidence-Based Complementary and Alternative Medicine, 2011,* 1–6.

Matthews, K., & Glass, D. (1981). Type A behavior, stressful life events, and coronary heart disease. In B. Dohrenwend & B. Dohrenwend (Eds.), *Stressful life events and their context.* New York, NY: Prodist.

McEwen, B. S. (1998). Protective and damaging effects of stress mediators. *New England Journal of Medicine, 338,* 171–179.

McEwen, B. S. (2000). Allostasis and allostatic load: Implications for neuropsychopharmacology. *Neuropsychopharmacology, 22*(2), 108–124.

McEwen, B. S., & Mendelson, S. (1983). Effects of stress on the neurochemistry and morphology of the brain: Counterregulation versus damage. In L. Goldberger & S. Breznitz (Eds.), *Handbook of stress: Theoretical and clinical aspects* (3rd ed.). New York, NY: Free Press.

McEwen, B. S., & Wingfield, J. C. (2003). The concept of allostasis in biology and biomedicine. *Hormone Behavior, 43*(1), 2–15.

McKay, K. A., Buen, J. E., Bohan, K. J., & Maye, J. P. (2010). Determining the relationship of acute stress, anxiety, and salivary alpha-amylase level with performance of student nurse anesthetists during human-based anesthesia simulator training. *Journal of the American Association of Nurse Anesthetists, 78*(4), 301–309.

McVicar, A. (2003). Workplace stress in nursing: a literature review. *Journal of Advanced Nursing, 44*(6), 633–642.

Melnyk, B. M., & Fineout-Overholt, E. (2010). *Evidence-based practice in nursing & healthcare: A guide to best practice* (2nd edition). Philadelphia: Wolters Kluwer/Lippincott, Williams & Wilkins.

Mertin, S., Sawatzky, J. V., Diehl-Jones, W. L., & Lee, T. (2007). Roadblock to recovery: The surgical stress response. *Dynamics, 18*(1), 14–22.

Mikosch, P., Hadrawa, T., Laubreiter, K., Brandl, J., Jurgen, P., Stettner, H., & Grimm, G. (2010). Effectiveness of respiratory-sinus-arrhythmia biofeedback on state-anxiety in patients undergoing coronary angiography. *Journal of Advanced Nursing, 66*(5), 1101–1110.

Mitchell, G., & Pilkington, B. (1990). Theoretical approaches to nursing practice: A comparison of Roy and Parse. *Nursing Science Quarterly, 3,* 81–87.

Motzer, S. A., & Hertig, V. (2004). Stress, stress response, and health. *Nursing Clinics of North America, 39*(1), 1–17.

Neuman, B. (1982). *The Neuman Systems Model.* Norwalk, CT: Appleton-Century-Crofts.

Nicholson, N. R. (2009). Social isolation in older adults: An evolutionary concept analysis. *Journal of Advanced Nursing, 65*(6), 1342–1352.

Nightingale, F. (1969). *Notes on nursing: What it is and what it is not.* New York, NY: Dover. (Original work published 1860)

Nilsson, U., Rawal, N., & Unosson, M. (2003). A comparison of intra-operative or postoperative exposure to music—a controlled trial of the effect on postoperative pain. *Anaesthesia, 58,* 699– 673.

Page, G. G., & Ben-Eliyahu, S. (1997). The immune-suppressive nature of pain. *Seminars in Oncology Nursing, 13,* 10–15.

Papathanassoglou, E. D. (2010). Psychological support and outcomes for ICU patients. *Nursing Critical Care, 15*, 118–128.

Park, N., & Kang, D. (2008). Breast cancer risk, distress, and natural killer cell activity (NKCA) in healthy women. *Southern Online Journal of Nursing Research, 8*(2).

Peled, R., Carmil, D., Siboni-Samocha, O., & Shoham-Vardi, I. (2008). Breast cancer, psychological distress and life events among young women. *BMC Cancer, 8*, 245.

Rambo, B. (1983). *Adaptation nursing: Assessment and intervention.* Philadelphia: W. B. Saunders.

Ramelet, A., Abu-Saad, H. H., Rees, N., & McDonald, S. (2004). The challenges of pain measurement in critically ill young children: A comprehensive review. *Australian Critical Care, 17*(1), 33–34.

Robley, L., Ballard, N., Holtzman, D., & Cooper, W. (2010). The experience of stress for open heart surgery patients and their caregivers. *Western Journal of Nursing Research, 32*(6), 794–813.

Roy, C. (1984). *Introduction to nursing: An adaptation model* (2nd ed.). Englewood Cliffs, NJ: Prentice Hall.

Roy, C., & Andrews, H. (1991). *The Roy Adaptation Model: The definitive statement.* Norwalk, CT: Appleton & Lange.

Ruiz, R. J., Fullerton, J., Guerrero, L. C., Garcia-Atwater, M., & Dolbier, C. L. (2006). Development of a culturally sensitive stress instrument for pregnant Hispanic women. *Hispanic Health Care International, 4*(1), 27–35.

Ruotsalainen, J. H., & Verbeek, J. H. (2006). Preventing occupational stress in healthcare workers. *Cochrane Database of Systematic Reviews,* Issue 4, Art. No.: CD002892. doi:10.1002/14651858.CD002892.pub2

Ryan, M. (1996). Loneliness, social support, and depression as interactive variables with cognitive status: Testing Roy's model. *Nursing Science Quarterly, 9*, 107–114.

Santamaria, N. (2001). The relationship between nurses' personality and stress levels reported when caring for interpersonally difficult patients. *Australian Journal of Advanced Nursing, 18*(2), 20–26.

Selye, H. (1936). A syndrome produced by diverse nocuous agents. *Nature, 138,* 32.

Selye, H. (1950). Forty years of stress research: Principal remaining problems and misconceptions. *CMA Journal, 115,* 53–55.

Selye, H. (1956). *The stress of life.* New York, NY: McGraw-Hill.

Selye, H. (1974). *Stress without distress.* Philadelphia, PA: J. B. Lippincott.

Selye, H. (1976a). *Stress in health and disease.* Reading, MA: Butterworth's.

Selye, H. (1976b). *The stress of life* (Rev. ed.). New York, NY: McGraw-Hill.

Selye, H. (1976c). Forty years of stress research: Principal remaining problems and misconceptions. *CMA Journal, 115,* 53–55.

Selye, H. (1979). *The stress of my life: A scientist's memoirs.* New York, NY: Van Nostrand.

Selye, H. (1980). *Selye's guide to stress research.* New York, NY: Van Nostrand Reinhold.

Sercekus, P., & Mete, S. (2010). Effects of antenatal education on maternal prenatal and postpartum adaptation. *Journal of Advanced Nursing, 66*(5), 999–1010.

Shannon, M. T., King, T. L., & Kennedy, H. P. (2007). Allostasis: A theoretical framework for understanding and evaluating perinatal health outcomes. *Journal of Obstetric, Gynecologic, and Neonatal Nursing, 36*(2), 125–134.

Sherwood, L. (2010). *Human physiology: From cell to system* (7th ed.). London, England: Cengage Learning.

Simonton, C., Simonton, S., & Creighton, J. (1978). *Getting well again.* Los Angeles, CA: Tarcher.

Slater, R. (2010). Impact of an enhanced recovery programme in colorectal surgery. *British Journal of Nursing, 23,* 19–21.

Solà, I., Thompson, E. M., Casacuberta, M., Lopez, C., & Pascual, A. (2004). Non-invasive interventions for improving well-being and quality of life in patients with lung cancer. *Cochrane Database of Systematic Reviews,* Issue 4.

Sterling, P., & Eyer, J. (1988). Allostasis: A new paradigm to explain arousal pathology. In S. Fisher & J. Reason (Eds.), *Handbook of life stress, cognition and health* (pp. 629–649). New York, NY: J. Wiley & Sons.

Strahler, J., Berndt, C., Kirschbaum, C., & Rohleder, N. (2010). Aging diurnal rhythms and chronic stress: Distinct alteration of diurnal rhythmicity of salivary alpha-amylase and cortisol. *Biological Psychology, 84,* 248–256.

Strahler, J., Mueller, A., Rosenloecher, F., Kirschbaum, C., & Rohleder, N. (2010). Salivary alpha-amylase stress reactivity across different age groups. *Psychophysiology, 47,* 587–595.

Symes, L., McFarlane, J., Frazier, L., Henderson-Everhardus, M., McGlory, G., Watson, K. B., . . . Hoogeveen, R. C. (2010). Exploring violence against women and adverse health outcomes in middle age to promote women's health. *Critical Care Nursing Quarterly, 33*(3), 233–243.

Tache, J., & Selye, H. (1985). On stress and coping mechanisms. *Issues in Mental Health Nursing, 7,* 3–24.

Thompson, R. L., Lewis, S. L., Murphy, M. R., Hale, J. M., Blackwell, P. H., Acton, G. J., . . . Bonner, P. N. (2004). Are there sex differences in emotional and biological responses in spousal caregivers of patients with Alzheimer's disease? *Biological Research for Nursing, 5*(4), 319–330.

Toth, J. (1984). *Variables associated with the stressful experience of hospital discharge during acute myocardial infarction* (Doctoral dissertation). The Catholic University of America, Washington, DC. Retrieved from Dissertation Abstracts International. (A82857)

Toth, J. (1987). Stressors affecting older versus younger AMI patients. *Dimensions of Critical Care Nursing, 6,* 147–157.

Toth, J. (1988). Measuring the stressful experience of hospital discharge following acute myocardial infarction. In C. Waltz & O. Strickland (Eds.), *Measurement of nursing outcomes* (pp. 3–23). New York, NY: Springer.

Toth, J. (1993). Is stress at hospital discharge after acute myocardial infarction greater in women than in men? *American Journal of Critical Care, 2,* 35–40.

Ulrich, C. M., Taylor, C., Soeken, K., O'Donnell, P., Farrar, A., Danis, M., & Grady, C. (2010). Everyday ethics: Ethical issues and stress in nursing practice. *Journal of Advanced Nursing, 66*(11), 2510–2519.

Uman, L. S., Chambers, C. T., McGrath, P. J., & Kisely, S. R. (2006). Psychological interventions for needle-related procedural pain and distress in children and adolescents. *Cochrane Database of Systematic Reviews,* Issue 4.

Van den Berghe, G. (2001). The neuroendocrine response to stress is a dynamic process. *Clinical Endrocrinology & Metabolism, 15*(4), 405–419.

van den Tooren, M., & de Jonge, J. (2008). Managing job stress in nursing: What kind of resources do we need? *Journal of Advanced Nursing, 63*(1), 75–84.

Vitaliano, P., Scanlan, J., Ochs, H., Siegler, I., & Snyder, E. (1998). Psychosocial stress moderates the relationship of cancer history with natural killer cell activity. *Annals of Behavioral Medicine, 20,* 199–208.

Walker, L. O. (1994). *Strategies for theory construction in nursing* (3rd ed.). Norwalk, CT: Appleton & Lange.

Walker, L. O., & Avant, K. C. (1988). *Strategies for theory construction in nursing.* Norwalk, CT: Appleton & Lange.

Washington, T. D. (2009). Psychological stress and anxiety in middle to late childhood and early adolescence: Manifestations and management. *Journal of Pediatric Nursing, 24*(4), 302–313.

Watson, M., Pettingale, K., & Greer, S. (1984). Emotional control and autonomic arousal in breast cancer patients. *Journal of Psychosomatic Research, 28,* 467–474.

Weiland, S. (2010). Integrating spirituality into critical care: An APN perspective using Roy's Adaptation Model. *Critical Care Nursing Quarterly, 33*(3), 282–291.

Weiss, R., Cali, A. M., Dziura, J., Burgert, T. S., Tamborlane, W. V., & Caprio, S. (2007). Degree of obesity and glucose allostasis are major effectors of glucose tolerance dynamics in obese youth. *Diabetes Care, 30*(7), 1845–1850.

Werner, J. S. (1993). Stressors and health outcomes: Synthesis of nursing research, 1980–1990. In J. Barnfather & B. Lyon (Eds.), *Stress and coping: State of the science and implications for nursing theory, research, and practice* (pp. 11–38). Indianapolis, IN: Sigma Theta Tau International.

White, N. E., Richter, J. M., & Fry, C. (1992). Coping, social support, and adaptation to chronic illness. *Western Journal of Nursing Research, 14*(2), 211–224.

Yeh, C. H. (2001). Adaptation in children with cancer: Research with Roy's model. *Nursing Science Quarterly, 14*(2), 141–148.

Yeh, C. H. (2003). Psychological distress: Testing hypotheses based on Roy's Adaptation Model. *Nursing Science Quarterly, 16*(3), 255–263.

Zhan, L. (2000). Cognitive adaptation and self-consistency in hearing-impaired older persons: Testing Roy's Adaptation Model. *Nursing Science Quarterly, 13*(2), 158–165.

Zolten, A. (1989). Constructive integration of learning theory and phenomenological approaches to biofeedback training. *Biofeedback Self Regulation, 14,* 89–99.

3

STRESS, IMMUNITY, AND HEALTH OUTCOMES

LINDA WITEK JANUSEK, DINA TELL COOPER, AND
HERBERT L. MATHEWS

For many years, anecdotal evidence suggested that psychological and physical stress, mood, and behavior modulate the immune system and predispose an individual to immune-related disorders, like autoimmune disease, infection, and cancer. Yet empirical evidence supporting these observations was lacking. It is only within recent years that the biological linkages that connect the brain with the cells and tissues of the immune system have been discovered. These discoveries form the foundation of psychoneuroimmunology (Irwin, 2008; Kemeny & Schedlowski, 2007). *Psychoneuroimmunology (PNI) is defined as the study of the interactions among behavioral, neural, endocrine (neuroendocrine), and immunological processes of adaptation* (Ader, 1980).

The central premise of PNI is that an individual's adaptive response to the environment involves coordinated interactions among the nervous, endocrine, and immune systems. The biological pathways that connect the brain with the cells and tissues of the immune system include direct innervation of lymphatic tissue by the central nervous system and a shared communication network in which cells of the nervous, endocrine, and immune systems use common molecules and receptors to reciprocally modulate biologic activity. Stressors, thoughts, and behavior are known to activate these anatomical and biochemical pathways and in turn modulate immune function. Moreover, an expanding body of evidence suggests that emotions play an important role in the development and/or progression of disorders that involve immune processes (Irwin, 2008; Kemeny & Schedlowski, 2007; Wrona, 2006). Given this evidence, this chapter focuses on the role that PNI plays in health and illness.

The first part of the chapter describes the mechanisms whereby the nervous system (including the brain, neurotransmitters, and the neuroendocrine system) and the immune system (including lymphoid organs and tissues, circulating immune cells, and cytokines) communicate with one another. This forms the biological basis by which to understand the effects of psychological constructs (including feelings, emotions, behavior, personality, and mind) on the immune system. The second part of the chapter exemplifies how PNI influences the expression and/or progression of human disease. Lastly, the contributions of nurse scientists to PNI are highlighted.

AUTHORS' NOTE: This chapter is dedicated to the memory of my (LWJ) mentor and my friend, Dr. Sabath F. Marotta (1929–1996), who introduced me and numerous other nurses to scientific inquiry and stress physiology; may his memory live on in our collective contributions to the field of stress. This preparation of this chapter was supported, in part, by the National Cancer Institute grants, R01CA125455.

The Brain and the Immune System

Two major biological pathways link the brain with the immune system and provide a communication network whereby one's behavior and emotions influence immune function and affect the course of immune-related disease. These are the autonomic nervous system (ANS), which provides direct innervation of immune cells, and the neuroendocrine system, which releases immunomodulatory stress hormones and other mediators that enter the circulation. These systems serve as the major stress-response systems of the body in that they are activated by environmental events that are appraised and perceived as threatening (Elenkov & Chrousos, 2006). The following describes how these systems bridge the brain with the immune system.

Autonomic Nervous System (ANS)-Immune Interactions. Activation of the sympathetic division of the ANS leads to the release of catecholamines (e.g., norepinephrine) from postganglionic nerve endings that terminate in target tissues, as well as the secretion of catecholamines (primarily epinephrine) directly into the circulation from the adrenal medulla, whereas activation of the parasympathetic division of the autonomic nervous system releases acetylcholine at target tissues. Lymphoid tissues of the immune system, such as the bone marrow, spleen, thymus gland, and lymph nodes, are innervated by nerve fibers of both sympathetic and parasympathetic origin, however, the extent and type of innervation varies based on the tissue affected. This is key to PNI as it provides the "hard-wiring" that connects the brain with the immune system.

As a result, ANS activation is capable of influencing immune function during stressful situations that are processed in the brain and provoke emotions and/or arousal. In turn, immune cells are capable of responding to and altering their function in response to neurotransmitters released by the nerve fibers of the autonomic nervous system because they possess adrenergic and cholinergic receptors, as well as receptors for various neuropeptide hormones, including vasoactive intestinal polypeptide, somatostatin, calcitonin gene-related peptide, substance P, and opioids. The presence of such receptors on immune cells provides a mechanism whereby the immune system can respond to biochemical signals from the brain. Activation of these receptors leads to functional changes in the immune response (i.e., lymphocyte proliferation, cytotoxicity, antibody production, and cytokine secretion) (Elenkov & Chrousos, 2006; Wrona, 2006).

Similar to glucocorticoids, catecholamines were initially believed to suppress the immune response. However, recent evidence demonstrates that both catecholamines and glucocorticoids, at physiologic levels or at levels observed during stress, modulate the immune response in a more complex manner. That is, certain aspects of the immune response may be up-regulated, while other aspects can be down-regulated. It is now more correct to view stress as producing immune dysregulation, as opposed to simply producing a monochromatic immunosuppressive response (Elenkov & Chrousos, 2006). This insight has assisted in explaining the often contradictory observations of the effects of stress on immunity and the onset and the course of common stress-related conditions, such as autoimmune and inflammatory disease, allergy, and cancer. This is discussed further below.

Emerging work has demonstrated that vagal parasympathetic pathways play a role in the suppression of pro-inflammatory cytokine release from the spleen (Czura & Tracey, 2005; Thayer & Sternberg, 2010). These studies show that activation of the parasympathetic nervous system results in the down-regulation of inflammatory responses (Bernik et al., 2002; Borovikova et al., 2000; Tracey, 2002). For instance, a higher vagal (i.e., reflective of greater parasympathetic activity) control of heart rate has been associated with lower production of TNF-alpha and IL-6 (Marsland et al., 2007). These associations are independent of demographic, health characteristics, and blood cell counts and provide support for a cholinergic anti-inflammatory pathway (Borovikova et al., 2000). The neural cholinergic, anti-inflammatory pathway is a means by which inflammation activates the afferent (sensory) fibers of the vagus nerve to signal the brain to trigger an anti-inflammatory response through firing of the efferent vagus nerve. Acetylcholine released by stimulation of the vagus nerve binds to acetylcholine receptors expressed by cells of the immune system to suppress proinflammatory cytokine production (Metz & Tracey, 2005). The cholinergic anti-inflammatory pathway serves as an adaptive pathway to attenuate the inflammatory response to stress, preventing untoward effects as might occur with excessive inflammation (Elenkov, Iezzoni, Daly, Harris, & Chrousos, 2005; Sternberg, 2006).

Neuroendocrine-Immune Connections. The major neuroendocrine axis that communicates with the immune system is the hypothalamic-pituitary-adrenocortical (HPA) axis. In response to psychological stress, the hypothalamus releases corticotrophin-releasing hormone (CRH), which stimulates the release of adrenocorticotropic hormone (ACTH) from the anterior pituitary gland. ACTH, in turn, stimulates cortisol secretion from the adrenal cortex. (See Figure 3.1.) Cortisol is the major glucocorticoid in humans, and it mediates a wide array of effects on the immune and inflammatory response.

Other classic pituitary hormones and neuropeptides are secreted in response to stressful stimuli and include hormones such as growth hormone, thyroid-stimulating hormone, prolactin, endorphins, as well as neuropeptides, like somatostatin, Substance P, and calcitonin gene–related peptide. The molecules released in response to emotions can alter immune function because immune cells display complementary receptors for all of these molecules. The most studied neuroendocrine axis in psychoneuroimmunology is the HPA axis, and more is known about how cortisol, released in response to stress, alters immune function and influences immune-based disease. The following describes this relationship as these are the key molecules secreted upon activation of the major stress systems.

Effects of Glucocorticoids and Catecholamines on Cytokine Balance. One of the most important effects of glucocorticoids and catecholamines on the immune response is their ability to influence the activity of T helper (Th) lymphocytes. Th1 lymphocytes provide cellular immunity by the production of cytokines, which promote protection against intracellular bacteria, protozoa, fungi, and several viruses. In contrast, Th2 lymphocytes produce cytokines that promote humoral immunity, which, in turn, provide protection against multicellular parasites, extracellular bacteria, some viruses, soluble toxins, and allergens by their production of antibodies. Cytokines are key regulators of the immune response and act in an autocrine, paracrine, or endocrine fashion to control the proliferation,

differentiation, and activity of immune cells. For instance, Th1 lymphocytes primarily secrete interferon (IFN) gamma, interleukin (IL)-2, and tumor necrosis factor (TNF), which promote cellular immunity; Th2 cells secrete a different set of cytokines, primarily IL-4, IL-10, and IL-13, which promote humoral immunity (Elenkov & Chrousos, 1999; Mosmann & Sad, 1996). In general, cortisol and catecholamines promote a shift in the Th1 to Th2 cytokine balance, so that there is an increase in the production of Th2 cytokines and a decrease in the production of Th1 cytokines. For example, glucocorticoids (i.e., cortisol), norepinephrine, and epinephrine suppress the production of IL-12 by antigen-presenting cells. IL-12 promotes a Th1 response to antigen and in its absence a shift to a Th2 profile of cytokine production results. Glucocorticoids activate Th2 cells to increase production of Th1 cytokines. Further, glucocorticoids and catecholamines inhibit the production of IL-1 and TNF by antigen-presenting cells and IFN gamma by Th1 lymphocytes. Catecholamines directly reduce cytokine production by Th1 cells in that Th1 lymphocytes express surface beta 2 adrenergic receptors, which are not expressed by Th2 cells. Glucocorticoids are well known for their strong anti-inflammatory actions, and stress is accompanied by the release of proinflammatory molecules, like IL-1, IL-6, and TNF. An important role of glucocorticoids, as well as catecholamines, during the stress response is to counter the effects of proinflammatory molecules and to prevent these molecules from causing tissue damage and disease when they are produced in excess or at low levels over long periods of time (i.e., low-grade inflammation) (Sternberg, 2006). This is described below.

PNI and the Inflammatory Response. Complex and finely tuned interactions must exist among glucocorticoids, catecholamines, proinflammatory cytokines, inflammation, and the immune system to maintain homeostasis, health, and well-being. An important adaptive role of stress-activated increases in glucocorticoids and catecholamines is to help protect an individual from systemic overproduction of proinflammatory cytokines, as inflammation is meant to be tailored to the stimulus and to be time-limited. Certain situations, like illness or chronic stress, can lead to a dysfunctional neuroendocrine-immune axis, characterized by abnormalities of this anti-inflammatory

Figure 3.1   Biological Pathways That Link the Brain, Neuroendocrine, and Immune Systems

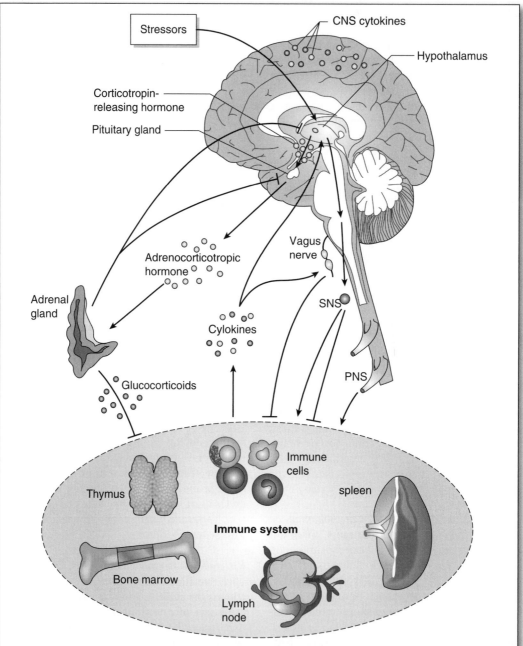

Illustration of pathways that link the brain, neuroendocrine, and immune systems. Perceived environmental stress is mediated by the central nervous system and triggers neuroendocrine and autonomic nervous system activation. The immune response can be altered by signals from autonomic nerve fibers that directly synapse with immune cells and by circulating catecholamines released from the adrenal medulla. Further alteration can be produced by secretory products (hormones and neuropeptides) released from the pituitary and endocrine target glands (adrenal cortex, thyroid, ovaries, and testes). In turn, feedback (dashed lines) from immune cell products (cytokines) can modulate endocrine and central nervous system activity by either humoral or neural communication networks.

PNS = Parasympathetic Nervous System; SNS = Sympathetic Nervous System.

feedback mechanism. The result is a hyperactive proinflammatory state marked by excess production of proinflammatory cytokines like IL-1, IL-6, and TNF and IFN gamma. The resulting excessive inflammatory condition may contribute to the pathogenesis of various human diseases such as allergy, autoimmunity, obesity, depression, and atherosclerosis (Sternberg, 2006). In contrast, an excess of circulating glucocorticoids, which can occur as a result of chronic stress, is associated with increased susceptibility to viral infections.

IMMUNE-TO-BRAIN COMMUNICATION

The next section describes how the brain can influence immune function. The reverse is also true in that secretions from the immune system influence brain function and, in turn, alter one's behavior and emotional state. Animal studies showed that when certain cytokines, like IL-1, were injected into the brain they not only caused fever, but they also triggered behaviors associated with being sick (Dantzer, O'Connor, Freund, Johnson, & Kelley, 2008). These so-called sickness behaviors included fatigue, loss of appetite, sleepiness, aching joints, sore muscles, and apathy or lack of interest in one's environment. It is theorized that cytokines released in response to infection or inflammation alert the brain of any real or potential threats and initiate behaviors that are thought to be important for survival. Some even refer to the ability of the immune system to alert or communicate with the brain as a "sixth sense" (Blalock & Smith, 2007).

Sickness behavior is believed to be adaptive in that it forces an individual to rest and withdraw from activities so that physiological processes can more effectively produce healing. These behavioral changes redirect metabolism and energy expenditure, so that a sick person's physiological resources are used to maintain the febrile response and energy utilization is reserved for processes aimed at defending against the foreign invader or pathogen. It is now known that proinflammatory cytokines (IL-1 beta, IL-alpha, and TNF-alpha) released during infection, inflammation, injury, and even psychological stress can signal the brain to initiate behavioral changes that facilitate adaptation to these threats. Cytokine-to-brain signaling has been implicated in mood disorders, particularly the depression that accompanies illness (Dantzer, 2009; Dantzer et al., 2008).

Although cytokines are large protein molecules, they are capable of entering the brain through the circumventricular organs (CVO). The CVO consist of areas of the brain that are located around the margin of the ventricular system and are devoid of a functional blood-brain barrier. As a result, these areas can "sense" the levels of various signaling molecules within the bloodstream, such as those released in response to infection or inflammation. In response to the detection of peripheral circulating proinflammatory cytokines or other byproducts of infectious microorganisms, cells within the CVO increase the synthesis of centrally produced proinflammatory cytokines within the brain, which in turn move into the areas of the brain that mediate behavior and neurovegetative functions (i.e., appetite, sleep, thirst, etc.).

Secondly, investigators have described specialized transporter mechanisms that are capable of moving peripherally produced cytokines into the brain. They, in turn, trigger brain production of cytokines that alter behavior during infection and/or inflammation. Finally, a more rapid system of immune-to-brain communication occurs through afferent neural pathways. Afferent nerve fibers, such as vagal afferents, located within the site of inflammation or infection can be activated by the local release of proinflammatory cytokines. Once activated, these nerves will transmit nervous impulses to areas of the brain that mediate the behavioral changes that accompany sickness.

In summary, immune-to-brain signaling results from peripherally produced cytokines that are released from macrophages at the site of injury, infection, and/or inflammation. These in turn signal the brain to increase the local production of cytokines in key areas of the brain that mediate behavioral responses and neurovegetative functions commonly referred to as sickness behavior. Sickness behavior is believed to be part of a central motivational state that orchestrates the individual's bio-behavioral priorities in order to successfully cope with and survive physical stressors like infection, inflammation, and/or injury (Dantzer & Kelley, 2007; Dantzer et al., 2008).

Investigators continue to evaluate the consequences of unchecked inflammatory responses that persist beyond the adaptive response. Evidence suggests that when inflammation is not "turned off" after a stress response, there is increased risk for conditions like chronic fatigue syndrome, fibromyalgia, and depressive illness. As such, cytokines are a "double-edged sword" in that they are vital to the adaptive response that promotes healing from injury, infection, or inflammation, but if produced at high levels over prolonged periods of time they may lead to mood and cognitive disorders, as well as neuronal cell death (Dantzer & Kelley, 2007).

Salubrious Effects of Stress on Immunity

Although the word stress generally has negative connotations, it is a familiar aspect of life, being a stimulant for some but a burden for others. It is often overlooked that an acute stress response can have salubrious (health promoting) effects. Differences exist in the ways that acute (short-term) and chronic (long-term) stressors affect the immune system. For example, chronic stress significantly suppresses delayed-type hypersensitivity (DTH) responses (e.g., to skin test) and decreases leukocyte mobilization to the skin. Acute stress enhances the DTH response and increases leukocyte mobilization (Dhabhar et al., 2010; Viswanathan, Daugherty, & Dhabhar, 2005). So although stress is typically thought to be immunosuppressive, acute stress can result in immune enhancement that can promote protection from infections, but alternatively can contribute to the exacerbation of immunopathology. In response to immunological challenges, acutely stressed individuals show significantly greater leukocyte infiltration, enhanced production of chemokines (chemoattractant proteins for leukocytes), and cytokines such as IL-1, IL-6, TNF, and IFN gamma (proinflammatory and Th1). Further, acute stress enhances maturation and trafficking of dendritic cells (DCs) to sites of antigenic challenge. DCs are efficient antigen-presenting cells (APCs), and these APCs effectively promote the activation and recruitment of T lymphocytes during initial antigen challenge, inducing a long-term increase in immunologic memory. The result would be subsequent augmentation of the immune response during secondary antigen exposure. Thus, the evolutionarily adaptive fight-or-flight stress response will prepare the immune system for impending danger (e.g., infection and wounding by a predator). The result would be enhanced immunological protection from the infectious agent and more rapid healing of the wound.

Stress could also exacerbate a pathological condition that is worsened by an increased immune response (e.g., autoimmune or inflammatory disease). However, an acute stress-induced enhancement of immune function provides a selective advantage when viewed from an evolutionary perspective. The brain perceives a stressor, warns of danger, and promotes survival. Stress-responsive neurotransmitters and hormones are the brain's signals to the body. In the case of a physical stressor, such an encounter that results in wounding and infection, such a stress response would promote a beneficial antigen-specific immune response. During such an immune response, factors such as leukocyte trafficking, antigen presentation, helper T-cell function, leukocyte proliferation, cytokine and chemokine function, and effector cell function would all be receptive to stress hormone–mediated immune enhancement. In contrast, at a later stage, these components may be more receptive to immune suppression. Thus, acute stress has adaptive immune responses enhancing effects that are beneficial. The effects of stress (acute or chronic) on immune function are especially important to understand because stress is a ubiquitous fact of life, and stress hormones are important components of an individual's physiological response to the environment.

Section Summary. Strong empirical evidence supports the existence of a communication network linking the nervous, endocrine, and immune systems. Psychological stimuli modulate the immune response either through direct activation of neural pathways that terminate in lymphoid tissue or by activation of neuroendocrine circuits leading to the release of molecules that bind to immunologically competent cells. Conversely, the immune system recognizes noncognitive stimuli, such as bacteria, fungi, and viruses, resulting in the secretion of an array of cytokines that act on receptors of the neuroendocrine system. Collectively, cognitive and noncognitive stimuli form a network, which is the basis for behaviorally induced alterations in immune function (Dantzer & Kelley, 2007; Dantzer et al., 2008). It is likely that this neuroendocrine-immune network mediates the effect of stress on the development, progression, or both of immune-based diseases (Irwin, 2008; Kemeny & Schedlowski, 2007; Wrona, 2006).

STRESS-IMMUNITY AND HEALTH OUTCOMES

One fundamental question that remains of high interest in the field of psychoneuroimmunology and the health professions—like nursing—is whether stress-induced alteration in immune function plays a role in disease development, disease progression, and healing. The following section describes evidence for the role of stress-immune mechanisms in selected clinical conditions and disorders.

Cancer and Stress

For many years, scientists have deliberated whether stress-related psychosocial factors play a role in cancer onset and disease progression (Reiche, Nunes, & Morimoto, 2004). At this time, evidence for the role of psychosocial factors in cancer initiation is limited and inconclusive. However, there is growing evidence supporting a role for psychological factors, like stress perception, depression, and social isolation in cancer progression, as reviewed in Antoni, Lutgendorf et al., 2006; S. K. Lutgendorf, Sood, and Antoni, 2010; and Thaker and Sood, 2008. The following section will focus on evidence that implicates psychosocial stress in cancer progression and metastasis, especially given that metastasis is responsible for most of the cancer-related deaths.

Metastasis involves reciprocal signaling between the tumor and its microenvironment, which consists of the extracellular matrix, fibroblasts, inflammatory and immune cells, and vascular cells (Fidler, 2003). This complex process involves a series of interrelated events that allow cells to escape the primary tumor site and to seed and proliferate in distant organ(s). As the primary tumor enlarges, angiogenic factors stimulate the in-growth of blood vessels, which provide a path for tumor cells to disseminate and embolize into the circulation. Circulating tumor cells may arrest in capillary beds of organs, extravasate out of the blood stream, and invade surrounding tissue. During tumor cell escape and invasion, their metastatic potential requires that these nascent tumor cells successfully evade immune defense mechanisms (Dunn, Bruce, Ikeda, Old, & Schreiber, 2002). Psychosocial stress has been found to affect many of the events that promote or limit metastatic spread (Thaker & Sood, 2008). This may occur through stress-responsive neuroendocrine and immune processes, which are capable of influencing biological pathways involved in cancer progression, including angiogenesis, invasion, and immune defense mechanisms (Antoni, Lutgendorf et al., 2006; S. K. Lutgendorf et al., 2010; Thaker & Sood, 2008).

Stress and Tumor Metastasis. Stress activation of the sympathetic nervous system and release of catecholamines has been linked to tumor blood vessel development or angiogenesis by elevating angiogenic factors like vascular endothelium growth factor (VEGF) and IL-6. Evaluations performed using cancer cell lines have demonstrated that beta adrenergic pathways stimulate tumor angiogenesis by increasing expression of VEGF (S. K. Lutgendorf et al., 2003). As well, when animals that are implanted with ovarian tumors are subjected to chronic restraint stress, tumor burden and invasiveness are increased through adrenergic receptor mediated elevations in VEGF and angiogenesis (Thaker et al., 2006). These findings are corroborated by clinical studies that show that women with ovarian cancer who report poor social support have higher IL-6 (an angiogenic factor) in their plasma, as well as in tumor ascites fluid (Costanzo et al., 2005).

To escape the primary tumor a tumor cell must invade through the tissue matrix (i.e., basement membrane) and enter the blood vessel. Evidence shows that this process is facilitated by stress-related beta adrenergic pathways, which increase matrix metalloprotineases (MMP) within tumor cells and facilitate their ability to penetrate the extracellular matrix. Ovarian tumors from women who report stress and depression were shown to have greater secretion of MMP by tumor-associated macrophages (Sood et al., 2006). Interestingly, social isolation in mice was found to be associated with an increase in mammary gland expression of genes involved in human tumorigenesis and an increase in tumor growth in a murine breast cancer model (Williams et al., 2009). In women with ovarian cancer, high depression and low social support was associated with upregulation of gene transcripts linked to signaling pathways involved in tumor growth and progression (S. K. Lutgendorf et al., 2009). As a whole, these studies demonstrate that stress and its accompanying emotions and behavioral states are associated with crucial processes that favor metastatic cancer progression.

Stress, Cancer, and Immune Defense. The immune system participates in surveillance and destruction of malignant cells and is key to defense against cancer and cancer metastasis. In humans, an altered cellular immune response, especially impaired natural killer (NK) cell activity (NKCA), and dysregulation of cytokines has been the focus of investigations in psycho-oncology. Such immune dysregulation is significant in that NK cells and cytokines, like IFN gamma, contribute to host protection from cancer by defending against tumor metastasis, tumor initiation, and primary tumor growth (Curcio et al., 2003; Diefenbach & Raulet, 2002; Street, Cretney, & Smyth, 2001; van den Broek et al., 1996). This is clinically relevant, as low peripheral NK-cell counts have been shown to be prognostic for early breast cancer mortality, and reduced NKCA is predictive of a poor clinical outcome in patients with carcinoma (Sephton, Sapolsky, Kraemer, & Spiegel, 2000). As well, excessive and chronically produced pro-inflammatory mediators, like IL-6, weaken immunity within the tumor microenvironment (Ben-Baruch, 2006; Kim, Emi, Tanabe, & Arihiro, 2006) and may contribute to tumor promotion and progression (Balkwill, Charles, & Mantovani, 2005; Ben-Baruch, 2006; Coussens & Werb, 2002; Smyth, Cretney, Kershaw, & Hayakawa, 2004; Van der Auwera et al., 2004).

A strong literature demonstrates that psychological stress or negative mood states, like depression, reduce natural killer cell activity against tumor cells (Biondi, 2001; Kiecolt-Glaser et al., 1987; Witek-Janusek, Gabram, & Mathews, 2007) and dysregulates cytokine production (Maes et al., 1999; Marshall et al., 1998; Witek-Janusek et al., 2007). Such immune dysregulation likely results from alterations of neuroendocrine stress-response systems, as individuals with cancer exhibit aberrant patterns of cortisol secretion (Bower et al., 2005; Sephton et al., 2000). Importantly, stress-induced dysregulation of the neuroendocrine-immune network may weaken cancer control (Elenkov et al., 2005) For example, glucocorticoids, like cortisol, have strong immunomodulatory effects (Schoneveld & Cidlowski, 2007; Webster, Tonelli, & Sternberg, 2002). As mentioned before, cortisol switches cytokine production from a Th1 (IFN gamma) to a Th2 (IL-4, IL-10) pattern (Chrousos, 2000; Daynes, Araneo, Dowell, Huang, & Dudley, 1990; Rook,

Hernandez-Pando, & Lightman, 1994), which can depress NK cell activity against tumor cells (Targan & Dorey, 1980) and elevate pro-inflammatory cytokines, like IL-6 (Esterling, Kiecolt-Glaser, & Glaser, 1996; Maes et al., 1999; Marshall et al., 1998).

Cancer patients have marked impairment in IFN gamma production, a shift toward a Th2 profile of cytokine secretion, and increased production of proinflammatory cytokines (Caras et al., 2004). In women undergoing breast cancer diagnosis, the anticipation of malignancy was shown to result in reductions in peripheral blood mononuclear cell (PBMC) NKCA, as well as reductions in PBMC production of IFN gamma (Witek-Janusek et al., 2007). And women with greater subjective stress after breast cancer surgery, but prior to adjuvant therapy, exhibited lower basal and interferon (IFN) augmented NK cell activity and reduced T-cell proliferative responses to mitogens (Andersen et al., 1998; Andersen et al., 2004).

Interestingly, the trajectory of the stress response to a diagnosis of breast cancer was reported to covary with NK cell activity. Women who reported greater subjective stress at diagnosis exhibited the greatest reduction in NK cell activity, while those women who showed an early decline in stress during cancer recovery also showed the most rapid recovery of NK cell activity (Thornton, Andersen, Crespin, & Carson, 2007). Recently, an evaluation of women stressed by a diagnosis of breast cancer showed that the stress-associated reduction in NK cell activity was related to epigenetic modification (i.e., histone modification) of effector molecules needed for NK cell function (Mathews et al., 2011).

In women with ovarian cancer, greater distress was associated with poorer NK cell activity in tumor-infiltrating lymphocytes (TIL) and reduced T-cell production of Th1 versus Th2 cytokines in both peripheral blood and in TIL (S. K. Lutgendorf et al., 2008). In contrast, women with ovarian cancer who reported greater social support had greater NK cell activity in peripheral blood and in TIL (S. K. Lutgendorf et al., 2005). Men undergoing radical prostatectomy for prostate cancer were found to exhibit reductions in NK cell activity that was related to surgical stress, rather than mood disturbance (Yermal, Witek-Janusek, Peterson, & Mathews, 2009). Because NK cells and IFN are key to the surveillance and destruction of tumor cells (Khakoo et al., 2004; Orange, 2002), stress-induced immune dysregulation may jeopardize cancer control, especially at critical times marked by risk of tumor dissemination, such as during the post-operative period or treatment (Avraham & Ben-Eliyahu, 2007; S. Lutgendorf, Costanzo, & Siegel, 2007).

Stress Reduction and Cancer Control. Evidence for the role of stress-related immune dysregulation in cancer control is also provided by studies that have evaluated the effect of stress-reduction interventions on psycho-immune outcomes in individuals with cancer. Most of these studies enrolled women with breast cancer. For example, within recent years cognitive behavioral therapy (CBT) and mindfulness-based stress-reduction programs have provided emerging evidence demonstrating these interventions to reduce psychological stress, improve quality of life and coping, reduce cortisol levels, and restore immune function in women with breast cancer (McGregor & Antoni, 2009; Witek-Janusek et al., 2008). Improvements in immune parameters included increased NKCA, increased T-cell lymphoproliferative response, and restoration of the Th1/Th2 cytokine balance (Antoni et al., 2009; McGregor et al., 2004; Thornton et al., 2007; Witek-Janusek et al., 2008). Moreover, recent randomized controlled trials evaluated whether psychological interventions aimed to reduce stress provided a survival advantage.

A randomized control trial enrolled women with stage 3 and 4 breast cancer into a 4-month group CBT intervention (e.g., relaxation, coping skills training) and demonstrated a reduction in overall and breast cancer–specific mortality rates, as well as reduced risk of breast cancer recurrence (Andersen et al., 2008). Yet this study did not provide evidence that linked a survival advantage to improvements in immune defense against cancer. In contrast, two other studies that enrolled women with metastatic breast cancer into a 12-month course of group supportive expressive therapy found no survival advantage attributable to the intervention (Kissane et al., 2007; Spiegel et al., 2007). It is likely that many factors contribute to the differences in survival outcomes among these studies, including differences in disease stage (i.e., metastatic versus nonmetastatic), as well as variations in the form of interventions employed and control of covariates.

Stress and Wound Healing

Substantial evidence demonstrates that stress delays wound healing and tissue repair and places individuals at risk for complications, such as wound infections (Christian, Graham, Padgett, Glaser, & Kiecolt-Glaser, 2006). Meta-analysis of studies evaluating the relationship of psychological stress with wound healing revealed a strong relationship. Studies meeting criteria for inclusion in the meta-analysis examined healing of a variety of wound types in different clinical contexts, and in experimentally inflicted wounds created by punch biopsy and blister wounds, as well as minor skin damage produced by tape stripping (Walburn, Vedhara, Hankins, Rixon, & Weinman, 2009).

An early study showed that chronic psychosocial stress associated with providing care for a spouse with Alzheimer's disease delayed healing of experimentally placed punch biopsy wounds by 9 days compared to an age-matched control group (Kiecolt-Glaser, Marucha, Malarkey, Mercado, & Glaser, 1995). Also, stressed caregivers produced less systemic IL-1 (an inflammatory cytokine important in the early inflammatory phase of wound healing). An evaluation of healing of experimentally placed wounds on the oral mucosa of dental students also found healing took longer during the stress of final exam week when compared to students who were on vacation (Marucha, Kiecolt-Glaser, & Favagehi, 1998). Likewise, others showed that punch biopsy wounds healed more slowly in healthy young males who reported greater levels of perceived psychosocial stress, lower trait optimism, and higher salivary cortisol levels. Differences in health behaviors, like poor sleep, alcohol intake, or poor diet, did not explain the observed differences in wound healing and strengthened the conclusion that stress was a key factor that delayed healing (Ebrecht et al., 2004). An assessment of a naturalistic stressor—marital discord—found that couples with more discord marked by hostility had a 60% slower healing of experimentally placed blister wounds and lower levels of local wound cytokine production (Kiecolt-Glaser et al., 2005).

In order to understand whether stress alters the local production of mediators important in the orchestration of wound healing, investigators devised a wounding model that involved the infliction of blister wounds that were fitted with a special covering that allowed sequential sampling of blister fluid as healing progressed. Using this wound model, it was found that individuals who reported greater levels of perceived stress also had lower levels of IL-1 and IL-8 in the blister fluid. These are proinflammatory cytokines which are needed in the early phase of wound healing (Glaser et al., 1999). Likewise, wound fluid collected post-operatively from inguinal hernia patients who reported greater pre-operative stress had decreased levels of inflammatory molecules in their wound fluid. Collectively these studies demonstrate that the psychosocial stress of both acute and chronic duration can slow wound healing, and this occurs, in part, by decreasing the production of inflammatory molecules needed for the early phase of wound healing (Marucha & Engeland, 2007).

Evidence supports a role for cortisol and catecholamines as mediators of the effect of psychosocial stress on wound healing. Glucocoticoids, like cortisol, induce a variety of anti-inflammatory and immunosuppressive effects, which can delay wound healing and increase risk of wound infection. For instance, cortisol suppresses the release of proinflammatory cytokines needed in the early phase of wound healing and reduces the recruitment of macrophages and neutrophils and decreases bacterial killing by these phagocytic cells (Marucha & Engeland, 2007). Such effects will impair containment and elimination of microorganisms and clearance of debris within the wound. Glucocorticoids also impair the re-epithelialization of the wound which decreases wound strength and slows wound closure and increases the chances for wound dehiscence. Thus, glucocorticoids suppress the levels of inflammatory cytokines and growth factors essential to successful wound closure and healing and likely contribute to stress-induced impairment of wound healing (Marucha & Engeland, 2007).

The role of psychoneuroimmunology in wound healing has clear clinical relevance, as delayed wound healing and wound infections can increase post-surgical length of hospital stay and the cost of health care, let alone the risk for poor patient outcomes. Most studies of psychoneuroimmunology-based mechanisms on wound healing have evaluated acute wounds. Less attention has been given to chronic wounds, such as diabetic venous leg ulcers, which present a major clinical challenge. Many patients with such wounds develop feelings of depression and this may impair wound healing.

For example, experimentally placed wounds on the oral hard palate healed more slowly in young adults who reported more depressive symptoms (Bosch, Engeland, Cacioppo, & Marucha, 2007). Whether reduction of psychosocial stress or improvement of mood can facilitate wound healing is a clinically relevant area of investigation. One study showed that wound healing (experimental punch biopsy) was enhanced by use of an emotional disclosure intervention (i.e., writing about a traumatic event) (Weinman, Ebrecht, Scott, Walburn, & Dyson, 2008). Nurses are in a pivotal position to recognize and reduce stress and to teach stress-management skills. This has the potential to promote healing and enhance health outcomes.

Stress, Immunity, and Inflammatory Joint Conditions

Psychosocial factors are implicated in the pathogenesis of several autoimmune diseases; however, PNI mechanisms have been most thoroughly investigated in juvenile idiopathic arthritis (JIA) and rheumatoid arthritis (RA). Inflammatory joint conditions, like RA and JIA, are autoimmune disorders whose etiology involves a genetic predisposition combined with an environmental trigger(s) (Gorby & Sternberg, 2007). Proinflammatory cytokines contribute to the pathogenesis of these inflammatory joint conditions as individuals with RA exhibit elevations in TNF and IL-1 (Chikanza, Kingsley, & Panayi, 1995), while agents that block TNF lead to clinical improvement (Maini et al., 2004). Studies support a role for psychological-induced immune alterations in the pathogenesis of inflammatory joint disease in genetically susceptible individuals (Gorby & Sternberg, 2007).

During the early asymptomatic phase of inflammatory conditions, like JIA and RA, stress plays a permissive role in disease development; however, during the symptomatic phase of disease, there is an imbalance of neuroendocrine-immune processes, such that psychosocial stress leads to an increased proinflammatory state and disease exacerbation (Straub, Dhabhar, Bijlsma, & Cutolo, 2005). Patients with RA who have greater daily stress levels also have greater bony erosions over time (Feigenbaum, Masi, & Kaplan, 1979). Disease flare-ups in women with RA were found to be associated with more interpersonal stressors occurring on the days prior to a clinic visit, and these women also had greater levels of immune markers (Zautra et al., 1997; Zautra et al., 2004). Depression is prevalent in individuals with RA (Dickens, McGowan, Clark-Carter, & Creed, 2002), and RA patients experiencing stress and depression have increased circulating levels of IL-6, a proinflammatory cytokine (Davis et al., 2008; Hirano, Nagashima, Ogawa, & Yoshino, 2001). Since IL-6 is implicated in depressive symptoms, it is not clear whether the elevations in IL-6 are a result of the depression or the cause of the depression. It is also likely that the chronic pain that RA patients endure may lead to depressive symptoms. Nevertheless, elevations of IL-6 can promote inflammatory processes and aggravate or precipitate symptoms in inflammatory joint disease.

The effect of psychosocial stress on inflammatory processes that underlie RA and JIA is best understood by examining the presymptomatic early phase of these conditions separately from the symptomatic phase. The presymptomatic phase of RA and JIA involves T and B cells and dendritic cells, and even though these individuals may have detectable autoantigens they are asymptomatic. During this phase, stress is believed to play a permissive role in disease initiation. The reasoning for this is as follows. In the early asymptomatic phase of inflammatory conditions, acute minor stressors will promote immune activation and inflammatory processes similar to what occurs in healthy individuals. As a result, acute stressors may serve as a permissive factor in disease development, as children who develop JIA are able to produce a more robust immune response to stress (as opposed to more elderly individuals who develop RA) (Straub et al., 2005). During the symptomatic phase of RA and JIA, inflammatory cells (i.e., neutrophils, macrophages, fibroblasts, osteoclasts), invade the affected joints and mediate the inflammation and joint destruction. It is during the symptomatic phase of RA or JIA that an imbalance in neuroendocrine-immune processes leads to a proinflammatory response to acute psychological stressors. This is manifested as disease exacerbation or flare-up during stressful situations.

A neuroendocrine-immune imbalance is believed to underlie the mechanism whereby stress leads to disease flare-up in individuals with RA and JIA. RA patients exhibit a reduced HPA response to environmental stressors leading to reduced cortisol levels (Dekkers et al., 2001).

This results from the continuous inflammatory stimulus to the HPA axis, which causes it to habituate or stop responding over time. Also, patients with RA exhibit a reduced number of glucocorticoid receptors (needed for target cells to respond to cortisol), hence their body cells are less responsive to effects of glucocorticoids, like cortisol. This leads to glucocorticoid resistance (Silverman & Sternberg, 2008). Given that cortisol has anti-inflammatory properties, the reduced cortisol response allows the proinflammatory chronic symptomatic phase of the disease to continue unabated (Straub et al., 2005).

In addition to the reduction in glucocorticoid receptors, patients with RA and JIA exhibit a beta to alpha adrenergic receptor shift characterized by fewer beta receptors and more alpha receptors. Typically, sympathetic stimulation of beta receptors leads to suppression of proinflammatory mediators from cells like macrophages, whereas activation of alpha receptors leads to increased release of proinflammatory mediators, like TNF. As a result of the beta to alpha adrenoreceptor shift, individuals with RA have a greater local proinflammatory situation marked by a greater production of TNF. Overall, this will exacerbate the inflammatory condition and symptoms. Hence, stress activation of the sympathetic nervous system promotes more inflammation and exacerbation of RA (i.e., a greater alpha adrenergic proinflammatory response). This, coupled with a reduction in the HPA release of the anti-inflammatory glucocorticoid cortisol, will lead to symptom exacerbation during periods of psychosocial stress (Straub et al., 2005). Clearly, these stress-initiated processes worsen the inflammatory condition and exacerbate symptom distress. This explains why disease expression varies with the experience of stressful events. Nurse-directed stress-management programs may serve as complementary approaches to decreasing symptom distress and disease progression in these patients.

Stress, Immune Processes, and Asthma

Immunologically, individuals with allergic disease and asthma exhibit a Th1/Th2 imbalance that is characterized by increased Th2 cytokines (IL-4, IL-5, and IL-13) and decreased Th1 cytokines (IFN-gamma). Psychosocial stress produces an imbalance of cytokines and this may trigger allergic symptoms and or exacerbations of allergic disease, like asthma (Chen & Miller, 2007). An 18-month prospective study of children with asthma showed that both chronic and acute stress increased the risk of a subsequent asthmatic attack. However, the risk of an asthmatic attack was 3 times greater in children who experienced an acute episode of stress (such as death of a family member) against a backdrop of chronic life stress. This typically occurred within 2 weeks of the negative event but could also occur for as long as 5 to 7 weeks later (Sandberg, Jarvenpaa, Penttinen, Paton, & McCann, 2004). Evidence shows that psychosocial stress contributes to asthma by altering immune mechanisms that mediate the inflammatory processes that characterize asthma. For example, the stress of school examinations was shown to increase IL-5 production in adolescents with asthma compared to that observed in adolescents without asthma (Kang et al., 1997). Also the stress of final examinations in asthmatic college students was shown to lead to higher sputum eosinophil counts and IL-5 production after antigen challenge (inhalation of an allergen to which the individual is sensitized immunologically) compared to that observed during a low stress period (mid-semester) (Liu et al., 2002).

It is well known that there is a greater prevalence of asthma and asthma-related events, including hospitalizations, in children with low socioeconomic status (SES). Although this may be explained by factors such as reduced access to care and greater exposure to asthma triggers, psychosocial factors also contribute to the greater prevalence of asthma in children from low SES backgrounds (Chen, Fisher, Bacharier, & Strunk, 2003; Chen et al., 2006). Growing up in a lower SES family is associated with greater life stress and threat of violence both at home and at school (Finkelhor & Dziuba-Leatherman, 1994; McLoyd, 1990). Clougherty et al. reported an association between traffic-related pollution and asthma diagnosis among children living in East Boston who had greater exposure to violence (Clougherty et al., 2007). Children with asthma from low SES neighborhoods not only report greater levels of chronic stress and perception of threat but also have heightened production of IL-5 and IL-13 (Th2 cytokines) and a higher eosinophil count than those from high SES neighborhoods. Importantly, chronic stress and threat perception mediated the association of low SES on these asthma-related immune

processes, and this effect was independent of other asthma triggers (Chen et al., 2006). These results indicate that chronic stress is a key mediator that links SES and immune processes (cytokines and eosinophilia) implicated in asthma. Thus, psychosocial stress, by tipping the cytokine balance toward a Th2 profile, may contribute to greater asthma morbidity and worse outcomes for asthmatic children exposed to chronic life stress associated with low SES. The mechanism underlying stress-induced cytokine dysregulation is linked to increased levels of cortisol and catecholamines. Cortisol will increase IL-4 and suppresses IFN-gamma, while norepinephrine activates beta receptors to inhibit IL-2, IFN-gamma, and IL-12 and stimulate IL-6 and IL-10 (Agarwal & Marshall, 2001). Norepinephrine also increases IL-4-stimulated IgE production (Paul-Eugene et al., 1993). These neuroendocrine-mediated immune alterations are thought to account for the effects of psychosocial stress on the progression and exacerbation of allergic disease.

Psychosocial stress does not independently trigger a flare-up of asthma (Chen & Miller, 2007). Rather, stress interacts with environmental triggers, such as exposure to animal dander, infection, or inhaled smoke, to intensify the inflammatory response to these triggers. In the presence of stress there is a greater production of Th2 cytokines, IgE, and eosinophilia; hence, stress increases the risk for and the intensity of disease exacerbation. However, considering that psychosocial stress increases both cortisol and catecholamine secretion, a paradox needs to be addressed. That is, glucocorticoids, like cortisol, have anti-inflammatory effects and beta adrenergic agonists, like epinephrine and norepinephrine, produce bronchodilation and these effects are beneficial to asthmatics. To reconcile this paradox, the following argument is proposed. Glucocorticoids promote a Th2 cytokine response (which promotes asthma and allergic responses); however, over time chronic stress leads to an adaptive down-regulation of glucocorticoid receptors on immune cells, hence producing resistance to the anti-inflammatory effects of glucocorticoids. In support of this concept, children with asthma were shown to have a 5.5-fold reduction in glucocorticoid receptor mRNA, which would diminish the anti-inflammatory effect of these molecules on target cells. In addition, chronic stress leads to unresponsiveness of the HPA axis and decreased cortisol secretion. Adolescents with positive skin test reactivity and a history of allergic rhinitis, atopic dermatitis, or asthma were shown to have a diminished cortisol response compared to nonatopic adolescents (Wamboldt, Laudenslager, Wamboldt, Kelsay, & Hewitt, 2003). Further, chronic stress is associated with fewer beta-adrenergic receptors on leukocytes of children with asthma, which would lead to increased Th2 cytokines and mast cell degranulation, and less bronchodilatory effects of adrenergic stimuli (Chen & Miller, 2007). Hence, an individual with an allergic or asthmatic phenotype who is under chronic stress will respond to an acute stressor without the benefit of cortisol and adrenergic mechanisms that would typically serve to dampen or counter the inflammatory response responsible for allergic or asthmatic symptoms. Several studies have evaluated the use of psychological interventions, such as biofeedback, mental imagery, relaxation therapy, and massage, for the reduction of allergic episodes. The results of these intervention studies are promising but further study is needed using more rigorous research designs to confirm the benefits of such interventions (Marshall & Roy, 2007).

Stress, Immunity, and Infectious Disease

Humans exposed to chronic psychological or physical stress experience decreased resistance to microbial pathogens. This decreased resistance is thought to be due to stress-induced immune suppression and to result in increased susceptibility and frequency of disease, prolonged healing time, and a greater incidence of secondary health complications associated with infection (Godbout & Glaser, 2006). Stressors can induce significant effects on a host's immune response to microbial pathogens and the extent of these effects depends on stressor type, duration, and intensity. For example, psychological stress or negative affective states have been shown to reduce natural killer cell activity, alter cytokine production, decrease proliferative response to mitogens, reduce specific antibody responses, and reduce T-lymphocyte-mediated cellular responses. These effects result from activation of various central nervous system (CNS) pathways including the HPA, the sympathetic nervous system, and the endogenous opioid pathway. Activation of these pathways increases the level of neuroendocrine hormones, which subsequently lead to suppressed innate and adaptive immune responses. Chronic stress produces the most profound immune suppression and is due to increased production of glucocorticoids and catecholamines. These modulate lymphocyte trafficking (Dhabhar, Satoskar, Bluethmann, David, & McEwen, 2000) and immune function through leukocyte receptors for these stress mediators (Sanchez-Barcelo, Cos, Fernandez, & Mediavilla, 2003).

Examples of the Effect of Stress Upon the Immune Response to Microorganisms

One of the best-characterized immune functions, affected by exposure to chronic stress, is NKCA (Bosch, Berntson, Cacioppo, & Marucha, 2005). In addition to antitumor effects, NK cells constitute the body's first line of defense against virus infections. NK cells (CD56+) are a component of the innate immune system and play a key role in controlling and lysing virus-infected cells during the early phase of a viral infection. Greater NK cell number and/or cytolytic activity increase one's natural resistance to viruses. Protection against viral infections is also mediated by two arms of the adaptive immune system. These are the cell-mediated immune response, which against viral infections is primarily mediated by cytotoxic T lymphocytes (CD8+). The other arm of the adaptive immune system is the humoral immune response by B lymphocytes (CD19+), which produce antibodies. Chronic stress results in lowered innate and reduced adaptive immune responses in humans and is associated with increased incidence, duration, and severity of infection as well as decreased survival (Caserta et al., 2008; Glaser & Kiecolt-Glaser, 2005).

Another good example of the effect of stress upon the immune system is the reactivation of latent viral infections. The immune suppressive effect of stress promotes reactivation of latent viruses (e.g., herpes simplex virus [HSV]-1 that cause oral herpes labialis, and HSV-2 that causes genital herpes). Stressors as diverse as academic examination and marital distress have been linked to apparent latent virus reactivation, as judged by higher levels of circulating antibody specific for HSV-1, HSV-2, as well as cytomegalovirus and Epstein-Barr virus (Glaser & Kiecolt-Glaser, 1997; Pariante et al., 1997). Each of these viruses is latent in that the virus exists within the host in a quiescent state, and this quiescent state is a consequence of continued and specific cell-mediated immunity directed against virus-infected somatic cells. However, if cell-mediated immunity is reduced (e.g., by stress), these viruses reactivate and replicate, leading to viral shedding and stimulation of the humoral immune response. Shed virus is antigenic and stimulates B lymphocytes to respond to the virus with the production of antibody, resulting in a subsequent increase in antibody levels specific for that virus. Hence, an increase in specific antibody within the circulation is an indication of viral shedding, resultant from the effect of stress upon the cell-mediated immune function that normally controls viral replication and shedding (Gouin, Hantsoo, & Kiecolt-Glaser, 2008).

It is clearly established that suppression of the immune response increases mycotic and bacterial infections. However, unequivocal empirical evidence that psychological stress increases the incidence and severity of bacterial and mycotic human infections is lacking. Nevertheless, the association of emotional stress and infectious mycological disease is suspected. Fungal infections are well known to be associated with the stressful conditions of surgical trauma, cancer, organ transplants, long-term antibiotic use, corticosteroid therapy, diabetes mellitus, critical illness, and pregnancy. Stress hormones such as cortisol and catecholamines are known to enhance pathogenesis of experimental fungal disease. For example, *Candida albicans* and related fungi are endogenous opportunists and infections with these fungi are typically associated with debilitating and/or predisposing conditions. *Candida* infections have become the first symptom of active AIDS to appear in HIV-positive individuals. One factor shared by AIDS patients and other susceptible individuals is hormonal imbalance resulting from HPA and sympathetic nervous system activation. Candidiasis also appears frequently in people undergoing surgery, a complex form of stress that involves emotional stressors (anxiety), chemical stressors (anesthesia), physical stressors (surgery), and often the stress of pain. Similarly, emotional stress has been positively correlated with increased incidence of the carriage of *Candida* and has been implicated in vulvovaginitis caused by *Candida albicans* (Meyer, Goettlicher, & Mendling, 2006). Interestingly,

somatic factors did not influence the occurrence or relapse with this infectious agent and antimycotic treatment influenced only the symptoms of the illness, not its cause. Women with recurrent vulvovaginal *candidiasis* have been shown to have a blunted rise in morning cortisol levels and lower mean levels of salivary cortisol after awakening (Ehrstrom, Kornfeld, Thuresson, & Rylander, 2005), as well as locally compromised immune function (Mendling & Seebacher, 2003). These observations suggest a role for stress in the incidence and susceptibility of these women to this fungal infection.

Stress has also been associated with the pathogenesis of tuberculosis caused by the bacterium *Mycobacterium tuberculosis* (Biondi & Zannino, 1997). With the recent resurgence of tuberculosis, understanding the potential role of stress in susceptibility to and progression of this infectious disease has become even more important. High rates of tuberculosis have been reported among socially isolated individuals and in school children and their teachers during periods of emotional stress, such as war. Those studies showed a reduced capacity of the infected individuals to phagocytize the infectious agent and suggested that stressful situations might serve as cofactors in the development of tuberculosis. In an extensive study, tubercular patients were shown to have a dramatic increase in the number of stressful life events approximately 2 years prior to their hospitalization. Likewise, mortality due to tuberculosis has been shown to be higher in subjects who have experienced divorce. Therefore it is possible stress, via its effects mediated by neuroendocrine-immune interactions, may contribute to the incidence and severity of this serious health hazard (Biondi & Zannino, 1997).

It is worth noting that invasion of the body by disease-causing microorganisms is not necessarily sufficient to actually cause the disease. Disease occurs only when the infectious agent is pathogenic and the immune system is compromised or unable to recognize the invading microorganism. Psychological stress can alter the immune response, but it is unclear whether such an alteration is sufficient to influence the body's ability to fight infectious disease. To address this issue a series of human viral challenge studies were conducted in which psychological parameters were assessed and then volunteers were exposed to one of five viruses that cause the common cold (A. Pedersen, Zachariae, & Bovbjerg, 2010). The participants were monitored for infection and illness. The results showed that the greater the psychological stress the greater the probability for clinical manifestations of a viral infection. Two types of psychologically stressful life events were strongly associated with greater illness susceptibility: enduring (1-month or longer) interpersonal problems with family or friends, and enduring problems related to work (under- or unemployment). Moreover, across all types of events, the longer the stressful life event lasted, the greater was the risk for developing a clinical illness. In these studies, higher levels of epinephrine and norepinephrine were related to a greater risk of developing a cold. However, neither catecholamines nor immune effector mechanisms were associated with the duration or clinical manifestations of viral infection.

In a separate study, influenza virus challenge of volunteers showed that those with higher psychological stress had greater symptomatology, greater accumulation of nasal mucus, and higher amounts of the proinflammatory cytokine IL-6. The IL-6 response was temporally related to illness expression, indicating that IL-6 acted as a major mediator through which stress was associated with symptoms of illness (Cohen, 2005). The effect of stress in this highly controlled human challenge model did not appear to be due to stress-elicited suppression of immune function. Instead, chronic stress appeared to interfere with the immune system's ability to respond to hormonal signals that turn off the release of proinflammatory cytokines. Individuals under stress may overrespond (e.g., produce too much IL-6), which in turn triggers and prolongs the symptoms of upper respiratory infections. In other words, stress did not reduce the immune response to viral challenge, but rather it amplified the IL-6 response. It may be that adults facing a severe chronic stressor have a diminished capacity to suppress IL-6 production because of stressor-induced glucocorticoid resistance. It is important to note that such data are derived from a controlled but artificial challenge paradigm and the results are based on correlations and causation is unproven. However, it is valuable to note that the relationship of stress to immune outcome is a complex one in that further investigation has demonstrated positive emotional style

to be associated with a lower risk of developing an upper respiratory infection. Individuals with positive emotional style had fewer symptoms and signs of respiratory viral infection and with fewer upper respiratory tract symptoms. Understanding the contribution of positive emotions to immunity and protection from disease has become an active area of PNI research.

Since stress influences the immune system in healthy populations, it is plausible that stress and other psychosocial factors may play a role in the immune abnormalities associated with human immunodeficiency viral infections (Cole, 2008). HIV-infected individuals display physiological changes consistent with chronic elevations of resting levels of cortisol, as evidenced by muted cortisol responsivity (due to down-regulated receptors), and a flattened cortisol circadian rhythm. (Note: Cortisol is secreted in a circadian pattern with high levels in the morning that decrease to low levels at bedtime.) Elevated cortisol levels predict accelerated immune decline and development of AIDS in those who are HIV-positive. Further, HIV-positive men show signs of sympathetic nervous system activation and a diminished capacity to suppress HIV plasma viral load as well as a poorer CD4+ T-cell recovery when treated with highly active antiretroviral therapy. Sympathetic nervous system activation results in down-regulation of lymphocyte and NK cell function and chronic sympathetic nervous system activation with release of norepinephrine alters lymphocyte trafficking, cytokine production, and cytotoxicity and facilitates HIV replication.

It is worth noting that HIV-positive individuals assigned to cognitive behavior stress management (CBSM) demonstrate less activation of HPA axis-mediated stress responses, better immunologic control of virus, and increased immune system reconstitution with decreased HIV viral RNA in peripheral blood. These biological changes were associated with reductions in depression and increases in relaxation and social support during the stress-management intervention. CBSM reduces anxiety, depression, and social isolation by lowering physical tension, increasing a sense of control and self-efficacy, and builds interpersonal skills necessary to maintain adequate and effective social relationships (Antoni, Carrico et al., 2006). Others have also show preliminary evidence that mindfulness-based stress reduction also benefits HIV-positive individuals (Robinson, Mathews, & Witek-Janusek, 2003). These psychological effects are hypothesized to improve regulation of peripheral catecholamines and cortisol via changes in the sympathetic nervous system and HPA axis, respectively, and, in turn, lead to better immune control of the HIV virus.

PNI and Vaccination. Psychological stress can also modulate the humoral immune response to vaccination (A. F. Pedersen, Zachariae, & Bovbjerg, 2009). Prospective longitudinal studies demonstrate that people who report higher levels of stress exhibit lower levels of protective antibodies against microbial pathogens including influenza, hepatitis B, and pneumonia (Glaser, Sheridan, Malarkey, MacCallum, & Kiecolt-Glaser, 2000; Gouin et al., 2008; Vedhara et al., 1999). From a clinical perspective, these findings suggest that stress may diminish the efficacy of vaccination procedures and thereby increase vulnerability to pathogens that give rise to infectious disease. The most robust evidence is derived from studies of older adults who experienced chronic stress as caregivers for family members suffering from dementia. These caretakers exhibit blunted antibody responses to influenza and to bacterial pneumonia vaccines when compared to matched control individuals. The deficits in antibody response persist years after the family member had died, suggesting that chronic, severe stressors may have long-term adverse consequences on the immune system (Glaser et al., 2000; Gouin et al., 2008).

Stress, Inflammation, and Cardiovascular Disease

Psychological stress is a risk factor for cardiovascular disease. Given that inflammatory processes accelerate the clinical expression of cardiovascular disease (Libby, Ridker, & Maseri, 2002; Ross, 1999), it is likely that stress-induced increases in inflammatory molecules, like IL-6, contribute to the pathogenesis of cardiovascular disease. In fact, PNI mechanisms may explain why there are a number of individuals who develop cardiovascular disease or who experience an acute cardiac event despite the fact that they do not have standard cardiovascular risk factors, such as a family history, hyperlipidemia, obesity, hypertension, or diabetes. To understand the role of stress-induced immune alterations in

cardiovascular disease, it is important to distinguish between the effects of chronic stress versus that of acute stress. The link between chronic stress and cardiovascular disease is demonstrated most markedly in individuals with low socioeconomic status who have substandard income, limited education, and low-prestige occupations (Steptoe & Brydon, 2007). These individuals live under chronic stress, often in neighborhoods marked by violence and with few opportunities or resources to buffer stress. These living conditions produce chronic fear, social isolation, and depression, as well as an increase in standard cardiovascular risks, such as poor diet, little physical activity, obesity, and hypertension. Likewise, chronic stress is prevalent in the lives of individuals who have a hostile personality trait. Hostile individuals are quick to anger and tend to respond aggressively to life events. Given that the development of coronary artery disease (CAD) occurs over many years, chronic stress, rather than acute or episodic stress, is more likely to contribute to the initiation of CAD. By activating the sympathetic nervous system over many years, chronic stress will promote lipid deposition and inflammatory processes that increase plaque deposition. Chronic stress and hostility have been shown to alter macrophage function and increase the release of proinflammatory mediators, like IL-6. In fact, individuals under chronic stress due to low SES have a chronic low-grade inflammatory state, characterized by increased circulating levels of inflammatory molecules such as IL-6, TNF-alpha, C-reactive protein, fibrinogen, and homocysteine (Panagiotakos et al., 2005). This was true even when smoking, diet, physical activity, and medication compliance were controlled. The release of inflammatory molecules as a consequence of stress may contribute to the initiation of atherosclerotic lesions and their progression into more severe vascular damage. Further, individuals living with chronic stress also contract more infectious diseases, which stimulates immune mediator release and which can also activate latent viruses within established plaque (Kop & Cohen, 2007). As a result, this intensifies inflammatory processes that promote vascular damage and plaque instability, placing these individuals at greater risk for acute coronary events.

An acute stress experience, such as an outburst of anger or experiencing a terrifying event like an earthquake, may also lead to immune consequences that contribute to acute coronary syndromes (ACS). This is most relevant to an individual who has existing CAD and is likely mediated by autonomic nervous system activation and release of inflammatory molecules (Bhattacharyya & Steptoe, 2007). Activation of the sympathetic nervous system by acute stress leads to increased heart rate, increased cardiac contractility, and increased oxygen demand. Typically, the increase in metabolic products within the working myocardium will increase coronary artery vasodilatation. In contrast, in an individual with existing coronary disease, the acute stress leads to the release of inflammatory mediators that may disrupt endothelial function and promote vasoconstriction, as opposed to vasodilatation. As a result, the risk for ACS is increased. Interestingly, the cardiovascular and immune response to acute stress is enhanced in persons who have chronic stress in their lives or who have hostile personalities, both of which can further increase the risk of ACS (Steptoe & Brydon, 2007). Also, individuals with low SES show greater levels of the proinflammatory cytokine, IL-6, in response to an acute stress situation in the laboratory (Brydon, Edwards, Mohamed-Ali, & Steptoe, 2004). This is supported by results of other studies that show that individuals who present with ACS have often experienced stressful situations marked by anger within a critical two-hour window prior to the ACS (Strike & Steptoe, 2005).

Depression and exhaustion have been consistently linked to poor outcomes and increased risk of death from cardiovascular disease (Kop & Cohen, 2007; Steptoe & Brydon, 2007). Individuals with depression are also more likely to suffer first and recurrent myocardial infarction, as well as sudden cardiac death (Wulsin & Singal, 2003). An evaluation of patients who suffered ACS showed that there is a greater risk of ACS in those who experienced acute depressed mood prior to the cardiac event; also, depressed mood was more common in ACS patients with lower income (Steptoe, Strike, Perkins-Porras, McEwan, & Whitehead, 2006). Others showed that depressive mood increased the risk for recurrence of atrial fibrillation after cardioversion. This was attributed to heightened adrenergic tone, which promotes a proinflammatory state (Lange & Herrmann-Lingen, 2007). Further, individuals with depression exhibit early signs of nonsymptomatic cardiovascular

disease as revealed by intimal-medial thickness of the arterial wall or coronary artery calcification. Likewise, those who are extremely fatigued or exhausted are at greater risk for cardiac disease and death (Prescott et al., 2003). Both depression and fatigue are associated with a heightened proinflammatory state, which is believed to contribute to instability of atherosclerotic plaques and plaque rupture that eventually leads to ACS (Kop & Cohen, 2007). Overall, these mechanisms explain the current thinking as to how a "brain-to-immune" or PNI process might promote cardiovascular disease. Individuals who have few social resources and little social support are at greater risk for cardiovascular disease and have a worse prognosis (Eng, Rimm, Fitzmaurice, & Kawachi, 2002; Rosengren, Wilhelmsen, & Orth-Gomer, 2004). This may be related to a heightened proinflammatory state, as others have shown that men who have larger social networks have lower circulating levels of IL-6 (Loucks et al., 2006). On the other hand, social support can decrease the stress-induced release of inflammatory mediators and may offer a way to lessen the adverse effects of psychosocial factors on cardiovascular disease. Currently, studies are underway to determine whether stress-reduction programs might decrease the risk for initial or recurrent cardiac events by reducing stress-induced inflammatory processes.

STRESS-IMMUNITY AND NURSING SCIENCE

The holistic view of human nature ascribed to by the discipline of nursing is consistent with the philosophical underpinnings of PNI (McCain & Smith, 1994; Robinson, Mathews, & Witek-Janusek, 2002; A. Starkweather, Witek-Janusek, & Mathews, 2005a; Zeller, McCain, & Swanson, 1996). It is therefore not surprising that nurse researchers have readily adopted the PNI framework, applying it to multiple scientific foci and in so doing have made significant contributions to the scientific growth of this field. Nurse investigators have examined stress-immune interactions in a variety of immune-based illnesses, including asthma (Kang & Weaver, 2009), HIV (McCain et al., 2008; Robinson et al., 2003), herniated disc (A. Starkweather, Witek-Janusek, & Mathews, 2005b; A. R. Starkweather, Witek-Janusek, Nockels,

Peterson, & Mathews, 2006), multiple sclerosis (Sorenson, Witek-Janusek, & Mathews, 2006), and cancer (Kang et al., 2009; Witek-Janusek et al., 2008). In addition, nurse scientists have documented the immunosuppressive nature of pain (Page, Blakely, & Kim, 2005) and post-operative stress (Yermal et al., 2009). A PNI framework has also been used to understand the immunologic implications of child birth, breast-feeding, and postpartal stress on maternal–infant well-being (M. Groer, El-Badri, Djeu, Harrington, & Van Eepoel, 2010; M. W. Groer & Davis, 2006). Some of these studies are elaborated upon in the following discussion.

As described earlier in this chapter, asthmatic symptoms are often initiated and potentiated by stressful life events, and the stress–asthma linkage has been assessed by nurse investigators. In this regard, Kang and colleagues reported that in adolescents, examination stress produced significant alterations in circulating immune cell subsets and in both proliferative and cytolytic activities, with males showing higher NK cell activity and greater lymphocyte proliferation than females. However, no differences in stress and changes in immune function were observed between healthy and asthmatic adolescents, which was attributed to the well-managed nature of the asthmatic sample (Kang, Coe, Karaszewski, & McCarthy, 1998; Kang, Coe, & McCarthy, 1996; Kang, Kim, & Suh, 2004). More recently, in asthmatic mice, Kang and Weaver (2009) found that exposure to acute stress produced a Th2-like pattern of cytokine production, suggesting a possible mechanism for stress-induced exacerbation of asthmatic symptoms. These studies are suggestive and need to be replicated in asthmatics with less stable disease and more intense or chronic stress.

Significant research has evaluated immune factors in response to the stress of pain in animal models and human conditions. Research from the laboratory of Gayle Page spans several such studies, which are linked by a PNI framework. Early experiments in rodents showed that untreated postoperative pain led to impaired NK cell activity and enhanced tumor metastases (Ben-Eliyahu, Page, Yirmiya, & Shakhar, 1999; Page & Ben-Eliyahu, 1997; Page, Ben-Eliyahu, & Liebeskind, 1994). In this model, rats were subjected to laparotomy and injected with NK cell-sensitive radiolabeled tumor cells. Rats that were treated with morphine, and that exhibited

signs of pain relief, had significantly less radio-labeled tumor and fewer metastatic lesions on the lung, and higher postoperative NK cell activity (Page et al., 1994). These results suggest that untreated postoperative pain leads to impaired immune function and potentially increased organ localization of tumor emboli. Experience of physical pain (i.e., needle paw prick) has also been demonstrated to affect immune function and impair cancer control (Page et al., 2005). Exposure to a paw needle prick for 7 postnatal days resulted in a greater tumor susceptibility and a weaker NK cell activity in male—but not in female—rats. Although these observations are limited to animal models, others nurse scientists evaluated postoperative stress and pain in men undergoing prostatectomy for cancer of the prostate. That study showed that the stress associated with surgery resulted in a postoperative reduction in NK cell activity compared to preoperative levels. Due to good pain management in the postoperative period no associations of NK cell activity were observed (Yermal et al., 2009). These studies indicate that the treatment of physical pain and psychological stress associated with pain is necessary not only to alleviate suffering but also to prevent pain-induced immunosuppression and possible tumor metastatic spread. Nurse investigators have also evaluated stress-immune processes in other human conditions marked by chronic and unrelenting pain. Angela Starkweather reported her findings, which described the complexity of pre- and post-operative interactions among stress-pain-immune mechanisms in individuals experiencing chronic back pain and sciatica due to herniated disc (A. Starkweather et al., 2005b; A. R. Starkweather et al., 2006).

Chronic systemic inflammation has also been associated with age-related conditions, and a growing body of evidence suggests that there is an immune-to-brain communication. Marsland et al. have demonstrated an inverse relationship between IL-6 and memory function in a community sample of healthy middle-aged adults (Marsland et al., 2006). Furthermore, utilizing a cross-sectional neuro-imaging procedure, peripheral levels of IL-6 were shown to inversely associate with the hippocampal gray matter volume. This relationship persisted after controlling for various demographic and health factors (e.g., physical activity, smoking), raising the possibility that IL-6 can serve as a novel bio-marker for risk of age-related cognitive decline (Marsland, Gianaros, Abramowitch, Manuck, & Hariri, 2008). Such exciting findings present future nursing scientists with an opportunity to investigate the role of anti-inflammatory inter-vention in the progression of memory decline in dementia and Alzheimer's disease patients.

Living with HIV is replete with multiple stressors, and nurse scientists have contributed to the supposition that the stress-endocrine-immune axis is implicated in HIV disease pro-gression (McCain & Cella, 1995; McCain & Gramling, 1992). Stress-induced neuroendo-crine activation leads to elevations in plasma cortisol and *in vitro,* physiological concentra-tions of cortisol increase HIV replication in monocyte-derived macrophages. This observa-tion suggests a potential role for stress hor-mones in HIV disease activation and progression (Swanson, Zeller, & Spear, 1998). To counter these effects of stress, the effectiveness of stress-reducing interventions in HIV disease has been extensively evaluated by McCain et al. In a com-prehensive randomized clinical trial McCain and colleagues (2008) examined the efficacy of three stress-management programs (cognitive-behavioral relaxation [CBR], focused tai chi [TC], and spiritual growth [SG]) on psychoim-mune variables. Both CBR and TC programs improved quality of life, while lymphocyte prolif-eration capacity was found to increase between pre- and postintervention in all treatment approaches. An investigation of another interven-tion, a mindfulness-based stress-reduction pro-gram in HIV-positive individuals, revealed NK cell activity and NK cell number to be signifi-cantly higher in the intervention group than the comparison group (Robinson et al., 2003). NK cell activity is an important host defense mecha-nism against viral and opportunistic microbial infections, which cause significant morbidity and mortality in HIV-positive patients.

Stress-induced immunosuppression may have special relevance to the nursing care of cancer patients who are at risk for dysregulated immune function. Immune dysregulation asso-ciated with cancer begins well before cancer treatment, as demonstrated in an evaluation of emotional stress and immune function in women undergoing breast biopsy for cancer diagnosis. Witek-Janusek et al. showed the stress of biopsy results in time-sensitive reductions of NK cell activity and dysregulation of cytokines no matter whether the results were benign or malignant biopsy. Stress-immune dysregulation continued in both groups well beyond the biopsy results (Witek-Janusek et al., 2007). That work led to a study which demonstrated that a mindfulness-based stress reduction (MBSR) intervention improved quality of life, increased coping effectiveness, and facilitated restoration of immune function after cancer diagnosis and treatment (Witek-Janusek et al., 2008). Moreover, at the molecular level, nuclear localization in lymphocytes of two transcription factors, NF-kappa B and AP-1, was shown to be decreased in women experiencing significant emotional stress as a result of diagnostic breast biopsy, whereas when stress was relieved (post-biopsy) the nuclear localization of these gene transcrip-tion factors was similar to those of age-matched control women (Nagabhushan, Mathews, & Witek-Janusek, 2001). Recent *in vitro* work in NK cell lines suggests that stress-induced reduc-tions in NKCA may be related to glucocorticoid-mediated epigenetic modification of NK cell function (Krukowski et al., in press). The newest direction of research of this group is to evaluate whether epigenetic modification mediates psy-chological distress-induced immune dysregula-tion, as an emerging body of evidence suggests that the psychosocial environment can trigger epigenetic modification for genes that regulate stress reactivity and possibly immune function. (See Chapter 4 [reviewed in Mathews & Witek Janusek, 2011].)

Nurse researchers have used a PNI approach toward understanding the impact of prenatal maternal stress and childbirth postpartal stress on maternal–child health. Groer et al. demonstrated that childbirth stress leads to a reduction in maternal secretory immuno-globulin A (sIgA). This reduction was most pronounced in women who reported an increased state of anxiety. Women with very low or undetectable levels of sIgA had a greater incidence of postpartal com-plications, and their infants had more illnesses. Examination of maternal postpartum immune function showed that NK cell activity was sup-pressed through the fifth month, reaching a nadir at two months. Although NK cell activity sup-pression is normal during pregnancy, why this persists into the postpartum period is unknown (M. Groer et al., 2010). As well, maternal stress may adversely affect the infant immune response, as glucocorticoid hormones have been shown to alter the pattern of cytokine production from neonatal mononuclear cells, which can increase the newborn's risk for infection (Witek-Janusek & Mathews, 1999).

The dysregulation of the innate immune system and the HPA axis may also be implicated in the development and the insidious nature of the postpartum depression (Corwin & Pajer, 2008). For example, women with elevated levels of IL1-beta have been shown to report higher levels of depressive symptoms and fatigue 2 weeks later than women who did not (Corwin, Johnston, & Pugh, 2008). Thus, stress during and after childbirth can have profound effects on maternal immune function, which can alter the clinical course of mothers and their infants.

The unique psychological and immunologic relationship between a breastfeeding mother and her infant is an intriguing paradigm in which to evaluate the stress–immune relationship. Stress-induced alterations in maternal immunity in breastfeeding mothers could potentially alter their capability to provide optimal levels of immunoglobulins for their infants. Although many factors influence maternal production of sIgA, high levels of perceived stress, anger, and infectious symptoms have been associated with higher milk sIgA (M. Groer, Davis, & Steele, 2004). Interestingly, a decreased IFN-gamma/IL-10 ratio was observed for women who experienced dysphoric mood, but only if they were formula feeding and not breastfeeding (M. W. Groer & Davis, 2006). A prolactin-mediated pathway was suggested as prolactin has been shown to relate to positive affect, decreased stress (M. Groer et al., 2005), and fatigue (M. W. Groer et al., 2005) in postpartum mothers. Such stress-induced alterations in breast milk endocrine and immune composition may potentially impact the immunologic benefits that infants receive from breast milk. This is especially relevant to premature and low-birth-weight infants, who are at high risk for infectious illness.

FUTURE DIRECTIONS AND NURSING IMPLICATIONS

A wealth of evidence has now established that stressors, of both a physical and psychological nature, can profoundly alter immune function. This body of work now forms the scientific grounding for the interdisciplinary field of PNI. Moreover, the guiding premise of PNI is that stress-induced impairment of immune function influences disease progression or response to therapy or both. As reviewed, investigations in PNI are directed toward understanding the effect of the psychoendocrine stress response on the immune system, particularly within the context of cancer, autoimmune disease, pain syndromes, infectious disease, and maternal–child health. Nurses must recognize the potential effectiveness of biobehavioral approaches to the care of patients with immune-based disease. Such approaches to stress management may not only improve the quality of life and emotional well-being of targeted populations but also halt disease progression or complications that arise as a result of immune dysregulation.

Future emphasis needs to be placed on understanding the mechanism(s) of stress-induced immune dysregulation and this may include understanding epigenetic effects of a stressful environment (see Chapter 4). Insight into the molecular mechanisms and physiological role of the links that connect the immune system with the brain and behavior will provide more definitive evidence that these interactions have important roles in health and disease. This knowledge can guide the development of behavioral interventions to prevent and manage stress-related disease and/or reduce symptoms associated with stress. Yet, critical questions remain that require intensive empirical investigations using human paradigms of stress and rigorous controlled research designs. Such approaches will lead to a better understanding of disease and to better diagnosis, treatment, or both of stress-induced immune dysfunction. It is anticipated that future investigations will provide the scientific foundation that will lead to the identification of individuals "at risk" for psychological distress, altered immune reactivity, and disease risk. New approaches to assessment of stress risk and timely intervention may prove to be cost-effective additions to health care. Nurse scientists have already contributed immensely to PNI and stand poised to provide scientific leadership in the future, as PNI enters a new era of discovery.

REFERENCES

Ader, R. (1980). Presidential address—1980. Psychosomatic and psychoimmunologic research. *Psychosomatic Medicine, 42*(3), 307–321.

Agarwal, S. K., & Marshall, Jr., G. D. (2001). Dexamethasone promotes type 2 cytokine production primarily through inhibition of type 1 cytokines. *Journal of Interferon & Cytokine Research, 21*(3), 147–155.

Andersen, B. L., Farrar, W. B., Golden-Kreutz, D., Kutz, L. A., MacCallum, R., Courtney, M. E., et al. (1998). Stress and immune responses after surgical treatment for regional breast cancer. *Journal of the National Cancer Institute, 90*(1), 30–36.

Andersen, B. L., Farrar, W. B., Golden-Kreutz, D. M., Glaser, R., Emery, C. F., Crespin, T. R., et al. (2004). Psychological, behavioral, and immune changes after a psychological intervention: a clinical trial. *Journal of Clinical Oncology, 22*(17), 3570–3580.

Andersen, B. L., Yang, H. C., Farrar, W. B., Golden-Kreutz, D. M., Emery, C. F., Thornton, L. M., et al. (2008). Psychologic intervention improves survival for breast cancer patients: a randomized clinical trial. *Cancer, 113*(12), 3450–3458.

Antoni, M. H., Carrico, A. W., Duran, R. E., Spitzer, S., Penedo, F., Ironson, G., et al. (2006). Randomized clinical trial of cognitive behavioral stress management on human immunodeficiency virus viral load in gay men treated with highly active antiretroviral therapy. *Psychosomatic Medicine, 68*(1), 143–151.

Antoni, M. H., Lechner, S., Diaz, A., Vargas, S., Holley, H., Phillips, K., et al. (2009). Cognitive behavioral stress management effects on psychosocial and physiological adaptation in women undergoing treatment for breast cancer. *Brain, Behavior, and Immunity, 23*(5), 580–591.

Antoni, M. H., Lutgendorf, S. K., Cole, S. W., Dhabhar, F. S., Sephton, S. E., McDonald, P. G., et al. (2006). The influence of bio-behavioural factors on tumour biology: Pathways and mechanisms. *Nature Reviews Cancer, 6*(3), 240–248.

Avraham, R., & Ben-Eliyahu, S. (2007). Neuroendocrine regulation of cancer progression: II. Immunological mechanisms, clinical relevance, and prophylactic measures. In R. Ader (Ed.), *Psychoneuroimmunology* (4th ed., Vol. 1, pp. 251–265). Burlington, MA: Elsevier Academic Press.

Balkwill, F., Charles, K. A., & Mantovani, A. (2005). Smoldering and polarized inflammation in the initiation and promotion of malignant disease. *Cancer Cell, 7*(3), 211–217.

Ben-Baruch, A. (2006). Inflammation-associated immune suppression in cancer: The roles played by cytokines, chemokines and additional mediators. *Seminars in Cancer Biology, 16*(1), 38–52.

Ben-Eliyahu, S., Page, G. G., Yirmiya, R., & Shakhar, G. (1999). Evidence that stress and surgical interventions promote tumor development by suppressing natural killer cell activity. *International Journal of Cancer, 80*(6), 880–888.

Bernik, T. R., Friedman, S. G., Ochani, M., DiRaimo, R., Ulloa, L., Yang, H., et al. (2002). Pharmacological stimulation of the cholinergic antiinflammatory pathway. *Journal of Experimental Medicine, 195*(6), 781–788.

Bhattacharyya, M. R., & Steptoe, A. (2007). Emotional triggers of acute coronary syndromes: strength of evidence, biological processes, and clinical implications. *Progress in Cardiovascular Diseases, 49*(5), 353–365.

Biondi, M. (2001). Effects of stress on immune functions: An overview. In R. Ader & N. Cohen (Eds.), *Psychoneuroimmunology* (3rd ed., Vol. 2, pp. 189–226). New York, NY: Academic Press.

Biondi, M., & Zannino, L. G. (1997). Psychological stress, neuroimmunomodulation, and susceptibility to infectious diseases in animals and man: A review. *Psychotherapy and Psychosomatics, 66*(1), 3–26.

Blalock, J. E., & Smith, E. M. (2007). Conceptual development of the immune system as a sixth sense. *Brain, Behavior, and Immunity, 21*(1), 23–33.

Borovikova, L. V., Ivanova, S., Zhang, M., Yang, H., Botchkina, G. I., Watkins, L. R., et al. (2000). Vagus nerve stimulation attenuates the systemic inflammatory response to endotoxin. *Nature, 405*(6785), 458–462.

Bosch, J. A., Berntson, G. G., Cacioppo, J. T., & Marucha, P. T. (2005). Differential mobilization of functionally distinct natural killer subsets during acute psychologic stress. *Psychosomatic Medicine, 67*(3), 366–375.

Bosch, J. A., Engeland, C. G., Cacioppo, J. T., & Marucha, P. T. (2007). Depressive symptoms predict mucosal wound healing. *Psychosomatic Medicine, 69*(7), 597–605.

Bower, J. E., Ganz, P. A., Dickerson, S. S., Petersen, L., Aziz, N., & Fahey, J. L. (2005). Diurnal cortisol rhythm and fatigue in breast cancer survivors. *Psychoneuroendocrinology, 30*(1), 92–100.

Brydon, L., Edwards, S., Mohamed-Ali, V., & Steptoe, A. (2004). Socioeconomic status and stress-induced increases in interleukin-6. *Brain, Behavior, and Immunity, 18*(3), 281–290.

Caras, I., Grigorescu, A., Stavaru, C., Radu, D. L., Mogos, I., Szegli, G., et al. (2004). Evidence for immune defects in breast and lung cancer patients. *Cancer Immunology, Immunotherapy, 53*(12), 1146–1152.

Caserta, M. T., O'Connor, T. G., Wyman, P. A., Wang, H., Moynihan, J., Cross, W., et al. (2008). The associations between psychosocial stress and the frequency of illness, and innate and adaptive immune function in children. *Brain, Behavior, and Immunity, 22*(6), 933–940.

Chen, E., Fisher, E. B., Bacharier, L. B., & Strunk, R. C. (2003). Socioeconomic status, stress, and immune markers in adolescents with asthma. *Psychosomatic Medicine, 65*(6), 984–992.

Chen, E., Hanson, M. D., Paterson, L. Q., Griffin, M. J., Walker, H. A., & Miller, G. E. (2006). Socioeconomic status and inflammatory processes in childhood asthma: the role of psychological stress. *Journal of Allergy and Clinical Immunology, 117*(5), 1014–1020.

Chen, E., & Miller, G. E. (2007). Stress and inflammation in exacerbations of asthma. *Brain, Behavior, and Immunity, 21*(8), 993–999.

Chikanza, I. C., Kingsley, G., & Panayi, G. S. (1995). Peripheral blood and synovial fluid monocyte expression of interleukin 1 alpha and 1 beta during active rheumatoid arthritis. *Journal of Rheumatology, 22*(4), 600–606.

Christian, L. M., Graham, J. E., Padgett, D. A., Glaser, R., & Kiecolt-Glaser, J. K. (2006). Stress and wound healing. *Neuroimmunomodulation, 13*(5–6), 337–346.

Chrousos, G. P. (2000). The stress response and immune function: clinical implications. The 1999 Novera H. Spector Lecture. *Annals of the New York Academy of Sciences, 917*, 38–67.

Clougherty, J. E., Levy, J. I., Kubzansky, L. D., Ryan, P. B., Suglia, S. F., Canner, M. J., et al. (2007). Synergistic effects of traffic-related air pollution and exposure to violence on urban asthma etiology. *Environmental Health Perspectives, 115*(8), 1140–1146.

Cohen, S. (2005). Keynote presentation at the eighth International Congress of Behavioral Medicine: The Pittsburgh common cold studies— Psychosocial predictors of susceptibility to respiratory infectious illness. *International Journal of Behavior Medicine, 12*(3), 123–131.

Cole, S. W. (2008). Psychosocial influences on HIV-1 disease progression: neural, endocrine, and virologic mechanisms. *Psychosomatic Medicine, 70*(5), 562–568.

Corwin, E. J., Johnston, N., & Pugh, L. (2008). Symptoms of postpartum depression associated with elevated levels of interleukin-1 beta during the first month postpartum. *Biological Research for Nursing, 10*(2), 128–133.

Corwin, E. J., & Pajer, K. (2008). The psychoneuroimmunology of postpartum depression. *Journal of Women's Health (Larchmt), 17*(9), 1529–1534.

Costanzo, E. S., Lutgendorf, S. K., Sood, A. K., Anderson, B., Sorosky, J., & Lubaroff, D. M. (2005). Psychosocial factors and interleukin-6 among women with advanced ovarian cancer. *Cancer, 104*(2), 305–313.

Coussens, L. M., & Werb, Z. (2002). Inflammation and cancer. *Nature, 420*(6917), 860–867.

Curcio, C., Di Carlo, E., Clynes, R., Smyth, M. J., Boggio, K., Quaglino, E., et al. (2003). Nonredundant roles of antibody, cytokines, and perforin in the eradication of established Her-2/neu carcinomas. *Journal of Clinical Investigation, 111*(8), 1161–1170.

Czura, C. J., & Tracey, K. J. (2005). Autonomic neural regulation of immunity. *Journal of Internal Medicine, 257*(2), 156–166.

Dantzer, R. (2009). Cytokine, sickness behavior, and depression. *Immunology and Allergy Clinics North America, 29*(2), 247–264.

Dantzer, R., & Kelley, K. W. (2007). Twenty years of research on cytokine-induced sickness behavior. *Brain, Behavior, and Immunity, 21*(2), 153–160.

Dantzer, R., O'Connor, J. C., Freund, G. G., Johnson, R. W., & Kelley, K. W. (2008). From inflammation to sickness and depression: When the immune system subjugates the brain. *Nature Reviews Neuroscience, 9*(1), 46–56.

Davis, M. C., Zautra, A. J., Younger, J., Motivala, S. J., Attrep, J., & Irwin, M. R. (2008). Chronic stress and regulation of cellular markers of inflammation in rheumatoid arthritis: Implications for fatigue. *Brain, Behavior, and Immunity, 22*(1), 24–32.

Daynes, R. A., Araneo, B. A., Dowell, T. A., Huang, K., & Dudley, D. (1990). Regulation of murine lymphokine production in vivo. III. The lymphoid tissue microenvironment exerts regulatory influences over T helper cell function. *Journal of Experimental Medicine, 171*(4), 979–996.

Dekkers, J. C., Geenen, R., Godaert, G. L., Glaudemans, K. A., Lafeber, F. P., van Doornen, L. J., et al. (2001). Experimentally challenged reactivity of the hypothalamic pituitary adrenal axis in patients with recently diagnosed rheumatoid arthritis. *Journal of Rheumatology, 28*(7), 1496–1504.

Dhabhar, F. S., Satoskar, A. R., Bluethmann, H., David, J. R., & McEwen, B. S. (2000). Stress-induced enhancement of skin immune function: A role for gamma interferon. *Proceedings of the National Academy of Sciences USA, 97*(6), 2846–2851.

Dhabhar, F. S., Saul, A. N., Daugherty, C., Holmes, T. H., Bouley, D. M., & Oberyszyn, T. M. (2010). Short-term stress enhances cellular immunity and increases early resistance to squamous cell carcinoma. *Brain, Behavior, and Immunity, 24*(1), 127–137.

Dickens, C., McGowan, L., Clark-Carter, D., & Creed, F. (2002). Depression in rheumatoid arthritis: a systematic review of the literature with meta-analysis. *Psychosomatic Medicine, 64*(1), 52–60.

Diefenbach, A., & Raulet, D. H. (2002). The innate immune response to tumors and its role in the induction of T-cell immunity. *Immunological Reviews, 188*, 9–21.

Dunn, G. P., Bruce, A. T., Ikeda, H., Old, L. J., & Schreiber, R. D. (2002). Cancer immunoediting: From immunosurveillance to tumor escape. *Nature Immunology, 3*(11), 991–998.

Ebrecht, M., Hextall, J., Kirtley, L. G., Taylor, A., Dyson, M., & Weinman, J. (2004). Perceived stress and cortisol levels predict speed of wound healing in healthy male adults. *Psychoneuroendocrinology, 29*(6), 798–809.

Ehrstrom, S. M., Kornfeld, D., Thuresson, J., & Rylander, E. (2005). Signs of chronic stress in women with recurrent candida vulvovaginitis. *American Journal of Obstetrics & Gynecology, 193*(4), 1376–1381.

Elenkov, I. J., & Chrousos, G. P. (1999). Stress hormones, Th1/Th2 patterns, pro/anti-inflammatory cytokines and susceptibility to disease. *Trends in Endocrinology and Metabolism, 10*(9), 359–368.

Elenkov, I. J., & Chrousos, G. P. (2006). Stress system—organization, physiology and immunoregulation. *Neuroimmunomodulation, 13*(5-6), 257–267.

Elenkov, I. J., Iezzoni, D. G., Daly, A., Harris, A. G., & Chrousos, G. P. (2005). Cytokine dysregulation, inflammation and well-being. *Neuroimmunomodulation, 12*(5), 255–269.

Eng, P. M., Rimm, E. B., Fitzmaurice, G., & Kawachi, I. (2002). Social ties and change in social ties in relation to subsequent total and cause-specific mortality and coronary heart disease incidence in men. *American Journal of Epidemiology, 155*(8), 700–709.

Esterling, B. A., Kiecolt-Glaser, J. K., & Glaser, R. (1996). Psychosocial modulation of cytokine-induced natural killer cell activity in older adults. *Psychosomatic Medicine, 58*(3), 264–272.

Feigenbaum, S. L., Masi, A. T., & Kaplan, S. B. (1979). Prognosis in rheumatoid arthritis. A longitudinal study of newly diagnosed younger adult patients. *American Journal of Medicine, 66*(3), 377–384.

Fidler, I. J. (2003). The pathogenesis of cancer metastasis: the "seed and soil" hypothesis revisited. *Nature Reviews Cancer, 3*(6), 453–458.

Finkelhor, D., & Dziuba-Leatherman, J. (1994). Children as victims of violence: a national survey. *Pediatrics, 94*(4, Pt 1), 413–420.

Glaser, R., & Kiecolt-Glaser, J. K. (1997). Chronic stress modulates the virus-specific immune response to latent herpes simplex virus type 1. *Annals of Behavioral Medicine, 19*(2), 78–82.

Glaser, R., & Kiecolt-Glaser, J. K. (2005). Stress-induced immune dysfunction: implications for health. *Nature Reviews Immunology, 5*(3), 243–251.

Glaser, R., Kiecolt-Glaser, J. K., Marucha, P. T., MacCallum, R. C., Laskowski, B. F., & Malarkey, W. B. (1999). Stress-related changes in proinflammatory cytokine production in wounds. *Archives of General Psychiatry, 56*(5), 450–456.

Glaser, R., Sheridan, J., Malarkey, W. B., MacCallum, R. C., & Kiecolt-Glaser, J. K. (2000). Chronic stress modulates the immune response to a pneumococcal pneumonia vaccine. *Psychosomatic Medicine, 62*(6), 804–807.

Godbout, J. P., & Glaser, R. (2006). Stress-induced immune dysregulation: Implications for wound healing, infectious disease and cancer. *Journal of Neuroimmune Pharmacology, 1*(4), 421–427.

Gorby, H. E., & Sternberg, E. M. (2007). The neuroendocrine system and rheumatoid arthritis: focus on the hypothalamic pituitary-adrenal axis. In R. Ader (Ed.), *Psychoneuroendocrinology* (4th ed., pp. 193–205). Amsterdam, Netherlands: Elsevier.

Gouin, J. P., Hantsoo, L., & Kiecolt-Glaser, J. K. (2008). Immune dysregulation and chronic stress among older adults: A review. *Neuroimmunomodulation, 15*(4–6), 251–259.

Groer, M., Davis, M., Casey, K., Short, B., Smith, K., & Groer, S. (2005). Neuroendocrine and immune relationships in postpartum fatigue. *MCN: The American Journal of Maternal/Child Nursing, 30*(2), 133–138.

Groer, M., Davis, M., & Steele, K. (2004). Associations between human milk SIgA and maternal immune, infectious, endocrine, and stress variables. *Journal of Human Lactation, 20*(2), 153–158; quiz 159–163.

Groer, M., El-Badri, N., Djeu, J., Harrington, M., & Van Eepoel, J. (2010). Suppression of natural killer cell cytotoxicity in postpartum women. *American Journal of Reproductive Immunology, 63*(3), 209–213.

Groer, M. W., & Davis, M. W. (2006). Cytokines, infections, stress, and dysphoric moods in breastfeeders and formula feeders. *Journal of Obstetric, Gynecologic, & Neonatal Nursing, 35*(5), 599–607.

Groer, M. W., Davis, M. W., Smith, K., Casey, K., Kramer, V., & Bukovsky, E. (2005). Immunity, inflammation and infection in post-partum breast and formula feeders. *American Journal of Reproductive Immunology, 54*(4), 222–231.

Hirano, D., Nagashima, M., Ogawa, R., & Yoshino, S. (2001). Serum levels of interleukin 6 and stress related substances indicate mental stress condition in patients with rheumatoid arthritis. *Journal of Rheumatology, 28*(3), 490–495.

Irwin, M. R. (2008). Human psychoneuroimmunology: 20 years of discovery. *Brain, Behavior, and Immunity, 22*(2), 129–139.

Kang, D. H., Coe, C. L., Karaszewski, J., & McCarthy, D. O. (1998). Relationship of social support to stress responses and immune function in healthy and asthmatic adolescents. *Research in Nursing & Health, 21*(2), 117–128.

Kang, D. H., Coe, C. L., & McCarthy, D. O. (1996). Academic examinations significantly impact immune responses, but not lung function, in healthy and well-managed asthmatic adolescents. *Brain, Behavior, and Immunity, 10*(2), 164–181.

Kang, D. H., Coe, C. L., McCarthy, D. O., Jarjour, N. N., Kelly, E. A., Rodriguez, R. R., et al. (1997). Cytokine profiles of stimulated blood lymphocytes in asthmatic and healthy adolescents across the school year. *Journal of Interferon & Cytokine Research, 17*(8), 481–487.

Kang, D. H., Kim, C. J., & Suh, Y. (2004). Sex differences in immune responses and immune reactivity to stress in adolescents. *Biological Research for Nursing, 5*(4), 243–254.

Kang, D. H., & Weaver, M. T. (2009). Airway cytokine responses to acute and repeated stress in a murine model of allergic asthma. *Biological Psychology, 84*, 66–73.

Kang, D. H., Weaver, M. T., Park, N. J., Smith, B., McArdle, T., & Carpenter, J. (2009). Significant impairment in immune recovery after cancer treatment. *Nursing Research, 58*(2), 105–114.

Kemeny, M. E., & Schedlowski, M. (2007). Understanding the interaction between psychosocial stress and immune-related diseases: A stepwise progression. *Brain, Behavior, and Immunity, 21*(8), 1009–1018.

Khakoo, S. I., Thio, C. L., Martin, M. P., Brooks, C. R., Gao, X., Astemborski, J., et al. (2004). HLA and NK cell inhibitory receptor genes in resolving hepatitis C virus infection. *Science, 305*(5685), 872–874.

Kiecolt-Glaser, J. K., Glaser, R., Shuttleworth, E. C., Dyer, C. S., Ogrocki, P., & Speicher, C. E. (1987). Chronic stress and immunity in family caregivers of Alzheimer's disease victims. *Psychosomatic Medicine, 49*(5), 523–535.

Kiecolt-Glaser, J. K., Loving, T. J., Stowell, J. R., Malarkey, W. B., Lemeshow, S., Dickinson, S. L., et al. (2005). Hostile marital interactions, proinflammatory cytokine production, and wound healing. *Archives of General Psychiatry, 62*(12), 1377–1384.

Kiecolt-Glaser, J. K., Marucha, P. T., Malarkey, W. B., Mercado, A. M., & Glaser, R. (1995). Slowing of wound healing by psychological stress. *Lancet, 346*(8984), 1194–1196.

Kim, R., Emi, M., Tanabe, K., & Arihiro, K. (2006). Tumor-driven evolution of immunosuppressive networks during malignant progression. *Cancer Research, 66*(11), 5527–5536.

Kissane, D. W., Grabsch, B., Clarke, D. M., Smith, G. C., Love, A. W., Bloch, S., et al. (2007). Supportive-expressive group therapy for women with metastatic breast cancer: Survival and psychosocial outcome from a randomized controlled trial. *Psycho-Oncology, 16*(4), 277–286.

Kop, W. J., & Cohen, N. (2007). Psychoneuro immunological pathways involved in acute coronary syndromes. In R. Ader (Ed.), *Psychoneuroimmunology* (4th ed., Vol. 2, pp. 921–944.). Amsterdam: Elsevier.

Krukowski, K., Eddy, J., Kosik, K. L., Konley, T., Janusek, L. W., & Mathews, H. L. (2010). Glucocorticoid dysregulation of natural killer cell function through epigenetic modification. *Brain, Behavior, and Immunity, 25*(5), 830–839.

Lange, H. W., & Herrmann-Lingen, C. (2007). Depressive symptoms predict recurrence of atrial fibrillation after cardioversion. *Journal of Psychosomatic Research, 63*(5), 509–513.

Libby, P., Ridker, P. M., & Maseri, A. (2002). Inflammation and atherosclerosis. *Circulation, 105*(9), 1135–1143.

Liu, L. Y., Coe, C. L., Swenson, C. A., Kelly, E. A., Kita, H., & Busse, W. W. (2002). School examinations enhance airway inflammation to antigen challenge. *American Journal of Respiratory and Critical Care Medicine, 165*(8), 1062–1067.

Loucks, E. B., Sullivan, L. M., D'Agostino, R. B., Sr., Larson, M. G., Berkman, L. F., & Benjamin, E. J. (2006). Social networks and inflammatory markers in the Framingham Heart Study. *Journal of Biosocial Science, 38*(6), 835–842.

Lutgendorf, S., Costanzo, E., & Siegel, S. (2007). Psychosocial influences on oncology: An expanded model of biobehavioral mechanisms. In R. Ader (Ed.), *Psychoneuroimmunology* (4th ed., Vol. 2, pp. 869–895). Burlington, MA: Elsevier Academic Press.

Lutgendorf, S. K., Cole, S., Costanzo, E., Bradley, S., Coffin, J., Jabbari, S., et al. (2003). Stress-related mediators stimulate vascular endothelial growth factor secretion by two ovarian cancer cell lines. *Clinical Cancer Research, 9*(12), 4514–4521.

Lutgendorf, S. K., DeGeest, K., Sung, C. Y., Arevalo, J. M., Penedo, F., Lucci, J., 3rd, et al. (2009). Depression, social support, and beta-adrenergic transcription control in human ovarian cancer. *Brain, Behavior, and Immunity, 23*(2), 176–183.

Lutgendorf, S. K., Lamkin, D. M., DeGeest, K., Anderson, B., Dao, M., McGinn, S., et al. (2008). Depressed and anxious mood and T-cell cytokine producing populations in ovarian cancer patients. *Brain, Behavior, and Immunity, 22*(6), 890–900.

Lutgendorf, S. K., Sood, A. K., Anderson, B., McGinn, S., Maiseri, H., Dao, M., et al. (2005). Social support, psychological distress, and natural killer cell activity in ovarian cancer. *Journal of Clinical Oncology, 23*(28), 7105–7113.

Lutgendorf, S. K., Sood, A. K., & Antoni, M. H. (2010). Host factors and cancer progression: Biobehavioral signaling pathways and interventions. *Journal of Clinical Oncology, 28*(26), 4094–4099.

Maes, M., Lin, A. H., Delmeire, L., Van Gastel, A., Kenis, G., De Jongh, R., et al. (1999). Elevated serum interleukin-6 (IL-6) and IL-6 receptor concentrations in posttraumatic stress disorder following accidental man-made traumatic events. *Biological Psychiatry, 45*(7), 833–839.

Maini, R. N., Breedveld, F. C., Kalden, J. R., Smolen, J. S., Furst, D., Weisman, M. H., et al. (2004). Sustained improvement over two years in physical function, structural damage, and signs and symptoms among patients with rheumatoid arthritis treated with infliximab and methotrexate. *Arthritis & Rheumatism, 50*(4), 1051–1065.

Marshall, G. D., Jr., Agarwal, S. K., Lloyd, C., Cohen, L., Henninger, E. M., & Morris, G. J. (1998). Cytokine dysregulation associated with exam stress in healthy medical students. *Brain, Behavior, and Immunity, 12*(4), 297–307.

Marshall, G. D., & Roy, S. R. (2007). Stress and allergic disease. In R. Ader (Ed.), *Psychoneuroimmunology* (4th ed., Vol. 2, pp. 799–824). Boston, MA: Elsevier.

Marsland, A. L., Gianaros, P. J., Abramowitch, S. M., Manuck, S. B., & Hariri, A. R. (2008). Interleukin-6 covaries inversely with hippocampal grey matter volume in middle-aged adults. *Biological Psychiatry, 64*(6), 484–490.

Marsland, A. L., Gianaros, P. J., Prather, A. A., Jennings, J. R., Neumann, S. A., & Manuck, S. B. (2007). Stimulated production of proinflammatory cytokines covaries inversely with heart rate variability. *Psychosomatic Medicine, 69*(8), 709–716.

Marsland, A. L., Petersen, K. L., Sathanoori, R., Muldoon, M. F., Neumann, S. A., Ryan, C., et al. (2006). Interleukin-6 covaries inversely with cognitive performance among middle-aged community volunteers. *Psychosomatic Medicine, 68*(6), 895–903.

Marucha, P. T., & Engeland, C. G. (2007). Stress, neuroendocrine hormones, and wound healing; Human models. In R. Ader (Ed.), *Psychoneuroimmunology* (4th ed., pp. 825–835). Amsterdam: Elsevier.

Marucha, P. T., Kiecolt-Glaser, J. K., & Favagehi, M. (1998). Mucosal wound healing is impaired by examination stress. *Psychosomatic Medicine, 60*(3), 362–365.

Mathews, H. L., Konley, T., Kosik, K. L., Krukowski, K., Eddy, J., Albuquerque, K., & Janusek, L. W. (2011). Epigenetic patterns associated with the immune dysregulation that accompanies psychosocial distress. *Brain, Behavior, and Immunity, 25*(5), 830–839.

Mathews, H. L., & Janusek, L. W. (2011). Epigenetics and psychoneuroimmunology: Mechanisms and models. *Brain, Behavior, and Immunity, 25*(1), 25–39.

McCain, N. L., & Cella, D. F. (1995). Correlates of stress in HIV disease. *Western Journal of Nursing Research, 17*(2), 141–155.

McCain, N. L., & Gramling, L. F. (1992). Living with dying: Coping with HIV disease. *Issues in Mental Health Nursing, 13*(3), 271–284.

McCain, N. L., Gray, D. P., Elswick, R. K., Robins, J. W., Tuck, I., Walter, J. M., et al. (2008). A randomized clinical trial of alternative stress management interventions in persons with HIV infection. *Journal of Consulting and Clinical Psychology, 76*(3), 431–441.

McCain, N. L., & Smith, J. C. (1994). Stress and coping in the context of psychoneuroimmunology: A holistic framework for nursing practice and research. *Archives of Psychiatric Nursing, 8*(4), 221–227.

McGregor, B. A., & Antoni, M. H. (2009). Psychological intervention and health outcomes among women treated for breast cancer: A review of stress pathways and biological mediators. *Brain, Behavior, and Immunity, 23*(2), 159–166.

McGregor, B. A., Antoni, M. H., Boyers, A., Alferi, S. M., Blomberg, B. B., & Carver, C. S. (2004). Cognitive-behavioral stress management increases benefit finding and immune function among women with early-stage breast cancer. *Journal of Psychosomatic Research, 56*(1), 1–8.

McLoyd, V. C. (1990). The impact of economic hardship on black families and children: psychological distress, parenting, and socioemotional development. *Child Development, 61*(2), 311–346.

Mendling, W., & Seebacher, C. (2003). Guideline vulvovaginal candidosis: Guideline of the German Dermatological Society, the German Speaking Mycological Society and the Working Group for Infections and Infectimmunology of the German Society for Gynecology and Obstetrics. *Mycoses, 46*(9–10), 365–369.

Metz, C. N., & Tracey, K. J. (2005). It takes nerve to dampen inflammation. *Nature Immunology, 6*(8), 756–757.

Meyer, H., Goettlicher, S., & Mendling, W. (2006). Stress as a cause of chronic recurrent vulvovaginal candidosis and the effectiveness of the conventional antimycotic therapy. *Mycoses, 49*(3), 202–209.

Mosmann, T. R., & Sad, S. (1996). The expanding universe of T-cell subsets: Th1, Th2 and more. *Immunology Today, 17*(3), 138–146.

Nagabhushan, M., Mathews, H. L., & Witek-Janusek, L. (2001). Aberrant nuclear expression of ap-1 and nfkb in lymphocytes of women stressed by the experience of breast biopsy. *Brain, Behavior, and Immunity, 15*(1), 78–84.

Orange, J. S. (2002). Human natural killer cell deficiencies and susceptibility to infection. *Microbes and Infection, 4*(15), 1545–1558.

Page, G. G., & Ben-Eliyahu, S. (1997). The immune-suppressive nature of pain. *Seminars in Oncology Nursing, 13*(1), 10–15.

Page, G. G., Ben-Eliyahu, S., & Liebeskind, J. C. (1994). The role of LGL/NK cells in surgery-induced promotion of metastasis and its attenuation by morphine. *Brain, Behavior, and Immunity, 8*(3), 241–250.

Page, G. G., Blakely, W. P., & Kim, M. (2005). The impact of early repeated pain experiences on stress responsiveness and emotionality at maturity in rats. *Brain, Behavior, and Immunity, 19*(1), 78–87.

Panagiotakos, D. B., Pitsavos, C., Manios, Y., Polychronopoulos, E., Chrysohoou, C. A., & Stefanadis, C. (2005). Socio-economic status in relation to risk factors associated with cardiovascular disease, in healthy individuals from the ATTICA study. *European Journal of Cardiovascular Prevention and Rehabilitation, 12*(1), 68–74.

Pariante, C. M., Carpiniello, B., Orru, M. G., Sitzia, R., Piras, A., Farci, A. M., et al. (1997). Chronic caregiving stress alters peripheral blood immune parameters: The role of age and severity of stress. *Psychotherapy and Psychosomatics, 66*(4), 199–207.

Paul-Eugene, N., Dugas, B., Gordon, J., Kolb, J. P., Cairns, J. A., Paubert-Braquet, M., et al. (1993). Beta 2-adrenoceptor stimulation augments the IL-4-induced CD23 expression and release and the expression of differentiation markers (CD14, CD18) by the human monocytic cell line, U 937. *Clinical & Experimental Allergy, 23*(4), 317–325.

Pedersen, A., Zachariae, R., & Bovbjerg, D. H. (2010). Influence of psychological stress on upper respiratory infection—a meta-analysis of prospective studies. *Psychosomatic Medicine, 72*(8), 823–832.

Pedersen, A. F., Zachariae, R., & Bovbjerg, D. H. (2009). Psychological stress and antibody response to influenza vaccination: A meta-analysis. *Brain, Behavior, and Immunity, 23*(4), 427–433.

Prescott, E., Holst, C., Gronbaek, M., Schnohr, P., Jensen, G., & Barefoot, J. (2003). Vital exhaustion as a risk factor for ischaemic heart disease and all-cause mortality in a community sample. A prospective study of 4084 men and 5479 women in the Copenhagen City Heart Study. *International Journal of Epidemiology, 32*(6), 990–997.

Reiche, E. M., Nunes, S. O., & Morimoto, H. K. (2004). Stress, depression, the immune system, and cancer. *Lancet Oncology, 5*(10), 617–625.

Robinson, F. P., Mathews, H. L., & Witek-Janusek, L. (2002). Issues in the design and implementation of psychoneuroimmunology research. *Biological Research for Nursing, 3*(4), 165–175.

Robinson, F. P., Mathews, H. L., & Witek-Janusek, L. (2003). Psycho-endocrine-immune response to mindfulness-based stress reduction in individuals infected with the human immunodeficiency virus: A quasiexperimental study. *Journal of Alternative and Complementary Medicine, 9*(5), 683–694.

Rook, G. A., Hernandez-Pando, R., & Lightman, S. L. (1994). Hormones, peripherally activated prohormones and regulation of the Th1/Th2 balance. *Immunology Today, 15*(7), 301–303.

Rosengren, A., Wilhelmsen, L., & Orth-Gomer, K. (2004). Coronary disease in relation to social support and social class in Swedish men. A 15 year follow-up in the study of men born in 1933. *European Heart Journal, 25*(1), 56–63.

Ross, R. (1999). Atherosclerosis—an inflammatory disease. *New England Journal of Medicine, 340*(2), 115–126.

Sanchez-Barcelo, E. J., Cos, S., Fernandez, R., & Mediavilla, M. D. (2003). Melatonin and mammary cancer: A short review. *Endocrine-Related Cancer, 10*(2), 153–159.

Sandberg, S., Jarvenpaa, S., Penttinen, A., Paton, J. Y., & McCann, D. C. (2004). Asthma exacerbations in children immediately following stressful life events: A Cox's hierarchical regression. *Thorax, 59*(12), 1046-1051.

Schoneveld, O., & Cidlowski, J. A. (2007). Glucocorticoids and immunity: mechanisms of regulation. In R. Ader (Ed.), *Psychoneuroimmunology* (4th ed., Vol. 1, pp. 45–61). Burlington, MA: Elsevier Academic Press.

Sephton, S. E., Sapolsky, R. M., Kraemer, H. C., & Spiegel, D. (2000). Diurnal cortisol rhythm as a predictor of breast cancer survival. *Journal of the National Cancer Institute, 92*(12), 994–1000.

Silverman, M. N., & Sternberg, E. M. (2008). Neuroendocrine-immune interactions in rheumatoid arthritis: Mechanisms of glucocorticoid resistance. *Neuroimmunomodulation, 15*(1), 19–28.

Smyth, M. J., Cretney, E., Kershaw, M. H., & Hayakawa, Y. (2004). Cytokines in cancer immunity and immunotherapy. *Immunological Reviews, 202*, 275–293.

Sood, A. K., Bhatty, R., Kamat, A. A., Landen, C. N., Han, L., Thaker, P. H., et al. (2006). Stress hormone-mediated invasion of ovarian cancer cells. *Clinical Cancer Research, 12*(2), 369–375.

Sorenson, M. R., Witek-Janusek, L., & Mathews, H. L. (2006). Perceived stress, illness uncertainty, and disease symptomatology in multiple sclerosis. *Spinal Cord Injury Journal, 23*, 1–10.

Spiegel, D., Butler, L. D., Giese-Davis, J., Koopman, C., Miller, E., DiMiceli, S., et al. (2007). Effects of supportive-expressive group therapy on survival of patients with metastatic breast cancer: A randomized prospective trial. *Cancer, 110*(5), 1130–1138.

Starkweather, A., Witek-Janusek, L., & Mathews, H. L. (2005a). Applying the psychoneuroimmunology framework to nursing research. *Journal of Neuroscience Nursing, 37*(1), 56–62.

Starkweather, A., Witek-Janusek, L., & Mathews, H. L. (2005b). Neural-immune interactions: Implications for pain management in patients with low-back pain and sciatica. *Biological Research for Nursing, 6*(3), 196–206.

Starkweather, A. R., Witek-Janusek, L., Nockels, R. P., Peterson, J., & Mathews, H. L. (2006). Immune function, pain, and psychological stress in patients undergoing spinal surgery. *Spine (Phila Pa 1976), 31*(18), E641–647.

Steptoe, A., & Brydon, L. (2007). Psychosocial factors and coronary heart disease: The role of psychoneuroimmunological processes. In R. Ader (Ed.), *Psychoneuroimmunology* (4th ed., Vol. 2, pp. 945–974). Amsterdam, Netherlands: Elsevier.

Steptoe, A., Strike, P. C., Perkins-Porras, L., McEwan, J. R., & Whitehead, D. L. (2006). Acute depressed mood as a trigger of acute coronary syndromes. *Biological Psychiatry, 60*(8), 837–842.

Sternberg, E. M. (2006). Neural regulation of innate immunity: A coordinated nonspecific host response to pathogens. *Nature Reviews Immunology, 6*(4), 318–328.

Straub, R. H., Dhabhar, F. S., Bijlsma, J. W., & Cutolo, M. (2005). How psychological stress via hormones and nerve fibers may exacerbate rheumatoid arthritis. *Arthritis and Rheumatism, 52*(1), 16–26.

Street, S. E., Cretney, E., & Smyth, M. J. (2001). Perforin and interferon-gamma activities independently control tumor initiation, growth, and metastasis. *Blood, 97*(1), 192–197.

Strike, P. C., & Steptoe, A. (2005). Behavioral and emotional triggers of acute coronary syndromes: A systematic review and critique. *Psychosomatic Medicine, 67*(2), 179–186.

Swanson, B., Zeller, J. M., & Spear, G. T. (1998). Cortisol upregulates HIV p24 antigen production in cultured human monocyte-derived macrophages. *Journal of the Association of Nurses in AIDS Care, 9*(4), 78–83.

Targan, S., & Dorey, F. (1980). Dual mechanism of interferon augmentation of natural killer cytotoxicity (NKCC). *Annals of the New York Academy of Sciences, 350*, 121–129.

Thaker, P. H., Han, L. Y., Kamat, A. A., Arevalo, J. M., Takahashi, R., Lu, C., et al. (2006). Chronic stress promotes tumor growth and angiogenesis in a mouse model of ovarian carcinoma. *Nature Medicine, 12*(8), 939–944.

Thaker, P. H., & Sood, A. K. (2008). Neuroendocrine influences on cancer biology. *Seminars in Cancer Biology, 18*(3), 164–170.

Thayer, J. F., & Sternberg, E. M. (2010). Neural aspects of immunomodulation: Focus on the vagus nerve. *Brain, Behavior, and Immunity, 24*(8), 1223–1228.

Thornton, L. M., Andersen, B. L., Crespin, T. R., & Carson, W. E. (2007). Individual trajectories in stress covary with immunity during recovery from cancer diagnosis and treatments. *Brain, Behavior, and Immunity, 21*(2), 185–194.

Tracey, K. J. (2002). The inflammatory reflex. *Nature, 420*(6917), 853–859.

van den Broek, M. E., Kagi, D., Ossendorp, F., Toes, R., Vamvakas, S., Lutz, W. K., et al. (1996). Decreased tumor surveillance in perforin-deficient mice. *Journal of Experimental Medicine, 184*(5), 1781–1790.

Van der Auwera, I., Van Laere, S. J., Van den Eynden, G. G., Benoy, I., van Dam, P., Colpaert, C. G., et al. (2004). Increased angiogenesis and lymphangiogenesis in inflammatory versus noninflammatory breast cancer by real-time reverse transcriptase-PCR gene expression quantification. *Clinical Cancer Research, 10*(23), 7965–7971.

Vedhara, K., Cox, N. K., Wilcock, G. K., Perks, P., Hunt, M., Anderson, S., et al. (1999). Chronic stress in elderly carers of dementia patients and antibody response to influenza vaccination. *Lancet, 353*(9153), 627–631.

Viswanathan, K., Daugherty, C., & Dhabhar, F. S. (2005). Stress as an endogenous adjuvant: Augmentation of the immunization phase of cell-mediated immunity. *International Immunology, 17*(8), 1059–1069.

Walburn, J., Vedhara, K., Hankins, M., Rixon, L., & Weinman, J. (2009). Psychological stress and wound healing in humans: A systematic review and meta-analysis. *Journal of Psychosomatic Research, 67*(3), 253–271.

Wamboldt, M. Z., Laudenslager, M., Wamboldt, F. S., Kelsay, K., & Hewitt, J. (2003). Adolescents with atopic disorders have an attenuated cortisol response to laboratory stress. *Journal of Allergy and Clinical Immunology, 111*(3), 509–514.

Webster, J. I., Tonelli, L., & Sternberg, E. M. (2002). Neuroendocrine regulation of immunity. *Annual Review of Immunology, 20*, 125–163.

Weinman, J., Ebrecht, M., Scott, S., Walburn, J., & Dyson, M. (2008). Enhanced wound healing after emotional disclosure intervention. *British Journal of Health Psychology, 13*(Pt 1), 95–102.

Williams, J. B., Pang, D., Delgado, B., Kocherginsky, M., Tretiakova, M., Krausz, T., et al. (2009). A model of gene-environment interaction reveals altered mammary gland gene expression and increased tumor growth following social isolation. *Cancer Prevention Research (Phila), 2*(10), 850–861.

Witek-Janusek, L., Albuquerque, K., Chroniak, K. R., Chroniak, C., Durazo-Arvizu, R., & Mathews, H. L. (2008). Effect of mindfulness based stress reduction on immune function, quality of life and coping in women newly diagnosed with early stage breast cancer. *Brain, Behavior, and Immunity, 22*(6), 969–981.

Witek-Janusek, L., Gabram, S., & Mathews, H. L. (2007). Psychologic stress, reduced NK cell activity, and cytokine dysregulation in women experiencing diagnostic breast biopsy. *Psychoneuroendocrinology, 32*(1), 22–35.

Witek-Janusek, L., & Mathews, H. L. (1999). Differential effects of glucocorticoids on colony stimulating factors produced by neonatal mononuclear cells. *Pediatric Research, 45*(2), 224–229.

Wrona, D. (2006). Neural-immune interactions: an integrative view of the bidirectional relationship between the brain and immune systems. *Journal of Neuroimmunology, 172*(1–2), 38–58.

Wulsin, L. R., & Singal, B. M. (2003). Do depressive symptoms increase the risk for the onset of coronary disease? A systematic quantitative review. *Psychosomatic Medicine, 65*(2), 201–210.

Yermal, S. J., Witek-Janusek, L., Peterson, J., & Mathews, H. L. (2009). Perioperative pain, psychological distress, and immune function in men undergoing prostatectomy for cancer of the prostate. *Biological Research for Nursing, 11*(4), 351–362.

Zautra, A. J., Hoffman, J., Potter, P., Matt, K. S., Yocum, D., & Castro, L. (1997). Examination of changes in interpersonal stress as a factor in disease exacerbations among women with rheumatoid arthritis. *Annals of Behavioral Medicine, 19*(3), 279–286.

Zautra, A. J., Yocum, D. C., Villanueva, I., Smith, B., Davis, M. C., Attrep, J., et al. (2004). Immune activation and depression in women with rheumatoid arthritis. *Journal of Rheumatology, 31*(3), 457–463.

Zeller, J. M., McCain, N. L., & Swanson, B. (1996). Psychoneuroimmunology: An emerging framework for nursing research. *Journal of Advanced Nursing, 23*(4), 657–664.

4

Epigenetics and Stress

A Life Course Perspective

Linda Witek Janusek, Dina Tell Cooper, and
Herbert L. Mathews

For nearly a century, stress has captured the attention of diverse scientific disciplines, ranging from the biological to the behavioral sciences. Currently, this interest has intensified as scientists gain new insight into the molecular processes that link a stressful environment with gene expression. In particular, the field of epigenetics is transforming the conceptualization of how environment–gene interactions influence our vulnerability or resistance to stressful life events and health (Feinberg, 2008).

Epigenetics is defined as the study of functional alterations in gene expression that do not result from alterations in the basic DNA (deoxyribonucleic acid) sequence but arise during development and from the influence of the environment. Advances in behavioral epigenetics demonstrate that stressful environments can affect gene expression by altering the epigenetic pattern of DNA methylation and/or chromatin structure (Mathews & Janusek, 2011). This work is largely based on investigations of early-life adversity that produces epigenetic modifications within relevant brain regions that impact adult behavior and response to stressors (T. Y. Zhang & Meaney, 2010). Yet evolving evidence demonstrates

that adults also respond epigenetically to environmental cues. Moreover, epigenetic modifications have been demonstrated to be reversible (Feinberg, 2008; Zhang & Meaney, 2010).

This insight places a new emphasis on the role of the environment in health and the potential for novel approaches to diminish the impact of adverse environments. Although the field of epigenetics is evolving rapidly, it is still in its infancy. At this time, much of the work evaluating epigenetic–environment interactions has been accomplished in animal models, predominately focusing on adverse early-life experiences. Yet there is tremendous potential to translate these findings to human conditions that are shaped by epigenetic influences. Such translational science, particularly in behavioral epigenetics, is consistent with the mission of nursing research and will likely influence the direction of nursing science and practice in years to come. With this in mind, this chapter provides an overview of epigenetic processes, presents examples of relevant research that exemplify the importance of epigenetics to the field of stress, and finally provides a perspective on future applications of this emerging field to the understanding of the role of stress in health outcomes.

AUTHORS' NOTE: The preparation of this chapter was supported, in part, by the National Cancer Institute grants R21CA117261, R01 CA134736, and R01CA125455.

EPIGENETICS AND THE EPIGENOME

Epigenetics refers to processes that regulate a person's expression of genes or sets of genes, completely independent of their DNA sequence. What epigenetic information does is determine how, where, and when DNA will be used. Whereas DNA encodes for genes by use of a sequence of nucleotide bases (adenine, thymine, guanine and cytosine [ATGC, respectively], epigenetic information (i.e., the *epigenetic code*) is characterized by the variation in chemical tags or epigenetic modifications that govern gene expression. In effect, epigenetic information regulates gene expression and determines whether genes are expressed or silenced (http://nihroadmap.nih.gov/epigenomics/index.asp).

On a larger scale, the term *epigenomics* refers to epigenetic patterns on a genome-wide scale. While all nucleated human cells contain the same DNA sequence or genome, cells express different genes based on cell type, that is, a cardiac cell will express a unique set of genes relative to nerve or other cells. DNA expression is regulated by the epigenome, which determines if genes are silenced or expressed. The epigenome is complex and dependent upon cell type, developmental stage, sex, age, and, most likely, other factors not yet determined. This complexity presents a challenge but characterization of the epigenome is underway as part of The Human Epigenome Project (HEP) (Human Epigenome Consortium, n.d.). HEP is an international consortium of academic centers and private enterprises established in 1999 to identify, catalogue, and interpret DNA methylation patterns across the genome of all major tissues. Just as the characterization of the human genome has led to gene expression arrays and analysis of individual genes, it is anticipated that HEP will yield a new era of epigenomic profiling with opportunity to transform health in the post-genomic era (Feinberg, 2010).

To appreciate epigenetic processes, it is important to understand the organization of genetic material. Within the nucleus of each cell there are two meters of DNA that contain all of the genes of an individual packaged into chromatin, which is further condensed into chromosomes. Chromatin refers to DNA and its associated proteins, which are known as histones. Each histone is a double quartet of proteins that serve as "spools" for DNA to wrap around, which is essential to efficiently package the long strands of DNA into chromosomes. Approximately 146 base pairs of DNA are coiled around the histone proteins, and a single histone spool with its associated DNA forms a nucleosome. Nucleosomes are interspersed along DNA similar to beads on a string. (See Figure 4.1.) The accessibility of DNA depends upon how tightly packaged the nucleosomal structure is and, as such, determines whether DNA is accessible for transcription or not. Thus the accessibility of DNA determines appropriate gene expression and DNA accessibility is determined by epigenetic processes.

Regulated gene expression is a consequence of small epigenetic chemical modifications. These modifications epigenetically "mark" the genome and turn genes on or off (Kouzarides, 2007). One such epigenetic mark is DNA methylation, which refers to the attachment of methyl groups to the backbone of the DNA molecule. This attachment occurs at adjacent cytosine and guanine dinucleotides, which are linked by a phosphate; hence these dinucleotides are called CpG (Razin, 1998). Such methylation typically turns genes off by reducing the accessibility of DNA. (See Figure 4.1.) Another epigenetic mark occurs by histone modification, which also affects DNA accessibility. Histones are modified by the attachment of small chemicals to amino acids at the amino terminus of histone tails. These small chemical modifications are best described for acetylation, methylation, and phosphorylation of specific amino acids, and facilitate the attachment of acetyl, methyl, or phosphate groups, respectively. (See Figure 4.2.)

The attachment of these chemicals changes the net charge of the amino acids and, as a result, determines how tightly or loosely DNA is packaged. If the packing is tight, a gene is hidden from the cell's protein-making machinery and less accessible and, hence, silenced. In contrast, if the packaging is loosened, a gene that was formerly inaccessible becomes accessible. For example, histone deacetylation of amino acids (i.e., removing an acetyl group) results in transcriptional repression and gene silencing. Conversely, histone acetylation of amino acids (i.e., adding an acetyl group) results in transcriptional activation and gene expression. (*Transcription* refers to the process of mRNA synthesis, which requires the enzyme RNA polymerase and ultimately permits the translation of the mRNA into protein.)

Figure 4.1 Overview of Epigenetic Processes

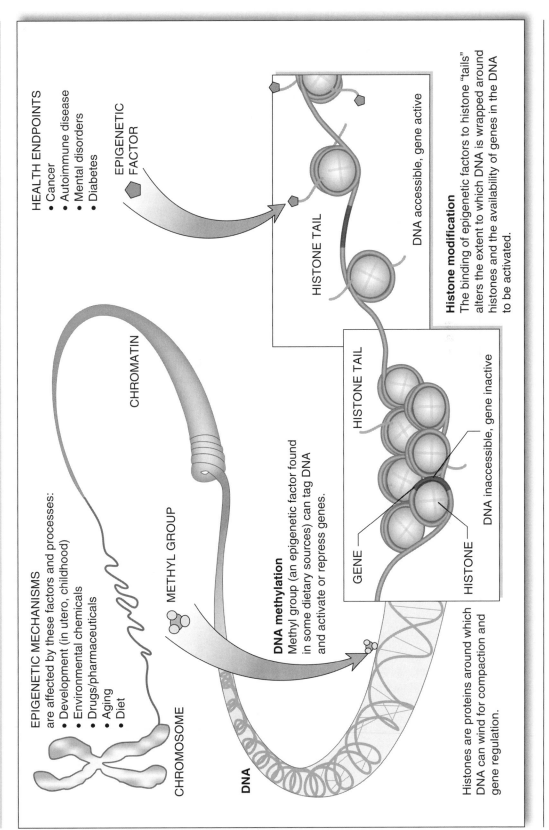

EPIGENETIC MECHANISMS
are affected by these factors and processes:
- Development (in utero, childhood)
- Environmental chemicals
- Drugs/pharmaceuticals
- Aging
- Diet

HEALTH ENDPOINTS
- Cancer
- Autoimmune disease
- Mental disorders
- Diabetes

EPIGENETIC FACTOR

CHROMOSOME

CHROMATIN

METHYL GROUP

DNA

Histones are proteins around which DNA can wind for compaction and gene regulation.

DNA methylation
Methyl group (an epigenetic factor found in some dietary sources) can tag DNA and activate or repress genes.

GENE

HISTONE TAIL

HISTONE

DNA inaccessible, gene inactive

HISTONE TAIL

DNA accessible, gene active

Histone modification
The binding of epigenetic factors to histone "tails" alters the extent to which DNA is wrapped around histones and the availability of genes in the DNA to be activated.

(Continued)

73

Figure 4.1 (Continued)

DNA methylation and histone modification is illustrated. DNA methylation is an epigenetic mark which represses gene transcription. Histones are proteins around which DNA is packaged, and histone modifications can either repress or enhance gene transcription. Histone modifications occur when epigenetic factors are bound to histone "tails" and alter the extent to which DNA is wrapped around the histones; this alters the availability of DNA for transcription. DNA methylation and histone modification can impact health and may contribute to diseases, such as cancer, autoimmune manifestations, mental disorders, or diabetes (Sedvi, 2009, #3672). Epigenetic mechanisms are affected by several factors and processes, including development *in utero* and in childhood, environmental stress and toxins, pharmaceuticals, aging, and diet (http://nihroadmap.nih.gov/epigenomics/index.asp).

Figure 4.2   Cross-Sectional Ribbon Diagram of a Nucleosome With Central Histones, Their Amino Terminal Tails, With DNA Wrapped About the Exterior Surface

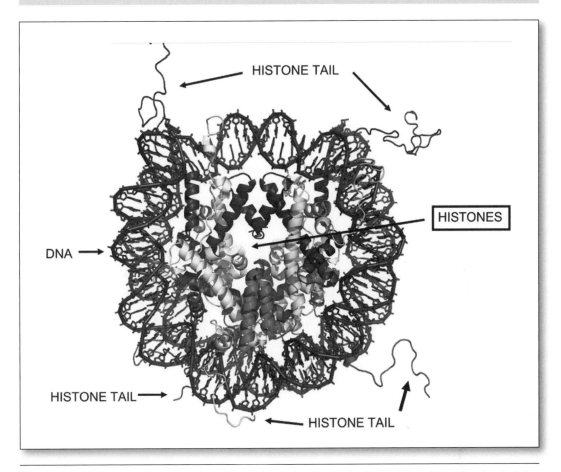

SOURCE: The figure is by Richard Wheeler (Zephyris), Sir William Dunn School of Pathology, University of Oxford, UK. Permission for its use has been obtained from Richard Wheeler, Zephyris.

The term *histone code* describes these modifications and the histone code hypothesis (Jenuwein & Allis, 2001; Strahl & Allis, 2000) proposes that epigenetic marks or histone modification patterns regulate functional expression of the genome. This hypothesis proposes a pattern of histone modifications that vary based on the cell type and the developmental stage of the organism. The pattern of histone modification comes about by a series of *writing* and *erasing* events induced by enzymes that chemically modify the amino acids of histone tails. The *writers* of histone modification refers to enzymes (e.g., acetyltransferases, methylases, and phosphorylases) that catalyze the addition of chemicals (acetyl, methyl, or phosphate groups) to the histone tails. In contrast, the *erasers* of histone modification refers to enzymes (e.g., deacetylase, demethylase, and phosphatases) that remove these chemicals from the histone tails (Jenuwein & Allis, 2001; Klose & Zhang, 2007; Strahl & Allis, 2000). For example, histone acetyltransferases are enzymes that acetylate or add acetyl groups to a given histone tail, whereas, a histone deacetylase refers to enzymes that remove acetyl groups from histone tails. The specific interpretation or the *reading* of the histone code is accomplished by effector proteins known as *readers*, which are proteins that bind chromatin. These proteins bind to specific epigenetic modifications (e.g., methylation and/or acetylation) and either silence or enhance the transcription of the histone code to produce a meaningful biological response. Depending upon the binding protein (i.e, *reader*) and the epigenetic modification, the interaction of this binding protein with the chromatin will either activate or silence gene transcription (Jenuwein & Allis, 2001; Strahl & Allis, 2000). Hence, modification of histones per se does not alter gene expression but requires the participation of binding proteins that permit the reading of the histone code. The activation or silencing can be achieved by direct physical modulation of chromatin structure or alteration of DNA and histone protein interactions within an individual chromosome or chromosomal segment (Jenuwein & Allis, 2001; Strahl & Allis, 2000). Such interactions result in genes that are either accessible for transcription or, alternatively, inaccessible for transcription. These complex interactions are the regulatory mechanisms that function to create an epigenetic landscape (i.e., the full array of epigenetic modifications within the epigenome of a cell), which ultimately determines that cell's fate during embryogenesis and development (Mikkelsen et al., 2007) as well as during gene transcription throughout the life span (Shi et al., 2006). The best-characterized forms of epigenetic regulation are DNA methylation, histone modification, conformational chromatin modification, and RNA associated gene silencing. These are described in more detail below.

DNA Methylation

The first form of epigenetic modification described was DNA methylation. This process involves the attachment of a methyl group to DNA at Cytosine (C) and Guanine (G) in locations known as CpG islands. CpG islands have a higher frequency of C-G base pairs than in other stretches of DNA. In fact, 40% of genes contain regions of DNA with CpG islands located prior to (i.e., upstream) their transcriptional initiation sites. Methylated CpG islands silence genes by blocking access to DNA (Li, 2002) or by recruiting chromatin binding proteins that complex with other proteins to repress gene transcription in a methylation dependent manner (Nan et al., 1998; Zhang et al., 1999). In mature cells, up to 80% of CpG islands are methylated and hence repressed (Bird, 2002).

DNA methylation is functionally important as it contributes to the regulation of gene control during embryogenesis and X-chromosome inactivation in females. The latter is required so that females do not express twice the number of X chromosome encoded genes (Delcuve, Rastegar, & Davie, 2009; Miranda & Jones, 2007). DNA methylation patterns in most cell types result from the balance of methylating and demethylating enzymes (Delcuve et al., 2009; Turek-Plewa & Jagodzinski, 2005) and these enzymatic activities are very important in that not all CpG islands are methylated in any given cell type (Razin, 1998). In other words, CpG island methylation is cell-type specific and the DNA methylation pattern confers upon the cell its functional identity and a particular tissue's functional identity. Simplistically, these epigenetic marks allow cells and organs to express a specific gene profile related to that cell's function despite the fact that all body cells contain the same DNA. Since DNA methylation is part of the chemical structure of the DNA itself it is more stable than other epigenetic marks and as such is an important marker relevant to environmental effects upon the genome (Beck, Olek, & Walter, 1999). Significant progress has been made in understanding the influence of environmental stressors on epigenetic modulation of chromatin structure and gene accessibility, as summarized below in *Stress and Epigenetic Modification*.

Histone Modification

The basic unit for the packaging of chromatin is the nucleosome, which is comprised of four core histone proteins—H3, H4, H2A, and H2B—two of each to form an octet. The core histones are predominantly globular proteins except for their amino terminal tails. (See Figure 4.2.) A striking feature of histones, and particularly of their tails, is the large number and types of amino acid residues that can be modified epigenetically. Over 60 different amino acid residues can be modified predominately by acetylation, methylation, or phosphorylation (Kouzarides, 2007). Such modification is even more complex in that mono-, di-, or trimethyl groups can also be added to these amino acids. This array of modifications provides for enormous potential to change functional responsiveness and the plasticity of the epigenome to environmental challenges.

Chromatin Remodeling

When histones are modified they can influence how the chromatin is arranged. This rearrangement of chromatin is referred to as *chromatin remodeling*. Chromatin remodeling is required for the efficient expression of genes necessary to the function of an individual cell. The process of chromatin remodeling involves shifting of the nucleosome's core along the length of the DNA molecule (i.e., nucleosome sliding). Studies suggest that this shift may involve the actual disassembly and reassembly of the nucleosome core (Lorch, Maier-Davis, & Kornberg, 2006). When this occurs it alters the position of the nucleosomes around transcription initiation sites and permits accessibility of the genes for transcription. There are direct relationships among epigenetic modifications (acetylation, methylation, and phosphorylation) and chromatin remodeling complexes (Bultman, Gebuhr, & Magnuson, 2005). For example, a change in acetylation status forms a molecular mark for the recruitment of chromatin-remodeling enzymes that function as transcriptional co-activating proteins (Hebbar & Archer, 2007). These co-activating proteins allow for local chromatin unwinding and the recruitment of the basal transcriptional complex and RNA (ribonucleic acid) polymerase that enzymatically catalyze the production of mRNA (Trotter & Archer, 2007). It is the combination of histone modification and chromatin remodeling that allows for transcription of a DNA sequence by the transcriptional machinery necessary for mRNA production.

Functional Significance of Histone Modifications

Histone acetylation is generally associated with regions of actively transcribed chromatin. For example, the addition of an acetyl group within the histone tail neutralizes the positive charge of specific amino acids, thereby disrupting interaction of those amino acids with the negatively charged DNA. This loosens the chromatin structure and the genes become more accessible for transcription (i.e., chromatin remodeling). This is an orderly process and permits the recruitment of transcriptional co-activating proteins that bind the acetylated amino acids, resulting in enhanced gene expression through chromatin remodeling (Haberland

et al., 2009). In contrast to acetylation, methylation of histone residues results in either activation or repression of genes depending upon which amino acids are methylated. As such, histone acetylation—along with some forms of methylation—is associated with accessibility of DNA for transcription, whereas histone hypo-acetylation and some forms of methylation constitute repressive marks and contribute to chromatin condensation and transcriptional repression (Cosgrove & Wolberger, 2005; Peterson & Laniel, 2004).

Noncoding RNAs

Other relevant regulators of chromatin structure and gene expression are noncoding (nc) RNAs. The ncRNAs are transcripts that are not translated into protein (Costa, 2008). ncRNA is thought to affect gene expression by DNA methylation and histone modification. A prominent member of the large ncRNAs is the *Xist* RNA, which mediates epigenetic inactivation of one X chromosome in females (Ng, Pullirsch, Leeb, & Wutz, 2007). *Xist* is transcribed from the future inactivated X chromosome and initiates silencing by direct interaction with the chromosome (Wutz, 2007). Stable silencing is finalized by enzymatic addition of repressive DNA methylation and histone marks. Small ncRNAs can mediate both transcriptional and post-transcriptional gene silencing (post-transcription silencing is that form of mRNA repression that occurs after transcription) (Bernstein & Allis, 2005). MicroRNAs (miRNAs) are a group of small ncRNA molecules (18–22 nucleotides) that function as post-transcriptional regulators of gene expression (Moazed, 2009). These miRNAs are transcribed in the nucleus by the action of RNA polymerases (which synthesize RNA), forming long precursor transcripts of RNA (Faller & Guo, 2008). These precursor RNA molecules are cleaved sequentially in the nucleus and the cytoplasm by endonucleases. The resulting mature miRNAs bind to other target mRNAs by base pairing at distinct regions and, thus, alter mRNA function (Mendell, 2005). It is posited that the histone code is affected by these small RNAs. The potential impact of miRNA-mediated biological regulation is estimated to be considerable in that for the over 1,000 cloned or predicted human miRNAs, thousands of potential targets have been estimated. Since the transcriptional regulation of miRNAs is incompletely understood, it is not known how epigenetic changes will affect the regulation of miRNAs. However, epigenetic pattern modifications brought on by the environment do have the potential to affect miRNA expression (Lewis, Burge, & Bartel, 2005).

STRESS AND EPIGENETIC MODIFICATION

Adverse Early-Life Experiences and Epigenetic Modification

During the fetal and early neonatal periods of life, there are critical windows of time in which early-life experiences can profoundly influence brain function and alter the regulation of the neuroendocrine stress systems. Recent developments in epigenetics have demonstrated the impact of early-life experiences on neuro-behavioral development that is mediated through alterations in the epigenetic pattern. Much of the evidence originates from studies that have evaluated the effect of variations in maternal care behavior (Zhang & Meaney, 2010). The fetal and early postnatal periods represent times when developing organs are especially vulnerable to environmental influence. During these critical periods exposure to stress can more easily elicit epigenetic modifications. The implications are significant as these alterations persist and may adversely affect health through adulthood (Fumagalli, Molteni, Racagni, & Riva, 2007).

To appreciate the epigenetic effects of maternal care behavior, it is important to understand regulation of the hypothalamic pituitary adrenocortical (HPA) axis, the body's major stress-response system. Physical or psychosocial stressors activate neural circuits that trigger secretion of corticotrophin-releasing hormone (CRH) from the hypothalamus. CRH then activates the anterior pituitary to secrete adrenocorticotrophic hormone (ACTH), and ACTH, in turn, stimulates the adrenal cortex to secrete the glucocorticoid hormone, cortisol. Normally, upon termination of a stressor, negative feedback processes operate to halt the HPA stress response. Negative feedback involves the binding of glucocorticoids to glucocorticoid receptors (GR) primarily in the hippocampus. When glucocorticoids are bound to these receptors, the HPA stress response is turned off (Sapolsky, Krey, & McEwen, 1984). Although other brain areas participate in the HPA negative feedback regulation, the hippocampus expresses the highest level of GR within the brain and is crucial to the HPA stress response (Aronsson et al., 1988). Also, the hippocampus is particularly vulnerable to the effects of stressful experiences, as the hippocampus shows a substantial capacity for structural and functional reorganization (i.e., neuro-plasticity) in response to environmental stimuli (Conrad, 2008; Lee, Ogle, & Sapolsky, 2002; McEwen, Gould, & Sakai, 1992; Sapolsky, 2000). As described below, stress may influence this neuro-plasticity through chromatin modification.

Rodent models of maternal care have provided valuable insight as to how epigenetic modification of GR gene expression within the brain results from environmental cues and, in turn, shapes stress responsivity and behavior in adult offspring. For example, lactating rats nurture their pups by licking and grooming (LG), the major source of tactile stimulation for the pups. Moreover, rodents display natural variations in the amount of LG provided to the pups. Such variation in LG gives rise to enduring differences in the HPA stress responsiveness and behavior of the offspring, which persists into adulthood (as reviewed in T. Y. Zhang & Meaney, 2010). That is, adult offspring of mothers who provided high levels of LG (HLG) during the first postnatal week show elevated hippocampal GR expression, enhanced glucocorticoid feedback sensitivity, and reduced hypothalamic CRH expression. In addition, offspring of HLG mothers exhibit a more moderate behavioral and hormonal reaction to stressors compared to offspring of mothers who provided low levels of LG (LLG). Interestingly, these neuro-behavioral effects are reversed by cross-fostering pups from an HLG mother to an LLG mother during the first postnatal week, or vice versa, demonstrating that the resulting stress-phenotype is derived from maternal nurturing behavior (Francis, Diorio, Liu, & Meaney, 1999; Liu et al., 1997). Important to the focus of this chapter are recent investigations that have demonstrated that variations in maternal LG confer unique DNA methylation patterns of genes that encode for GR within the hippocampus. Specifically, adult offspring of LLG mothers exhibit greater methylation of the GR promoter compared to offspring of HLG mothers. This reduces gene activity and decreases GR expression within the hippocampus. (A gene promoter is a segment of DNA that controls expression of a gene.) The reduced GR diminishes the effectiveness of feedback mechanisms that function to attenuate the HPA response to stress, leading to greater HPA responsivity and a heightened behavioral response to stress (i.e., increased anxiety) (Zhang & Meaney, 2010). These studies of rodent maternal care have contributed key evidence demonstrating that epigenetic processes (i.e., hippocampal methylation pattern) provide a bridge between the maternal/infant environment and the genome, thus shaping the stress response and behavior of adult offspring.

Interestingly, maternal care behavior patterns are passed to the next generation in such a manner that female offspring of HLG mothers also provide HLG to their young, whereas female offspring of LLG mothers provide LLG to their young. The transgenerational transfer of maternal LG behavior has been linked to epigenetic processes that regulate brain levels of the transcription factor, estrogen receptor alpha (ER-α). ER-α normally increases in response to the estrogen surge at birth and triggers expression of oxytocin receptors, which promotes oxytocin binding in pivotal brain regions that mediate the expression of maternal behavior. For offspring of LLG mothers the expression of brain ER-α is low due to greater DNA methylation of the ER-α promoter. Whereas, HLG offspring exhibit reduced methylation of the ER-α promoter and hence have greater transcription of ER-α (Champagne, 2008; Champagne et al., 2006). As a result, offspring of HLG mothers have greater transcription of the oxytocin receptor in the brain and greater oxytocin receptor binding. This promotes maternal nurturing behavior (i.e., HLG) whereas the opposite is true for female offspring of LLG mothers (Champagne, 2008; Champagne et al., 2006). This work demonstrates that maternal behavior induces an epigenetic modification that is instilled across generations. It should be emphasized, however, that the resultant epigenetic marks are not transmitted through the germ line but rather depend on maternal behavior which reinstates the epigenetic modification to the next generation. These findings in rodents are similar to observations in humans that show individual differences in infant care behaviors are transferred across generations from mother to daughter (Miller, Kramer, Warner, Wickramaratne, & Weissman, 1997).

Remarkably, the epigenetic imprint conferred by maternal care behavior can be reversed during adulthood by injecting drugs into the brain that alter hippocampal DNA methylation. When adult rats raised by LLG mothers are infused centrally with a drug that decreases hippocampal DNA methylation, GR expression is reset so that these rats now display the more moderate stress-sensitive phenotype, similar to pups raised by HLG mothers. As a result, their stress reactivity and stress-related behavior is normalized (Weaver et al., 2004). In contrast, increasing brain DNA methylation by infusing a drug directly into the brains of adult rats that received HLG as pups reduces expression of GR and confers a more stress-sensitive phenotype (Weaver et al., 2005; Weaver, Meaney, & Szyf, 2006). These results established a causal association among epigenetic modification, maternal care behavior, GR expression, and subsequent adult stress response and behavior. Also, these results showed that in adults, DNA epigenetic pattern, although relatively stable, is capable of modification. This implies that early life-induced unfavorable epigenetic marks may be altered, although there may be critical windows of time to diminish or reverse unfavorable epigenetic marks.

The preceding emphasizes that maternal care can exert long-lasting effects on HPA stress reactivity. This is clinically relevant in that dysregulated HPA reactivity contributes to disorders of mood and cognition (de Kloet, Joels, & Holsboer, 2005; Lupien, McEwen, Gunnar, & Heim, 2009). Additionally, long-term elevations in glucocorticoids resulting from heightened HPA activity may contribute to complex diseases in adulthood (e.g., coronary artery disease or type II diabetes) (Cottrell & Seckl, 2009). It is intriguing that the impetus for epigenetic modification of stress responsivity was maternal tactile stimulation (i.e., LG behavior). The psycho-biological benefits of maternal touch on infant development are well documented (Ferber, Feldman, & Makhoul, 2008; Moszkowski, Stack, & Chiarella, 2009). This was demonstrated by Harlow's early studies of infant monkeys who were removed from their natural mothers and "raised" by surrogate mothers constructed of either soft cloth or wire. Infant monkeys raised with cloth surrogate mothers spent more time with their mother and had better psychological outcomes compared to those raised with wire surrogates (Harlow, 1958). Furthermore, others showed that maternal-infant touch in humans reduces the infants' cortisol response to environmental stimuli. Similar to the rodent cross-fostering model, touch provided by others also diminishes an infants' cortisol stress response (Feldman, Singer, & Zagoory, 2010). The importance of human touch to infant development has led to the implementation of skin-to-skin care for premature infants. Research documents that skin-to-skin care benefits infant development, including blunting an infant's cortisol response to pain (Feldman, Eidelman, Sirota, & Weller, 2002; Morelius, Theodorsson, & Nelson, 2005). For premature infants, significant brain development takes places *ex-utero,* placing the premature brain at greater risk for stress-induced epigenetic modification. Thus, implementation of skin-to-skin care or infant massage may prevent or reduce imprinting of unfavorable epigenetic marks. Understanding the role of epigenetic processes that shape adult stress sensitivity may provide insight into disturbances in cognition and behavior that arise from disturbed maternal-infant attachment (Sroufe, 2005; Winberg, 2005). Whether moderation of HPA reactivity in response to human touch (or other positive care behaviors) is mediated by epigenetic modification will be challenging to establish in humans. Yet, intriguing findings have revealed that prenatal depressed mood can influence epigenetic programming of genes that regulate the expression of GR in cord blood mononuclear cells (described below) (Oberlander et al., 2008). Future evaluation of how maternal–child interactions modulate the epigenetic pattern of adult offspring has potential to contribute to the understanding of vulnerable versus resilient stress phenotypes.

Early-Life Abuse and Epigenetic Modification of Brain-Derived Neurotrophic Factor (BDNF)

Brain development involves nerve growth factors, like brain-derived neurotrophic factor (BDNF). BDNF fosters neural plasticity by facilitating the development of new synaptic connections among neurons (Cohen-Cory, Kidane, Shirkey, & Marshak, 2010). Negative early-life events have been linked to altered expression of BDNF, and this is thought to adversely impact brain development and increase risk for behavioral disorders later in life (De Bellis, 2005; Liu, 2010). Such environmentally induced alterations in BDNF may result from epigenetic modification (Roth, Lubin, Funk, & Sweatt, 2009; Roth & Sweatt, 2010). For instance,

subjecting rat pups to an abusive foster mother over the first week of life resulted in decreased BDNF mRNA in the prefrontal cortex and hippocampus of adult offspring. This reduction in BDNF mRNA was subsequent to increased DNA methylation of the promoter regions of the BDNF gene. Moreover, the aberrant DNA methylation pattern was reversed when a DNA methylation inhibitor was infused into the brains of adult rats that were previously abused as pups, demonstrating a causal relationship between early-life abuse and methylation for gene regions that encode for BDNF. This provides evidence that DNA methylation can be modified in adults. Additionally, the impact of maternal abuse was transferred across generations as females who were abused as pups became abusive mothers (Roth et al., 2009). This corresponds with the known perpetuation of child abuse across generations in humans (Bifulco et al., 2002; Noll, Trickett, Harris, & Putnam, 2009).

Child Abuse and Brain Epigenetic Modification in Suicide Victims

Child abuse results in a long-lasting heightened HPA stress response ·(Heim, Newport, Mletzko, Miller, & Nemeroff, 2008; Plotsky et al., 2005). Moreover, individuals with a history of child abuse have a greater risk for the development of affective disorders, including a greater suicidal risk (Heim & Nemeroff, 2001; Pruessner, Champagne, Meaney, & Dagher, 2004). The neurobiological mechanism remains unclear. However, recent evaluation of postmortem brain hippocampal samples suggests that epigenetic modification of brain GR expression is linked to suicide risk (McGowan et al., 2009). That study found that post-mortem brain specimens from suicide victims who had a history of childhood abuse had significantly reduced RNA message for GR and increased GR gene DNA methylation. Child abuse was the critical factor in the expression of this suicide-linked epigenetic profile, as it was not observed in hippocampal samples from suicide victims who had no history of child abuse, nor was it observed in samples from individuals who died from accidental causes. Because the epigenetic findings were restricted to suicide cases with a history of child abuse, the observed epigenetic modification is likely derived from childhood adversity rather than from suicide per se. What is most intriguing is that the observed changes in DNA methylation are consistent with the changes found in the hippocampus of rats subjected to low levels of maternal care (i.e., LLG). Moreover, humans with a history of child abuse have reduced hippocampal volume, indicating that the hippocampus is vulnerable to early-life adversity (Heim et al., 2009). These findings highlight the potential long-lasting impact of parental care on offspring epigenetic pattern and risk for psycho-pathology. The conclusions drawn from the study of suicide victims' brains, however, must be viewed cautiously as the retrospective study design does not "prove" that childhood abuse directly caused the differential pattern in hippocampal methylation (McGowan et al., 2009).

Epigenetics and Prenatal Depression

Maternal mood disorders, especially depression, can profoundly affect fetal neurodevelopment and behavioral outcomes for the child and adolescent (Field, Diego, & Hernandez-Reif, 2006). Altered neuroendocrine stress responsiveness may contribute to these adverse outcomes as infants of mothers with prenatal depression show an intensified cortisol response to stress and, furthermore, these infants have greater risk for behavioral disorders (Field et al., 2004; Field et al., 2006). Recently, maternal prenatal depressed mood was linked to epigenetic modification of the GR in leukocytes derived from umbilical cord blood. Specifically, the cord blood leukocytes showed increased methylation of DNA at the binding site for transcription factors necessary for transcription of GR. The increased DNA methylation resulted in reduced GR and was associated with an increased infant salivary cortisol response. These findings suggest that infants whose mothers suffered from prenatal depression developed disturbed central regulation of the HPA axis (Oberlander et al., 2008). It is tempting to conjecture that such peripheral (i.e., leukocyte) changes in the GR transcription machinery may reflect similar changes in hippocampal epigenetic regulation of GR expression, which in turn, increases stress responsivity. Such an interpretation, although intriguing, is not only speculative but difficult to prove given that the "epigenetic code" varies among tissues and cells. Nevertheless, these findings represent one of few studies in humans that bridge epigenetic modification to GR expression, psychological state (i.e., prenatal depressive mood), and

infant cortisol secretion. The exact mechanism by which maternal mood influences epigenetic pattern and stress responsivity of offspring is currently unknown. However, elevated maternal cortisol in women with prenatal depression was shown to predict adverse neonatal outcomes (Field et al., 2006). Hypothetically, it is possible that depression-induced dysregulation of maternal hormones might trigger adverse epigenetic modifications in the neonate. Such linkages remain to be evaluated.

Early-Life Physical Stressors and Epigenetic Modification

The above summarizes evidence that psychosocial stressors (i.e, maternal behavior and mood) induce long-lasting epigenetic modification. In addition to psychosocial stressors, physical stressors during early life also can shape the epigenetic imprint. For example, infants with intrauterine growth retardation (IUGR) are at risk for impaired neurological development. Such impairment has been linked to dysregulated neuroendocrine functioning, particularly altered HPA stress responsiveness (Cianfarani, Geremia, Scott, & Germani, 2002). A rat model of uteroplacental insufficiency showed that such impairments may originate from epigenetic modification subsequent to hypoxic stress or altered nutrient delivery. In this model, uteroplacental insufficiency produced growth retardation of the pups and increased risk for neuroendocrine dysregulation. This was accompanied by epigenetic modification as manifested by increased genome-wide DNA methylation in the hippocampus and periventricular white matter as well as increased histone acetylation. These results demonstrate that a physical insult can produce persistent changes in brain epigenetic patterns that can modify chromatin accessibility. Future studies are needed to determine whether such epigenetic modification contributes to the neurodevelopmental problems associated with IUGR.

Birth is accompanied by a barrage of stress hormones needed to facilitate the transition from fetal to neonatal life. Yet, the mode of birth delivery can modify this physiologic transition as infants delivered by Caesarean section (C-section) lack exposure to parturition-induced surges in stress hormones. This may even impact future health, as infants born by C-section have greater risk for a variety of diseases including immune-based disorders. (See references in Schlinzig,

Johansson, Gunnar, Ekstrom, & Norman, 2009.) A recent study showed differential epigenetic patterns in cord blood leukocytes of healthy full-term infants born by C-section compared to vaginally delivered infants; notably, leukocytes of C-section infants exhibited higher global DNA methylation than those of vaginally delivered infants (Schlinzig et al., 2009). It is possible that the differential global methylation was triggered by differences in stress hormones based on mode of delivery. Although the results of this small study are preliminary, it shows that leukocyte DNA methylation pattern is responsive to the birth process and that birth-related alterations in the epigenetic signature could conceivably contribute to the increased disease risk observed in infants born by C-section.

Section Summary

For many years adverse early-life experiences have been viewed as a source of adult mental health disorders. As reviewed above, recent evidence suggests that epigenetic modification may mediate these poor outcomes. Collectively, the studies reviewed demonstrate that the quality of maternal–child interaction is capable of imprinting stable epigenetic modifications that determine the adult gene transcription potential. Along with genomic variation, such epigenetic variation can contribute to individual differences in behavior, neuroendocrine stress reactivity, neural plasticity, and physiologic function throughout life. The accrual of this evidence builds an epigenetic framework that can explicate how the early-life environment shapes an individual's vulnerability or resistance to stressors and stress-induced illnesses throughout life. Most important, early-life-induced epigenetic modifications can be reversed. This opens up amazing opportunities to reduce or alleviate the impact of unfavorable epigenetic signatures and, thus, prevent or treat health problems rooted in early-life adversity.

STRESS-INDUCED DEPRESSION AND EPIGENETIC MODIFICATION OF BRAIN-DERIVED NEUROTROPHIC FACTOR (BDNF)

Depression commonly occurs in the aftermath of chronic stress (Sheline, Gado, & Kraemer, 2003). Chromatin remodeling of the BDNF gene in the hippocampus may contribute to stress-induced depression by altering neural plasticity. Evidence for this was derived using a mouse model of depression produced by chronic social defeat stress that involved exposing mice to a highly aggressive resident mouse. Such treatment induces depressive symptomatology characterized by subordination and greater avoidance behaviors and less social interaction. Mice displaying the depressive-like phenotype exhibit reductions in hippocampal BDNF gene expression that is accompanied by persistent histone modifications of the BDNF gene (Tsankova et al., 2006). These findings illustrate that chronic stress can confer enduring epigenetic modifications that contribute to depression.

Depression modeled in mice (produced by chronic social defeat or social isolation) can also lead to histone modification in the nucleus accumbens, which is a chief brain reward center implicated in depression in animals (Nestler & Carlezon, 2006) and humans (Tremblay et al., 2005). Both chronic social defeat and social isolation lead to depressive behavior that is accompanied by epigenetic modification of a variety of genes, including those that regulate inflammation. This suggests that such epigenetic modification may increase inflammatory mediators within the brain. Previous work has demonstrated that proinflammatory mediators within the brain are associated with depressive behavior in animals (Dantzer, O'Connor, Freund, Johnson, & Kelley, 2008). It is possible that epigenetic modification of genes involved in brain inflammatory pathways might contribute to the depressive behavior associated with chronic defeat stress and social isolation. Also, these forms of stress produced differences in genes that regulate actin. Stress-induced actin remodeling may relate to structural changes in the brain, specifically reduced hippocampal volume as observed in humans plagued by chronic stress and depression (Egger et al., 2008; Magarinos, McEwen, Flugge, & Fuchs, 1996). Another gene epigenetically affected in depression was a gene that encodes a slenoprotein, a molecule implicated in neurodegenerative diseases, like Alzheimer's disease (Chen & Berry, 2003). Although speculative, these findings raise the possibility that an epigenetic process might link chronic stress to an increased risk for neurodegenerative disease. Such a possibility is consistent with research that implicates epigenetic mechanisms in memory formation, as well as age-associated decline in memory, cognition, and learning (Roth & Sweatt, 2009).

Psychological Stress and Chromatin Remodeling

The hippocampus participates in memory formation and the behavioral and adaptive response to stress (McEwen, 2001). In response to environmental stimuli, the hippocampus, and especially the area of the hippocampus called the dentate gyrus, possess great capacity for structural and functional changes (i.e., neuro-plasticity) (Gould, Tanapat, McEwen, Flugge, & Fuchs, 1998; Malberg, Eisch, Nestler, & Duman, 2000). Evidence obtained from animal models indicates that psychological stress–induced changes in neuro-plasticity within the dentate gyrus result from chromatin remodeling. Notably, subjecting mice to psychological stressors (exposure to a predator or forced swimming), resulted in increased phosphorylation of histones in neurons within the dentate gyrus. The increased histone phosphorylation was specific to psychological stress as physical stressors had no effect on histone status. Remarkably, rats who had access to a running wheel, and hence greater physical activity prior to stress exposure, were found to be resistant to stress-induced chromatin remodeling within the dentate gyrus (Bilang-Bleuel et al., 2005). This finding is consistent with the positive effects exercise has on psycho-biological coping with stress in humans and raises the possibility that exercise may offer a way to attenuate chromatin remodeling associated with chronic stress (Morgan, Tobar, & Snyder, 2010).

Adaptive responses to stressful events may involve epigenetic processes that orchestrate the transcription of brain proteins associated with the consolidation of memory. The forced swim test is used as a model to study stress-related memory formation. When rodents are forced to swim in a closed basin with no escape, they exhibit immobilization behavior upon re-testing. The acquired immobility results from having learned from their previous experience that escape is not possible (De Pablo, Parra, Segovia, & Guillanon, 1989). Hence, they reduce their attempts to escape (i.e., learned immobility). Learned immobility was shown to be dependent upon chromatin remodeling in the dentate gyrus (Bilang-Bleuel et al., 2005), which required co-signaling through the GR and glutamate receptors (Chandramohan, Droste, Arthur, & Reul, 2008). These findings demonstrate that stress-related learning results in hippocampal chromatin remodeling, which may facilitate behavioral adaptation to environmental challenge.

Novelty Stress and Hippocampal Chromatin Remodeling

Forcing rodents to swim has a strong psychological component (anxiety, despair); however, swimming also involves physical exertion and loss of body heat. In contrast, exposure of rodents to a novel environment is an exclusive mild psychological stressor without physical burden. For rodents, who are nocturnal and prefer dark spaces, exposure to light provokes anxiety. Thus, subjecting rodents to increasing levels of light intensity serves as a model of novelty and a means by which to evoke a mild psychological stress response. The hippocampus contributes to stress-related adaptation and novelty detection. Exposure of rats to a novel environment of escalating light intensity was shown to result in histone modification within the hippocampus. In particular, this novel experience resulted in increased phosphorylation and acetylation of histones associated with local opening of condensed chromatin, thus allowing transcription of formerly silent genes (Cheung, Allis, & Sassone-Corsi, 2000). Further, the response was amplified with increasing gradations in light intensity; it occurred rapidly (within 30 minutes) and was followed by a return to pre-stress levels 2 hours later. Functionally, the changes in hippocampal chromatin remodeling were accompanied by c-fos gene transcription (a gene marker of recent neuronal activity) and were mediated by receptors (GR and glutamate) known to be implicated in neuro-plasticity. This investigation provides further evidence that epigenetic processes play a role in steering adaptive responses within the brain subsequent to an acute, albeit mild, psychological stressor.

Epigenetics and Aging-Associated Memory Impairment

An epigenetic theory of aging-related cognitive dysfunction proposes that dysregulation of epigenetic processes leads to the accumulation of abnormal epigenetic marks that disrupt neural plasticity and memory formation (Penner, Roth, Barnes, & Sweatt, 2010). The hippocampus is crucial to memory formation and is affected early on in dementia (Mesulam, 1999). Recently, age-associated memory impairment was shown to result from altered chromatin remodeling within the hippocampus (Peleg et al., 2010). When tested in a contextual fear conditioning/learning paradigm, aged mice exhibited memory impairment that was associated with their inability to upregulate histone acetylation within the hippocampus, as compared to young mice. This was functionally linked to a decrease in the expression of learning-induced genes, as the young mice exhibited differential regulation of a large number of hippocampal genes linked to associative learning, whereas aged mice exhibited essentially no change in their hippocampal gene expression profile. This implies that the aged mice have marked impairment in regulatory gene expression when exposed to situations that promote learning behavior. Remarkably, the delivery of a histone deacetylase inhibitor into the hippocampus of aged mice increased hippocampal histone acetylation in response to the learning paradigm and restored expression of learning-regulated genes and recovery of cognitive abilities. These findings indicate that deregulated histone acetylation plays a causal role in age-associated memory impairment and suggests that certain histone marks may serve as an "early biomarker for an impaired genome-environment interaction in the aging brain" (Peleg et al., 2010). These results are consistent with findings which show that the administration of histone deacetylases completely reverses contextual memory deficits in a mouse model of Alzheimer's disease (Kilgore et al., 2010). Although it is plausible that epigenetic-based therapeutics might prevent or re-establish memory in the elderly, agents currently available are not tissue-specific and may have untoward effects. Furthermore, the agents evaluated were delivered directly into the animal's brain and it is unclear, if administered peripherally, whether they can reach brain targets.

Epigenetic and Resilience to Stressful Challenge

Resilience is the capacity of an individual who, in the face of adversity, continues to mobilize adaptive responses and resists developing affective disorders, like depression (Charney, 2004). The psycho-neurobiological mechanisms underlying resilience are complex. However, a mouse model demonstrates that the resilient phenotype is linked to a unique chromatin pattern for gene expression within the brain (Wilkinson et al., 2009). Approximately one third of inbred mice naturally display a stress-resilient phenotype, as these mice do not develop adverse neuro-behavioral consequences when

subjected to chronic social defeat. This dichotomous response (susceptible versus resilient) has been associated with a unique histone methylation pattern. When subjected to chronic social defeat, resilient mice exhibit a brain histone methylation pattern that is more similar to that of the unstressed mice. Yet, despite the general similarity in brain histone methylation between the resilient and the unstressed mice, unique differences in methylation pattern existed between these two groups. This implies that resilience is an *active process*. That is, the stress paradigm actively induced changes in gene expression and chromatin modifications unique to the resilient phenotype. This suggests that "resilience genes" may respond to challenge in a manner that imparts protection and guards against the development of depression. This may contribute to individual differences in a person's ability to withstand or succumb to chronic stress. In contrast, other unique genes may mediate vulnerability to depression that emerges with chronic stress (i.e., a susceptible phenotype). Key overlap between epigenetic mechanisms of resilience and those of antidepressants was also observed, indicating that antidepressants may work, in part, by generating epigenetic-based changes in gene expression that occur naturally in more resilient individuals. However, a number of genes remained differentially regulated in the resilient compared to the antidepressant-treated mice. This suggests that other novel genes are implicated in resilience, which could be exploited as targets for new classes of antidepressants (Feder, Nestler, & Charney, 2009; Wilkinson et al., 2009).

Stressor Duration and Epigenetic Modification

Successful adaptation to stress involves maintaining homeostasis through change, which is termed *allostasis*. Chronic stress can exert a toll on one's adaptive capacity, producing allostatic load. Allostatic load is characterized by dysregulation of the body's stress response systems. In fact, brain regions involved in the stress response undergo structural changes upon exposure to unrelenting stress, as manifested by reduced dendritic arborization (Magarinos & McEwen, 1995) and reduced hippocampal neurogenesis (Gould, McEwen, Tanapat, Galea, & Fuchs, 1997). The hippocampus is most vulnerable to chronic stress, and in humans allostatic load is associated with reductions in hippocampal volume

(McEwen, 2001). Recently, brain epigenetic modification was shown to be temporally sensitive to stressor duration and may, thus, contribute to adaptation to stress (Hunter, McCarthy, Milne, Pfaff, & McEwen, 2009). Acute restraint stress produced rapid and large chromatin modifications in rat hippocampi, whereas chronic restraint produced less dramatic effects. The observed temporal sensitivity of hippocampal chromatin remodeling provides insight into the process of adaptation to a stressor and could relate to the known habituation of the HPA response that occurs with repeated stress (Uchida et al., 2008). It is possible that hippocampal chromatin remodeling may presage the transition from allostasis to allostatic load and contribute to the neuro-pathogenic effects of unrelenting stress (Hunter et al., 2009).

Post-Traumatic Stress Disorder, Depression, and Epigenetic Modification of Immune-Related Genes

Neuroendocrine stress hormones may signal epigenetic modification in the immune system given that the brain and neuroendocrine system regulate immune function. Stress hormones, like glucocorticoids, have strong immunomodulatory effects and influence the epigenetic pattern for genes that regulate immune function (Krukowski et al., 2011). Hence, it is possible for stressful or traumatic events to induce epigenetic modification of genes that encode immunoregulatory proteins. For instance, individuals with post-traumatic stress disorder (PTSD) are known to not only have heightened stress reactivity, but also to exhibit a distinct expression profile for genes that influence immune function (Segman et al., 2005). New evidence demonstrates that for individuals with PTSD, the experience of a traumatic event triggers downstream alterations in immune function by decreasing methylation of immune-related genes (Uddin et al., 2010). That study identified a set of uniquely unmethylated genes that encode for immune function in individuals with PTSD. Moreover, the PTSD epigenetic profile negatively correlated with traumatic burden (i.e., number of traumatic event exposures). These findings demonstrate the capacity of a traumatic event to trigger long-lasting epigenetic-induced alterations in immune function, possibly through brain–immune interactions. Nevertheless, this study is limited by its cross-sectional design, which prevents determining

whether the PTSD methylation pattern was present prior to the traumatic exposure, hence representing a pre-existing biologic vulnerability. Furthermore, the whole blood epigenetic analyses prevented determination of cell-specific epigenetic profiles. The results, however, raise the intriguing possibility that a traumatic life event induces long-lasting alterations in immune function through epigenetic modification.

Evidence linking epigenetics, mood disorder, and inflammatory mediators was recently reported in a community-based sample. A genome-wide evaluation of whole blood DNA from individuals with a lifetime history of depression revealed a unique set of methylated and unmethylated genes compared to nondepressed individuals. The depression-related methylation profile was functionally relevant in that circulating levels of inflammatory markers, IL-6 and C-reactive protein (CRP), were elevated in the individuals with lifetime depression, and, importantly, IL-6 methylation showed an inverse correlation with circulating IL-6 (but not CRP) in depressed individuals only (Uddin et al., in press). These findings have implications for the pathogenesis of depression, as inflammatory mediators have been previously linked to the etiology of depressive symptoms (Dantzer et al., 2008). Yet, similar to the above-described study of DNA methylation profiles and individuals with PTSD, this study is also limited by its small sample, cross-sectional design, and lack of distinguishing methylation status for specific blood cells. Despite these limitations, the findings are intriguing in that a community sample of individuals was evaluated and the findings functionally link peripheral blood DNA methylation status of depressed individuals with the inflammatory cytokine, IL-6 (Uddin et al., in press).

Section Summary

The foregoing provides considerable evidence, predominately in animal models, that stress exposure in adults results in epigenetic modification in brain regions that regulate the neuroendocrine stress response (mainly in the hippocampus and the nucleus accumbens). These results build on evidence derived from studies of the effects of early-life experiences on epigenetic modification and demonstrate the plasticity of the epigenome across the lifespan. A variety of stress models in rodents, including those with depression induced by chronic social defeat and social isolation, forced swim, novelty stress, restraint stress, stress-related memory paradigms, and age-associated memory impairment, have been evaluated. The findings emphasize that stress-induced epigenetic modification is sensitive to psychological stress, even if it is mild, and furthermore, such epigenetic modification is sensitive to the duration of stressor exposure and can be reversed. Moreover, intriguing evidence demonstrates a unique epigenetic profile that characterizes resilience to stress (i.e., resilient phenotype) and this may contribute to individual differences in stress vulnerability. Although currently there is little evaluation of stress-related epigenetic modification in humans, the findings in individuals with PTSD and individuals with lifetime depression provides preliminary evidence suggesting that the experience of a traumatic event results in epigenetic imprinting of genes that encode for immune function, including inflammatory mediators (Uddin et al., 2010; Uddin et al., in press). Collectively, these findings provide impetus for further exploration in human stress paradigms, as well as in disorders for which stress has been established as a vulnerability factor.

IMPLICATIONS

Epigenetics has engendered a renewed enthusiasm and appreciation for the effect of the environment on gene expression. As reviewed, evidence is accruing which demonstrates that epigenetic processes bridge the environment with the expression of genes that regulate neuroendocrine stress activation, behavior, emotions, and physiological function. This fresh insight offers real potential to yield myriad implications for identification, treatment, and prevention of a wide range of disorders across the lifespan, particularly those associated with stress reactivity. (See Figure 4.3.) Understanding how the environment modulates gene expression to impact health outcomes through epigenetic modification is highly germane to nursing. Of particular importance to nursing is the linkage between stress-related emotions and behavior as a consequence of epigenetic modification. Although the field is new, discovery is moving at a rapid pace and, as noted in the discussion below, there is ample opportunity for nurse scientists to

contribute to this field, especially as the preclinical animal research moves toward translation in human paradigms. The sequencing of the human genome has transformed nursing science, education, and practice; now, in the postgenomic era, the mapping of the epigenome will do likewise.

Given the evidence that implicates epigenetic modifications as mediators of early-life experiences, it is essential to extend these investigations to further the understanding of the influence of the psychosocial environment on human development. This is not only highly significant to perinatal, neonatal, and pediatric nursing practice, but also to the practice of nurses who work with populations of adults afflicted by disorders rooted in adverse early experiences. Child development studies consistently demonstrate that pre- and postnatal maternal stress and early caregiving behaviors contribute to long-term health outcomes in adults (Clavarino et al., 2010; Gutteling et al., 2006; Moeller, Bachmann, & Moeller, 1993). It is clear that there are vulnerable periods during gestation and postnatal care when exposure to environmental stress may result in increased risk for developing psychological and physical problems. For instance, gestational periods between 19 and 26 weeks, and the last several weeks of gestation, have been identified as periods when the developing fetus is most sensitive to stress-induced elevations in maternal glucocorticoids (Seckl & Meaney, 2006). It is possible that stress-induced stimulation of neuroendocrine secretory products, like glucocorticoids, may induce epigenetic modification, especially during critical developmental periods. Greater insight into the molecular machinery of epigenetic processes may identify molecular mechanisms that underlie periods of biological vulnerability. Because epigenetic modifications appear to be reversible, epigenetic-based interventions could be targeted to these critical periods to guard the infant and child from the deleterious effects of stress. Epigenetic-based assessment and management of health disorders will likely become part of the future of clinical practice in the post-genomic era.

Epigenetics holds substantial promise to predict and/or explain how early childhood experiences shape individuals' behavioral and affective responses to stress and why some of these responses may be maladaptive (Foley et al., 2009). Early childhood exposure to adversity

Figure 4.3 The Epigenetic Profile Responds to the Environment Across the Lifespan

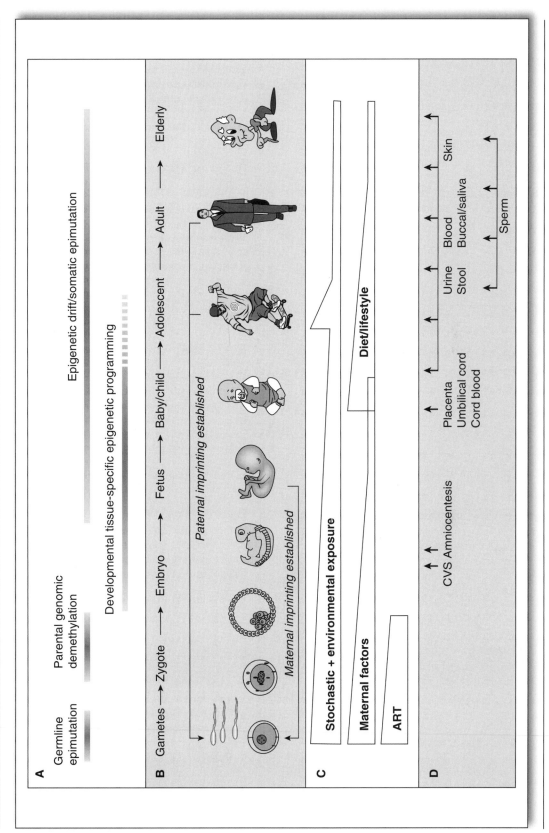

(Continued)

Figure 4.3 (Continued)

The epigenetic profile is dynamic and responsive to the environment across the lifespan. A. Epigenetic modification may involve both genome-wide remodeling and tissue-specific programming events. After fertilization, maternal and paternal DNA is demethylated, with the exception of imprinted genes, which are selectively marked with either a maternal or paternal epigenetic pattern. B. Cell differentiation during early development involves epigenetic modification to produce epigenetic marks that are unique to that cell type. C. Over one's lifetime, stochastic and environmentally induced epigenetic modifications accumulate and may be passed through the germ line to subsequent generations, or reinstated subsequent to maternal behavior or other environmental cues. Critical periods of development are likely more sensitive to environmental insults such as maternal diet and behavior, environmental stress or toxic exposure, assisted reproductive technologies (ART), and a person's lifestyle. D. Biological specimens accessible for epigenetic evaluation include cerebrovascular system (CVS) and amniocentesis cells, placenta, umbilical cord/cord blood, sperm, body secretions, and cells, such as buccal/skin samples.

SOURCE: Figure is used with permission and is from "Prospects for Epigenetic Epidemiology," by D. L. Foley, J. M. Craig, R. Morley, C. A. Olsson, T. Dwyer, K. Smith et al., 2009, *American Journal of Epidemiology*, *169*, pp. 389–400. Copyright 2009 by Oxford University Press.

(e.g., neglect, abuse) has been linked to increased risk for internalizing and externalizing problems, including conduct disorder, antisocial behavior, anxiety, and depression (Barber, 1996; Chorpita & Barlow, 1998; Johnson, Cohen, Kasen, Smailes, & Brook, 2001), as well as adult onset of diseases of the heart, lung, and gastrointestinal system (Felitti et al., 1998). In children as young as 7 years, early-life exposure to physical and sexual abuse was shown to result in disrupted cortisol secretion (Pendry & Adam, 2007; Trickett, Noll, Susman, Shenk, & Putnam, 2010). Furthermore, aberration in the HPA stress response observed during early life persists into adulthood (Trickett et al., 2010), highlighting the capacity for early-life adversity to imprint enduring changes in psycho-biological function. This is of particular interest because childhood exposure to mild conditions such as a marital conflict, lack of social support, and unaffectionate exchanges is associated with abnormal cortisol response profiles, weakened immunity, and recurrent illness (Flinn, 1999). Recent advancements in behavioral epigenetics offer promise for the development of sophisticated epigenetic-based interventions designed to circumvent the environmental effects on the epigenome, especially if implemented during critical windows of development. There are many challenges ahead, as it remains unclear whether peripheral administration of a pharmacological agent can target affected brain areas.

The vast majority of research in behavioral epigenetics has focused on the effects of adversity during early life, a period when the brain is more susceptible to environmental insult, as significant neurobiological development is taking place. Yet, it is also likely that other vulnerable periods exist throughout the lifespan, such as puberty (Foley et al., 2009). Notably, at the onset of puberty there is a second wave of neuronal growth (i.e., synaptogenesis) in several parts of the brain. Also, following puberty, selective synapse elimination occurs, a process which refines brain networks. These processes are sensitive to environmental influences and may represent a period of vulnerability for epigenetic-induced modulation of brain plasticity (Giedd et al., 1999). Moreover, biological sensitivity to stress, mainly evidenced by increased cortisol secretion, has been shown in adolescents (Spear, 2000; Walker, Walder, & Reynolds, 2001). It is well documented that certain psychiatric disorders (e.g., schizophrenia) have their onset during or shortly after adolescence (First, 2000) and may relate to the effects of stress on the changing physiological and neurobiological networks characteristic of puberty. In addition, emerging evidence in rodent models suggests that exposure to high levels of stress during adolescence can result in permanent changes in future cognitive functioning (Teicher et al., 2003), possibly resulting in a more rapid age-related memory decline. It is likely that some of the environmental effects on the developing brain are epigenetically driven. Thus, using a lifespan approach to understand vulnerability to epigenetic modification will yield valuable insight regarding when unfavorable epigenetic modifications are more likely to be induced, and thus more effectively prevented or diminished. Investigating environmental-based vulnerability factors such as pubertal timing, adolescent drug use, or physical abuse during early childhood, within the context of epigenetics, can enrich future understanding as to how environmental factors contribute to disorders that emerge during these vulnerable periods. These are fertile areas of investigation that would benefit from a multidisciplinary team approach consisting of molecular biologists, psychologists, and nurse scientists.

Interestingly, women with a history of childhood abuse not only have greater HPA stress responsiveness but also a decrease in cerebral spinal fluid levels of oxytocin (a hormone that promotes empathy and maternal bonding behavior) (Heim et al., 2009). Indeed, behavioral studies demonstrate that children who form a secure attachment bond with a parent are more likely to do so with their own offspring (Main, Kaplan, & Cassidy, 1985). In addition, children whose primary caregiver was emotionally unavailable (i.e., depressed) are more likely to become parents who experience difficulties caring for their own children. The relationship between developmental history and future parenting practices is highlighted in the literature on child abuse, showing that parents are more likely to abuse their children if they have experienced abuse during their own childhood (e.g., Belsky, 1984). Undeniably, behavioral and physiological transmission of the cross-generational effects of stress is multifaceted, yet it is possible that epigenetic mechanisms are an important part of this process. As described earlier, epigenetic mechanisms are implicated in the reduction of brain oxytocin receptor expression in offspring exposed to early-life stress. These alterations may endure across the lifespan and may explain intergenerational transmission of psychopathology and persistence of maladaptive behaviors beyond genetic factors.

Insight regarding the pathogenesis of autism spectrum disorders (ASD) may also benefit from the recent discoveries of epigenetic modifications to the oxytocin and glucocorticoid receptor genes, in that ASD has been associated with decreased production of oxytocin (Yamasue, Kuwabara, Kawakubo, & Kasai, 2009) and hypersensitivity to stress (Corbett, Mendoza, Abdullah, Wegelin, & Levine, 2006). Treatment of autistic individuals with oxytocin reduced repetitive behaviors and increased retention of social cognition and affective speech comprehension (Hollander et al., 2007; Hollander et al., 2003). Moreover, it has been hypothesized that hypersensitivity to stress in infants may contribute to the development of autism (Zelazo, 2001). The trajectory starts with a young child's inability to sustain normal patterns of social interaction and behavioral compliance due to low stress tolerance. These patterns disrupt child–caretaker interactions needed for acquisition of socio-emotional and communicative skills. Although underlying mechanisms for this connection have not been elucidated, emerging evidence suggests that epigenetic, as opposed to genetic influences, may account for the recent increased prevalence of ASD (Previc, 2007) and the disproportionate number of males affected (Kaminsky, Wang, & Petronis, 2006). This opens a window for a variety of new interventions targeting epigenetic alterations.

The consequences of stress-induced epigenetic modification may emerge during aging. (See Figure 4.3.) As reviewed, generalized decreases in DNA methylation accumulate with aging (Foley et al., 2009). This may be unique to tissues and/or genes and may contribute to diseases in the elderly. Cumulative effects of chronic exposure to stress may lead to unfavorable epigenetic marks that increase the vulnerability of the aging brain and body to disease. A lifetime of exposure to endogenous or exogenous factors (e.g., diet, stress, inflammation) may trigger changes in disease-associated gene expression that are then epigenetically maintained and manifested in pathology considerably later in life (Lahiri, Maloney, & Zawia, 2009). For example, cognitive impairment and memory decline are characteristics of aging that are a result of deterioration of the hippocampus and the frontal cortex of the brain. In late adulthood these brain areas may be most vulnerable to the effects of stress hormones. Indeed, exposure to stress and high levels of glucocorticoids is associated with memory impairments and hippocampal atrophy (Landfield, Blalock, Chen, & Porter, 2007), as well as increased levels of beta-amyloid protein, which is implicated in Alzheimer's disease progression (LaFerla, Green, & Oddo, 2007). These brain changes may be epigenetically mediated, as animal studies show that epigenetic mechanisms are involved in long-term memory formation and associative learning (Levenson & Sweatt, 2005; Peleg et al., 2010), that can be reversed by the administration of histone deacetylases (Kilgore et al., 2010). This indicates the prospect for epigenetic-based intervention(s). Such a possibility awaits the development of more specific agents capable of targeting discrete brain regions. Equally important will be preventive measures that incorporate stress reduction to limit the accumulation of adverse epigenetic marks.

The stochastic nature of the underlying biochemistry of epigenetic alterations has been suggested to be a contributing factor in the cellular breakdown, characteristic of aging and age-associated diseases (Sedivy, Banumathy, & Adams, 2008). Given that the epigenome is sensitive to environmental influences, it is possible that disease can be induced or exacerbated by stress and/or lifestyle (e.g., diet). Variations in intake of micronutrients, like folate, can alter availability of methyl donors and affect DNA methylation levels (Foley et al., 2009). Environmental-induced epigenetic modification would be especially relevant to those diseases for which stress is an established risk factor. Both animal and clinical studies demonstrate that immunological and cardiovascular disease and cancer involve epigenetic mechanisms. Moreover, epigenetic modification may mediate the immune dysregulation that accompanies psychosocial stress in individuals with cancer. A recent evaluation of women stressed by breast cancer diagnosis showed that the reduction in natural killer cell lytic activity against tumor cells was linked to modification of histone proteins (Mathews et al., 2011). As well, epigenetics has been demonstrated to contribute to the pathogenesis of systemic lupus erythematosus and rheumatoid arthritis (Trenkmann, Brock, Ospelt, & Gay, 2010); type 1 diabetes, celiac disease, and idiopathic thrombocytopenia (Brooks, Le Dantec, Jaques-Olivier, Youinou, & Renaudineau, 2010); multiple sclerosis (Lincoln & Cook, 2009); asthma and allergy (Martino & Prescott, 2010); as well as atherosclerosis (Turunen, Aavik, & Yla-Herttuala, 2009). Accordingly, epigenetics is a promising area of science that can explain the interaction between nature and nurture in the development of diseases where stress is a risk factor and help create new ways to prevent and manage these conditions.

In conclusion, evidence supports the concept that an epigenetic code serves to translate the relationship between the environment and the genome, and in this manner influences health. Rapid advances in this field have the potential to transform the conceptualization of the origin of many diseases, especially those for which stress is a risk factor. This knowledge can guide the development of new therapeutic approaches, including lifestyle approaches that take advantage of the plasticity of the epigenome and its dynamic responsivity to the environment. Epigenetic-based therapies are currently underway for many hematological malignancies and this will only escalate in the future (Feinberg, 2008). Epigenetics is a field that integrates the biological and behavioral sciences and requires investigation in basic, translational, and clinical research that cuts across multiple levels of inquiry, from molecular to psychosocial. Much of the research accomplished in animal models of stress paradigms raises clinically relevant questions, which await exploration and application to the human condition. Nurse scientists are well poised to move this field forward at multiple levels of inquiry, from translational knowledge discovery to developing and testing innovative approaches to assess, prevent, and manage health conditions linked to stress-induced epigenetic modification. Such discovery will contribute to the body of knowledge that will form the future foundation for epigenetic-based nursing practice.

REFERENCES

Aronsson, M., Fuxe, K., Dong, Y., Agnati, L. F., Okret, S., & Gustafsson, J. A. (1988). Localization of glucocorticoid receptor mRNA in the male rat brain by in situ hybridization. *Proceedings of the National Academy of Sciences USA, 85*(23), 9331–9335.

Barber, B. K. (1996). Parental psychological control: Revisiting a neglected construct. *Child Development, 67*(6), 3296–3319.

Beck, S., Olek, A., & Walter, J. (1999). From genomics to epigenomics: A loftier view of life. *Nature Biotechnology, 17*(12), 1144.

Belsky, J. (1984). The determinants of parenting: A process model. *Child Development, 55*(1), 83–96.

Bernstein, E., & Allis, C. D. (2005). RNA meets chromatin. *Genes & Development, 19*(14), 1635–1655.

Bifulco, A., Moran, P. M., Ball, C., Jacobs, C., Baines, R., Bunn, A., et al. (2002). Childhood adversity, parental vulnerability and disorder: Examining inter-generational transmission of risk. *Journal of Child Psychology and Psychiatry, 43*(8), 1075–1086.

Bilang-Bleuel, A., Ulbricht, S., Chandramohan, Y., De Carli, S., Droste, S. K., & Reul, J. M. (2005). Psychological stress increases histone H3 phosphorylation in adult dentate gyrus granule neurons: Involvement in a glucocorticoid receptor-dependent behavioural response. *European Journal of Neuroscience, 22*(7), 1691–1700.

Bird, A. (2002). DNA methylation patterns and epigenetic memory. *Genes & Development, 16*(1), 6–21.

Brooks, W. H., Le Dantec, C., Jaques-Olivier, P., Youinou, P., & Renaudineau, Y. (2010). Epigenetics and autoimmunity. *Journal of Autoimmunity, 34*(3), J207–J219.

Bultman, S. J., Gebuhr, T. C., & Magnuson, T. (2005). A Brg1 mutation that uncouples ATPase activity from chromatin remodeling reveals an essential role for SWI/SNF-related complexes in beta-globin expression and erythroid development. *Genes & Development, 19*(23), 2849–2861.

Champagne, F. A. (2008). Epigenetic mechanisms and the transgenerational effects of maternal care. *Frontiers in Neuroendocrinology, 29*(3), 386–397.

Champagne, F. A., Weaver, I. C., Diorio, J., Dymov, S., Szyf, M., & Meaney, M. J. (2006). Maternal care associated with methylation of the estrogen receptor-alpha1b promoter and estrogen receptor-alpha expression in the medial preoptic area of female offspring. *Endocrinology, 147*(6), 2909–2915.

Chandramohan, Y., Droste, S. K., Arthur, J. S., & Reul, J. M. (2008). The forced swimming-induced behavioural immobility response involves histone H3 phospho-acetylation and c-Fos induction in dentate gyrus granule neurons via activation of the N-methyl-D-aspartate/extracellular signal-regulated kinase/mitogen- and stress-activated kinase signalling pathway. *European Journal of Neuroscience, 27*(10), 2701–2713.

Charney, D. S. (2004). Psychobiological mechanisms of resilience and vulnerability: Implications for successful adaptation to extreme stress. *American Journal of Psychiatry, 161*(2), 195–216.

Chen, J., & Berry, M. J. (2003). Selenium and selenoproteins in the brain and brain diseases. *Journal of Neurochemistry, 86*(1), 1–12.

Cheung, P., Allis, C. D., & Sassone-Corsi, P. (2000). Signaling to chromatin through histone modifications. *Cell, 103*(2), 263–271.

Chorpita, B. F., & Barlow, D. H. (1998). The development of anxiety: The role of control in the early environment. *Psychology Bulletin, 124*(1), 3–21.

Cianfarani, S., Geremia, C., Scott, C. D., & Germani, D. (2002). Growth, IGF system, and cortisol in children with intrauterine growth retardation: Is catch-up growth affected by reprogramming of the hypothalamic-pituitary-adrenal axis? *Pediatric Research, 51*(1), 94–99.

Clavarino, A. M., Mamun, A. A., O'Callaghan, M., Aird, R., Bor, W., O'Callaghan, F., et al. (2010). Maternal anxiety and attention problems in children at 5 and 14 years. *Journal of Attention Disorders, 13*(6), 658–667.

Cohen-Cory, S., Kidane, A. H., Shirkey, N. J., & Marshak, S. (2010). Brain-derived neurotrophic factor and the development of structural neuronal connectivity. *Developmental Neurobiology, 70*(5), 271–288.

Conrad, C. D. (2008). Chronic stress-induced hippocampal vulnerability: The glucocorticoid vulnerability hypothesis. *Reviews in the Neurosciences, 19*(6), 395–411.

Corbett, B. A., Mendoza, S., Abdullah, M., Wegelin, J. A., & Levine, S. (2006). Cortisol circadian rhythms and response to stress in children with autism. *Psychoneuroendocrinology, 31*(1), 59–68.

Cosgrove, M. S., & Wolberger, C. (2005). How does the histone code work? *Biochemistry and Cell Biology, 83*(4), 468–476.

Costa, F. F. (2008). Non-coding RNAs, epigenetics and complexity. *Gene, 410*(1), 9–17.

Cottrell, E. C., & Seckl, J. R. (2009). Prenatal stress, glucocorticoids and the programming of adult disease. *Frontiers in Behavioral Neuroscience, 3*, 1–9.

Dantzer, R., O'Connor, J. C., Freund, G. G., Johnson, R. W., & Kelley, K. W. (2008). From inflammation to sickness and depression: When the immune system subjugates the brain. *Nature Reviews Neuroscience, 9*(1), 46–56.

De Bellis, M. D. (2005). The psychobiology of neglect. *Child Maltreatment, 10*(2), 150–172.

de Kloet, E. R., Joels, M., & Holsboer, F. (2005). Stress and the brain: From adaptation to disease. *Nature Reviews Neuroscience, 6*(6), 463–475.

Delcuve, G. P., Rastegar, M., & Davie, J. R. (2009). Epigenetic control. *Journal of Cellular Physiology, 219*(2), 243–250.

De Pablo, J. M., Parra, A., Segovia, S., & Guillanon, A. (1989). Learned immobility explains the behavior of rats in the forced swim test. *Physiology & Behavior, 46*, 229–237.

Egger, K., Schocke, M., Weiss, E., Auffinger, S., Esterhammer, R., Goebel, G., et al. (2008). Pattern of brain atrophy in elderly patients with depression revealed by voxel-based morphometry. *Psychiatry Research, 164*(3), 237–244.

Faller, M., & Guo, F. (2008). MicroRNA biogenesis: There's more than one way to skin a cat. *Biochimica et Biophysica Acta, 1779*(11), 663–667.

Feder, A., Nestler, E. J., & Charney, D. S. (2009). Psychobiology and molecular genetics of resilience. *Nature Reviews Neuroscience, 10*(6), 446–457.

Feinberg, A. P. (2008). Epigenetics at the epicenter of modern medicine. *Journal of the American Medical Association, 299*(11), 1345–1350.

Feinberg, A. P. (2010). Genome-scale approaches to the epigenetics of common human disease. *Virchows Archiv, 456*(1), 13–21.

Feldman, R., Eidelman, A. I., Sirota, L., & Weller, A. (2002). Comparison of skin-to-skin (kangaroo) and traditional care: Parenting outcomes and preterm infant development. *Pediatrics, 110*(1 Pt 1), 16–26.

Feldman, R., Singer, M., & Zagoory, O. (2010). Touch attenuates infants' physiological reactivity to stress. *Developmental Science, 13*(2), 271–278.

Felitti, V. J., Anda, R. F., Nordenberg, D., Williamson, D. F., Spitz, A. M., Edwards, V., et al. (1998). Relationship of childhood abuse and household dysfunction to many of the leading causes of death in adults. The Adverse Childhood Experiences (ACE) Study. *American Journal of Preventive Medicine, 14*(4), 245–258.

Ferber, S. G., Feldman, R., & Makhoul, I. R. (2008). The development of maternal touch across the first year of life. *Early Human Development, 84*(6), 363–370.

Field, T., Diego, M., Dieter, J., Hernandez-Reif, M., Schanberg, S., Kuhn, C., et al. (2004). Prenatal depression effects on the fetus and neonate. *Infant Behavior and Development, 27*, 216–229.

Field, T., Diego, M., & Hernandez-Reif, M. (2006). Prenatal depression effects on the fetus and newborn: A review. *Infant Behavior and Development, 29*(3), 445–455.

First, M. B. (Ed.). (2000). *Diagnostic and statistical manual of mental disorders* (4th ed.). Washington, DC: American Psychiatric Association.

Flinn, M. V. (1999). Family environment, stress, and health during childhood. In C. Panter-Brick & C. Worthman (Eds.), *Hormones, health, and behavior* (pp. 105–138). Cambridge, UK: Cambridge University Press.

Foley, D. L., Craig, J. M., Morley, R., Olsson, C. A., Dwyer, T., Smith, K., et al. (2009). Prospects for epigenetic epidemiology. *American Journal of Epidemiology, 169*(4), 389–400.

Francis, D., Diorio, J., Liu, D., & Meaney, M. J. (1999). Nongenomic transmission across generations of maternal behavior and stress responses in the rat. *Science, 286*(5442), 1155–1158.

Fumagalli, F., Molteni, R., Racagni, G., & Riva, M. A. (2007). Stress during development: Impact on neuroplasticity and relevance to psychopathology. *Progress in Neurobiology, 81*(4), 197–217.

Giedd, J. N., Blumenthal, J., Jeffries, N. O., Rajapakse, J. C., Vaituzis, A. C., Liu, H., et al. (1999). Development of the human corpus callosum during childhood and adolescence: A longitudinal MRI study. *Progress in Neuro-Psychopharmacology & Biological Psychiatry, 23*(4), 571–588.

Gould, E., McEwen, B. S., Tanapat, P., Galea, L. A., & Fuchs, E. (1997). Neurogenesis in the dentate gyrus of the adult tree shrew is regulated by psychosocial stress and NMDA receptor activation. *Journal of Neuroscience, 17*(7), 2492–2498.

Gould, E., Tanapat, P., McEwen, B. S., Flugge, G., & Fuchs, E. (1998). Proliferation of granule cell precursors in the dentate gyrus of adult monkeys is diminished by stress. *Proceedings of the National Academy of Science USA, 95*(6), 3168–3171.

Gutteling, B. M., de Weerth, C., Zandbelt, N., Mulder, E. J., Visser, G. H., & Buitelaar, J. K. (2006). Does maternal prenatal stress adversely affect the child's learning and memory at age six? *Journal of Abnormal Child Psychology, 34*(6), 789–798.

Haberland, M., Montgomery, R. L., & Olson, E. N. (2009). The many roles of histone deacetylases in development and physiology: Implications for disease and therapy. *Nature Reviews Genetics, 10*(1), 32–42.

Harlow, H. (1958). The nature of love. *American Psychologist, 13,* 673–685.

Hebbar, P. B., & Archer, T. K. (2007). Chromatin-dependent cooperativity between site-specific transcription factors in vivo. *Journal of Biological Chemistry, 282*(11), 8284–8291.

Heim, C., & Nemeroff, C. B. (2001). The role of childhood trauma in the neurobiology of mood and anxiety disorders: Preclinical and clinical studies. *Biological Psychiatry, 49*(12), 1023–1039.

Heim, C., Newport, D. J., Mletzko, T., Miller, A. H., & Nemeroff, C. B. (2008). The link between childhood trauma and depression: Insights from HPA axis studies in humans. *Psychoneuroendocrinology, 33*(6), 693–710.

Heim, C., Young, L. J., Newport, D. J., Mletzko, T., Miller, A. H., & Nemeroff, C. B. (2009). Lower CSF oxytocin concentrations in women with a history of childhood abuse. *Molecular Psychiatry, 14*(10), 954–958.

Hollander, E., Bartz, J., Chaplin, W., Phillips, A., Sumner, J., Soorya, L., et al. (2007). Oxytocin increases retention of social cognition in autism. *Biological Psychiatry, 61*(4), 498–503.

Hollander, E., Novotny, S., Hanratty, M., Yaffe, R., DeCaria, C. M., Aronowitz, B. R., et al. (2003). Oxytocin infusion reduces repetitive behaviors in adults with autistic and Asperger's disorders. *Neuropsychopharmacology, 28*(1), 193–198.

Human Epigenome Consortium. (n.d.). *Human Epigenome Project.* Retrieved July 15, 2010, from http://www.epigenome.org/

Hunter, R. G., McCarthy, K. J., Milne, T. A., Pfaff, D. W., & McEwen, B. S. (2009). Regulation of hippocampal H3 histone methylation by acute and chronic stress. *Proceedings of the National Academy of Sciences USA, 106*(49), 20912–20917.

Jenuwein, T., & Allis, C. D. (2001). Translating the histone code. *Science, 293*(5532), 1074–1080.

Johnson, J. G., Cohen, P., Kasen, S., Smailes, E., & Brook, J. S. (2001). Association of maladaptive parental behavior with psychiatric disorder among parents and their offspring. *Archives of General Psychiatry, 58*(5), 453–460.

Kaminsky, Z., Wang, S. C., & Petronis, A. (2006). Complex disease, gender and epigenetics. *Annals of Medicine, 38*(8), 530–544.

Kilgore, M., Miller, C. A., Fass, D. M., Hennig, K. M., Haggarty, S. J., Sweatt, J. D., et al. (2010). Inhibitors of class 1 histone deacetylases reverse contextual memory deficits in a mouse model of Alzheimer's disease. *Neuropsychopharmacology, 35*(4), 870–880.

Klose, R. J., & Zhang, Y. (2007). Regulation of histone methylation by demethylimination and demethylation. *Nature Reviews Molecular Cell Biology, 8*(4), 307–318.

Kouzarides, T. (2007). Chromatin modifications and their function. *Cell, 128*(4), 693–705.

Krukowski, K., Eddy, J., Kosik, K. L., Konley, T., Janusek, L. W., & Mathews, H. L. (2011). Glucocorticoid dysregulation of natural killer cell function through epigenetic modification. *Brain, Behavior, and Immunity, 25*(2), 239–249.

LaFerla, F. M., Green, K. N., & Oddo, S. (2007). Intracellular amyloid-beta in Alzheimer's disease. *Nature Reviews Neuroscience, 8*(7), 499–509.

Lahiri, D. K., Maloney, B., & Zawia, N. H. (2009). The LEARn model: An epigenetic explanation for idiopathic neurobiological diseases. *Molecular Psychiatry, 14*(11), 992–1003.

Landfield, P. W., Blalock, E. M., Chen, K. C., & Porter, N. M. (2007). A new glucocorticoid hypothesis of brain aging: Implications for Alzheimer's disease. *Current Alzheimer Research, 4*(2), 205–212.

Lee, A. L., Ogle, W. O., & Sapolsky, R. M. (2002). Stress and depression: Possible links to neuron death in the hippocampus. *Bipolar Disorders, 4*(2), 117–128.

Levenson, J. M., & Sweatt, J. D. (2005). Epigenetic mechanisms in memory formation. *Nature Reviews Neuroscience, 6*(2), 108–118.

Lewis, B. P., Burge, C. B., & Bartel, D. P. (2005). Conserved seed pairing, often flanked by adenosines, indicates that thousands of human genes are microRNA targets. *Cell, 120*(1), 15–20.

Li, E. (2002). Chromatin modification and epigenetic reprogramming in mammalian development. *Nature Reviews Genetics, 3*(9), 662–673.

Lincoln, J. A., & Cook, S. D. (2009). An overview of gene-epigenetic-environmental contributions to MS causation. *Journal of the Neurological Sciences, 286*(1–2), 54–57.

Liu, D., Diorio, J., Tannenbaum, B., Caldji, C., Francis, D., Freedman, A., et al. (1997). Maternal care, hippocampal glucocorticoid receptors, and hypothalamic-pituitary-adrenal responses to stress. *Science, 277*(5332), 1659–1662.

Liu, R. T. (2010). Early life stressors and genetic influences on the development of bipolar disorder: The roles of childhood abuse and brain-derived neurotrophic factor. *Child Abuse & Neglect, 34*(7), 516–522.

Lorch, Y., Maier-Davis, B., & Kornberg, R. D. (2006). Chromatin remodeling by nucleosome disassembly in vitro. *Proceedings of the National Academy of Sciences USA, 103*(9), 3090–3093.

Lupien, S. J., McEwen, B. S., Gunnar, M. R., & Heim, C. (2009). Effects of stress throughout the lifespan on the brain, behaviour and cognition. *Nature Reviews Neuroscience, 10*(6), 434–445.

Magarinos, A. M., & McEwen, B. S. (1995). Stress-induced atrophy of apical dendrites of hippocampal CA3c neurons: Comparison of stressors. *Neuroscience, 69*(1), 83–88.

Magarinos, A. M., McEwen, B. S., Flugge, G., & Fuchs, E. (1996). Chronic psychosocial stress causes apical dendritic atrophy of hippocampal CA3 pyramidal neurons in subordinate tree shrews. *Journal of Neuroscience, 16*(10), 3534–3540.

Main, M., Kaplan, N., & Cassidy, J. (1985). Security in infancy, childhood, and adulthood: A move to the level of representation. In I. Bretherton & E. Waters (Eds.), *Growing points of attachment theory and research: Monographs of the society for research in child development* (Vol. 50, pp. 66–104).

Malberg, J. E., Eisch, A. J., Nestler, E. J., & Duman, R. S. (2000). Chronic antidepressant treatment increases neurogenesis in adult rat hippocampus. *Journal of Neuroscience, 20*(24), 9104–9110.

Martino, D. J., & Prescott, S. L. (2010). Silent mysteries: Epigenetic paradigms could hold the key to conquering the epidemic of allergy and immune disease. *Allergy, 65*(1), 7–15.

Mathews, H. L., & Witek Janusek, L. (2011). Epigenetics and psychoneuroimmunology: Mechanisms and models. *Brain, Behavior, and Immunity, 25*(1), 25–39.

Mathews, H. L., Konley, T., Kosik, K. L., Krukowski, K., Eddy, J., Albuquerque, K., & Janusek, L. W. (2011). Epigenetic patterns associated with the immune dysregulation that accompanies psychosocial distress. *Brain, Behavior, and Immunity, 25*(5), 830–839.

McEwen, B. S. (2001). Plasticity of the hippocampus: Adaptation to chronic stress and allostatic load. *Annals of the New York Academy of Sciences, 933*, 265–277.

McEwen, B. S., Gould, E. A., & Sakai, R. R. (1992). The vulnerability of the hippocampus to protective and destructive effects of glucocorticoids in relation to stress. *British Journal of Psychiatry Supplement, 15*, 18–23.

McGowan, P. O., Sasaki, A., D'Alessio, A. C., Dymov, S., Labonte, B., Szyf, M., et al. (2009). Epigenetic regulation of the glucocorticoid receptor in human brain associates with childhood abuse. *Nature Neuroscience, 12*(3), 342–348.

Mendell, J. T. (2005). MicroRNAs: Critical regulators of development, cellular physiology and malignancy. *Cell Cycle, 4*(9), 1179–1184.

Mesulam, M. M. (1999). Neuroplasticity failure in Alzheimer's disease: Bridging the gap between plaques and tangles. *Neuron, 24*(3), 521–529.

Mikkelsen, T. S., Ku, M., Jaffe, D. B., Issac, B., Lieberman, E., Giannoukos, G., et al. (2007). Genome-wide maps of chromatin state in pluripotent and lineage-committed cells. *Nature, 448*(7153), 553–560.

Miller, L., Kramer, R., Warner, V., Wickramaratne, P., & Weissman, M. (1997). Intergenerational transmission of parental bonding among women. *Journal of the American Academy of Child and Adolescent Psychiatry, 36*(8), 1134–1139.

Miranda, T. B., & Jones, P. A. (2007). DNA methylation: The nuts and bolts of repression. *Journal of Cellular Physiology, 213*(2), 384–390.

Moazed, D. (2009). Small RNAs in transcriptional gene silencing and genome defence. *Nature, 457*(7228), 413–420.

Moeller, T. P., Bachmann, G. A., & Moeller, J. R. (1993). The combined effects of physical, sexual, and emotional abuse during childhood: Long-term health consequences for women. *Child Abuse & Neglect, 17*(5), 623–640.

Morelius, E., Theodorsson, E., & Nelson, N. (2005). Salivary cortisol and mood and pain profiles during skin-to-skin care for an unselected group of mothers and infants in neonatal intensive care. *Pediatrics, 116*(5), 1105–1113.

Morgan, A. L., Tobar, D. A., & Snyder, L. (2010). Walking toward a new me: The impact of prescribed walking 10,000 steps/day on physical and psychological well-being. *Journal of Physical Activity & Health, 7*(3), 299–307.

Moszkowski, R. J., Stack, D. M., & Chiarella, S. S. (2009). Infant touch with gaze and affective behaviors during mother-infant still-face interactions: Co-occurrence and functions of touch. *Infant Behavior and Development, 32*(4), 392–403.

Nan, X., Ng, H. H., Johnson, C. A., Laherty, C. D., Turner, B. M., Eisenman, R. N., et al. (1998). Transcriptional repression by the methyl-CpG-binding protein MeCP2 involves a histone deacetylase complex. *Nature, 393*(6683), 386–389.

Nestler, E. J., & Carlezon, W. A., Jr. (2006). The mesolimbic dopamine reward circuit in depression. *Biological Psychiatry, 59*(12), 1151–1159.

Ng, K., Pullirsch, D., Leeb, M., & Wutz, A. (2007). Xist and the order of silencing. *EMBO Reports, 8*(1), 34–39.

Noll, J. G., Trickett, P. K., Harris, W. W., & Putnam, F. W. (2009). The cumulative burden borne by offspring whose mothers were sexually abused as children: Descriptive results from a multigenerational study. *Journal of Interpersonal Violence, 24*(3), 424–449.

Oberlander, T. F., Weinberg, J., Papsdorf, M., Grunau, R., Misri, S., & Devlin, A. M. (2008). Prenatal exposure to maternal depression, neonatal methylation of human glucocorticoid receptor gene (NR3C1) and infant cortisol stress responses. *Epigenetics, 3*(2), 97–106.

Peleg, S., Sananbenesi, F., Zovoilis, A., Burkhardt, S., Bahari-Javan, S., Agis-Balboa, R. C., et al. (2010). Altered histone acetylation is associated with age-dependent memory impairment in mice. *Science, 328*(5979), 753–756.

Pendry, P., & Adam, E. K. (2007). Associations between Parents' Marital Functioning, Maternal Parenting Quality, Maternal Emotion and Child Cortisol Levels. *International Journal of Behavioral Development, 31*(3), 218–231.

Penner, M. R., Roth, T. L., Barnes, C. A., & Sweatt, J. D. (2010). An epigenetic hypothesis of aging-related cognitive dysfunction. *Frontiers in Aging Neuroscience, 2*, 9.

Peterson, C. L., & Laniel, M. A. (2004). Histones and histone modifications. *Current Biology, 14*(14), R546–551.

Plotsky, P. M., Thrivikraman, K. V., Nemeroff, C. B., Caldji, C., Sharma, S., & Meaney, M. J. (2005). Long-term consequences of neonatal rearing on central corticotropin-releasing factor systems in adult male rat offspring. *Neuropsychopharmacology, 30*(12), 2192–2204.

Previc, F. H. (2007). Prenatal influences on brain dopamine and their relevance to the rising incidence of autism. *Medical Hypotheses, 68*(1), 46–60.

Pruessner, J. C., Champagne, F., Meaney, M. J., & Dagher, A. (2004). Dopamine release in response to a psychological stress in humans and its relationship to early life maternal care: A positron emission tomography study using [11C]raclopride. *Journal of Neuroscience, 24*(11), 2825–2831.

Razin, A. (1998). CpG methylation, chromatin structure and gene silencing—A three-way connection. *EMBO Journal, 17*(17), 4905–4908.

Roth, T. L., Lubin, F. D., Funk, A. J., & Sweatt, J. D. (2009). Lasting epigenetic influence of early-life adversity on the BDNF gene. *Biological Psychiatry, 65*(9), 760–769.

Roth, T. L., & Sweatt, J. D. (2009). Regulation of chromatin structure in memory formation. *Current Opinion in Neurobiology, 19*(3), 336–342.

Roth, T. L., & Sweatt, J. D. (2010). Epigenetic marking of the BDNF gene by early-life adverse experiences. *Hormones and Behavior.*

Sapolsky, R. M. (2000). Glucocorticoids and hippocampal atrophy in neuropsychiatric disorders. *Arch Gen Psychiatry, 57*(10), 925–935.

Sapolsky, R. M., Krey, L. C., & McEwen, B. S. (1984). Glucocorticoid-sensitive hippocampal neurons are involved in terminating the adrenocortical stress response. *Proceedings of the National Academy of the Sciences USA, 81*(19), 6174–6177.

Schlinzig, T., Johansson, S., Gunnar, A., Ekstrom, T. J., & Norman, M. (2009). Epigenetic modulation at birth—altered DNA-methylation in white blood cells after Caesarean section. *Acta Paediatrica, 98*(7), 1096–1099.

Seckl, J. R., & Meaney, M. J. (2006). Glucocorticoid "programming" and PTSD risk. *Annals of the New York Academy of Sciences, 1071*, 351–378.

Sedivy, J. M., Banumathy, G., & Adams, P. D. (2008). Aging by epigenetics—a consequence of chromatin damage? *Experimental Cell Research, 314*(9), 1909–1917.

Segman, R. H., Shefi, N., Goltser-Dubner, T., Friedman, N., Kaminski, N., & Shalev, A. Y. (2005). Peripheral blood mononuclear cell gene expression profiles identify emergent post-traumatic stress disorder among trauma survivors. *Molecular Psychiatry, 10*(5), 500–513, 425.

Sheline, Y. I., Gado, M. H., & Kraemer, H. C. (2003). Untreated depression and hippocampal volume loss. *American Journal of Psychiatry, 160*(8), 1516–1518.

Shi, X., Hong, T., Walter, K. L., Ewalt, M., Michishita, E., Hung, T., et al. (2006). ING2 PHD domain links histone H3 lysine 4 methylation to active gene repression. *Nature, 442*(7098), 96–99.

Spear, L. P. (2000). Neurobehavioral changes in adolescence. *Current Directions in Psychological Science, 9*(4), 111–114.

Sroufe, L. A. (2005). Attachment and development: A prospective, longitudinal study from birth to adulthood. *Attachment and Human Development, 7*(4), 349–367.

Strahl, B. D., & Allis, C. D. (2000). The language of covalent histone modifications. *Nature, 403*(6765), 41–45.

Teicher, M. H., Andersen, S. L., Polcari, A., Anderson, C. M., Navalta, C. P., & Kim, D. M. (2003). The neurobiological consequences of early stress and childhood maltreatment. *Neuroscience & Biobehavioral Reviews, 27*(1–2), 33–44.

Tremblay, L. K., Naranjo, C. A., Graham, S. J., Herrmann, N., Mayberg, H. S., Hevenor, S., et al. (2005). Functional neuroanatomical substrates of altered reward processing in major depressive disorder revealed by a dopaminergic probe. *Archives of General Psychiatry, 62*(11), 1228–1236.

Trenkmann, M., Brock, M., Ospelt, C., & Gay, S. (2010). Epigenetics in rheumatoid arthritis. *Clinical Reviews in Allergy and Immunology, 39*(1), 10–19.

Trickett, P. K., Noll, J. G., Susman, E. J., Shenk, C. E., & Putnam, F. W. (2010). Attenuation of cortisol across development for victims of sexual abuse. *Developmental Psychopathology, 22*(1), 165–175.

Trotter, K. W., & Archer, T. K. (2007). Nuclear receptors and chromatin remodeling machinery. *Molecular and Cellular Endocrinology, 265–266*, 162–167.

Tsankova, N. M., Berton, O., Renthal, W., Kumar, A., Neve, R. L., & Nestler, E. J. (2006). Sustained hippocampal chromatin regulation in a mouse model of depression and antidepressant action. *Nature Neuroscience, 9*(4), 519–525.

Turek-Plewa, J., & Jagodzinski, P. P. (2005). The role of mammalian DNA methyltransferases in the regulation of gene expression. *Cellular and Molecular Biology Letters, 10*(4), 631–647.

Turunen, M. P., Aavik, E., & Yla-Herttuala, S. (2009). Epigenetics and atherosclerosis. *Biochimica et Biophysica Acta, 1790*(9), 886–891.

Uchida, S., Nishida, A., Hara, K., Kamemoto, T., Suetsugi, M., Fujimoto, M., et al. (2008). Characterization of the vulnerability to repeated stress in Fischer 344 rats: Possible involvement of microRNA-mediated down-regulation of the glucocorticoid receptor. *Eur Journal of Neuroscience, 27*(9), 2250–2261.

Uddin, M., Aiello, A. E., Wildman, D. E., Koenen, K. C., Pawelec, G., de Los Santos, R., et al. (2010). Epigenetic and immune function profiles associated with posttraumatic stress disorder. *Proceedings of the National Academy of Sciences of the United States of America, 107*(20), 9470–9475.

Uddin, M., Koenen, K.C., Aiello, A.E., Wildman, D.E., de los Santos, R., & Galea, S. (in press). Epigenetic and inflammatory marker profiles associated with depression in a community-based epidemiologic sample. *Psychological Medicine.*

Walker, E. F., Walder, D. J., & Reynolds, F. (2001). Developmental changes in cortisol secretion in normal and at-risk youth. *Development and Psychopathology, 13*(3), 721–732.

Weaver, I. C., Cervoni, N., Champagne, F. A., D'Alessio, A. C., Sharma, S., Seckl, J. R., et al. (2004). Epigenetic programming by maternal behavior. *Nature Neuroscience, 7*(8), 847–854.

Weaver, I. C., Champagne, F. A., Brown, S. E., Dymov, S., Sharma, S., Meaney, M. J., et al. (2005). Reversal of maternal programming of stress responses in adult offspring through methyl supplementation: Altering epigenetic marking later in life. *Journal of Neuroscience, 25*(47), 11045–11054.

Weaver, I. C., Meaney, M. J., & Szyf, M. (2006). Maternal care effects on the hippocampal transcriptome and anxiety-mediated behaviors in the offspring that are reversible in adulthood. *Proceedings of the National Academy of Sciences USA, 103*(9), 3480–3485.

Wilkinson, M. B., Xiao, G., Kumar, A., LaPlant, Q., Renthal, W., Sikder, D., et al. (2009). Imipramine treatment and resiliency exhibit similar chromatin regulation in the mouse nucleus accumbens in depression models. *Journal of Neuroscience, 29*(24), 7820–7832.

Winberg, J. (2005). Mother and newborn baby: Mutual regulation of physiology and behavior—a selective review. *Developmental Psychobiology, 47*(3), 217–229.

Wutz, A. (2007). Xist function: Bridging chromatin and stem cells. *Trends in Genetics, 23*(9), 457–464.

Yamasue, H., Kuwabara, H., Kawakubo, Y., & Kasai, K. (2009). Oxytocin, sexually dimorphic features of the social brain, and autism. *Psychiatry and Clinical Neurosciences, 63*(2), 129–140.

Zelazo, P. R. (2001). A Developmental Perspective on Early Autism: Affective, Behavioral, and Cognitive Factors. In J. A. Burack, T. Charman, N. Yirmiya & P. R. Zelazo (Eds.), *The Development of Autism: Perspectives from Theory and Research* (pp. 39–60). Mahwah, NJ: Lawrence Erlbaum Associates.

Zhang, T. Y., & Meaney, M. J. (2010). Epigenetics and the environmental regulation of the genome and its function. *Annual Review of Psychology, 61*, 439–466, C431–433.

Zhang, Y., Ng, H. H., Erdjument-Bromage, H., Tempst, P., Bird, A., & Reinberg, D. (1999). Analysis of the NuRD subunits reveals a histone deacetylase core complex and a connection with DNA methylation. *Genes & Development, 13*(15), 1924–1935.

5

Physiological Measurement(s) of the Stress Response

Jill M. Winters

Many renowned scholars have attempted to describe and delineate stress. Although Cannon (1939) did not directly define it, he discussed stress as the results of increased sympathetic nervous system activity and a compensatory process in response to aversive or threatening situations. This increased sympathetic nervous system activity reflects an effort to regain a sense of homeostasis. Years later, Hans Selye, a world-renowned endocrinologist, popularized stress as a scientific and medical phenomenon. He described stress as *the nonspecific response of the body to any demands placed on it* (Selye, 1974). This response enables the body to resist stressors by enhancing the adaptive function of its systems. Changes from the normal resting state can occur in cognitions, emotions, behaviors, physiologic functioning, or all of these. This chapter addresses a variety of means to measure the stress response.

A normally functioning stress-response system interprets and integrates numerous incoming signals and responds accordingly. These signals may originate from the external environment or the internal milieu. When these signals are interpreted as threatening to the organism, a stress response ensues with resultant activation of the autonomic nervous system, the sympatho-adreno-medullary system, the hypothalamic-pituitary-adrenal-cortical

system, the immune system, or all of these (Guyton & Hall, 2006; Porth & Mattfin, 2009) (Figure 5.1). This response results in hypothalamic neurons containing corticotrophin-releasing factor increasing the release of corticotropin (ACTH), β-endorphin, and other pro-opiomalancortin products from the anterior pituitary gland (Musselman, Rudisch, McDonald, & Nemeroff, 2004). The effects are further modulated by various neuropeptides, vagal (parasympathetic) outflow, circadian influences, adaptive strategies, genetic factors, and the presence of disease or defects.

Three categories of human reaction have been described: (a) effort without distress, (b) effort with distress, and (c) distress without effort (Frankenhaeuser, 1983; Peters et al., 1998). Effort without distress occurs during complex coping attempts with a stressor (Frankenhaeuser, 1983). The sympathoadreno-medullary system is activated with increases in heart rate and blood pressure, as well as releases of epinephrine and norepinephrine (Frankenhaeuser, 1983; Henry, 1992; Peters et al., 1998). In contrast, activation of the hypothalamic-pituitary-adrenal-cortical system is associated with distress without effort. In this situation, the individual's inability to cope, feelings of helplessness, and perceptions of powerlessness (Peters et al., 1998; Weiner, 1992) result in the release of adrenocorticotrophic hormone (ACTH) and cortisol (Weiner, 1992), with associated increases in blood pressure and total peripheral resistance and reductions in heart rate and cardiac output. Situations involving effort with distress would activate both systems simultaneously (Frankenhaeuser, 1983).

Physiologic manifestations of the stress response can be measured by a variety of methods, many of which include the use of bioinstrumentation techniques or biochemical analyses. Bioinstrumentation methods such as electrocardiograph recording equipment or blood pressure monitoring machines are commonly used to measure cardiovascular responses to stress. Many of the biochemical analyses incorporate the use of chromatography, radioimmunoassay, or enzyme-linked immunoabsorbent assay to study neuroendocrine or immune system manifestations of stress. Many of these methods require expensive supplies and equipment. Some methods involve invasive procedures and can introduce additional stress to the experimental situation. The insertion of a needle to draw blood, for example, can introduce an element of both physiological and psychological stress. All techniques require thorough understanding of the procedure and underlying theoretical base of the measure employed.

Although many authors have extolled the high degree of objectivity, reliability, and validity associated with physiological measures (Polit & Beck, 2007; Waltz, Strickland, & Lenz, 2010; Woods & Cantanzaro, 1988), measurement error remains a prominent concern. Investigators choosing to use physiological measures of the stress response must attend closely to issues of validity, reliability, selectivity, sensitivity, specificity, cost, and availability.

When physiological measures are employed, reliability is directly related to the precision of the method, consistency of the measurements with repeated sampling, and the reproducibility of the measurements made by the method. Measures of reliability reflect the amount of random error introduced into the measurements (Waltz et al., 2010). *Validity* reflects the difference

Figure 5.1   Stress Response

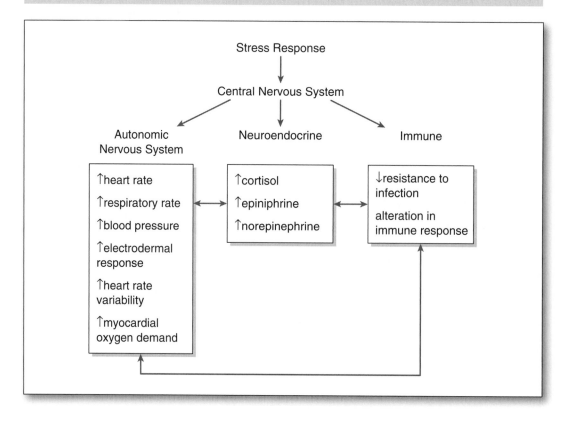

between a given value and the true value and whether the measure is carrying out its intended purpose. Closely related to validity are the concepts of selectivity, sensitivity, and specificity. The ability of an instrument to identify signals under study correctly and to distinguish them from all other signals is known as *selectivity* (Rubin, 1987). *Sensitivity* can be interpreted two different ways, depending on the type of physiological measurement being used. For example, when bioinstrumentation is used, sensitivity refers to the smallest amount of change in a parameter or variable that can be detected or measured precisely (Cromwell, Weibell, & Pfeiffer, 1980). In a clinical laboratory situation, sensitivity generally is defined as the likelihood that an individual with a given condition will have a positive test result (Waltz et al., 2010). In contrast, *specificity* refers to the probability that an individual without a specified condition will have a negative test result. The levels of validity, selectivity, sensitivity, and specificity provide information about systematic error introduced by a particular method of measurement. For additional reading with respect to these factors, several authors have provided excellent discussions (Burns, 2009; Shadish, Cook, & Campbell, 2001; Cromwell et al., 1980; Polit & Beck, 2007; Rubin, 1987; Waltz et al., 2010; Woods & Cantanzaro, 1988).

AUTONOMIC NERVOUS SYSTEM MEASURES OF THE STRESS RESPONSE

The first physiological axis to become activated during the stress response is the autonomic nervous system. During a stress response, the balance between sympathetic and parasympathetic activity is disrupted, with sympathetic nervous system activity being dominant. Activation of the sympathetic nervous system is oriented toward performance, with little regard to the physiological "costs" of this demand. The primary neurotransmitter that is released is norepinephrine, resulting in increased heart rate, blood pressure, blood glucose levels, pupil dilation, bronchial dilation and respiratory rate, and myocardial oxygen (MVO_2) consumption. At the same time, reductions in heart rate variability, gastric motility, pancreatic activity, and blood flow to the skin, stomach, and kidneys occur.

The primary autonomic nervous system indicators of the stress response used in research are heart rate, respiratory rate, blood pressure, heart rate variability, cardiac output, and electrodermal activity. In addition, rate pressure product has been used as a reliable noninvasive indicator of myocardial oxygen demand. Recently, impedance cardiography has been employed to determine noninvasive estimates of cardiac output and peripheral vascular resistance.

Measurement of Heart Rate

Heart rate refers to the number of ventricular contractions per minute. Measurement of heart rate can be accomplished by use of electrocardiographic equipment that records the electrical events associated with cardiac contraction or through methods that trace the pulse wave that is generated as blood is ejected from the heart with each contraction. Heart rate also can be determined by auscultation with a stethoscope over the chest wall. Accuracy of this method depends on correct detection of heart sounds and time keeping. Another approach to measuring heart rate is palpation of peripheral pulses. Reliability of this method is dependent on perfusion of ventricular contractions to the periphery and on precise identification and counting of pulse waves. In human stress research, heart rate should be regarded as a highly labile state-dependent measure. When using heart rate as an indicator of autonomic nervous system activity in stress research, consideration must be given to the impact of circadian variation, body position, environmental conditions, and medications.

Electrocardiographic Methods

Passive electrocardiogram (ECG) provides a graphic display or recording or both of the time-variant voltages produced by the myocardium during the cardiac cycle. To record ECG data, electrodes are affixed to the body. The electrodes are connected to an ECG machine, telemetry box, or Holter recorder by means of lead wires. When examining the ECG recording, the QRS complex corresponds with ventricular depolarization. In a normally functioning heart, ventricular depolarization results in contraction of the ventricles. Under pathological conditions, QRS complexes may not have a corresponding peripheral pulse wave. Many types of ECG monitoring equipment provide a digital display of heart rate. The computer-generated digitally displayed heart rate, however, is dependent on accurate detection of QRS complexes, and the displayed numbers represent an average heart rate from a given sampling period. A more reliable method involves generating a hard copy of one minute of ECG data and having the investigator identify and tabulate the number of ventricular depolarizations recorded during a given time frame. A decision must be made regarding inclusion of ectopic complexes. Placement of electrodes, condition of lead wires, and movement of the individual under study can produce artifact, making interpretation of the ECG complexes more difficult (LeWinter & Osol, 2004).

Pulse Wave Methods

Examination of the pulse wave can be accomplished in a variety of ways: (a) photoplysmography, (b) audiometry, and (c) oscillometry. Photoelectric plethysmography involves the application of a light source in an opaque chamber that transmits light through a fingertip or other body region to which the transducer is applied. Light is scattered and transmitted through the capillaries of the region and sensed by the photocell, which is shielded from all other light. With each pulse wave, the capillaries are filled with blood and the blood density increases, thereby reducing the amount of light reaching the photocell. Resistance changes are sensed by the photocell and can be measured and recorded. This type of measurement is limited primarily to detecting pulsations in the finger. In addition, the slightest movement of the finger with respect to the photocell or light source results in a severe amount of movement artifact. Moreover, if the light source produces heat, changes in local circulation beneath the light source and photocell may occur (Cromwell et al., 1980).

When audiometric methods are employed, a microphone is positioned over an artery to detect each pulse wave. In contrast, the oscillometric approach to measuring heart rate employs a pressure sensor that detects the distention of the arterial wall as a pulse wave moves through it. The brachial artery is the most frequently used artery for these purposes. These approaches generally are used in conjunction with blood pressure measurements, whereby the artery being sampled is compressed by an inflatable cuff. Compression of the artery produces more accurate sensing of the Korotkoff sounds

and arterial distentions (Everly & Sobelman, 1987). These methods introduce the potential for movement artifact. In addition, if the microphone or pressure sensor is not placed directly over the artery, pulse waves may not be detected accurately.

The optimal method for determining heart rate is by means of an ECG recording. This approach provides a hard copy of heart rate and allows for intrarater or interrater reliability checks or both. Because heart rate is a reflection of state-dependent changes, test-retest reliability is not appropriate. Heart rate measures have been used as indicators of psychological and physiological stress in many studies (Matsubara et al., 2011; McKay, Buen, Bohan, & Maye, 2010; Trappe, 2010).

Heart Rate Variability Measurement

In the absence of any neurohumoral influences, normal intrinsic heart rate is approximately 100 to 120 beats per minute (Hainsworth, 1995). With an intact, unblocked autonomic nervous system, heart rate provides a representation of the net effect of parasympathetic nervous system and sympathetic nervous system influences on the sinoatrial (SA) node. During normal resting periods, heart rate is primarily controlled by vagal (parasympathetic) influences (LeWinter & Osol, 2004). As vagal outflow increases, greater cardiac interbeat variability is evident. Conversely, with increased sympathetic nervous system arousal, a reduction in cardiac variability occurs (Fuller, 1992).

Traditionally, it has been suggested that normal sinus rhythm (NSR), with all intervals between successive QRS complexes (R-R intervals) nearly identical in duration, is the optimal cardiac rhythm. Respiratory sinus arrhythmia is an alteration in NSR that reflects the cholinergic influences on waxing and waning of SA node activity that is entrained to the respiratory rate as a result of afferent input from bronchopulmonary receptors (Grossman, vanBeek, & Wientjes, 1990). Today, it is accepted that respiratory sinus arrhythmia is the optimal heart rhythm, and beat-to-beat heart rate should not be completely regular.

Respiratory sinus arrhythmia is a major component of heart rate variability, and it reflects alterations in vagal function (Berntson, Cacioppo, & Quigley, 1993; Grossman et al., 1990; Saul &

Cohen, 1994). Heart rate varies in a phase relationship with inspiration and expiration. Vagal cardiometer neurons are inhibited during inspiration and appear to be mildly activated during the expiratory phase of respiration. In contrast, excitation of sympathetic motor neurons occurs during the inspiratory phase, whereas mild inhibition occurs during expiration (Richter & Spyer, 1990; Saul & Cohen, 1994). Therefore, heart rate is increased during inspiration and reduced during expiration. Both voluntary and involuntary alterations in respiratory patterns influence heart rate variability (Hirsch & Bishop, 1981).

Analysis of heart rate variability produces indirect measures of cardiovascular responsiveness to alterations in autonomic nervous system reactivity. Heart rate variability measures provide quantification of modulations in heart periods, or R-R intervals, resulting from cyclical fluctuations in autonomic nervous system control of the SA node. That is, heart rate variability analysis yields information about the variation from one cardiac cycle to the next. Distinct changes in heart rate are expected in response to physiological and mental stressors (Pagani et al., 1995).

To perform heart rate variability analyses, a continuous ECG recording and sophisticated computer software are required. The ECG recording must be examined, and the morphology of each QRS complex must be identified and categorized. Identification is accomplished by computer program, and data are edited by trained personnel. Then, either instantaneous heart rate or intervals between successive sinus QRS complexes are determined. When performing heart rate variability analysis, only sinus complexes are used. In the event that ECG complexes are generated from other areas of the cardiac conduction system, or short sequences of bad or missing data are identified, interpolation techniques generally are employed in heart rate variability determinations. Although other methods of heart rate variability analysis are sometimes used, time and frequency domain measures are employed most frequently.

Time Domain Measures of Heart Rate Variability

Time domain measures of heart rate variability are perhaps the simplest to perform and involve determination of either instantaneous heart rate or interval lengths between successive ECG complexes originating from depolarization of the SA node. Simple time domain measures generally are examined in many ways, including measurements of variance, standard deviations, log units, counts, and percentages.

Most time domain variables can be categorized into two classes—one based on interbeat intervals and the other on comparisons of adjacent cycle lengths (Hatch, Borcherding, & Norris, 1990). Interbeat interval-based measures are broad based and are influenced by both short-term (e.g., respiratory) and long-term (e.g., circadian) factors. Comparisons of adjacent cycle lengths are virtually independent of long-term trends and predominantly reflective of vagal tone (Kleiger et al., 1991). Measures based on interbeat intervals include standard deviation of all normal sinus R-R intervals (SDNN) and the standard deviation of 5-minute mean heart periods during a 24-hour period (SDANN). SDNN is sensitive to both short- and long-term variations, whereas SDANN is insensitive to short-term sources of variation.

The second category of time domain measures is based on the differences between lengths of adjacent cycles. This category includes the pNN50 and rMSSD. The pNN50 is a measure of the proportion of adjacent normal sinus R-R intervals of more than 50 ms. It is computed by examining triplets of normal complexes. Each triplet defines two adjacent coupling intervals. The difference between the two coupling intervals is compared to 50 ms, and a count is maintained. When the analysis has been completed, a proportion is computed and is expressed as a percentage. The rMSSD is the root mean square difference of successive normal sinus R-R intervals. It is determined by examining triplets of normal complexes as well. In this analysis, the difference between the two coupling intervals is squared and summed. Then, the sum is divided by the number of triplets, and the square root is determined. Both pNN50 and rMSSD are most sensitive to vagal influences.

Two other commonly employed time domain measures are the mean of all coupling intervals between normal complexes (mean NN) and the mean standard deviations of normal sinus R-R intervals of successive 5-minute blocks during a 24-hour period *(SD)*. The mean NN interval is determined by using only coupling intervals that contain no ectopy or noise. *SD* is less sensitive to posture and activity changes than SDANN but is sensitive to all other vagal influences. Furthermore, SDANN is sensitive to long-term changes, whereas *SD* is insensitive to circadian variations.

Frequency Domain Measures of Heart Rate Variability

Data analysis in the frequency domain is mathematically more complex than in the time domain. Frequency domain measurement, also known as power spectral analysis, provides information about the amount of overall variance in heart rate resulting from periodic oscillations of heart rate at various frequencies (Stein, Bosner, Kleiger, & Conger, 1994). Power spectral analysis breaks down the natural oscillations of heart rate into their component frequencies, and the amplitude or power of each oscillation is plotted over a range of frequencies. From the resultant frequency components, inferences can be drawn regarding the influence of physical activity, baroreceptors, and circadian rhythms (Akselrod et al., 1981; Ebert, 1992; Task Force, 1996).

When power spectral analysis is performed, the power of each contributing component is generally displayed over the frequency range of 0 to 0.5 Hz (Figure 5.2). When displayed in this manner, there are three primary frequencies of heart rate oscillations that contain the majority of the heart rate power: very-low-frequency (VLF), low-frequency (LF), and high-frequency (HF) bands. Power spectral densities can be examined over specified time periods, such as 2-minute, 1-hour, or 24-hour epochs. The VLF oscillations occur at frequencies ranging from 0 to 0.04 Hz. This band is the least understood of the three regions and is believed to reflect thermoregulatory feedback mechanisms (Hyndman, Kitney, & Sayers, 1971), reninangiotensin activity (Akselrod et al., 1981), and circulating neurohormone levels (Saul, 1990).

The LF component extends over the range of 0.04 to 0.15 Hz. This band reflects both sympathetic and vagal input to the heart (Akselrod et al., 1981; Ebert, 1992; Task Force, 1996). Both chemoreceptors and baroreceptors are involved in generating these oscillations.

The HF band appears to originate from the parasympathetic nervous system exclusively (Akselrod et al., 1981; Appel, Berger, Saul, Smith, & Cohen, 1989; Pagani et al., 1986; Pomeranz et al., 1985). Respiratory sinus arrhythmia is contained within this band. Heart rate oscillations

Figure 5.2   Power Spectrum of Instantaneous Heart Rate Fluctuations Featuring Three Main Peaks: Very Low Frequency (0–0.04 Hz), Low Frequency (0.04–0.15 Hz), and High Frequency (0.15–0.40 Hz).

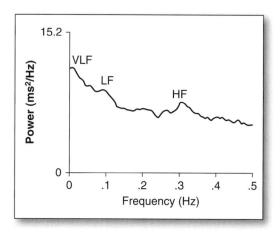

occurring with respiration are believed to be controlled by the medullary respiratory centers, baroreceptors in the large thoracic capacitance vessels, and the Bainbridge reflex (Ebert, 1992).

Power spectral analysis is generally performed by either fast Fourier transform (FFT) (nonparametric) or autoregressive (AR) (parametric) spectral models. When both methods have been employed on the same data set, correlations of the integral of the power spectral density between AR and FFT techniques within LF and HF bands ranged from $r = .97$ to $r = .99$, when 4-minute, 1-hour, and 24-hour segments were analyzed (Cowan, Kogan, Burr, Hendershot, & Buchanan, 1990). Therefore, both methods appear to provide comparable results.

Spectral density of the HF component of heart rate variability provides a reliable estimate of parasympathetic nervous system influence on the SA node. As parasympathetic nervous system influences dominate, HF heart rate variability increases. Sympathetic nervous system activity is more difficult to display and quantify (Akselrod, 1995). Some have suggested that the ratio of power of LF:HF heart rate variability may provide a measure of sympathovagal balance (Malliani, Pagani, Lombardi, & Cerutti, 1991). It may be a valid estimate in a variety of physiological situations, particularly when the purpose of evaluation is to determine changes in sympathovagal balance under various conditions (Akselrod, 1995).

Although heart rate variability measures may provide valuable insights into autonomic outflow, many extraneous variables or conditions may impact the reliability of these measures. The magnitude of heart rate variability decreases with age (Hrushesky, Fader, Schmitt, & Gilbertsen, 1984; I. O'Brien, O'Hare, & Corrall, 1985; Schwartz, Gibb, & Tran, 1991). In addition, changes in body position can have a profound effect on short-term measures of heart rate variability (Malliani et al., 1991; Vybiral, Bryg, Maddens, & Boden, 1989). As with other cardiovascular measures, consideration must be given to the possible impact medications might have on measures of heart rate variability, particularly beta-adrenergic blocking agents. In addition, these measures are generally performed only on individuals whose underlying cardiac rhythm is sinus in origin. When more than 10% of the ECG data in any segment are not sinus complexes, or are unreadable, the segment should be discarded from the analysis. Heart rate variability measures have been used as indicators of psychological and physiological stress in many studies (Bradley et al., 2010; Matsubara et al., 2011; Tang, Tegeler, Larrimore, Cowgill, & Kemper, 2010; Trappe, 2010).

Blood Pressure Measurement

Blood pressure is a product of cardiac output and tone of the peripheral resistance vessels in the arterial system. Both heart rate, a determinant of cardiac output, and peripheral vascular resistance are regulated by the autonomic nervous system; as a result, they are strongly influenced by both physiological and psychological stressors. During periods of acute stress, the systolic blood pressure changes more rapidly than diastolic blood pressure. For example, changes in systolic blood pressure can be observed within 1 or 2 minutes of the cold-pressor stress test in which the hand is immersed in cold water (Porth, 1976; Tassorelli, Micieli, Osipova, Rossi, & Nappi, 1995). Thus, methods that can detect rapid changes in blood pressure are often needed to demonstrate the effect of acute stress. The effects of chronic stress on blood pressure are less obvious, presumably

because there is an adaptation of blood pressure control mechanisms.

Blood pressure can be measured directly using an arterial catheter and a pressure transducer or indirectly using a blood pressure cuff and a method for detecting the arterial pressure wave as it travels through the arterial system (Andrew & Scott, 1985; Gorny, 1993; E. O'Brien, Fitzgerald, & O'Malley, 1985). Direct and indirect methods of blood pressure monitoring measure different phenomenon. Direct monitoring methods use the arterial pressure wave to determine the blood pressure. Because these methods require insertion of an arterial catheter, they are seldom used in stress studies. Indirect methods, which are noninvasive, determine blood pressure by volume displacement or by flow detection. Noninvasive blood pressure measurement methods include the auscultatory method, oscillometric method, Doppler technique, and the finger blood pressure cuff. A modification of the auscultatory method uses a microphone to detect the auscultatory sounds during cuff inflation and deflation.

The accuracy of blood pressure measurements obtained by the different methods of measurement are subject to user-related and instrumentation-related errors that correspond to the technique and measurement assumptions of each type of instrumentation. Noninvasive blood pressure equipment should meet Standards of the Association of Advancement of Medical Instrumentations (www.aami.org/standards/). Most noninvasive blood pressure machines that are purchased by patients for home blood pressure monitoring are not adequate for use in research studies.

The Auscultatory Method of Blood Pressure Measurement

The auscultatory method relies on arterial occlusion by an inflated cuff and, as the cuff is deflated, detection of the auscultatory sounds by means of a stethoscope. Accurate measurement of blood pressure requires that the cuff be deflated at a rate of 2 mm/second. Investigators are referred to the American Heart Association or British Hypertension Society guidelines for blood pressure measurement (Working Party, 1997). This method generally limits the frequency with which blood pressure measurements can be obtained to every 2 or 3 minutes and may be inadequate for studies that require beat-by-beat measurements of blood pressure. The use of proper cuff size as determined by the arm circumference of the subject is essential for accurate measurements (Banner & Gavenstein, 1991). Because this method requires listening to auscultatory sounds, data collectors need to be trained in the skills of blood pressure monitoring, and observer accuracy must be established if more than one investigator is involved in data collection (E. O'Brien, Mee, Tan, Atkins, & O'Malley, 1991). The mercury sphygmomanometer is usually considered more accurate than the anaeroid manometer. If an anaeroid manometer is used, frequent calibration checks are required.

The Oscillometric Method of Blood Pressure Measurement

The oscillometric method employs a cuff that compresses the limb and underlying vasculature and measures blood pressure by sensing arterial pulsations as a function of cuff pressure. This is the method used with many of the automatic noninvasive blood pressure machines. Cuff deflation usually is determined by heart rate. The oscillometric devices have the advantage of serial measurement capabilities through automatic cycling without investigator intervention. As with the auscultatory method, accuracy of measurement depends on use of proper cuff size and instrument calibration.

Doppler Techniques of Blood Pressure Measurement

Doppler techniques require placement of a sensor over an artery distal to an inflatable cuff or between the cuff and the limb. The sensor consists of a transmitter that projects ultrasound waves into the limb and a transducer that picks up the reflected ultrasound from the various soft tissue interfaces. The sound transmitted from the blood moving through the artery is converted to an audible sound from which the listener can determine maximum cuff pressure for blood flow distal to the cuff. As with other noninvasive blood pressure methods, the accuracy of blood pressure measurements is dependent on proper cuff size. Systolic measurements are more accurate than diastolic.

Finger Arterial Measurement of Blood Pressure

The finger arterial blood pressure monitoring method (Finapres, Datex Ohmeda) facilitates continuous finger arterial pressure waveform (Imholz, Wieling, van Montfrans, & Wessling, 1998). The equipment is easy to use and provides a method for continuous measurement of blood pressure changes. Although there are conflicting reports regarding their utility in the clinical setting in which treatment options are determined by blood pressure measurements (Jagomägi, Talts, Raamat, & Lansimes, 1996; Latman, 1992; Lyew & Jamieson, 1994; Nesselroad, Flacco, Phillips, & Kruse, 1996; Ristuccia, Grossman, Watkins, & Lown, 1997), they provide a noninvasive method for tracking momentary blood pressure changes in stress studies (Imholz et al., 1988). Blood pressure measures have been used as indicators of psychological and physiological stress in many studies (Han et al., 2010; Jefferson, 2010; Mikosch et al., 2010; Tõru et al., 2010).

Rate Pressure Product

When a stress response is elicited, there is a concomitant increased release of epinephrine and norepinephrine. Increased circulating levels of epinephrine and norepinephrine result in increases in heart rate, peripheral vascular resistance, and force of myocardial contraction. These protective mechanisms are initiated to meet the increased demands of the body, but they are accompanied by an increase in the myocardial oxygen demand of the heart (MVO_2 demand).

Rate pressure product (RPP) is a reliable noninvasive indicator of myocardial oxygen demand (Amsterdam, Hughes, DeMaria, Zelis, & Mason, 1974; Gobel, Nordstrom, Nelson, Jorgenson, & Wang, 1978). It is calculated by multiplying heart rate by systolic blood pressure. Gobel et al. (1978) reported a correlation of $r = .83$ when calculated RPPs were compared to direct measures of myocardial oxygen demand. Measures of RPP are only as reliable as the measures of heart rate and systolic blood pressure obtained to calculate this value. RPP has been used as a noninvasive measure of myocardial oxygen demand in response to physiologic and psychological stressors in numerous studies (Bairey Merz et al., 1998; Belkic, Emdad, & Theorell, 1998; Hattori et al., 1998; Jain et al.,

1998; Kavanagh, Matosevic, Thacker, Belliard, & Shephard, 1998; Villella, Villella, Barlera, Franzosi, & Maggioni, 1999; White, 1999).

Cardiac Output Measurements

Impedance cardiography provides a noninvasive method for obtaining data related to cardiac function (Jensen, Yakimets, & Teo, 1995; Woltjer, Bogaard, & deVries, 1997). This method uses the electrical impedance or resistance changes that occur as a low-voltage (2.5–4.0 mA), high-frequency (70–100 kHz), alternating electrical current is passed through the thorax using spot or band electrodes. The electrical impedance changes are detected by sensing electrodes. Pulsatile blood flow through the thoracic aorta causes shifts in the thoracic impedance as a function of changes in blood volume. There is a decrease in electrical impedance as the blood volume in the aorta increases; as blood volume decreases, electrical impedance increases.

The impedance cardiac output method was originally developed by Kubicek and colleagues (Kubicek, Karnegis, Patterson, Witssoe, & Mattson, 1966). Assumptions of the impedance cardiograph include that the thorax acts as a cylinder that is homogeneously perfused with blood of specific resistivity (p) in ohms, which can vary with hematocrit. The thorax is thought to have a steady-state base impedance (Z_0) between the electrodes (ohms) with pulsatile variations in aortic blood flow and electrical impedance (ΔZ), which is further expressed as its first derivative (dZ/dt). This derivative has been shown to be proportional to the stroke volume (SV) of the heart. When the heart rate is known, cardiac output can be derived. According to Kubicek et al. (1996), stroke volume can be determined using the following equation:

$$SV = \frac{p \cdot L^2 \cdot (dZ/dt)\max \cdot LVET}{Z_0^2},$$

where L^2 is the length between the sensing electrodes (cm), and $LVET$ (seconds) is the left ventricular ejection time. The LVET is determined from an ECG tracing. Heart sounds are often used to confirm the markings for LVET.

Computerized methods of impedance cardiograph monitoring have been developed that provide a means for continuous measurement of stoke volume and cardiac output during research of the stress response. Measurement of blood pressure permits determination of changes in peripheral vascular resistance. Impedance cardiography has been used to study the cardiovascular responses to both physical and emotional stress (Bosch et al., 2009; Knepp & Friedman, 2008; Oosterman & Schuengel, 2007; Yu, Nelesen, Ziegler, & Dimsdale, 2001).

Respiratory Rate Measurement

Respiratory rate is controlled by brain stem sensors that monitor blood oxygen and carbon dioxide levels. The pattern of breathing can also be altered by emotional responses to conditions such as fear and anxiety by other parts of the brain, including the limbic system and hypothalamus.

Respiratory rate can be measured by means of impedance pneumography, visual inspection, or auscultation with a stethoscope over the chest wall. An impedance pneumograph senses changes in resistance across the chest that are caused by the act of breathing. Reliability of this measure is dependent on accurate placement of the electrodes. Visual inspection of the act of breathing is more accurate when both the chest and abdomen can be viewed directly. Combining visual inspection with chest auscultation may provide a better alternative to either visual inspection or auscultation alone. Some impedance pneumographs are capable of providing a hard copy of respirations, but the expense of this equipment makes visual inspection and auscultation a viable option for consideration.

Electrodermal Activity Measurement

The notion that changes in electrical activity of the skin can be produced by a variety of physical and emotional stimuli was first reported by Charles Fere in 1888 (Woodworth & Schlosberg, 1954). He passed a small current between two electrodes on the surface of the skin and noted changes in electrodermal activity when individuals were presented with various stimuli.

From a psychophysiological perspective, electrodermal activity refers to the bioelectrical attributes of the skin or the neurons directly associated with the skin. The skin is supplied by two types of sweat glands: the eccrine and apocrine sweat glands. The eccrine sweat glands are particularly abundant on the palms of the hands, the soles of the feet, and the forehead. Eccrine gland secretion, which is a hypotonic electrolyte solution, functions in regulation of body temperature. In contrast, the apocrine sweat glands secrete more fatty acids and proteins, empty into hair follicles, and are more abundant in the axillary and anogenital areas. The eccrine sweat glands located in the soles of the feet and the palms of the hands are believed to respond to psychological stimulation rather than to temperature changes (Everly & Sobelman, 1987). The sympathetic fibers innervating these glands are adrenergic in nature (Guyton & Hall, 2006), making skin conductance (SC) and skin potential (SP) indices of sympathetic nervous system activity. A delay time between the time stimulation occurs and the actual response of electrodermal activity has been estimated to range from 1.5 to 2.5 seconds (Edelberg, 1972). The activity of sympathetic neurons innervating the sweat glands and the moisture produced by eccrine gland sweating form the physiological basis for measurement of electrodermal activity.

There are two basic techniques for measuring electrodermal activity: exosomatic and endosomatic (Everly & Sobelman, 1987). The exosomatic approach involves introduction of a mild electrical current to the skin. This technique is sometimes referred to as *galvanic skin response.* The measurement obtained is that of SC. Because moist skin conducts current more readily than dry skin, skin conductance varies with eccrine gland sweating. In contrast, the endosomatic method consists of passive reception of the electrical activity of sympathetic neurons of the dermal substrate (skin). This approach is referred to as SP.

There are two basic types of circuits used to measure skin conductance: those that apply a constant voltage and those that employ a constant current (Andreassi, 1989). The SC method uses bipolar placement of electrodes placed on the medial phalanxes of two adjacent fingers (either the second and third or the fourth and fifth) (Venables & Christie, 1973). This approach maintains constant voltage across the electrodes, and the current through the skin varies with changes in conductance. As sympathetic nervous system activity increases, sweat production increases and thus SC increases. The changes in conductance are recorded. When current through the skin is held constant, the voltage necessary to maintain this current varies with resistance. Increased sweat production reduces resistance. When this method is employed, changes in resistance are recorded. With increased sympathetic nervous system activity, resistance is lowered and SC increases. For additional information with respect to these techniques, the reader is referred to Edelberg (1967, 1972), Venables and Christie (1973), and Venables and Martin (1967).

When SP is measured, a unipolar method is employed (Andreassi, 1989). The active electrode is placed on the palm of the hand and is referred to an essentially inactive site (reference) on the forearm. To prepare the site for the inactive electrode, the skin is abraded prior to electrode application. The active electrode must be placed in an area that is free from cuts or other skin lesions because their presence can interfere with the measured response. The SP may be measured by means of a sensitive DC amplifier.

Measures of electrodermal activity may be useful indicators of arousal states (Andreassi, 1989; Everly & Sobelman, 1987). Their utility in reflecting relaxation is questionable, however (Andreassi, 1989). In addition, electrodermal activity possesses both tonic status and phasic propensities (Everly & Sobelman, 1987). Therefore, it is critical that the investigator establish a reliable baseline (situational tone) prior to attempting to determine any reactionary states (phasic activity). In addition, electrode size can affect skin potential and skin conductance measures. Electrodermal response has been used to evaluate responses to physiological and psychological stress in many studies (Guzzetta, 1989; Rief, Shaw, & Fichter, 1998; Seibt, Boucsein, & Schuech, 1998; Steptoe, Cropley, & Joekes, 1999; Steptoe, Evans, & Fieldman, 1997; Vogele, 1998).

NEUROENDOCRINE MEASURES OF THE STRESS RESPONSE

It has long been recognized that the psychoneuroendocrine manifestations of stress reflect the activity of the hypothalamic-pituitary-adrenal-cortical and sympatho-adreno-medullary systems. Thus, methods for studying the stress response often focus on measurement of cortisol, which can be used as a marker of hypothalamic-pituitary-adrenal-cortical activity, and on the catecholamines as measures of sympatho-adreno-medullary activity. Cortisol is the primary natural glucocorticoid in humans, with most of it circulating bound to cortico-steroid-binding globulin and albumin (Perogamvros, Keevil, Ray, & Trainer, 2010). Stress is commonly considered a generalized response; as such, there is interaction among other hormones (e.g., prolactin and growth hormone) and with other neurotransmitters (e.g., dopamine and serotonin). In stress studies, cortisol levels are commonly obtained from saliva samples, whereas catecholamines are generally measured from plasma samples or urine specimens.

Because of their invasive nature, tests used in the diagnosis of clinical disease may be inappropriate for research studies. For example, introduction of a venipuncture procedure introduces a stress of its own, thereby imposing extraneous influences on measures obtained in this manner. Intraindividual variations such as changes in body position and baroreflex activity, as well as circadian influences, affect cortisol and catecholamine levels.

Salivary Cortisol

Cortisol, which is produced by the adrenal cortex, is commonly regarded as a marker of activity in the hypothalamic-pituitary-adrenal-cortical system. The measurement of cortisol in saliva has become an acceptable alternative to blood analysis (Kirschbaum & Hellhammer, 1994; Kirschbaum, Read, & Hellhammer, 1992). Because cortisol is thought to enter the saliva by passive diffusion or other means independent of active transport mechanisms, it approximates the level of free cortisol in the plasma and is not affected by the salivary flow rate. Also, the ease of sample collection allows for almost unlimited frequency of sample collection in a variety of research settings. The cortisol response to acute psychological stress is thought to peak after 20 to 30 minutes; thus, momentary changes in cortisol can be measured using this method (Kirschbaum & Hellhammer, 1989). This measure has been used for studying stress in infants (Azar, Paquette, & Stewart, 2010) and children (McCarthy et al., 2010), adults (Zoccola, Quas,

& Yim, 2010), and the elderly (Minton, Hertzog, Barron, French, & Reiter-Palmon, 2009; Strahler, Berndt, Kirschbaum, & Rohleder, 2010).

Salivary α-Amylase

Salivary α-amylase has been proposed as a marker for stress-induced sympathetic nervous system activation (Rohleder, Wolf, Maldonado, & Kirschbaum, 2006). Alpha-amylase is a major protein component of saliva. Enzymatic digestion of carbohydrates is the main function of salivary α-amylase, but it is also important for mucosal immunity in the oral cavity, as it inhibits the adherence and growth of bacteria (Bosch, de Geus, Veerman, Hoogstraten, & Nieuw Amerongen, 2003; Scannapieco, Torres, & Levine, 1993). Alpha-amylase is one of several proteins synthesized and secreted by acinar cells, which make up more than 80% of cells in the major salivary glands (Castle & Castle, 1998).

Elevated plasma catecholamine levels have been associated with increased secretion of salivary α-amylase in studies in which stressful physiological and/or psychological stressors have been introduced (Gilman, Fischer, Biersner, Thornton, & Miller, 1979). Gilman, Thornton, Miller, and Biersner (1979) reported that intense physical exercise increased salivary α-amylase levels, and this increase was attributed to adrenoceptor activation of salivary glands. Similarly, Chatterton, Vogelsong, Lu, Ellman, and Hudgens (1996) reported a significant positive correlation between salivary amylase and plasma norepinephrine in response to a 20-minute running exercise. A marked increase in α-amylase levels also was reported in response to a parachute jump (Chatterton, Vogelsong, Lu, & Hudgens, 1997) and to a stressful video game (Skosnik, Chatterton, Swisher, & Park, 2000). During psychological stress that was introduced my means of a written examination, correlations were much lower ($r = .64$ vs. $r = .17$) (Chatterton, Vogelsong, Lu, Ellman, & Hodgens, 1996). However, Bosch and colleagues (1996) reported higher salivary α-amylase levels on the day of an academic examination than those obtained on control days. In a later study, Bosch, de Geus, Veerman, Hoogstraten, and Nieuw Amerongen (2003) reported increased α-amylase levels during passive coping while watching a stressful video recording. Other studies have provided evidence that psychological stress results in increased α-amylase levels (Nater et al., 2005, 2006; Rohleder, Nater, Wolf, Ehlert, & Kirschbaum, 2004). Salivary α-amylase has exhibited a half-life of approximately 10 minutes after removal of the stressor, while heart rate response was quite similar. In contrast, salivary cortisol levels remained elevated much longer (Chatterton et al., 1996).

Relationships with plasma norepinephrine levels have been weaker in studies examining psychological stress when compared with exercise-related stress (Chatteron et al., 1996; Nater et al., 2006; Rohleder et al., 2004). Changes in salivary α-amylase level responses to stress also have been associated with increases in heart rate ($r = .56$) and decreases in heart rate variability ($r = -.36$) (Bosch et al., 2003). In addition, pharmacological approaches have been used to validate the association between salivary α-amylase and autonomic nervous system responses. Introduction of β-adrenergic receptor blockade (propanolol) was successful in reducing stress-induced α-amylase increases (van Stegeren, Rohleder, Everaerd, & Wolf, 2006). Further, stimulation of the sympathetic nervous system by introduction of an α-2 adrenergic receptor antagonist (yohimbine) resulted in a significant increase in salivary α-amylase levels (Ehlert, Erni, Hebisch, & Nater, 2006).

A key issue in determining the validity of salivary α-amylase measurements as an indicator of the stress response is whether these measures are independent of salivary flow rate. Salivary secretion generally is activated by tactile and gustatory stimuli in the mouth, as well as by visual and olfactory stimuli (Edgar, 1992; Losso, Singer, & Nicolau, 1997). It is known that a higher salivary flow rate results from mechanical stimulation and introduction of fluids, and it also occurs with lower pH (Guinard, Zoumas-Morse, & Walchak, 1997). It is commonly accepted that sympathetic stimulation results in secretion of salivary proteins and salivary flow rate is primarily mediated by parasympathetic influences (Anderson et al., 1984; Garrett, 1987). Rohleder et al. (2006) found that psychologically based, stress-induced increases in salivary α-amylase were correlated with increases of amylase output but not with salivary flow rate, providing evidence that salivary α-amylase is independent of salivary flow rate. Salivary α-amylase appears to be a valid marker for the stress response in adults, but it does not appear

to be a less robust measure in children (Strahler, Mueller, Rosenloecher, Kirschbaum, & Rohleder, 2010; Yim, Granger, & Quas, 2010).

Salivary Cortisone

Recently, the importance of measuring circulating free cortisol has been recognized (Perogamvros et al., 2010). Changes in binding proteins, particularly cortico-steroid-binding globulin (CBG), greatly affect total, but not free serum, cortisol levels (Coolens, VanBaelen, & Heyns, 1987). Measuring total cortisol also provides an underestimation of the cortisol response in stress, as it does not account for the exponential rise of free serum cortisol due to CBG saturation (Vogesor, Briegel, & Zachoval, 2002). It is widely recognized that individuals on estrogen replacement therapy, who have high CBG levels, may have to stop their treatment for 6 weeks prior to assessing HPA status. It is also important to consider that the binding protein is acutely regulated in sepsis and critical illness, leading to significant problems in interpreting HPA status in critical illness (Perogamvros et al., 2010).

Although the importance of bioavailable levels of circulating cortisol, free serum cortisol assays are rarely used, mostly because they are expensive, cumbersome, and time consuming. Salivary cortisol has been used as a surrogate for free serum cortisol, and it is widely accepted, particularly in stress research (Hellhammer, Wüst, & Kudielka, 2009). Recently, Perogamvros et al. (2010) provided evidence that salivary cortisone has the potential to be a useful surrogate for serum-free cortisol in research and clinical assessment, as it closely reflects free serum cortisol after adrenal stimulation and hydrocortisone administration, and it was unaffected by CBG changes. This measure has been used for studying stress in infants (Schäffer, Luzi, Burkhardt, Rauh, & Beinder, 2009; Schäffer, Müller-Vizentini et al., 2009). Most published studies with salivary cortisone studies have been for validation purposes.

Saliva Collection

Although there are saliva collection techniques for gland-specific saliva by either suction or cannulation, mixed saliva is the only practical collection method for most research and clinical settings. There are several methods for collecting mixed salivary samples. Whole saliva can be sampled in wide, disposable containers that provide adequate material for analysis. Participants are asked to spit or drool directly into the collection device. Active spitting is considered adequate stimulus, resulting in up to 1 ml/minute, whereas passive drooling is considered to provide nonstimulated saliva (Gröschl, 2008). This method of collection has several disadvantages, including the social stigma associated with spitting (Nguyen & Wong, 2006), particularly with geriatric populations. In addition, application of citric acid to the tongue has been used to increase salivary flow, but citric acid has been reported to interfere with immunoassay analysis by decreasing pH of the sample (Gallagher, Leitch, Massey, McAllister-Williams, & Young, 2006). Therefore, saliva is generally collected with absorbent tissues in the mouth and then extracted by centrifugation.

There are a number of commercially available collection devices for saliva. Because of the importance of not affecting salivary concentrations, any absorption or modification of the analytes must be avoided. Materials such as Parafilm (Chang & Chiou, 1976) and cotton (Höld, deBoer, Zuidema, & Maes, 1995) are known to absorb target molecules for saliva, resulting in falsely reduced measures. The most commonly used sampling methods are the Salivette, the Quantisal, Whatman, and the Intercept. All these systems use a collection pad that is inserted into the mouth, either in the cheek or under the tongue. This pad is maintained in the mouth to absorb saliva for a standardized period of time, generally 1 to 2 minutes. The pad is transferred to a storage container. Saliva is removed from the pad by centrifugation.

Recently, the reliability of a variety of saliva collection devices was tested. Pooled saliva was spiked with ascending concentrations of a variety of hormones and applied to a variety of absorbents, such as the cotton and the polyester Salivette, the foam-tip applicator, and strips of blood-spot collection paper. Analysis was performed by liquid chromatography with tandem mass spectrometry. Best results were obtained with the polyester Salivette (Gröschl & Rauh, 2006). They concluded that only the polyester version of the Salivette was suitable for salivary steroid analysis. The weakest recovery was achieved with the foam-tip applicator.

Another sampling device designed to facilitate the noninvasive measurement of adrenocortical activity is called the oral diffusion sink (ODS). It allows for the collection of time-integrated measures of cortisol (Wade & Haegele, 1991). It is worn in the mouth and continuously accumulates the compounds of interest as they diffuse into the device along a concentration gradient. This device consists of a rigid tubular shell of radio-opaque polycarbonate resin that is 2 mm by 15 mm, with 12 perforations (ports) that are covered by a membrane that allows salivary components to diffuse into the device according to their molecular weights. The ODS is secured to a tooth in the subject's mouth with dental floss. Cortisol molecules are bound inside the ODS by either specific antibodies (Wade & Haegele, 1991) or β-cyclodextrin (Wade, 1992). The binding capacity allows for sampling intervals of 1 to 8 hours, thus permitting measurement over prolonged periods. The validity of the ODS has been studied both *in vitro* (Shipley, Alessi, Wade, Haegele, & Helmbold, 1992) and *in vivo* (Gehris & Kathol, 1992).

In infants, saliva can be obtained by gently swabbing the baby's mouth with a cotton dental roll (Gunnar, Connors, & Isenee, 1989) or by aspirating saliva with a small pipette (Hanecke & Haeckel, 1992). Hanecke and Haeckel described a method in which modified feeding bottles containing absorption material within the nipple were used.

Stability of salivary hormones has been studied by a number of researchers (DePalo, Antonelli, Benetazzo, Prearo, & Gatti, 2009; Garde & Hansen, 2005; Gröschl, Wagner, Rauh, & Dörr, 2001; Wood, 2009). Salivary steroids have been shown to be stable at +4 °C for a month and at –20 °C for 3 months. Salivary cortisol has been shown to be stable for 1 year at –80 °C, and uncentrifuged samples have remained stable for 9 months at –20 °C.

Plasma and Urinary Measures of Catecholamines

The catecholamines, epinephrine and norepinephrine, are sympathetic neurotransmitters of the stress response. Norepinephrine is the neurotransmitter released at the postganglionic synapses of the sympathetic nervous system. The adrenal medulla, which is part of the sympathetic nervous system, secretes both epinephrine and norepinephrine in a ratio of approximately 3:1 (Dimsdale & Ziegler, 1991). Two methods have been used to measure catecholamine response to stress: One measures the catecholamines in the plasma and the other measures urinary catecholamines.

The measurement and interpretation of the catecholamine response to stress are complicated by the fact that most of the norepinephrine that is released from nerve endings is taken back up into the presynaptic neuron through the reuptake process, with only a small percentage making its way into the bloodstream. Once in the bloodstream, approximately 10% is filtered into the urine, but most is rapidly cleared from the body (Dimsdale & Ziegler, 1991). Each organ rapidly clears and adds norepinephrine to the plasma. Furthermore, the various organs add and remove norepinephrine from the blood at different rates. Organs with the largest blood flow contribute the largest amount of norepinephrine. The sampling site for blood has a marked effect on catecholamine levels. Arterial blood has higher epinephrine and lower norepinephrine levels. Catecholamine levels from venous blood more accurately reflect catecholamines released from all body organs.

Plasma venous catecholamines are exquisitely sensitive to stress. Venipuncture, however, can increase catecholamine levels by more than 50% (Carruthers, Taggart, Conway, Bates, & Somerville, 1990). Thus, venous catheterization is usually done when multiple samples are required. Plasma catecholamines also are affected by diet, caffeine, nicotine, posture, and the stress of the experimental protocol. Because of the assay variability, the numerous confounding variables, and the modest effect of the stressors, relatively large sample sizes may be needed to perceive stress effects of 100 pg/ml in venous epinephrine (Dimsdale & Ziegler, 1991).

Catecholamine levels are commonly measured using high-performance liquid chromatography (HPLC). Although radio-immunoassays (RIAs) can be performed on small blood volumes, and they are fairly sensitive, the methods are difficult to perform and require expensive agents. The HPLC methods use electrochemical detectors to quantify the catecholamines after HPLC separation. The detectors lack the sensitivity to measure low levels of epinephrine and suffer from instability and electrical interference at their most sensitive setting. Therefore, investigators using this method are advised to use an already established catecholamine laboratory.

Biochemical Measurement Methods

Among the biochemical methods used to measure the neuroendocrine responses to stress response are chromatography, RIA, and enzyme-linked immunoabsorbent assay (ELISA). These assays usually require sophisticated methods, and less experienced investigators often find it advantageous to collaborate with laboratories that are experienced in performing these tests. In the process of developing a research protocol that uses the services of any laboratory, it is recommended that the investigator understand the assay method that will be used and receive an assurance that the same method and reagents will be used for all samples that will be submitted. Research protocols frequently require that samples be collected, stored, and transported to the laboratory that has been contracted to carry out the studies.

Chromatography

Chromatography methods use differences in the solubility of compounds to achieve their separation. In all forms of chromatography, substances are introduced into a column containing an absorbent material that interacts with the compound passing through the column (Figure 5.3). When molecules of a compound are introduced in the top of the column, they are subjected to two opposing forces—that of the mobile forces that tend to move them through the column and that of the stationary phase that has a tendency to keep them within the column (DuFour, 1990). There are several types of chromatography separation methods, including thin layer and column chromatography, which separate polar and nonpolar substances; ion exchange, which separates cations and anions; molecular sieve column chromatography, which separates compounds based on differences in size; and gas-liquid chromatography, which separates an absorbed liquid into an inert support (stationary phase) and an inert gas (mobile phase).

Column chromatography is used for purification of urine vanillylmandelic acid and fractionalization of urine androgens; gas-liquid chromatography is used to separate estrogens and progestagins. In HPLC, the mobile phase is liquid (Allenmark, 1988). It is used to separate catecholamines and catecholamine metabolites

Figure 5.3   Column Chromatography

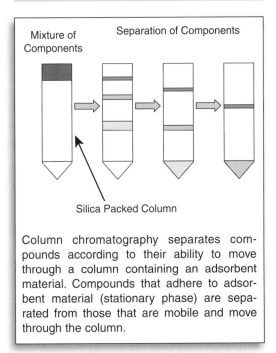

Column chromatography separates compounds according to their ability to move through a column containing an adsorbent material. Compounds that adhere to adsorbent material (stationary phase) are separated from those that are mobile and move through the column.

Figure 5.4   Radioimmunoassay

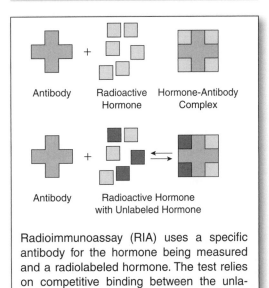

Radioimmunoassay (RIA) uses a specific antibody for the hormone being measured and a radiolabeled hormone. The test relies on competitive binding between the unlabeled hormone in the sample being tested and the radiolabeled hormone. The hormone-antibody complexes from samples containing a high concentration of unlabeled hormone will have a lower radiation count than samples containing a low concentration of hormone.

(DuFour, 1990). HPLC can be automated and has the advantage of relatively rapid separation, but it is more expensive than other methods and requires experience in performing the assays. Gas-liquid chromatography requires a high capital outlay and expert technical assistance as well.

Once separated, the substance being measured can be detected by monitoring specific physical or chemical properties of substances that remain in the column or by analyzing material removed by the mobile phase of the process. The ultraviolet spectrophotometer commonly is used for this purpose.

Radioimmunoassay

Radioimmunoassay, which was developed in the late 1950s and early 1960s, is a major tool in endocrine research (Rhoades & Tanner, 1995). Since its inception, RIA has revolutionized the quantification of hormone levels. It is a competitive binding assay that uses a specific antibody for the hormone being measured and a radioactively labeled hormone (Figure 5.4). The hormone is measured *in vitro* in a series of

test tubes. Fixed amounts of hormone antibody and the radiolabeled antibody are added to all the test tubes. A given volume of the sample to be tested (plasma, saliva, or urine) is then added to one series of tubes. Varying concentrations of the hormone being tested, added to a second series of test tubes, provide the standard for the test. In each series of test tubes, the amount of radioactive hormone bound to the antibody is measured. The response produced by the radiolabeled hormone in the standard series is used to generate a standard curve, and the response produced by the hormone level in the sample is compared to the standard curve.

The assay is based on the principle that the unlabeled hormone in the sample and the radiolabeled hormone in the test tube will compete for the limited number of binding sites present in the antibody that has been added to the test tubes. The amount of each hormone that is bound to the antibody is an indicator of the proportion present in the test tube solution. In a sample with a high concentration of hormone, less radioactive hormone will be bound to antibody and vice versa.

One of the limitations of the RIA is that it measures immunoreactivity rather than biologic activity. The presence of an immunologically related but different hormone or heterogeneous forms of the same hormone can complicate the interpretation of the results. The RIA generates radioactive waste that poses a disposal problem and adds to the expense of the test.

Enzyme-Linked Immunoabsorbent Assay

The enzyme-linked immunoabsorbent assay (ELISA) is a solid-phase, enzyme-based assay whose use and application have increased greatly during the past few years. A typical ELISA is a colorimetric or fluorometric assay that does not use radioactive materials and thus does not produce radioactive waste. This procedure eliminates the increasing environmental concerns and cost of radioactive waste disposal. Because the ELISA is a solid-phase assay, it can be automated to a great extent, which also has served to reduce the cost of this procedure.

The typical ELISA is performed on a 3-in. × 5-in. plastic plate containing small wells that are precoated with an antibody that is specific for the hormone being measured. A sample of the specimen being tested is introduced into the wells, followed by the addition of a second hormone-specific antibody that binds to the hormone contained in the specimen (Figure 5.5). A third antibody, which recognizes the second antibody, is then added. The third antibody is coupled to an enzyme that will convert an appropriate substrate into a colored or fluorometric product. The amount of product that is formed can be determined using optical methods. After addition of each antibody or sample to the wells, the plates are incubated for an appropriate amount of time to allow the antibodies and hormones to bind. Any unbound hormone is washed out of the well before the addition of the next reagent. The amount of colored or fluorometric product produced is directly proportional to the amount of hormone present in specimen. As with the RIA, this test is conducted using a standard sample. Concentrations are determined using a standard curve.

Figure 5.5   Enzyme-Linked Immunoabsorbent Assay

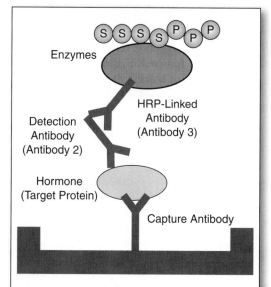

The ELISA relies on a change in color or fluorometric properties of a hormone (or antigen). The typical test uses a plastic plate containing small antibody (antibody 1)-coated wells that binds the hormone in the sample being tested. A second hormone (antibody 2) binds to the antibody-hormone complex and to a third antibody (antibody 3). Antibody 3, in turn, activates an enzyme that converts an appropriate substrate (S) to a colored or fluorometric product (P) that can be seen or measured.

IMMUNE MEASURES OF THE STRESS RESPONSE

The precise mechanism by which stress produces its effect on immune function is unknown. It has been suggested that immune and neuroendocrine cells share common signal pathways, and that hormones and neuropeptides can alter the function of immune cells. Furthermore, the immune system and its products can impact neuroendocrine function (Falaschi, Martocchia, Proietti, Pastore, & D'urso, 1994). The nervous and immune systems are comparable in several ways. Both systems are characterized by a diversity of cell types and by cell-to-cell transmission of information by soluble factors, including lymphokines (immune system) and neurotransmitters (nervous system) (Terr, Dubey, Yunis, Slavin, & Waldman, 1991). Lymphocytes and macrophages have receptors that are capable of responding to the neurotransmitters norepinephrine, acetylcholine, endorphins, enkephalins, ACTH, corticosteroids, insulin, prolactin, growth hormone, estradiol, and testosterone. Likewise, lymphocytes are capable of producing and secreting ACTH and endorphin-like compounds.

The human immune response can be divided into nonspecific and specific responses (Cacioppo, 1994). Nonspecific responses refer to general bodily defenses that result from pathogen exposure and include activation of natural killer (NK) cells, which monitor the body and destroy virally infected and tumor cells. Also included in this category is the activation of macrophages that engulf and destroy foreign substances. Specific immune responses include antibody production by B lymphocytes and T lymphocyte-mediated responses involving helper/inducer and suppressor/cytotoxic T lymphocytes.

There are five classes of antibodies or immunoglobulins (Igs): IgA, IgD, IgE, IgG, and IgM. IgA, a secretory immunoglobulin, is found in tears, saliva, breast milk, and bronchial, gastrointestinal, prostatic, and vaginal secretion. IgG (gamma globulin), the most abundant of the immunoglobulins, is present in body fluids and is the only immunoglobulin to cross the placenta. It displays antiviral, antitoxin, and antibacterial properties. IgM, a large antibody, is predominant in early immune responses. IgD is found on the cell membrane of B lymphocytes and functions in their maturation. IgE is involved in combating parasitic infections, inflammation, allergy, and hypersensitivity responses.

The technique of producing virtually unlimited quantities of a single antibody specific for a particular antigenic determinant has revolutionized immunology. Known as monoclonal antibodies, these laboratory-generated antibodies interact with specific antigenic markers or immune cells. The modern classification of immune cells is based on the development of population-specific monoclonal antibodies and on the discovery that functionally distinct subpopulations, such as helper T lymphocytes, express different cell membrane proteins called clusters of differentiation (CD).

Generally, two methods are employed to examine cellular immune status (Cacioppo, 1994). First, the percentage of various kinds of blood cells can be quantified in vitro by using commercially available monoclonal antibodies. Flow cytometry using monoclonal antibodies is used routinely for determination of NK, CD4+, and CD8+ cell counts. For example, the CD4+ marker on the cell surface identifies helper/inducer lymphocytes, whereas CD8+ markers identify suppressor/cytotoxic lymphocytes (Stites, 1991). Because the balance between helper/inducer and suppressor/cytotoxic T lymphocytes is important in mounting an effective immune response (Herbert & Cohen, 1993), the ratio of CD4+:CD8+ cells is also frequently reported.

The second method provides insight into the functional status of cellular immunity. This procedure involves quantification of the blasatogenic response to mitogens in vitro. Specific mitogens are introduced in an effort to stimulate B and T lymphocyte proliferation (Stites, 1991). In addition, NK cell function can be tested in vitro by means of radioactively labeled targets. Measurement of the radioactivity released from the lysed cells provides data about the NK cytotoxicity (Stites, 1991).

When examining measures of immune function, there are three issues that deserve consideration (Rabin, Kusnecov, Shurin, Zhou, & Rasnick, 1994). First, a laboratory value may indicate that a particular component is not functioning normally. However, it may only appear abnormal as a result of actions being exerted by another component of the interactive system that is functioning abnormally. For example, with common variable immunodeficiency, immunoglobulin production becomes markedly reduced when it previously had been normal. This situation is not caused by an abnormality of B lymphocytes but rather by increased activity of the T-suppressor lymphocyte population that acts to inhibit B lymphocytes from producing antibody (Ammann, 1991).

A second consideration demanding attention is that it may be difficult to determine when a statistical abnormality is biologically abnormal (Rabin et al., 1994). When the immune system is evaluated, a statistically significant reduction in immune measures may not be sufficient to have clinical relevance. For example, an IgG concentration of 300 mg/dl is markedly lower than the lower limits of normal range, but it remains adequate to protect an otherwise healthy individual from many infectious diseases.

The third concern that must be considered when evaluating measures of immune function is that a laboratory value that appears normal, and is an accumulation of multiple parts, actually may be abnormal (Rabin et al., 1994). An example of this situation is the analysis of IgG levels. There are four subclasses that comprise IgG: IgG_1, IgG_2, IgG_3, and IgG_4. Although the total IgG may appear to be normal, it may be composed of an abnormal subcomponent mixture. Therefore, a statistically normal value may be biologically abnormal.

Salivary IgA (sIgA) can be affected by chronic stress and mood. Salivary IgA concentrations or secretion rates or both have been reduced in conjunction with relatively high levels of stress or in the absence of positive mood states (Euler, Schimpf, Hennig, & Brosig, 2005; Evans, Bristow, Hucklebridge, Clow, & Walters, 1993; Gallagher et al., 2008; Graham, Chiron, Bartholomeusz, Taboonpong, & La Brooy, 1988; McClelland, Alexander, & Marks, 1982). In contrast, when the immunological response to acute stress has been investigated, almost invariably an increase in sIgA occurred during or immediately after the stressor was reported (Bristow, Hucklebridge, Clow, & Evans, 1997; Carroll et al., 1996; Deinzer & Schuller, 1998; Evans, Bristow, Hucklebridge, Clow, & Pang, 1994; Murphy, Denis, Ward, & Tartar, 2010; Okamura et al., 2010; Takatsuji et al., 2010; Willemsen et al., 1998; Zeier, Brauchli, & Joller-Jemelka, 1996). Results from these studies suggest that different mechanisms may control acute and chronic regulation of sIgA. Cacioppo (1994) suggested that reductions in sIgA in the long term may reflect involvement of the hypothalamic-pituitary-adrenal-cortical system, whereas short-term increases in sIgA may be a result of sympatho-adreno-medullary activation. In contrast, McClelland, Ross, and Patel (1985) proposed that reductions in sIgA associated with chronic stress may represent receptor downregulation resulting from repeated exposure to short-term challenges. Further investigation into the role of autonomic nervous system influences on sIgA is necessary to provide a better understanding of the meaningfulness of sIgA measures.

For sIgA measurement, saliva generally is collected by means of a Salivette. Before collection of the sample, subjects are asked to swallow until their mouths are dry. Then, a cotton wool swab is placed under the tongue for 2 to 5 minutes. Next, the swab is placed into a Salivette tube. The saliva can be analyzed within 48 hours of collection, or the Salivette can be sealed and frozen at −20° C for later analysis. Both sIgA secretion rate and concentration can be determined.

Until recently, the most commonly employed method for quantifying IgA was the radial immunodiffusion (RID) technique. Secretory IgA (11S) has different diffusion properties than those found in serum (7S), which is used as the standard for the RID assay. Therefore, results obtained from the RID assay for sIgA must be multiplied by a factor of three to correct for this difference in diffusion properties (Samson, McClelland, & Shearman, 1973). When there is a mixture of 7S, 9S, and 11S IgA, as well as IgA fragments, the correction factor method is less accurate (Sack, Neogi, & Alam, 1980).

The purpose of RID is to detect the reaction of antigen and antibody by the precipitation reaction (Stites & Rodgers, 1991). RID is based on the principle that a quantitative relationship exists between the amount of antigen placed in a well cut in an agar-antibody plate and the resulting ring of precipitation. The area circumscribed by the precipitation ring is proportionate to the concentration of antigen. This method requires that the precipitation ring be allowed to reach its maximal size. This method may require 48 to 72 hours of diffusion. A standard curve is experimentally determined with known antigen standards. The equation that describes the standard curve then can be used for determining the antigen concentration corresponding to any diameter size. The sensitivity of these methods ranges from 1 to 3 µ,g/ml of antigen.

Another method used to determine these measures is the nephelometric technique (Deinzer & Schuller, 1998). Using this technique, samples are spun for 2 minutes at 3,000 rpm. Specific human anti-IgA and a buffer are added to the sample. The suspension is stirred, and after 6 seconds, a blank value for determining diffuse light scattering is obtained. After a 30-minute incubation period, the solution is stirred again to obtain response values. To determine sIgA concentration, the difference between blank and response light scattering is compared with a previously calculated standard curve between 0.5 and 150 mg/dl. Concentration rate can then be determined by multiplying the concentration by one fifth of the sampled saliva volume.

ELISA methods, described previously, also are frequently used in the determination of sIgA concentrations. These methods produce rapid (same day), sensitive, and reproducible results, and they do not require a correction factor when measuring sIgA (Sack et al., 1980). When sIgA measures determined by ELISA methods have been compared with quantifications obtained by RID techniques, very high correlations have been reported ($r = .875$ to $r = .992$) (Miletic, Schiffman, Miletic, & Sattely-Miller, 1996; Sack et al., 1980). Likewise, when sIgA measures obtained by means of nephelometric techniques have been compared with quantifications determined by RID methods, correlations of $r = .93$ have been reported (Deinzer & Schuller, 1998).

Studies of stressor-induced alterations in human immune function have focused on activation of the sympathetic nervous system as the mediator of immune changes. In a meta-analysis of cardiovascular and immune responses to acute psychological stress in young and old women, a medium to large significant correlation between NK cell numbers and heart rate responses and small to medium correlations between NK cell number changes and blood pressure response were obtained (Benschop et al., 1998). The positive correlation between changes in heart rate and NK cell numbers was consistently observed across studies, independent of age or type of stressor. This finding was consistent with reports using male subjects (Benschop et al., 1994, 1995; Huang, Webb, Garten, Kamimori, & Acevedo, 2010; Naliboff et al., 1995).

RELIABILITY AND VALIDITY CONSIDERATIONS

Manifestations of the stress response can be measured in a variety of ways. Some methods require invasive procedures; many approaches demand expensive equipment; all techniques require thorough understanding of the procedure and underlying theoretical base of the measures employed. Many measurement methods can introduce additional stress to the experimental situation. The insertion of a needle to draw blood, for example, can introduce an element of both physiological and psychological stress.

Time

The time at which measurements are completed also demands consideration. Variables such as catecholamine release and heart rate undergo rapid changes during an acute stress challenge. In studies of acute stress, a beat-by-beat recording of heart rate may be required to ensure that the entire response is included in the analysis. Other variables such as changes in immune cells occur over a longer period of time. Thus, an understanding of the physiologic events being studied and the time sequence during which measurements should be made can be critical in designing a research protocol.

Many physiologic variables follow a circadian rhythm (Mathias & Alam, 1995; Moore, 1997). For example, cortisol peaks during early morning hours (Turton & Deegan, 1974). Other physiologic variables, such as norepinephrine and epinephrine, are influenced by the hypothalamic-pituitary-adrenal-cortical system. The body may be more susceptible to stresses imposed at certain phases of the circadian cycle than others. Thus, stress studies in which physiologic measurements are employed are best conducted at the same time each day to avoid variability among subject responses to circadian influences.

Although heart rate and blood pressure often are used in evaluating the effects of physical and emotional stressors, there are methodological challenges associated with using these variables in the laboratory setting (Parati et al., 1991). Blood pressure and heart rate responses to laboratory-induced stressors are limited by within-subject variability, poor correlation between blood pressure and heart rate responses to different stressors, and the fact that these responses bear only a limited relation to 24-hour patterns of variability in these measures.

Gender and Age

Both gender and age can influence physiologic responses to stress. Because of their different body size and composition and different hormonal profiles, women may recruit and use physiologic mechanisms differently than men (Frey & Porth, 1990). With aging, there is a general decline in adaptive capacity, in addition to changes in the ability to respond to stress.

The physiologic responses of women and men to physical and psychological stressors reflect the autonomic nervous system, central nervous system, responsiveness to hormones, and function of the cardiovascular system. For example, men reportedly secrete more catecholamines during mental and other exercise stresses, whereas women secrete more catecholamines during exercise (Frankenhaeuser, 1983). Until recently, published data about women were integrated into a study with data of men, and samples consisted predominantly of male subjects. As a result, many of the differences and similarities in the physiologic responses to stress between the sexes remain unclear.

Differences in hormones, particularly the reproductive hormones, provide one possible explanation for differences in responses of men and women to stress. When measuring effects of the stress response in women, consideration must be given to the women's station in the menstrual cycle (Heitkemper et al., 1996). Responses to experimental and naturally occurring stress in daily life can be influenced by these hormonal fluctuations. For example, heart rate and systolic blood pressure were reported to be significantly greater during the luteal phase of the menstrual cycle when compared to the follicular phase (Manhem & Jern, 1994). Ovulation can be determined by use of a 9-day test kit (OvuQuick) to track the urinary luteinizing hormone surge (Rudy & Estok, 1992).

There is a reported decline in autonomic nervous system and cardiovascular responsiveness to stress associated with advancing age (Smith & Porth, 1990). Effects of aging on cardiovascular responsiveness, reaction time, and ability to respond to stress are all factors that need to be addressed when designing a research study.

Many of these noninvasive measures require expensive equipment and a thorough understanding of their underlying scientific principles and of the physiologic phenomenon that they measure. Furthermore, many physiologic parameters that these methods measure are subject to the impact of circadian, gender, and age influences, changes in posture or body position, and investigator or operator error or both. In addition, proper use of the equipment requires special training. Interrater and intrarater variability can impose threats to the reliability of these measures. Controlling for time of day, body position, and phase of menstrual cycle can increase validity of these measures.

As with any laboratory tests, accuracy or validity of test results relies on use of proper procedures and reagents in the laboratory. It is advisable to determine the reliability of the laboratory, its personnel, and equipment in use. When multiple laboratories are used, the possibility of additional measurement error is introduced. Laboratory procedures are expensive. Frequently, venipuncture is involved, making these approaches less attractive to potential subjects. If repeated measures are employed, repeated venipuncture may be necessary. In addition, it is very important that careful consideration be given to the specificity and sensitivity of these measures in relation to the questions being posed. The cost–benefit ratio of using any physiological measures must also be examined.

The value of physiologic measures of the stress response will be enhanced by using multiple physiological measures in conjunction with psychometric instruments. Inclusion of interrater or intrarater reliability checks or both is imperative. All equipment used to determine physiological responses must meet professionally set specifications that ensure reliability and validity of determined measures.

Summary

Physiologic measures can be a reliable method for studying the consequences of physiological and psychological stress. Technologic advances that have led to development of noninvasive measurement methods favor their use in stress research. These measurements can be used singly, in combination, or as an adjunct to other more subjective methods of measuring the stress response.

References

Akselrod, S. (1995). Components of heart rate variability: Basic studies. In M. Malik & A. J. Camm (Eds.), *Heart rate variability* (pp. 147–163). Armonk, NY: Futura.

Akselrod, S., Gordon, D., Ubel, F. A., Shannon, D. C., Barger, A. C., & Cohen, R. J. (1981). Power spectrum analysis of heart rate fluctuation: A quantitative probe of beat-to-beat cardiovascular control. *Science, 213,* 220–222.

Allenmark, S. (1988). High-performance liquid chromatography of catecholamines and their metabolites in biological material. *Monographs in Endocrinology, 30*, 32–65.

Amsterdam, E. A., Hughes, J. L., DeMaria, A. N., Zelis, R., & Mason, D. T. (1974). Indirect assessment of myocardial oxygen consumption in the evaluation of mechanisms and therapy of angina pectoris. *American Journal of Cardiology, 33*, 737–743.

Ammann, A. J. (1991). Antibody (B cell) immunodeficiency disorders. In D. P. Stites & A. I. Terr (Eds.), *Basic and clinical immunology* (7th ed., pp. 322–334). Norwalk, CT: Appleton & Lange.

Anderson, L. C., Garrett, J. R., Johnson, D. A., Kauffman, D. L., Keller, P. J., & Thulin, A. (1984). Influence of circulating catecholamines on protein secretion into rat parotid saliva during parasympathetic stimulation. *Journal of Physiology, 353*, 163–171.

Andreassi, J. L. (1989). *Psychophysiology: Human behavior and physiological response* (2nd ed.). Hillsdale, NJ: Lawrence Erlbaum.

Andrew, W., & Scott, C. (1985). Haemodynamic monitoring: Measurement of system blood pressure. *Canadian Anaesthesia Society Journal, 32*, 294–298.

Appel, M. L., Berger, R. D., Saul, J. P., Smith, S. M., & Cohen, R. J. (1989). Beat to beat variability in cardiovascular variables: Noise or music? *Journal of the American College of Cardiology. 14*, 1139–1148.

Azar, R., Paquette, D., & Stewart, D. E. (2010). Prenatal tobacco exposure and cortisol levels in infants of teen mothers. *Journal of Perinatal Medicine, 38*, 689–692.

Bairey Merz, C. N., Kop, W., Krantz, D. S., Helmers, K. F., Berman, D. S., & Rozanski, A. (1998). Cardiovascular stress response and coronary artery disease: Evidence of an adverse postmenopausal effect in women. *American Heart Journal, 135* (5, Pt. 1). 881–887.

Banner, T. E., & Gavenstein, J. S. (1991). Comparative effects of cuff size and tightness of fit on accuracy of blood pressure measurements. *Journal of Clinical Monitoring, 7*, 281–284.

Belkic, K., Emdad, R., & Theorell, T. (1998). Occupational profile and cardiac risk: Possible mechanisms and implications for professional drivers. *International Journal of Occupational Medicine and Environmental Health, 11*, 37–57.

Benschop, R. J., Geenen, R., Mills, R. J., Naliboff, B. D., Giecoli-Glaser, J. K., Herbert, T. B., . . . Cacioppo, J. T. (1998). Cardiovascular and immune responses to acute psychological stress in young and old women: A meta-analysis. *Psychosomatic Medicine, 60*, 290–296.

Benschop, R. J., Godaert, G. L. R., Geenen, R., Brosschot, J. R., deSmet, J. B. M., Olff, M., . . . Ballieux, R. E. (1995). Relationships between cardiovascular and immunologic changes in an experimental stress model. *Psychological Medicine, 25*, 323–327.

Benschop, R. J., Nieuwenhuis, E. E. S., Tromp, E. A. M., Godaert, G. L. R., Ballieux, R. E., & van Doornen, L. J. P. (1994). Effects of beta-adrenergic blockade on immunologic and cardiovascular changes induced by mental stress. *Circulation, 89*, 762–769.

Berntson, G. G., Cacioppo, J. T., & Quigley, K. S. (1993). Respiratory sinus arrhythmia: Autonomic origins, physiological mechanisms, and psychophysiological implications. *Psychophysiology, 30*, 183–196.

Bosch, J. A., Brand, H. S., Ligtenberg, T. J., Bermond, B., Hoogstraten, J., & Nieuw Amerongen, A. V. (1996). Psychological stress as a determinant of protein levels and salivary-induced aggregation of Streptococcus gordonii in human whole saliva. *Psychosomatic Medicine, 58*, 374–382.

Bosch, J. A., de Geus, E. J., Carroll, D., Goedhart, A. D., Anane, L. A., van Zanten, J. J., . . . Edwards, K. M. (2009). A general enhancement of autonomic and cortisol responses during social evaluative threat. *Psychosomatic Medicine, 71*, 877–885.

Bosch, J. A., de Geus, E. J., Veerman, E. C., Hoogstraten, J., & Nieuw Amerongen, A. V. (2003). Innate secretory immunity in response to laboratory stressors that evoke distinct patterns of cardiac autonomic activity. *Psychosomatic Medicine, 65*, 245–258.

Bradley, R. T., McCraty, R., Atkinson, M., Tomasino, D., Daugherty, A., & Arguelles, L. (2010). Emotion self-regulation, psychophysiological coherence, and test anxiety: Results from an experiment using electrophysiological measures. *Psychophysiology & Biofeedback, 35*, 261–283.

Bristow, M., Hucklebridge, F., Clow, A., & Evans, P. (1997). Modulation of secretory immunoglobulin A in saliva in relation to an acute episode of stress and arousal. *Journal of Psychophysiology, 11*, 248–255.

Burns, N. (2009). *The practice of nursing research: Appraisal, synthesis, and generation of evidence (6th ed.).* St. Louis, MO: W. B. Saunders.

Cacioppo, J. T. (1994). Social neuroscience: Autonomic, neuroendocrine, and immune responses to stress. *Psychophysiology, 31*, 113–128.

Cannon, W. B. (1939). *The wisdom of the body.* New York, NY: Norton.

Carroll, D., Ring, C. L., Shrimpton, J., Evans, P., Willemsen, G., & Hucklebridge, F. (1996). Secretory immunoglobulin A and cardiovascular responses to acute psychological challenge. *International Journal of Internal Medicine, 3,* 266–279.

Carruthers, M., Taggart, P., Conway, N., Bates, D., & Somerville, W. (1990). Validity of plasma catecholamine estimation. *Lancet, 2,* 62–67.

Castle, D., & Castle, A. (1998). Intracellular transport and secretion of salivary proteins. *Critical Reviews in Oral Biology & Medicine, 9,* 4–22.

Chang, K., & Chiou, W. L. (1976). Interactions between drugs and saliva-stimulation parafilm and their implication in measurements of saliva drug levels. *Research Communications in Chemical Pathology and Pharmacology, 13,* 357–360.

Chatterton, R. T., Jr., Vogelsong, K. M., Lu, Y., Ellman, A. B., & Hudgens, G. A. (1996). Salivary α-amylase as a measure of endogenous adrenergic activity. *Clinical Physiology, 16,* 433–448.

Chatterton, R. T. Jr., Vogelsong, K. M., Lu, Y. C., & Hudgens, G. A. (1997). Hormonal responses to psychological stress in men preparing for skydiving. *Journal of Clinical Endocrinology & Metabolism, 82,* 2503–2509.

Coolens, J. L., Van Baelen, H., & Heyns, W. (1987). Clinical use of unbound plasma cortisol as calculated from total cortisol and corticosteroid-binding globulin. *Journal of Steroid Biochemistry, 26,* 197–202.

Cowan, M. J., Kogan, H., Burr, R., Hendershot, S., & Buchanan, L. (1990). Power spectral analysis of heart rate variability after biofeedback training. *Journal of Electrocardiology, 23 Supp,* 85–94.

Cromwell, L., Weibell, F. J., & Pfeiffer, E. A. (1980). *Biomedical instrumentation and measurements* (2nd ed.). Englewood Cliffs, NJ: Prentice Hall.

Deinzer, R., & Schuller, N. (1998). Dynamics of stress-related decrease in salivary immunoglobulin A (sIgA): Relationship to symptoms of the common cold and studying behavior. *Behavioral Medicine, 23,* 161–169.

DePalo, E. F., Antonelli, G., Benetazzo, A., Prearo, M., & Gatti, R. (2009). Human saliva cortisone and cortisol simultaneous analysis using reverse phase HPLC technique. *Clinica Chimica Acta, 405,* 60–65.

Dimsdale, J. E., & Ziegler, M. G. (1991). What do plasma and urinary measures of catecholamines tell us about human response to stressors? *Circulation, 83*(Suppl. II), II-36–II-42.

DuFour, D. R. (1990). Reference values in endocrinology. In K. L. Becker, J. P. Bilezikian, W. J. Bremmer, W. Hung, C. R. Kahn, D. L. Loriaux, R. W. Rebar, G. L. Robertson, & L. Wartofsky (Eds.), *Principles and practice of endocrinology and metabolism* (pp. 1723–1765). Philadelphia, PA: J. B. Lippincott.

Ebert, T. J. (1992). Autonomic balance and cardiac function. *Current Opinions in Anaesthesiology, 5,* 3–10.

Edelberg, R. (1967). Electrical properties of the skin. In C. C. Brown (Ed.), *Methods in psychophysiology* (pp. 1–53). Baltimore, MD: Williams & Wilkins.

Edelberg, R. (1972). Electrodermal activity of the skin. In N. S. Greenfield & R. A. Sternbach (Eds.), *Handbook of psychophysiology* (pp. 367–418). New York, NY: Holt, Rinehart & Winston.

Edgar, W. M. (1992). Saliva: Its secretion, composition and functions. *British Dental Journal, 172,* 305–312.

Ehlert, U., Erni, K., Hebisch, G., & Nater, U. (2006). Salivary alpha-amylase levels after yohimbine challenge in healthy men. *Journal of Clinical Endocrinology & Metabolism, 91,* 5130–5133.

Euler, S., Schimpf, H., Hennig, J., & Brosig, B. (2005). On psychobiology in psychoanalysis—salivary cortisol and secretory IgA as psychoanalytic process parameters. *Psycho-Social-Medicine, 2,* Doc05.

Evans, P., Bristow, M., Hucklebridge, F., Clow, A., & Pang, F. Y. (1994). Stress arousal, cortisol, and secretory immunoglobulin A in students undergoing assessment. *British Journal of Clinical Psychology, 33,* 575–576.

Evans, P., Bristow, M., Hucklebridge, F., Clow, A., & Walters, N. (1993). The relationship between secretory immunity, mood and life events. *British Journal of Clinical Psychology, 32,* 227–236.

Everly, G. S., Jr., & Sobelman, S. A. (1987). *Assessment of the human stress response: Neurological, biochemical, and psychological foundations.* New York, NY: AMS Press.

Falaschi, P., Martocchia, A., Proietti, A., Pastore, R., & D'urso, R. (1994). Immune system and the hypothalamus-pituitary-adrenal axis. *Annals of the New York Academy of Sciences, 741,* 223–231.

Frankenhaeuser, M. (1983). The sympathetic-adrenal and pituitary-adrenal response to challenge: Comparison between the sexes. In T. M. Dembroski, T. H. Schmidt, & G. Blumchen (Eds.), *Biobehavioral bases of coronary heart disease* (pp. 91–105). Basel, Switzerland: Karger.

Frey, M. A. B., & Porth, C. M. (1990). Sex differences in response to orthostatic and other stresses. In J. J. Smith (Ed.), *Circulatory response to the upright position* (pp. 141–167). Boca Raton, FL: CRC Press.

Fuller, B. F. (1992). The effects of stress—Anxiety and coping styles on heart rate variability. *International Journal of Psychophysiology, 12,* 81–86.

Gallagher, P., Leitch, M. M., Massey, A. E., McAllister-Williams, R. H., & Young, A. H. (2006). Assessing cortisol and dehydroepiandrosterone (DHEA) in saliva: Effects of collection method. *Journal of Psychopharmacology, 20,* 643–649.

Gallagher, S., Phillips, A. C., Evans, P., Der, G., Hunt, K., & Carroll, D. (2008). Caregiving is associated with low secretion rates of immunoglobulin A in saliva. *Brain, Behavior, and Immunity, 22,* 565–572.

Garde, A. H., & Hansen, A. M. (2005). Long-term stability of salivary cortisol. *Scandinavian Journal of Clinical and Laboratory Investigation, 65,* 433–436.

Garrett, J. R. (1987). The proper role of nerves in salivary secretion: A review. *Journal of Dental Research, 66,* 387–397.

Gehris, T. L., & Kathol, R. G. (1992). Comparison of time-integrated measurement of salivary corticosteroids by oral diffusion sink technology to plasma cortisol. *Endocrine Research, 18,* 77–89.

Gilman, S., Thornton, R., Miller, D., & Biersner, R. (1979). Effects of exercise stress on parotid gland secretion. *Hormone and Metabolic Research, 11,* 454.

Gilman, S. C., Fischer, G. J., Biersner, R. J., Thornton, R. D., & Miller, D. A. (1979). Human parotid gland alpha-amylase secretion as a function of chronic hyperbaric exposure. *Undersea Biomedical Research, 6,* 303–307.

Gobel, F. L., Nordstrom, L. A., Nelson, R. R., Jorgenson, C. R., & Wang, Y. (1978). The rate-pressure product as an index of myocardial oxygen consumption during exercise in patients with angina pectoris. *Circulation, 57,* 549–556.

Gorny, D. A. (1993). Arterial pressure measurement techniques. *AACN Clinical Issues in Critical Care Nursing, 4,* 66–78.

Graham, N. M. H., Chiron, R., Bartholomeusz, A., Taboonpong, N., & La Brooy, J. T. (1988). Does anxiety reduce the secretion rate of secretory IgA in saliva? *Medical Journal of Australia, 148,* 131–133.

Gröschl, M. (2008). Current status of salivary hormone analysis. *Clinical Chemistry, 54,* 1759–1769.

Gröschl, M., & Rauh, M. (2006). Influence of commercial collection devices for saliva on the reliability of salivary steroids analysis. *Steroids, 71,* 13–14.

Gröschl, M., Wagner, R., Rauh, M., & Dörr, H. G. (2001). Stability of salivary steroids: The influences of storage, food and dental care. *Steroids, 66*(10), 737–741.

Grossman, P., vanBeek, J., & Wientjes, C. (1990). A comparison of three quantification methods for estimation of respiratory sinus arrhythmia. *Psychophysiology, 27,* 702–714.

Guinard, J.-X., Zoumas-Morse, C., & Walchak, C. (1997). Relation between parotid saliva flow and composition and the perception of gustatory and trigeminal stimuli in foods. *Physiology & Behavior, 63,* 109–118.

Gunnar, M. R., Connors, J., & Isenee, J. (1989). Lack of stability in neonatal adrenocortical reactivity because of rapid habituation of the adrenocortical response. *Developmental Psychobiology, 22,* 221–233.

Guyton, A. C., & Hall, J. E. (2006). *Textbook of medical physiology* (11th ed.). Philadelphia, PA: Elsevier Saunders.

Guzzetta, C. E. (1989). Effects of relaxation and music therapy on patients in a coronary care unit with presumptive acute myocardial infarction. *Heart & Lung, 18,* 609–616.

Hainsworth, R. (1995). The control and physiological importance of heart rate. In M. Malik & A. J. Camm (Eds.), *Heart rate variability* (pp. 3–19). Armonk, NY: Futura.

Han, L., Li, J. P., Sit, J. W., Chung, L., Jiao, Z. Y., & Ma, W. G. (2010), Effects of music intervention on physiological stress response and anxiety level of mechanically ventilated patients in China: A randomised controlled trial. *Journal of Clinical Nursing, 19,* 978–987.

Hanecke, P., & Haeckel, R. (1992). A method to collect saliva from infants. In C. Kirschbaum, G. F. Read, & D. H. Hellhammer (Eds.), *Assessment of hormones and drugs in saliva in biobehavioral research* (pp. 33–35). Seattle, WA: Hogrefe & Huber.

Hatch, J. P., Borcherding, S., & Norris, L.K. (1990). Cardiopulmonary adjustments during operant heart rate control. *Psychophysiology, 27,* 641–648.

Hattori, N., Tamaki, N., Kudoh, T., Masuda, I., Magata, Y., Kitano, H., . . . Konishi, J. (1998). Abnormality of myocardial oxidative metabolism in noninsulin-dependent diabetes mellitus. *Journal of Nuclear Medicine, 39,* 1835–1840.

Heitkemper, M., Jarrett, M., Cain, K., Shaver, J., Bond, E., Woods, N. F., & Walker, E. (1996). Increased urine catecholamines and cortisol in women with irritable bowel syndrome. *American Journal of Gastroenterology, 91,* 906–913.

Hellhammer, D. H., Wüst, S., & Kudielka, B. M. (2009). Salivary cortisol as a biomarker in stress research. *Psychoneuroendocrinology, 34,* 163–171.

Henry, J. P. (1992). Biological basis of the stress response. *Integrative Physiology and Behavioural Science, 27,* 66–83.

Herbert, T. B., & Cohen, S. (1993). Stress and immunity in humans: A meta-analytic review. *Psychosomatic Medicine, 55,* 364–379.

Hirsch, J. A., & Bishop, B. (1981). Respiratory sinus arrhythmia in humans: How breathing pattern modulates heart rate. *American Journal of Physiology, 241,* H620–H629.

Höld, K. M., deBoer, D., Zuidema, J., & Maes, R. A. (1995). Evaluation of the Salivette as sampling device for monitoring beta-adrenoceptor blocking drugs in saliva. *Journal of Chromatography B: Biomedical Sciences and Applications, 663,* 103–110.

Hrushesky, W. J. M., Fader, D., Schmitt, O., & Gilbertsen, V. (1984). The respiratory sinus arrhythmia: A measure of cardiac age. *Science, 224,* 1001–1004.

Huang, C., Webb, H. E., Garten, R., Kamimori, G. H., & Acevedo, E. O. (2010). Psychological stress during exercise: Lymphocyte subset redistribution in firefighters. *Physiology & Behavior, 101,* 320–326.

Hyndman, B. W., Kitney, R. I., & Sayers, B. M. (1971). Spontaneous rhythms in physiological control systems. *Nature, 233,* 339–342.

Imholz, B. P. M., van Montfrans, G. A., Settels, J. J., Gerard, M. A., VanDerHoeven, G. M. A., Karemaker, J. M., & Wieling, W. (1988). Continuous non-invasive blood pressure monitoring: Reliability of Finapres device during the Valsalva maneuver. *Cardiovascular Research, 22,* 390–397.

Imholz, B. P., Wieling, W., van Montfrans, G. A., & Wessling, K. H. (1998). Fifteen years experience with finger arterial pressure monitoring: Assessment of the technology. *Cardiovascular Research, 38,* 605–616.

Jagomägi, K., Talts, J., Raamat, R., & Lansimes, E. (1996). Continuous non-invasive measurement of mean blood pressure in finger by volume-clamp and differential oscillometric method. *Clinical Physiology, 16,* 551–560.

Jain, D., Shaker, S. M., Burg, M., Wackers, F. J., Soufer, R., & Zaret, B. L. (1998). Effects of mental stress on left ventricular and peripheral vascular performance in patients with coronary artery disease. *Journal of the American College of Cardiology, 31,* 1314–1322.

Jefferson, L. L. (2010). Exploring effects of therapeutic massage and patient teaching in the practice of diaphragmatic breathing on blood pressure, stress, and anxiety in hypertensive African-American women: An intervention study. *Journal of National Black Nurses' Association, 21,* 17–24.

Jensen, L., Yakimets, J., & Teo, K. K. (1995). A review of impedance cardiography. *Heart & Lung, 24,* 183–193.

Kavanagh, T., Matosevic, V., Thacker, L., Belliard, R., & Shephard, R. J. (1998). On-site evaluation of bus drivers with coronary heart disease. *Journal of Cardiopulmonary Rehabilitation, 18,* 209–215.

Kirschbaum, C., & Hellhammer, D. H. (1989). Salivary control in psychobiological research. An overview. *Neuropsychology, 22,* 150–169.

Kirschbaum, C., & Hellhammer, D. H. (1994). Salivary cortisol in psychoneuroendocrine research: Recent developments and applications. *Psychoneuroendocrinology, 19,* 313–333.

Kirschbaum, C., Read, G. F., & Hellhammer, D. H. (1992). *Assessment of hormones and drugs in saliva in biobehavioral research.* Seattle, WA: Hogrefe & Huber.

Kleiger, R. E., Bigger, J. T., Bosner, M. S., Chung, M. K., Cook, J. R., Rolnitzky, L. M., . . . Fleiss, J. L. (1991). Stability over time of variables measuring heart rate variability in normal subjects. *American Journal of Cardiology, 68,* 626–630.

Knepp, M. M., & Friedman, B. H. (2008). Cardiovascular activity during laboratory tasks in women with high and low worry. *Biological Psychology, 79,* 287–293.

Kubicek, W. G., Karnegis, J. N., Patterson, R. P., Witssoe, D. A., & Mattson, R. H. (1966). Development and evaluation of an impedance cardiac output system. *Aerospace Medicine, 37,* 1208–1212.

Latman, N. S. (1992). Evaluation of finger blood pressure monitoring instruments. *Biomedical Instrumentation and Technology, 26,* 52–57.

LeWinter, M. M., & Osol, G. (2004). Normal physiology of the cardiovascular system. In V. Fuster, R. W. Alexander, R. A. O'Rourke, R. Roberts, S. B. King III, I. S. Nash, & E. N. Prystowsky (Eds.), *Hurst's the heart* (11th ed., pp. 87–112). New York, NY: McGraw-Hill.

Losso, E. M., Singer, J. M., & Nicolau, J. (1997). Effect of gustatory stimulation on flow rate and protein content of human parotid saliva according to the side of preferential mastication. *Archives of Oral Biology, 42,* 83–87.

Lyew, M. A., & Jamieson, J. W. (1994). Blood pressure measurement using oscillometric finger cuffs in children and young adults. *Anesthesia, 49,* 895–899.

Malliani, A., Pagani, M., Lombardi, F., & Cerutti, S. (1991). Cardiovascular neural regulation explored in the frequency domain. *Circulation, 84,* 482–492.

Manhem, K., & Jern, S. (1994). Influence of daily-life activation on pulse rate and blood pressure changes during the menstrual cycle. *Journal of Human Hypertension, 8,* 851–856.

Mathias, C. J., & Alam, M. (1995). Circadian changes of the cardiovascular system and the autonomic nervous system: Observations in autonomic disorders. In M. Malik & A. J. Camm (Eds.), *Heart rate variability* (pp. 21–30). Armonk, NY: Futura.

Matsubara, T., Arai, Y. C., Shiro, Y., Shimo, K., Nishihara, M., Sato, J., & Ushida, T. (2011). Comparative effects of acupressure at local and distal acupuncture points on pain conditions and autonomic function in females with chronic neck pain. *Evidence-Based Complementary and Alternative Medicine, 2011.* Retrieved from http://www.ncbi.nlm.nih.gov/pmc/articles/PMC2952311/?tool=pubmed

McCarthy, A. M., Kleiber, C., Hanrahan, K., Zimmerman, M. B., Westhus, N., & Allen, S. (2010). Factors explaining children's responses to intravenous needle insertions. *Nursing Research, 59,* 407–416.

McClelland, D. C., Alexander, C., & Marks, E. (1982). The need for power, stress, immune function and illness among male prisoners. *Journal of Abnormal Psychology, 91,* 61–70.

McClelland, D. C., Ross, G., & Patel, V. (1985). The effect of an academic examination on salivary norepinephrine and immunoglobulin levels. *Journal of Human Stress, 11,* 52–59.

McKay, K. A., Buen, J. E., Bohan, K. J., & Maye, J. P. (2010). Determining the relationship of acute stress, anxiety, and salivary alpha-amylase level with performance of student nurse anesthetists during human-based anesthesia simulator training. *American Association of Nurse Anesthetists Journal, 78,* 301–309.

Mikosch, P., Hadrawa, T., Laubreiter, K., Brandl, J., Pilz, J., Stettner, H., & Grimm, G. (2010). Effectiveness of respiratory-sinus-arrhythmia biofeedback on state-anxiety in patients undergoing coronary angiography. *Journal of Advanced Nursing, 66,* 1101–1110.

Miletic, I. D., Schiffman, S. S., Miletic, V. D., & Sattely-Miller, E. A. (1996). Salivary IgA secretion rate in young and elderly persons. *Physiology & Behavior, 60,* 243–248.

Minton, M. E., Hertzog, M., Barron, C. R., French, J. A., & Reiter-Palmon, R. (2009). The first anniversary: Stress, well-being, and optimism in older widows. *Western Journal of Nursing Research, 31,* 1035–1056.

Moore, R. Y. (1997). Circadian rhythms: Basic neurobiology and clinical applications. *Annual Review of Medicine, 48,* 253–260.

Murphy, L., Denis, R., Ward, C. P., & Tartar, J. L. (2010). Academic stress differentially influences perceived stress, salivary cortisol, and immunoglobulin-A in undergraduate students. *Stress, 13,* 365–370.

Musselman, D. L., Rudisch, B., McDonald, W. M., & Nemeroff, C.B. (2004). Effects of mood and anxiety disorders on the cardiovascular system. In V. Fuster, R. W. Alexander, R. A. O'Rourke, R. Roberts, S. B. King III, I. S. Nash, & E. N. Prystowsky (Eds.), *Hurst's the heart* (11th ed., pp. 2189–2209). New York, NY: McGraw-Hill.

Naliboff, B. D., Solomon, G. F., Gilmore, S. L., Fahey, J. L., Benton, D., & Pine, J. (1995). Rapid changes in cellular immunity following a confrontational role-play stressor. *Brain, Behavior, & Immunity, 9,* 207–219.

Nater, U. M., La Marca, R., Florin, L., Moses, A., Langhans, W., Koller, M. M., & Ehlert, U. (2006). Stress-induced changes in human salivary alpha-amylase activity—associations with adrenergic activity. *Psychoneuroendocrinology, 31,* 49–58.

Nater, U. M., Rohleder, N., Gaab, J., Berger, S., Jud, A., Kirschbaum, C., & Ehlert, U. (2005). Human salivary alpha-amylase reactivity in a psychosocial stress paradigm. *International Journal of Psychophysiology, 55,* 333–342.

Nesselroad, J. M., Flacco, V. A., Phillips, D. M., & Kruse, J. (1996). Accuracy of automated finger blood pressure devices. *Family Medicine, 28,* 189–192.

Nguyen, S., & Wong, D. T. (2006). Cultural, behavioral, social, and psychological perceptions of saliva: Relevance to clinical diagnostics. *Journal of the California Dental Association, 34,* 317–322.

O'Brien, E., Fitzgerald, D., & O'Malley, K. (1985). Blood pressure measurement: Current practice and future trends. *British Medical Journal, 290,* 729–734.

O'Brien, E., Mee, F., Tan, S., Atkins, N., & O'Malley, K. (1991). Training and assessment of observers for blood pressure measurement in hypertension research. *Journal of Human Hypertension, 5,* 7–10.

O'Brien, I. A. D., O'Hare, P., & Corrall, R. J. M. (1985). Heart rate variability in healthy subjects: Effects of age and the derivation of normal ranges for tests of autonomic function. *British Heart Journal, 55,* 348–354.

Okamura, H., Tsuda, A., Yajima, J., Mark, H., Horiuchi, S., Toyoshima, N., & Matsuishi, T. (2010). Short sleeping time and psychobiological responses to acute stress. *International Journal of Psychophysiology, 78,* 209–214.

Oosterman, M., & Schuengel, C. (2007). Autonomic reactivity of children to separation and reunion with foster parents. *Journal of the American Academy of Child & Adolescent Psychiatry, 46,* 1196–1203.

Pagani, M., Lombardi, F., Guzzetti, S., Rimoldi, U., Furlan, R., Pizzinelli, P., . . . Malliani, A. (1986). Power spectral analysis of heart rate and arterial pressure variabilities as a marker of sympatho-vagal interaction in man and conscious dog. *Circulation Research, 59,* 178–193.

Pagani, M., Lucini, D., Rimoldi, O., Furlan, R., Piazza, S., & Biancardi, L. (1995). Effects of physical and mental exercise on heart rate variability. In M. Malik & A. J. Camm (Eds.), *Heart rate variability* (pp. 245–266). Armonk, NY: Futura.

Parati, G., Trazzi, S., Ravogli, A., Casadei, R., Omboni, S., & Manacia, G. (1991). Methodological problems in evaluation of cardiovascular effects of stress in humans. *Hypertension, 17*(Suppl. III), III-50–III-55.

Perogamvros, I., Keevil, B. G., Ray, D. W., & Trainer, P. J. (2010). Salivary cortisone is a potential biomarker for serum free cortisol. *Journal of Clinical Endocrinology & Metabolism, 95*, 4951–4958.

Peters, M. L., Godaert, G. L. R., Ballieux, R. E., van Vliet, M., Willemsen, J. J., Sweep, F. C. G. J., & Heijnen, C. J. (1998). Cardiovascular and endocrine responses to experimental stress. *Psychophysiology, 23*, 1–17.

Pickering, T. (1995). Recommendations for use of home (self) and ambulatory blood-pressure monitoring. American Society for Blood Pressure Ad Hoc Panel. *American Journal of Hypertension, 9*, 1–11.

Polit, D. F., & Beck, C. T. (2007). *Nursing research: Generating and assessing evidence for nursing practice* (8th ed.). Philadelphia, PA: J. B. Lippincott.

Pomeranz, B., Macaulay, J. B., Caudill, M. A., Kutz, I., Adam, D., Gordon, D., . . . Benson, H. (1985). Assessment of autonomic function in humans by heart rate spectral analysis. *American Journal of Physiology, 17*, H151–H153.

Porth, C. M. (1976). A comparison of cardiovascular responses to cold pressor and isometric handgrip exercises in normal young males. Unpublished master's thesis, Medical College of Wisconsin, Milwaukee.

Porth, C. M., & Mattfin, G. (2009). Structure and function of the cardiovascular system. In C. M. Porth & G. Mattfin (Eds.), *Pathophysiology: Concepts of altered health states* (8th ed., pp. 450–476). Philadelphia, PA: J. B. Lippincott.

Rabin, B. S., Kusnecov, A., Shurin, M., Zhou, D., & Rasnick, S. (1994). Mechanistic aspects of stressor-induced immune alteration. In R. Glaser & J. Kiecolt-Glaser (Eds.), *Handbook of human stress and immunity* (pp. 23–51). San Diego, CA: Academic Press.

Rhoades, R. A., & Tanner, G. A. (1995). *Medical physiology.* Boston, MA: Little, Brown.

Richter, D. W., & Spyer, K. M. (1990). Cardiorespiratory control. In A. D. Loewy & K. M. Spyer (Eds.), *Central regulation of autonomic function* (pp. 189–207). New York, NY: Oxford University Press.

Rief, W., Shaw, R., & Fichter, M. M. (1998). Elevated levels of psychophysiological arousal and cortisol in patients with somatization syndrome. *Psychosomatic Medicine, 60,* 198–203.

Ristuccia, H. L., Grossman, P., Watkins, L. L., & Lown, B. (1997). Incremental bias in Finapres estimation of baseline blood pressure levels over time. *Hypertension, 19,* 1039–1043.

Rohleder, N., Nater, U. M., Wolf, J. M., Ehlert, U., & Kirschbaum, C. (2004). Psychosocial stress-induced activation of salivary alpha-amylase: An indicator of sympathetic activity? *Annals of the New York Academy of Sciences, 1032,* 258–263.

Rohleder, N., Wolf, J. M., Maldonado, E. F., & Kirschbaum, C. (2006). The psychosocial stress-induced increase in salivary alpha-amylase is independent of saliva flow rate. *Psychophysiology, 43,* 645–652.

Rubin, S. A. (1987). Measurement theory and instrument errors. In S. A. Rubin (Ed.), *The principles of biomedical instrumentation* (pp. 50–74). Chicago, IL: Year Book Medical.

Rudy, E. B., & Estok, P. (1992). Professional and lay interrater reliability of urinary luteinizing hormone surges measured by OvuQuick test. *Journal of Obstetrics and Gynecological and Neonatal Nursing, 21,* 407–411.

Sack, D. A., Neogi, P. K. B., & Alam, M. D. K. (1980). Immunobead enzyme-linked immunosorbent assay for quantifying immunoglobulin A in human secretions and serum. *Infection and Immunity, 29,* 281–283.

Samson, R. R., McClelland, D. B. L., & Shearman, D. J. C. (1973). Studies on the quantification of immunoglobulin in human intestinal secretions. *Gut, 14,* 616–626.

Saul, J. P. (1990). Beat-to-beat variations of heart rate reflect modulation of cardiac autonomic outflow. *NIPS, 5,* 32–37.

Saul, J. P., & Cohen, R. J. (1994). Respiratory sinus arrhythmia. In M. N. Levy & P. J. Schwartz (Eds.), *Vagal control of the heart: Experimental basis and clinical implications* (pp. 511–536). Armonk, NY: Futura.

Scannapieco, F. A., Torres, G., & Levine, M. J. (1993). Salivary alpha-amylase: Role in dental plaque and caries formation. *Critical Reviews in Oral Biology and Medicine, 4,* 301–307.

Schäffer, L., Luzi, F., Burkhardt, T., Rauh, M., & Beinder, E. (2009). Antenatal betamethasone administration alters stress physiology in healthy neonates. *Obstetrics & Gynecology, 113,* 1082–1088.

Schäffer, L., Müller-Vizentini, D., Burkhardt, T., Rauh, M., Ehlert, U., & Beinder, E. (2009). Blunted stress response in small for gestational age neonates. *Pediatric Research, 65,* 231–235.

Schwartz, J. B., Gibb, W. J., & Tran, T. (1991). Aging effects on heart rate variability. *Journal of Gerontology, 46,* M99–M106.

Seibt, R., Boucsein, W., & Schuech, K. (1998). Effects of different stress settings on cardiovascular parameters and their relationship to daily life blood pressure in normotensives, borderline hypertensives and hypertensives. *Ergonomics, 41,* 634–648.

Selye, H. (1974). *Stress without distress.* New York, NY: New American Library.

Shadish, W. R., Cook, T. D., & Campbell, D. T. (1979). *Experimental and quasi-experimental designs for generalized causal inference (2nd ed.).* Boston, MA: Houghton Mifflin.

Shipley, J. E., Alessi, N. E., Wade, S. E., Haegele, A. D., & Helmbold, B. (1992). Utility of an oral diffusion sink (ODS) device for quantification of saliva corticosteroids in human subject. *Journal of Clinical Endocrinology & Metabolism, 71,* 639–644.

Skosnik, P. D., Chatterton, R. T., Swisher, T., & Park, S. (2000). Modulation of attentional inhibition by norepinephrine and cortisol after psychological stress. *International Journal of Psychophysiology, 36,* 59–68.

Smith, J. J., & Porth, C. J. M. (1990). Age and the response to orthostatic stress. In J. J. Smith (Ed.), *Circulatory response to the upright posture* (pp. 121–139). Boca Raton, FL: CRC Press.

Stein, P. K., Bosner, M. S., Kleiger, R. E., & Conger, B. M. (1994). Heart rate variability: A measure of cardiac autonomic tone. *American Heart Journal, 127,* 1376–1381.

Steptoe, A., Cropley, M., & Joekes, K. (1999). Job strain, blood pressure and response to uncontrollable stress. *Journal of Hypertension, 17,* 193–200.

Steptoe, A., Evans, O., & Fieldman, G. (1997). Perceptions of control over work: Psychophysiological responses to self-paced and externally paced tasks in an adult population sample. *International Journal of Psychophysiology, 25,* 211–220.

Stites, D. P. (1991). Laboratory evaluation of immune competence. In D. P. Stites & A. I. Terr (Eds.), *Basic and clinical immunology* (7th ed., pp. 312–318). Norwalk, CT: Appleton & Lange.

Stites, D. P., & Rodgers, R. P. C. (1991). Clinical laboratory methods for detection of antigens and antibodies. In D. P. Stites & A. I. Terr (Eds.), *Basic and clinical immunology* (7th ed., pp. 217–262). Norwalk, CT: Appleton & Lange.

Strahler, J., Berndt, C., Kirschbaum, C., & Rohleder, N. (2010). Aging diurnal rhythms and chronic stress: Distinct alteration of diurnal rhythmicity of salivary alpha-amylase and cortisol. *Biological Psychology, 84,* 248–256.

Strahler, J., Mueller, A., Rosenloecher, F., Kirschbaum, C., & Rohleder, N. (2010). Salivary alpha-amylase stress reactivity across different age groups. *Psychophysiology, 47,* 587–595.

Tang, R., Tegeler, C., Larrimore, D., Cowgill, S., & Kemper, K. J. (2010). Improving the well-being of nursing leaders through healing touch training. *Journal of Alternative and Complementary Medicine, 16,* 837–841.

Takatsuji, K., Sugimoto, Y., Ishizaki, S., Ozaki, Y., Matsuyama, E., & Yamaguchi, Y. (2010). The effects of examination stress on salivary cortisol, immunoglobulin A, and chromogranin A in nursing students. *Biomedical Research (Tokyo, Japan), 29*(4), 221–224.

Task Force of the European Society of Cardiology and the North American Society of Pacing and Electrophysiology. (1996). Heart rate variability: Standards of measurement, physiological interpretation, and clinical use. *European Heart Journal, 60,* 1239–1245.

Tassorelli, C., Micieli, G., Osipova, V., Rossi, F., & Nappi, G. (1995). Pupillary and cardiovascular responses to cold-pressor test. *Journal of the Autonomic Nervous System, 55*(1/2), 45–49.

Terr, A. I., Dubey, D. P., Yunis, E. J., Slavin, R. G., & Waldman, R. H. (1991). Physiologic and environmental influences on the immune system. In D. P. Stites & A. I. Terr (Eds.), *Basic and clinical immunology* (7th ed., pp. 187–199). Norwalk, CT: Appleton & Lange.

Tõru, I., Aluoja, A., Võhma, U., Raag, M., Vasar, V., Maron, E., & Shlik, J. (2010). Associations between personality traits and CCK-4-induced panic attacks in healthy volunteers. *Psychiatry Research, 178,* 342–347.

Trappe, H. J. (2010). The effects of music on the cardiovascular system and cardiovascular health. *Heart, 96,* 1868–1871.

Turton, M. B., & Deegan, T. (1974). Circadian variations of plasma catecholamines, cortisol, and immunoreactive insulin concentrations in supine subjects. *Clinica Chimica Acta, 55,* 389–397.

van Stegeren, A., Rohleder, N., Everaerd, W., & Wolf, O. T. (2006). Salivary alpha amylase as marker for adrenergic activity during stress: Effect of betablockade. *Psychoneuroendocrinology, 31,* 137–141.

Venables, P. H., & Christie, M. J. (1973). Mechanism, instrumentation, recording techniques and quantification of responses. In W. F. Prokasy & D. C. Raskin (Eds.), *Electrodermal activity in psychological research* (pp. 1–124). New York, NY: Academic Press.

Venables, P. H., & Martin, I. (1967). Skin resistance and skin potential. In P. H. Venables & I. Martin

(Eds.), *Manual of psycho-physiological methods* (pp. 53–102). Amsterdam, Netherlands: North-Holland.

Villella, M., Villella, A., Barlera, S., Franzosi, M. G., & Maggioni, A. P. (1999). Prognostic significance of double product and inadequate double product response to maximal symptom-limited exercise stress testing after myocardial infarction in 6,296 patients treated with thrombolytic agents. *American Heart Journal, 137,* 443–452.

Vogele, C. (1998). Serum lipid concentrations, hostility and cardiovascular reactions to mental stress. *International Journal of Psychophysiology, 28,* 167–179.

Vogeser, M., Briegel, J., Zachoval, R. (2002). Dialyzable free cortisol after stimulation with Synacthen. *Clinical Biochemistry, 35,* 539–543.

Vybiral, T., Bryg, R. J., Maddens, M. E., & Boden, W. E. (1989). Effect of passive tilt on sympathetic and parasympathetic components of heart rate variability in normal subjects. *American Journal of Cardiology, 53,* 1117–1120.

Wade, S. E. (1992). An oral-diffusion-sink device for extended sampling of multiple steroid hormones from saliva. *Clinical Chemistry, 38,* 1878–1882.

Wade, S. E., & Haegele, A. D. (1991). Time-integrated measurement of corticosteroids in saliva by oral diffusion sink technology. *Clinical Chemistry, 37,* 1166–1172.

Waltz, C. F., Strickland, O. L., & Lenz, E. R. (2010). *Measurement in nursing and health research* (4th ed.). New York, NY: Springer.

Weiner, H. (1992). *Perturbing the organism: The biology of the stressful experience.* Chicago, IL: University of Chicago Press.

White, J. M. (1999). Effects of relaxing music on cardiac autonomic balance and anxiety after acute myocardial infarction. *American Journal of Critical Care, 8,* 220-230.

Willemsen, G., Ring, C., Carroll, D., Evans, P., Clow, A., & Hucklebridge, F. (1998). Secretory immunoglobulin A and cardiovascular reactions to mental arithmetic and cold pressor. *Psychobiology, 35,* 252–259.

Woltjer, H. H., Bogaard, H. J., & deVries, P. M. J. M. (1997). The technique of impedance cardiography. *European Heart Journal, 18,* 1396–1403.

Wood, P. (2009). Salivary steroid assays—research or routine? *Annals of Clinical Biochemistry, 46,* 183–196.

Woods, N. F., & Cantanzaro, M. (1988). *Nursing research: Theory and practice.* St. Louis, MO: C. V. Mosby.

Woodworth, R. S., & Schlosberg, H. (1954). *Experimental psychology.* New York, NY: Holt.

Working Party on Blood Pressure Measurement of the British Hypertension Society. (1997). *Blood pressure measurement: Recommendations of the British Hypertension Society* (3rd ed.). Plymouth, UK: British Medical Journal Publishing Group.

Yim, I. S., Granger, D. A., & Quas, J. A. (2010). Children's and adult's salivary alpha amylase responses to a laboratory stressor and to verbal recall of the stressor. *Developmental Psychobiology, 52,* 598–602.

Yu, B. H., Nelesen, R., Ziegler, M. G., & Dimsdale, J. E. (2001). Mood states and impedance cardiography-derived hemodynamics. *Annals of Behavioral Medicine, 23,* 21–25.

Zeier, H., Brauchli, P., & Joller-Jemelka, H. I. (1996). Effects of work demands on immunoglobulin A and cortisol in air traffic controllers. *Biological Psychology, 42,* 413–423.

Zoccola, P. M., Quas, J. A., & Yim, I. S. (2010). Salivary cortisol responses to psychological laboratory stressor and later verbal recall of the stressor: The role of trait and state rumination. *Stress, 13,* 435–443.

PART III

STIMULUS-ORIENTED STRESS

6

Major and Minor Life Stressors, Measures, and Health Outcomes

Joan Stehle Werner, Marlene Hanson Frost,
Carol L. Macnee*, Susan McCabe*, and Virginia Hill Rice

Stress is a broad area of study and knowledge development involving many disciplines in search of describing, understanding, and predicting major and minor life events and their consequences for health and well-being. Ultimately, for some disciplines such as nursing, the goal is to mitigate the ill effects of stress within individuals, families, communities, and societies.

Stress has been portrayed as a process, including a stimulus, individual characteristics and perception, a response, and long-term consequences (Elliott & Eisdorfer, 1982). Cohen, Kessler, and Gordon (1995) described a model they called the "unifying model of the stress process" (p. 10) that included the following: (a) environmental demands, (b) cognitive evaluation of the threat potential of the demand and coping abilities available, (c) perceptions of stress, (d) negative emotional reactions, and (e) behavioral and/or physiological responses that put a person at risk for psychiatric and physical illness (p. 10). Much has been studied to understand this process better, including genetic predisposition, personality, appraisal, resources, social support, personal control, vulnerability, and context.

Within the broad rubric of stress, three major traditions or spheres of scholarly work have historically flourished, each engendering voluminous amounts of research. Knowledge within these spheres has often been cultivated separately with little attention paid to other aspects of the overall process. Cohen and colleagues (1995), in discussing stress and disease risk, refer to these three traditions as the environmental, biological, and psychological stress perspectives (pp. 4–8).

- The environmental view emphasizes elements of the outside world or stressful events that happen to people that have an impact that brings about a need for adjustment.

- The biological perspective encompasses processes within the body following exposure to a stressor.

- The psychological standpoint focuses on perception, subjective meaning, and interpretation as crucial parts of the stress process.

Others have coined different labels for these points of view. In theoretical terms, they have been labeled stimulus, response, and relational or transactional (Cox, 1978; Derogatis & Coons, 1993; Lazarus & Folkman, 1984; Lyon & Werner, 1987). The stimulus-based orientation views stress as the initiator or spark of the process,

---

AUTHOR'S NOTE: Carol L. Macnee and Susan McCabe both died in an auto accident in December 2008.

where often stress is viewed as originating outside of the individual. The response-based orientation posits that stress occurs within the individual and consists of complicated physiological changes that essentially serve to bring about adaptation but, when over- or underused, produce ill effects. This maladaptive functioning is often conceptualized as a precursor to disease or disorder. The relational or transactional orientation focuses on individual differences, mainly through an emphasis on cognitive and emotional aspects of the person; the appraisal process is central to this perspective (Lazarus, 1966; Lazarus & Folkman, 1984).

In the first part of this chapter, we will focus on the environmental or stimulus-based orientation. The initiator of the stress process is termed a stressor or stress-as-stimulus. Several other terms have been used also to denote stress-as-stimulus and are often based on the underlying dimension of the stress portrayed. Examples include major life event, stressful life events, life-change events, life changes, and life events. The stress-as-stimulus view embraces the notion that stressors come from outside the individual and that stress is inherent in these events, regardless of individual responses and differences.

In the latter part of the chapter, the focus will be on the origin and evolution of the hassles and uplifts appraisal model of minor life events. Many researchers (e.g., DeLongis, Lazarus, & Folkman, 1988; Lazarus & Folkman, 1984) have argued that it is not the major life events and changes that weigh on people's minds and bodies and cause them stress and illness but rather the day-to-day chronic buildup of minor life demands or hassles. Hassles and uplifts reflect relatively "minor" daily experiences and conditions that have been appraised as salient to an individual. They can be perceived as potentially harmful or threatening (hassles) or they can be perceived as positive or favorable (uplifts) (Lazarus & Folkman, 1984). As such, hassles and uplifts are day-to-day irritants and momentary joys that reflect the stress of daily living in relation to how the individual psychologically and subjectively experiences a situation. Because hassles and uplifts depend on cognitive appraisal or assessment, the same event can be a hassle for one person and an uplift for another or even a hassle and a uplift for the same individual at different points in time. Theoretically, hassles and uplifts should equally affect health outcomes, such as somatic, psychological, and affective symptoms, because they are thought to potentially balance one another.

Section 1. Conceptualizations of Stress-as-Stimulus (Major Life Events)

No matter what the discipline or theoretical perspective of stress, all traditions include an *initiator* of the stress process. In the environmental or stimulus-based perspective, this initiator is presumed to be the stress itself. In addition to stress, this initiator is often alternately called the stressor (Breznitz & Goldberger, 1993; Elliott & Eisdorfer, 1982; Selye, 1956), the stimulus (Cox, 1978; Derogatis & Coons, 1993), the activator or potential activator (Elliott & Eisdorfer, 1982), and overstrain or fatigue (Johannisson, 2006). Stressors in the environmental or stress-as-stimulus perspective include both specific life events and environmental conditions (F. Cohen et al., 1982). On the basis of an extensive review of nursing research regarding stressors in patient-client populations, and Elliott and Eisdorfer's concept of reaction (1982, p. 20), Werner (1993) defined a *stressor* as *"an external or internal event, condition, situation, and/or cue, that has the potential to bring about, or actually activates significant physical or psychosocial reactions"* (p. 15).

The origins of the stress-as-stimulus conceptualization appear to have begun in ancient history. Lazarus and Folkman (1984) related that as early as the 1300s, the term *stress* was used to describe adversity or hardship. In the 1600s, Hooke employed the term stress to refer to an external force in the physical science sense of load that produced strain. These ideas are still employed in engineering today (Cox, 1978). Hinkle (1973) noted that in the 1800s in medicine, physicians such as Osler had observed that "intensity of life" was thought to contribute to angina pectoris or heart pain.

In the 20th century, Cannon (1932) was known for studying physical and emotional stimuli and the resulting disruption in the internal environment of the body in the form of the "fight-or-flight" response. From early in the last century to the 1930s, Adolf Meyer, a psychiatrist interested in the precursors of disease, developed a life chart that served as part of the medical examination and history interview with his patients (as cited in S. Cohen et al., 1995). His biographies suggested that patients became ill shortly after clusters of major changes in their lives more often than patients without such clusters. Additional work stemming from this type of stressor or event interview in medical practice led to research in the 1940s that began to illuminate the relationships between stressful life events and illness.

Also in the 1930s, Hans Selye began his work that led to a large body of physiological stress research. As a medical student, he observed the "syndrome of just being sick" in response to varying disease states (Selye, 1993, p. 9). He is best known for his response-based definition of stress.

Mason (1975), however, noted that Selye in his early writings appeared to use the term *stress in the stimulus* sense of the word and later changed his idea of stress to the *nonspecific bodily response* that has been his signature definition.

In 1950, Wolff, Wolff, and Hare investigated stressful aspects of the telephone operator occupation and documented periods of stress that were associated with various illnesses (as cited in S. Cohen et al., 1995). The researchers emphasized the dynamic state of the organism as a centerpiece of their conceptualization of stress. In the 1950s and 1960s, there were also several key pieces of research focusing on war and combat stemming from both the Korean and the Vietnamese conflicts. Effects of many major stressors were investigated, including bombing (Janis, 1951) and concentration camp experiences (Bettelheim, 1960).

Social sources of stress began to gain in importance in the 1970s. Levine and Scotch's (1970) book *Social Stress* laid out many social stressors, such as work organization, the family life cycle, race, social class, social isolation, and role conflict. Incorporated in Levine and Scotch's volume are life stressors, including marriage and divorce. These topics as social stressors were the forerunners of the current perspective of life transitions as significant stressors.

In most of these historical conceptualizations and examinations of stress-as-stimulus, the other important factor contributing to stress is the adaptive capability of the individual. Mechanic (1968) advocated that stress not only occurs in the presence of a stressor but also when the individual's adaptive capacities or resources either fail or are not able to completely

handle the threat. He defined stress as "a discrepancy between the demands impinging on a person—whether these demands be external or internal, whether challenges or goals—and the individual's potential responses to these demands" (p. 301). This view is one in which negative consequences such as illness occur when the adaptive response, or the ability to adjust or adapt, is inappropriate or insufficient in the face of a stressor.

The theme of adaptation or readjustment leads quite clearly to perhaps the most often investigated and cited work in the area of stressful life events—that of Holmes and his colleagues. Drawing on Meyers's use of the life chart to indicate major life disruptions that affected health status, Holmes and colleagues (Holmes & Masuda, 1974; Holmes & Rahe, 1967) *conceptualized stress as amount of life change, based on life experiences, that brings about the need for readjustment or further adaptation.*

Accordingly, their checklist measurement device was called the Social Readjustment Rating Scale (SRRS) (Holmes & Rahe, 1967). This tool is based on several assumptions concerning stress-as-stimulus. First, change, whether positive or negative, creates stress. Second, various life events result in different degrees of stress and necessary readjustment. Across individuals, however, these levels are relatively similar. To reflect this assumption in their measurement scale, the researchers used a panel of raters to establish average or normative levels of adjustment called life change units (LCUs) associated with each of 42 predetermined events. These values were then added to obtain a score representing stress as life change. This summation indicates the third assumption—that stress in the form of life changes is cumulative.

The stress-as-stimulus perspective previously described became the dominant paradigm of stress research from the early 1970s to the present. This, in part, resulted from the ease of using the checklist measurement device as a quick and easy way to measure stress. It also resulted from the viewpoint that the change associated with certain events was stressful to everyone who experienced them. This viewpoint is reflected in an often-quoted definition of stressful life events as "*objective occurrences of sufficient magnitude to bring about changes in the usual activities of most individuals who experience them*" (Dohrenwend, Krasnoff, Askenasy,

& Dohrenwend, 1982, p. 336). For the past three decades, the stressful life event or stress-as-stimulus theoretical underpinnings has changed very little. Measurement, however, has taken on many variations. There are many stressful and life change event instruments for children, adolescents, adults, the aging, families, the ill, and the healthy. (See Table 6.1.)

Probably the most important theoretical premise of this stress-as-stimulus tradition is that an accumulation of life changes or of stressors is associated with a subsequent probability of disease or negative health consequences. Cohen et al. (1995), in discussing the research immediately following the development of the SRRS, reported that there was "documentation of dramatic associations" (p. 5) with regard to stressful life events and illness. Most research in this area, however, has yielded modest associations, usually in the correlational range of .10 to .30. These results have accounted for up to 10% of the variance explained that otherwise might not be attributable. Although these correlations are too low to be considered extraordinary, they are consistently and most times substantially present in studies of stressful life events with many health outcome measures.

The body of knowledge regarding stressful life events and their effects on health and illness has been developed in and is important to many disciplines, including nursing. The reason for this widespread interest stems from the large body of evidence supporting the fact that stressful life events and environmental conditions do have an impact on physical and psychological reactions and, in some cases, on health and illness (Turner & Wheaton, 1995). They have been shown to influence the risk for, the initiation of, and the course of a wide range of physical and emotional disorders from colds and infections (Cohen, Tyrrell, & Smith, 1991) to major health crises such as the negative effects of birth trauma on breastfeeding (Beck, 2008), myocardial infarction (Hammoudeh & Alhaddad, 2009), asthma (Lietzen et al., 2010), heart disease in young adults (Twisk, Snel, de Vente, Kemper, & van Mechelen, 2000), and posttraumatic stress disorder (Goodman et al., 1998; Norris & Hamblen, 2004). Because of the substantial body of knowledge supporting this stress–illness relationship, it is no wonder many dimensions and aspects of stress-as-stimulus have been examined.

CLASSIFICATIONS OF STRESS-AS-STIMULUS

There are many categorization and classification schemes that detail organizing systems for stressors. Each is characterized by dimensions that underlie the classification schema. Consideration of the underlying dimensions is important as researchers attempt to identify characteristics of the environment or events that promote illness. For example, in a review of the nursing research on stressors, Werner (1993) discussed the dimensions of *locus, forecasting, tone, temporality, duration and frequency (repetitiveness),* and *impact* as representative of the underpinnings of many of the available classifications of stressors.

A key dimension that needs further explication is *impact*. It is a very important and the most often cited and studied characteristic of stressful life events and other stressors. It can have two connotations. First, it refers to the power, strength, or force of the event on the person(s). Second, it addresses the precise timing of the stress occurrence (Lazarus & Folkman, 1984) such as the "time of impact." In this section, impact is used to discuss the dimensions of force, influence, or stressfulness of the stimulus. Other terms for this connotation of impact are *intensity* and *severity.*

It is essentially the impact dimension or intensity that researchers attempt to measure when they obtain ratings of importance, seriousness, or stressfulness by judges, raters, or those affected. Observers' ratings of events in this regard estimate stressfulness across individuals and, therefore, yield an "average difference in impact potential" (Turner & Wheaton, 1995, p. 43). Paterson and Neufeld (1989) indicated that the severity of stressor impact is "one of the most fundamental considerations in the appraisal of a threat" (p. 26) and appears to be influenced by several subjective components including the goals or ideas of expected states, the importance of these goals, and the degree of threat engendered by goals not being attained. They conclude by explaining that greater stressfulness or severity can be affected by an increase in the "magnitude of impact" or longer duration (p. 28).

Most researchers and theorists agree that there is a threshold above which certain life events affect virtually everyone who experiences them (Costa, Somerfield, & McCrae, 1996; Eriksen & Ursin, 2005). Terms for this type of stress-as-stimulus include *extreme stressors* (Hobfoll, Freedy, Green, & Solomon, 1996, p. 322), *disasters* (Weisaeth, 1993, 2005), and *cataclysms* (Lepore & Evans, 1996). Hobfoll and colleagues (1996) noted the following properties of extreme stressors that differentiate them from less severe stressful events. They (a) attack people's most basic values (e.g., life and shelter); (b) make excessive demands; (c) occur without warning; (d) are outside the realm of which resource utilization strategies have been practiced and developed; and (e) leave a powerful mental image that is evoked by cues associated with the event (p. 328). These characteristics help conceptualize the dimension of severity of the stressor, or the dimension of impact, that may be thought of as occurring on a continuum from lesser to greater stressfulness or intensity.

A more global connotation of impact has been offered by family stress nursing theorists McCubbin and colleagues (Figley & McCubbin, 1983; McCubbin, 2002; McCubbin & Figley, 1983; McCubbin & Patterson, 1983). Instead of a continuum, their differentiation cites two qualitatively distinct types of events. These theorists separate major family stressors into normative life transitions and catastrophe. (See Table 1.1 in Chapter 1.)

They defined *normative life transitions* as changes or transitions that are expected and predictable that most, if not all, families will experience over the life cycle that require adjustment and adaptation (McCubbin & Figley, 1983). Examples include a family member leaving to go to college or to work and the addition of a new member. They define *catastrophe* as "an event which is sudden, unexpected, often life-threatening (to us or to someone we care deeply about), and due to the circumstances renders the survivors feeling an extreme sense of helplessness" (Figley & McCubbin, 1983, p. 6). Examples of catastrophe include death of a family member, severe illness, and natural disasters and other extreme changes and events. These theorists explain that both of these types of stressors can have a significant impact on families and family life.

The dimension of impact as discussed by McCubbin and Patterson (1983) was adapted by Werner (1993) and Werner, Frost, and Orth (2000) to describe groupings of stressors targeted in nursing research for 1980 to 1990 and the years 1991 to 1995, respectively. Stressors studied were found to focus in two broad areas.

The first included the more predictable and developmental life stress experiences and transitions, called life-related normative. The second overall grouping included catastrophic life stressors, or the unexpected and often life-threatening situations, termed life-related catastrophic. Two other categories were subsets of the previous two.

Because nursing is centrally concerned with health and departures from health, specific stressors related to health, illness, disease, and/or treatment were targeted, forming a subset within each major category. These subcategories were termed *health/illness-related normative* and *health/illness-related catastrophic* (Werner, 1993, p.17). An examination of the Cumulative Index of Nursing and Allied Health Literature (CINAHL) for the years 2000–2010 indicated 828 life-related normative stressor studies, 1,240 health/illness-related normative event studies, 155 life-related catastrophic event studies, and 783 health/illness-related catastrophic studies.

Another dimension that can be used to classify stressful life events is *context*. Context refers to "the whole situation, background, or environment relevance" (Neufeldt & Guralnik, 1996, p. 301). A classification of environmental stressors based on context has been developed by Lepore and Evans (1996), who proposed the following "general categories" (p. 352): (a) Cataclysms: These events are defined as "sudden, tumultuous, irrevocable events that impose great adaptive demands on many people" (p. 353) such as floods, earthquakes, hurricanes, and war; (b) Major life events: These events are defined as being severe in impact to most people. They are "episodic" and "irrevocable," calling for substantial adaptation (p. 353). Examples include death of partner, divorce, and unemployment; (c) Daily stressors: These stressors are the daily, ongoing, often minor stressors that occur repeatedly. They may, however, also be severe in nature. Often, they occur in tandem with other ongoing stressors. These stressors are similar to "daily hassles," a concept developed by Kanner, Coyne, Schaefer, and Lazarus (1981) that is discussed later in this chapter. Examples include lost car keys, "words" with the boss or partner, and lateness for an appointment; (d) Ambient stressors: Ambient stressors are characteristics of the environment that are difficult to change and that have an ongoing effect on those in the environment ranging from minor to severe. Examples include overcrowding, noise, and pollution; and (e) Role stressors: These stressors are related to the social obligations of the person experiencing them. When these stressors occur in important social roles, such as marriage or work, they can be severe (Lepore & Evans, 1996). Lepore and Evans noted that any of the stressors described above can interact with any of the other types, generating some of the stressor patterns previously mentioned. Often cataclysmic or major life events give way to a host of daily and role stressors, complicating the research conducted on and the understanding of the effects of the various stressor types (Weisaeth, 2005).

STRESS-AS-STIMULUS IN NURSING KNOWLEDGE

Nursing has a long tradition of studying stress and stressors as they relate to life, health, and illness. Studies date back to 1956, when the first indexed reference to stress appeared in the Cumulative Index for Nursing and Allied Health Literature (CINAHL). In a review and critical examination of nursing research regarding stress for the years 1974 to 1984, 28% ($n = 23$) of the 82 studies meeting inclusion criteria focused on stress-as-stimulus (Lyon & Werner, 1987). In a later comprehensive review and synthesis of findings in nursing for the years spanning 1980 through 1990, there were 133 studies focused on stressors, 81 of which met criteria for inclusion in the evaluation (Frost, 1993; Werner, 1993). Yet another review for the years 1991 through 1995 yielded an overall total of 362 studies fitting within the rubric of nursing research on stressors (Frost, Orth, & Werner, 2000; Werner, Frost, & Orth, 2000).

A recent review of the nursing research on stress as stimulus in the CINAHL literature between 1998 and 2010 resulted in 477 English-language citations. Stressors in these studies included workload and burnout (Jenkins & Elliot, 2004; Weitzel & McCahon, 2008); prematurity for infants (Turan, Başbakkal, & Ozbek, 2008); adolescence (Garcia, 2010); care of the critically ill (Schmelz, Bridges, Duong, & Ley, 2003); pain management (Lamb et al., 2010); pediatric oncology (Hinds, 2000); and aging (Stokes & Gordon, 1988, 2003). The growing number of stress-as-stimulus studies in nursing mirrors the large number of these studies in related disciplines and indicates nursing's continuous interest and contribution to stressors and life change.

Theoretical and Conceptual Development

Nursing has also included stress-as-stimulus in theoretical works of its discipline. Theories developed by Neuman (1989); Erickson, Tomlin, and Swain (1983); Roy (1984); and Johnson (1980) have all focused to differing degrees on stressors and stress. Neuman (1989) adapted a systems framework and incorporated primary, secondary, and tertiary prevention. The goal of her model is to guide nurses to protect and fortify the individual, family, and community from noxious stressors. Since 1995, there have been 10 research articles and 2 dissertations using the Neuman Systems Model that are referenced in CINAHL. Diverse study foci include stressors in cancer patients and caregivers (Skalski, DiGerolamo, & Gigliotti, 2006), stress and wellness in adolescence (Yarcheski, Mahon, Yarcheski, & Hanks, 2010), humor and slimming in Swedish women (Eilert-Petersson & Olsson, 2003), and chronic nonmalignant pain in adults (Gerstle, All, & Wallace, 2001).

Erickson, Tomlin, and Swain (1983) adapted Selye's view of stress as foundational to the development of a theory of modeling. They incorporated basic needs as described by Maslow and the theories of psychosocial and cognitive development, loss and attachment, and object relations to assist nurses in understanding clients and their health. Four studies from 2000 to 2010 were found in CINAHL that were guided by the theory of modeling and role modeling. One focused on role modeling excellence in clinical practice (Perry, 2009). A second targeted morbid obesity (Lombardo & Roof, 2005). A third looked at self-care as defined by members of the Amish community (Baldwin, Hibbein, Herr, Lohner, & Cire, 2002) and a fourth focused on systematic holistic nursing care in China (Li, Shi, & Zheng).

Roy's Adaptation Model (RAM) (1984), one of the most used theories for nursing, focuses on adaptation as a person–environment interaction, which if successful contributes to health. People are depicted as adjusting to internal and external stimuli called focal stimuli or stressors. Stressors, as explained by Roy, lead to a biological stress response that is explained by Selye's theory. The nurse's role is to promote effective adaptation. Since 1996 there have been 18 studies cited in

CINAHL using or testing Roy's model. Areas of focus have been the meaning of living with spinal cord injury (DeSanto-Madeya, 2006), cognitive adaptation and self-consistency in hearing-impaired older adults (Zhan, 2000), adaptation of children with cancer (Yeh, 2001), theory-guided interventions for heart failure (Bakan & Akyol, 2008), and urinary control adaptation (Jirovec, Jenkins, Isenberg, & Baiardi, 1999).

All the theoretical frameworks described above emphasize the importance of stress and stressors in the nursing care of patients. Their importance lies in the fact that they underscore the need for nurses to attend to the human experience of stress to promote health and to mitigate illness. None of them, however, were able to assist in understanding stressors or stress-as-stimulus at an empirical level. Blegen and Tripp-Reimer (1997) noted that these nursing models, although "essential in nursing's articulation of its identity . . . evolved parallel to, rather than interwoven with, research" (p. 38). In fact, much of the nursing research conducted to describe and explain stress-as-stimulus has been a-theoretical, underscoring Blegen and Tripp-Reimer's (1997) assertion that there is a need for middle-range theories to account for what is observed in a general way. This is occurring slowly, however, adaptations of stress theories focusing on other aspects of the stress process have been developed (e.g., Scott, Oberst, & Dropkin, 1980). Regarding stress-as-stimulus, nursing has largely at this point conducted research that stems from and contributes to the theoretical knowledge base from other disciplines, mainly psychology, sociology, and family studies.

In 1984, Norbeck asserted that the popularity of measuring stressful life events had not waned despite unresolved methodological and theoretical questions. This assertion continues to be true today. A recent search of the literature revealed that the research on stressful life events has increased dramatically in the past few years. Although there were 7,207 articles identified using a Medline search of life events between the years 1963 and 1998, less than 10% ($n = 515$) were published before 1980. In addition, there was an increase in the number of articles identified in the 9-year period 1990 to 1998 ($n = 3,611$) compared to the previous 10-year period of time ($n = 3,073$). This same trend was identified with a CINAHL search in which less than 1% of the stressful life event articles were published

before 1980. A larger number of articles were published from 1990 to 1998 ($n = 335$) compared to 1980 to 1989 ($n = 182$). In the 20-year period between 1990 and 2010, the number of stressful life event and health articles found in Medline was 8,915, and in CINAHL it was 7,364. The number of research articles for the same time period referenced in Medline is 655 and the number in CINAHL is 533.

Measurement

The initiation of stressful life event measurements, and the theoretical orientation of stress-as-stimulus as already addressed, is often credited to Holmes and Rahe with the development of the Social Readjustment Rating Scale (SRRS) in 1967. Work in the area of life events, however, began long before the development of the SRRS. As far back as 1949, Homes and Rahe used a life chart modeled after the work of Adolph Meyer. In the 1930s, Meyer, building on the science of psychobiology, used a life chart device to organize medical data that he envisioned as dynamic, involving a relationship between biological, psychological, and sociological phenomena (Holmes & Rahe, 1967). By the late 1940s, Meyer's data provided support for associations between stressful life events and physical health or illness outcomes (Wolff et al., 1950).

In 1957, Hawkins, Davies, and Holmes developed the Schedule of Recent Experiences (SRE) to systematize Meyer's life chart. In 1967, Holmes and Rahe modified the SRE by assigning weights to represent the amount of difficulty or change created by each event. Holmes and Rahe made this change because they believed the addition of estimating the magnitude of various life events would advance the precision of their research. They developed this aspect of their research by providing individuals a list of life changes and asking them to score each event using as a pivot point an arbitrary score of 500 for marriage. This methodology resulted in a weighted score, an average, referred to as a life change unit (LCU), for each event. The resulting SRRS measured changes in sleep, eating, social life, recreation, personal activities, and interpersonal habits as well as significant losses like the death of a spouse and divorce (Rahe, 1968, 1972). Adding LCUs for each event experienced yielded a total SRRS score, which was used as a predictor of illness in the next two years.

Interestingly, the process of developing the SRRS led Holmes and Rahe (1967) to note that "as expected, the psychological significance and emotions varied widely with the patient" (p. 216). They chose, however, to focus on what they termed the high degree of consensus in assigned scores to indicate the amount of stress created by each life change event, in turn sacrificing the individual perspective.

Several basic assumptions were used in the development of the SRRS: (a) life change events are normative, requiring a similar amount of adjustment across individuals and times; (b) the positive or negative tone of the event is irrelevant; (c) there is a common threshold beyond which disruption occurs; and (d) stress is an additive phenomenon (Rahe, 1977). These assumptions imply that individuals are passive recipients of stress.

The basic assumptions used in the development of the SRRS served as a basis for many life event instruments developed in the 1970s and even in the present. Various researchers have revised Holmes and Rahe's tool and measurement methodology by making changes in the weighting of items, the specific events included, and the significance of negative and positive events. Researchers have also placed emphasis on events that are unique to specific populations for whom stressors or life events may be different from those of the general population. For instance, Coddington (1972a, 1972b) modified the SRRS to measure stressful life events in childhood. Volicer and Bohannon (1975) based the development of the Hospital Stress Rating Scale for use with medical, surgical, and psychiatric patients on Holmes and Rahe's work. Lengthier life event scales were developed, such as the Psychiatric Epidemiological Research Interview—Life Events Scale developed by Dohrenwend, Krasnoff, Askenasy, and Dohrenwend (1978; 1982) for a psychiatric population, allowing individuals to assign their own weight or score. Also developed was the Universal and Group Specific Events Scale by Hough (as cited by Miller, 1981) to incorporate differences based on ethnicity. Numerous other life event and stressor instruments for adolescents, adults, children, family members, and the aging identified as a result of the recent search of the literature previously mentioned can be found in Table 6.1 below.

Table 6.1   Selected Measures of Stressful Life Events, Life Change Events, Hassles, Uplifts, and Minor Stressors

Populations	Instrument	Measurement focus
Adolescents	Adolescent-Family Inventory of Life Events and Changes (McCubbin, Patterson, Bauman, & Harris, 1981)	Recent family, adolescent, and youth life events and changes; chronic stressors and strains; the family's and youth's vulnerability and cumulative life events
	Adolescent Life Change Event Scale (Yeaworth, York, Hussey, Ingle, & Goodwin, 1980)	Adolescent life change events
	Adolescent Life Experiences (Towbes, Cohen, & Glyshaw, 1989)	Life stress inventory for adolescents
	Adolescent Perceived Events Scale (Compas, Davis, Forsythe, & Wagner, 1987)	Adolescents rate life events according to desirability, impact, and frequency
	High School Social Readjustment Scale (Tolor, Murphy, Wilson, & Clayton, 1983)	Stressful events in high school students
	Junior High Life Events Survey (Swearingen & Cohen, 1985)	Life events of junior high school students

(Continued)

Table 6.1   (Continued)

Populations	Instrument	Measurement focus
	Life Events Checklist (Johnson & McCutcheon 1980)	Life stress in older children and adolescents
	Life Events Inventory (Cochrane & Robertson, 1973)	Psychosocial stressors and the distress created
	Life Event Scale for Adolescents (Coddington & Troxell, 1980)	Life events of adolescents
Adults	Daily Hassles & Uplift Scale (Kanner, Coyne, Schaefer, & Lazarus, 1981)	Demands and rewards of daily living
	Detroit Couples Study Life Events Method (Kessler & Wethington, 1991)	Checklist of life events with semi-structured interview probes
	Hassles Scale, Uplift Scale (Elder, Wollin, Härtel, Spencer & Sanderson, 2003)	Nurses' experiences with cognitively impaired
	Hemodialysis Stressor Scale (Murphy, Powers, & Jalowiec, 1985)	Stressors associated with hemodialysis
	Henderson, Byrne, & Duncan-Jones List of Recent Experiences (Henderson, Byrne, & Duncan-Jones, 1981)	Interview to obtain life events
	Hospital Stress Rating Scale (Volicer & Bohannon, 1975)	Events related to the experience of hospitalization
	Impact of Event Scale (Horowitz, 1979)	Degree of subjective impact experienced during the preceding week as a result of a specific life event
	Interview for Recent Life Events (Paykel, 1997)	Semistructured interview to establish life events and month in which they occurred
	Interview Schedule for Events and Difficulties (Brown & Harris, 1978)	Life events and stressors
	Life Crisis History (Antonovsky & Kats, 1967)	Life crisis
	Life Events and Difficulties Schedule (Brown & Harris, 1982)	Interview to obtain life events
	Life Event Questionnaire (Norbeck, 1984)	Life event questionnaire modified for adult female population of child-bearing age
	Life Events Questionnaire (Horowitz, Schaefer, Hiroto, Wilner, & Levin, 1977)	Life events
	Life Experiences Survey (Sarason, Johnson, & Siegel, 1978)	Life events experienced in the past 12 months
	Psychiatric Epidemiological Research Interview—Life Events Scale (PERI-LES) (Dohrenwend, Krasnoff, Askenasy, & Dohrenwend, 1978)	Life events scale for psychiatric population
	Munich Events List (Wittchen, Essau, Hecht, Teder, & Pfister, 1989)	Life events interview in which context is explored
	Paykel Brief Life Event List (Paykel, 1983)	Interview of life events and difficulties with contextual probes

Populations	Instrument	Measurement focus
	Psoriasis Life Stress Index (Gupta & Gupta, 1995)	Checklist of psoriasis-related events and rating of effect of each event
	Questionnaire on Stress in Patients With Diabetes—Revised (Herschbach et al., 1997)	Sources of stress and the amount of distress experienced with each source
	Recent Life Change Questionnaire (Rahe, 1975)	Life changes
	Review of Life Events (Hurst, Jenkins, & Rose, 1978)	Life change stress
	Schedule of Recent Life Events (SRE) (Holmes & Rahe, 1967)	Life changes listed by year of occurrence
	Social Readjustment Rating Scale (Holmes & Rahe, 1967)	Quantification of experienced life events
	Sources of Stress in Nursing Students (Gibbons, Dempster, & Moutray, 2009)	Measures sources of eustress in nursing students
	Spouse Transplant Stressor Scale (Collins, White-Williams, & Jalowiec, 1996)	Stressors associated with heart transplant
	Standardized Self-Report Measures of Civilian Trauma and PTSD (Norris & Hamblen, 2004)	Experiences, witnesses, or confronts an event or events that involve actual or threatened death or serious injury, or a threat to the physical integrity of self or others (criterion AI), and the person's response involved intense fear, helplessness, or horror
	Stressful Life Events Screening Questionnaire (SLESQ) (Goodman, Corcoran, Turner, Yuan, & Green, 1998)	Assesses lifetime exposure to traumatic events, i.e., life-threatening accident, physical and sexual abuse
	Subjective Stress Scale (Bramston & Fogarty, 1995)	Stressors of people with intellectual disabilities
	Symptoms of Illness Checklist (Stowell, Hedges, Ghambaryan, Key, & Bloch, 2009)	Psychological influences on physical symptoms
	Symptom Severity Index (Black, Griffiths, & Pope, 1996)	Severity of stress incontinence and bothersome symptoms
	The Standardized Event Rating System (Dohrenwend, Raphael, Schwartz, Stueve, & Skodol, 1993)	Interview derived from the PERI and to be used with a variety of populations
	The Universal and Group-Specific Event Scale (Hough as cited in Miller, 1981)	Incorporated life event differences based on ethnic group
	War Events Scale (Unger, Gould, & Babich, 1998)	Experience with war-time atrocities and the distress associated with them
Children	Childhood Life Events and Family Characteristics Questionnaire (Byrne, Velamoor, Cernovsky, Cortese, & Losztyn, 1990)	Childhood life events and parent–child relationship
	Children's Life Event Questionnaire (Deutsch & Erickson, 1989)	Early childhood life events
	Childhood Unwanted Sexual Events (Lange, Kooiman, Huberts, & van Oostendorp, 1995)	Incidence of childhood experiences with sexual threat or abuse or both

(Continued)

Table 6.1   (Continued)

Populations	Instrument	Measurement focus
	Children's Headache Assessment Scale (Budd, Workman, Lemsky, & Quick, 1994)	Environmental events and variables associated with pediatric headache
	Chronicity Impact and Coping Instrument: Parent Questionnaire (Hymovich, 1983)	Parent concerns in caring for a child with a chronic health problem
	General Life Events Schedule for Children (Sandler, Nolichuk, Brauer, & Fogas, 1986)	Events of children of divorce
	Modified SRRQ (Coddington, 1972a)	Life events in children
	Psychosocial Assessment of Childhood Experiences (Glen, Simpson, Drinnan, McGuinness, & Sandberg, 1993)	Life events and experiences in childhood
	Life Stress Inventory (Cohen-Sandler, Berman, & King, 1982)	Life stress of children
	The Children of Alcoholics Life-Events Schedule (Roosa, Sandler, Gehring, Beals, & Cappo, 1988)	Life events and stressors of children of alcohol-abusing parents
	Social Readjustment Scale for Children (Coddington, 1972b)	Quantification of experienced life events of children
College Students	Life Change Inventory (Costantini, Braun, Davis, & Ivervolino, 1974)	Quantification of life events experienced by college students
	Student Life Stress Inventory (Gadzella, 1994)	Undergraduate college student stressors
	Undergraduate Stress Questionnaire (Crandall, Preisler, & Aussprung, 1992)	Life event stress in college students
Family	Family Inventory of Life Events and Changes (McCubbin, Patterson, & Wilson, 1980)	Life events and changes experienced by the family in the preceding year
	Questionnaire on Resources and Stress (Glidden, 1993)	Demands, stresses, strains, and resources of families raising children with developmental disabilities
Older Adults	Geriatric Social Readjustment Rating Scale (Amster & Krauss, 1974)	Life events of geriatric population
	Louisville Older Person Event Scale (Murrell, Norris, & Hutchins, 1984)	Life events in older adults
	Stokes-Gordon Stress Scale (Stokes & Gordon, 1988, 2003)	Stressors of adults 65 years old or older

More recently, life event measurements have focused on individuals' subjective appraisals of particular events. Instead of predetermined weights given to events, individuals are asked to rate the amount of stress that they have experienced as a result of a particular event or stressor. For example, Budd, Workman, Lemsky, and Quick (1994) focused on headaches in children,

whereas Gupta and Gupta (1995) emphasized stressors related to psoriasis.

Methodological Concerns

Several terms are used in the life events literature, including life events, life change events, and life change. The Medline and CINAHL search term is "life change events." It is not clear how life change differs from life events. These terms are used interchangeably at times. It is also not clear how use of the term *event* differs from use of the term *stressor* because many items on life change event inventories are of smaller magnitudes than one would associate with an event. For example, on the Hospital Stress Rating Scale (Volicer & Bohannon, 1975), "your call light answered" was considered an event. Cohen et al. (1995) assert the importance of distinguishing between events and other sources of stress. This is not possible if terminology is not consistent among researchers.

An examination of definitions reveals that an event is defined as something that happens, and change is defined as making something different (Kidney, 1993). Although obviously two different concepts, the interchangeable use of these terms is consistent with the stress-as-stimulus model, in which events are assumed to create change in individuals regardless of their appraisal of those situations. Life events were originally defined by Holmes and Rahe (1967) as changes that are indicative of or require significant readjustments. They accentuated change from a steady state and not the psychological meaning, emotion, or social desirability associated with the change. A favorable event was assumed to require as much of an adjustment as an unfavorable event, and similarity in individuals' responses was emphasized while ignoring the diversity that exists. Similar to Holmes and Rahe's definition, Dohrenwend and colleagues (1978, 1982) defined stressful life events as objective occurrences that are of a magnitude that require changes in the usual activities of most individuals.

Despite the continued use of terminology similar to that of Holmes and Rahe (1967), there is movement toward exploring life events as a concept influenced by individuals' appraisals of events and factors that influence life events. The theoretical underpinnings of stress-as-stimulus, however, still influence the methodology chosen by many researchers. This was apparent in the aforementioned 5-year review of identified stressors in nursing research in which very few researchers identified individuals' appraisals of how disruptive or significant identified stressors were to their lives (Frost et al., 2000).

Several other methodological concerns have also been posed. One is the single-dimensional nature of most of the life event scales, in which many of the factors that may affect the significance of a life event are ignored. For instance, potential factors often not measured include the individual's coping abilities, understanding of the event, social networks, cultural bias, personality, clustering with other events, biological variables, socioeconomic status, and interpersonal support system (Werner, 1996; Werner & O'Neill, 1992). The lack of examining life events from a multidimensional perspective may explain why the relationships between life events and illness onset are often weak (Lyon & Werner, 1987; Norbeck, 1984) and results among studies conflicting.

The significance of including positive events is not fully understood. Although correlations between negative events and health distress have been fairly consistent, the associations between positive events and health or distress have not (Zautra & Reich, 1983). It is possible that the effects of positive events are not captured with current theoretical models and measures that do not account for the multiple factors that influence outcomes.

Comparison of results across life event studies is difficult due to variations in the life events included in the instrument, the times referenced, weights given to each event, and decisions made regarding what is a positive compared to a negative event. Specifically, some of the life event instruments are very specific to a given population and thus not transferable to other populations. Even among the general life event instruments, there is a lack of consistency in the events measured and the inclusion of positive events. Items rated differently result in score differences. Likewise, omission of any significant event may result in the underestimation of an individual's risk for detrimental health outcomes. Some researchers have accounted for the potential omission of an event significant to the study participants through the addition of an opportunity for the participant to list additional events at the end of the scale.

Available instruments reference a variety of time intervals, such as last week, last month, and last year. The names of the instruments provide little if any guidance with regard to the time period that they reference. For instance, the Schedule of Recent Events (SRE) (Hawkins et al., 1957), the forerunner of the SRRS (Holmes & Rahe, 1967), actually measures events during the past 12 months and not the past week or past few days as the name suggests. The most appropriate time period for referencing of items is not clear. The 1-year time reference initially used in life event instruments was chosen because it was thought that it was the period of time needed to allow health outcomes to manifest or for adjustment to occur (e.g., for the loss of a partner) (Holmes, 1979; Holmes & Masuda, 1974).

The 12-month time interval, however, has been debated for a long time. Some researchers have reported that the time interval before health outcomes are manifested is approximately 6 months rather than 1 year (Rutter, 1989), whereas others note that a time interval of at least 12 months is important (Brown & Harris, 1978). Cohen and colleagues (1995) raised a related issue. They pointed out that it is very unclear how long events can have an effect on health outcomes. It is likely that events such as parental conflict, divorce, and physical or sexual abuse may leave lifelong scars. Other events have an effect for a much shorter period of time, and these effects may not even be evident one year after the event. Time of measurement is also important in terms of recall. A fallout rate of 1% to 5% per month has been identified with the recall of major events. When dealing with less important events, the forgetting may be even higher (Brown & Harris, 1982; Funch & Marshall, 1984).

Artificial differences between study findings can also be found as a result of researchers providing different weights for various events. Although some researchers weight undesirable events stronger than desirable events, others weigh them identically. Some researchers assign negative and positive valences to an event. It is generally the researcher who makes judgments regarding the positive or negative effect of various events (Levenstein et al., 1993). Another area of concern is that illness may influence the report of a real or artificially high number of events (Cohen et al., 1995). There is also evidence suggesting that individuals may report a stressor as a result of a relatively minor event as if it was a significant event (Dohrenwend, Link, Kern, Shrout, & Markowitz, 1990).

Another factor that is not always clear is the interrelationship and the complexity of a number of significant life events. For example, when a person is divorced or widowed (two of the highest-rated life change events) they not only lose their partner and their marriage, but they also may experience changes in finances and lost friendships connected to being part of a couple. Also he or she may have to move to another state, get a different job, and have a different relationship with their family members, children, and in-laws, etc. (Ben-Zur & Michael, 2009).

IMPLICATIONS FOR NURSING PRACTICE

Interventions

Nursing interventions vary for every stressor and with knowledge of the factors influencing individuals' appraisal of stressors. Therefore, it is not feasible to list all potential associated interventions. Obviously, there are some life change events and other stressors that are not predictable, avoidable, or changeable. Examples include death and weather-related catastrophic events. In these situations, focus needs to be placed on cognitive interventions that influence appraisal for reducing the threat or on supporting the individual(s) in obtaining resources to meet related challenges.

The level of stress experienced by individuals is dependent, in part, on all of the stressors they are currently experiencing and on their appraisal of any given situation. Assessment skills are needed to thoroughly evaluate not only the life change events or demands but also the person's perception of the stressors and the level of distress they are experiencing. Of great importance is the caveat that what may appear to be a benign or insignificant event or stressor to the health care professional may have great significance for others, and what health professionals view as most stressful may have little significance for patients.

In some situations, reframing can be used, in which the appraisal of the situation is refocused so that the situation is viewed from a more positive perspective. For situations that are obviously not positive, and cannot be reframed as such, stress-management techniques can be taught to mitigate the distress resulting from the stressor and stress process. Interventions shown to be effective include relaxation techniques (McCain, et al., 2003), massage therapy (Bost & Wallace, 2006), journaling (Ray, 2009), music therapy (Chou & Lin, 2006), art therapy (Chilcote, 2007; Reynolds, Lim, & Prior, 2008), guided imagery (Chou &

Lin, 2006), and "pleasant events" interventions in long-term care (Meeks, Shah, & Ramsey, 2009). Social support groups may be useful for individuals who have experienced similar types of stressors, and assisting individuals in seeking social support may be of assistance (e.g., Cropley & Steptoe, 2005; DeLongis, Holtzman, Puterman, & Lam, 2010; Jopp & Schmitt, 2010).

Purposeful priority setting and purposeful problem solving may be useful techniques for individuals who are overwhelmed by the number of life change events or stressors to which they are exposed. Another intervention with potential to assist persons facing one or more meaningful stressors or changes is values clarification. Assisting individuals to identify life changes that are best delayed until the level of stress they are experiencing diminishes may also be a useful intervention. Assisting individuals to proactively examine the number of planned significant events (such as the purchase of a house and marriage) or to anticipate foreseeable events (such as an expected death) may be useful in giving individuals some control over the number of events or stressors to which they are simultaneously exposed. At times when an individual is unable to prioritize for him or herself, such as when comatose, the health care provider will need to play a more active role in limiting the number of stressors that are impinging on the person.

There are literally thousands of texts and lay readings on managing and/or avoiding stress and stressors. One treatment or intervention does not fit all; they must be tailored to fit the needs of the individual and his or her significant others. A review of life events and nursing interventions research between 2000 and 2010 in CINAHL revealed 67 studies. Examples of areas of study included nursing home behavioral interventions (Meeks et al., 2009), medication management for the elderly (Travis et al., 2007), management of life-threatening events in infants (Scollan-Koliopoulos & Koliopoulos, 2010), asthma in adults (Lietzen et al., 2011), efforts to increase enrollment in cardiac care for post-coronary syndrome patients (Cossette, D'Aoust, Morin, Heppell, & Frasure-Smith, 2009), caregiver outcomes after client discharges from ICUs (Van Pelt, Schultz, Chelluri, & Pinsky, 2010), support groups for bereaved children (Mitchell et al., 2007), and enhanced spirituality in healthy adults (Cavendish et al., 2000). A very useful text is the recent Harvard Medical School Special Health Report on Stress Management's "Approaches for Preventing and Reducing Stress," by Benson and Casey (2008). It is prescriptive for reducing and/or managing life stress.

CONCLUSION

This section provided historical, theoretical, and background information on stress-as-stimulus definitions (including several types and dimensions) and selected findings from nursing research in this area. To some extent, this section reflects a fleeting glance of work in progress because there have been so many studies on stressors and presumably many more to come. Promising areas of stressor research include organizational stress, epigenetics, and information technology (see Chapters 4, 7, and 12 in this text). Despite the many questions that remain, it is clear that stressors (i.e., life events) do have an influence on the health and well-being of our clients and patients and, therefore, are worthy of nursing's dedicated research efforts.

SECTION 2. CONCEPTUALIZATIONS OF STRESS-AS-STIMULUS AND MINOR LIFE EVENTS

This section of the chapter focuses on the origin and evolution of the hassles and uplifts model of minor life events. Some researchers (e.g., Lazarus & Folkman, 1984) argued that it was not the major life events and changes that weigh on people's minds and bodies and cause them stress and illness but rather the day-to-day chronic buildup of minor life demands or hassles. Hassles and uplifts reflect relatively "minor" daily experiences and conditions that have been appraised as salient to an individual. They can be perceived as potentially harmful or threatening (hassles), or they can be perceived as positive or favorable (uplifts). As such, hassles and uplifts are day-to-day irritants and momentary joys that reflect daily living in relation to how the individual psychologically and subjectively experiences a situation. Within the hassles and uplifts theory, inputs are the day-to-day events and the outputs or health outcomes depend on the subjective saliency and threat of the inputs. Because hassles and uplifts depend on cognitive appraisal or assessment, the same event can be a hassle for one person and an uplift for another, or even change from a hassle to an uplift or vice versa for the same individual at different points in time. Theoretically, hassles and uplifts should equally affect health outcomes, such as somatic, psychological, and affective symptoms as they are thought to potentially balance one another (Lazarus & Folkman, 1984).

THE THEORETICAL CONTEXT FOR THE MODEL

The Hassles and Uplifts Model reflects a cognitive perceptual approach to understanding the effects of stress on health. The model derives from the broader transactional theory of stress and coping (TTSC), which was developed in the late 1960s and 1970s by Lazarus and his colleagues (Lazarus, 1993). The TTSC takes a psychological view of the effects of stress on health by considering individual differences in motivation and cognitive appraisal as intervening variables between a potential external stressor and the stress reaction. The theory takes a relational approach to understanding the effects of stress on health rather than the more linear perspective of inputs of stress as a stimulus and outputs of stress as a response, which is best reflected in the early work of Selye (1993, 1998).

According to Lazarus (1993), the TTSC has its origins in Lewin's (1935) writing about positively and negatively valenced situations, in which the environment is viewed as a product of perceptions and reactions rather than objective reality. The TTSC proposes that stress is the product of transactions between individuals and their environments, with two major concepts mediating the dynamics: (a) primary and secondary cognitive appraisal, and (b) coping. The TTSC is described in greater detail in Chapter 9.

Concurrent with the development of the TTSC, the theory of life events as stressors that affect health outcomes was proposed and broadly accepted (Holmes & Rahe, 1967). As described earlier in this chapter, life events theory is linear and stimulus oriented, and it assumes that major changes in life, whether positive or negative, are stressful and that the accumulation of life changes leads to changes in health (Holmes & Rahe, 1967). The Hassles and Uplifts Model reflects the view that micro-stressors, in the form of perceived minor irritations or demands, and pleasures have an impact on health outcomes as well. This view is in response to criticisms that life events theory ignores psychological mediators, such as the saliency of an event, and the individual's coping resources for dealing with the event.

Given the relational view of stress and coping, it was argued that the effects of life events on health outcomes vary depending on the meaning of the events to the individual. For example, divorce for one individual might be a major loss, whereas for another individual it might be a relief and an opportunity to grow and move forward in life. It was argued that a difference in cognitive appraisal of the same event would likely lead to the event having different effects on health outcomes. In addition, the Hassles and Uplifts Model proposes that events that are perceived as negative versus those perceived as positive will have different effects on health, and that day-to-day events that have positive tones or uplifts act as buffers for the negative effects of stressors on health. This is in contrast to the assumptions in life events theory that any change, no matter what its emotional tone, would negatively affect health outcomes.

Another criticism of the life events theory is that research using this conceptualization explains relatively small amounts of the variance in health outcomes (Lazarus & Folkman, 1984). Day-to-day events or micro-stressors are considered to be more proximal to health outcomes than life events, and therefore their cumulative effects can be greater than that of somewhat distant life events (DeLongis, Coyne, Dakof, Folkman, & Lazarus, 1982). Kanner and others (1981) suggested three possible explanations for how life events and daily micro-stressors relate to health outcomes. One explanation is that major life events moderate the effect of micro-stressors on health outcomes. For example, a major life event such as divorce can change the relative stressfulness of an individual's daily routine and pattern, such as meal preparation and household management, thus moderating the effects of these day-to-day events on health. As a moderating variable, life events could have an effect on health even when all the effects of micro-stressors are statistically removed.

An alternative idea is that the effects of major life events are mediated by more proximal day-to-day events that then affect health outcomes. For example, death of a partner can lead to actual changes in daily routines that then can directly alter health outcomes. If micro-stressors mediate the effect of major life events, then the effects of life events on health outcomes could occur solely because of and through their effects on day-to-day living. A third explanation is that life events and day-to-day hassles exert independent effects on health outcomes.

In addition to responding to theoretical criticism of life events theory, the Hassles and Uplifts Model responds to concerns that research using life event scales are psychometrically flawed by a lack of independence among the life event items surveyed. Another concern is the lack of culturally appropriate life event tools for different socio-demographic groups. It has been noted that items on most life event scales generally reflect White, middle-class life situations that might be irrelevant or too narrow for other cultural and economic groups (DeLongis et al., 1982).

Congruent with the theoretical model of hassles and uplifts as day-to-day events that affect health and because of the saliency and potential threat or positive experience of these events, the original Hassles scales listed a wide variety of day-to-day events, such as too many things to do, yard work, and outside home maintenance. Uplifts included using skills well at work, the health of a family member, praying, completing a task, and so on. Day-to-day events on the measures are diverse and considered to reflect issues and experiences that spanned the daily life of individuals from a wide range of backgrounds (Kanner et al., 1981). The separate Hassles and Uplifts scales were later combined into a single scale on which respondents rated their experiences as either a hassle or an uplift to better reflect the theoretical perspective that "perception" of events is central to their effects on health (e.g., Madu & DeJong, 2002).

Empirical Examination of the Effects of Micro-Stressors Versus Life Events on Health

Studies comparing the effects of hassles versus life events on health outcomes have consistently found hassles to be a better predictor of both psychological and somatic symptoms (Charles et al., 2010; DeLongis et al., 1982; Elder et al., 2003; Hunt, 2003; Ivancevich, 1986; Jandorf, Deblinger, Neale, & Stone, 1986; Kanner & Feldman, 1991; Madu & DeJong, 2002; Wagner, Compas, &

Howell, 1988; Weinberger, Hiner, & Tierney, 1987; Wolf, Elston, & Kissling, 1989).

A classic study (DeLongis et al., 1982) compared the effects of the two approaches to stress measurement using a repeated-measure, longitudinal design with 100 adults representing a probability sample of Alameda County residents. Subjects completed the Hassles and Uplifts scales monthly for 9 consecutive months. A Life Events Questionnaire and Health Status Questionnaire were administered twice during the same period. This study, reported in two separate publications, found that hassles were better predictors of concurrent and later psychological symptoms (Kanner et al., 1981) and somatic symptoms (DeLongis et al., 1982) than were life events. Furthermore, when the effects of life events on health outcomes were statistically removed, hassles remained significantly related to both somatic and psychological symptoms (DeLongis et al., 1982, 1988; Kanner et al., 1981).

Although there was evidence that hassles were better predictors of health outcomes than life events, two studies provided different results. Zarski (1984) found life experiences accounted for greater variance in somatic health than did hassles. A second study found that the number of life events directly affected hassles, which in turn affected perceived effects of life events and illness (Dykema, Bergbower, & Peterson, 1995). Zarski's (1984) descriptive study used a single cross-sectional measurement model with 397 subjects, and Dykema and colleagues (1995) used path analysis with cross-sectional data from a sample of 121 college students. It is important to note that the Life Experience Survey used in Zarski's (1984) study asked subjects to rate on a 7-point scale the stress degree of the positive or negative life event, and Dykema and others (1995) found that it was the nature of the life events, not their frequency, that directly affected health outcomes. Thus, subjective saliency was included in both of these measures, unlike the more traditional measures of life events.

Results from studies examining the relative roles of hassles and life events on health outcomes have supported the explanation that hassles can act as mediators of life events. Also some studies have found bivariate relationships among hassles, life events, and health outcomes. When the effects of hassles on health outcomes are partialed out statistically, life events do not significantly contribute to explained variance in health outcomes (DeLongis et al., 1982; Ivancevich, 1986; Ungar & Florian, 2004; Wagner et al., 1988; Weinberger et al., 1987). An exception is the findings of Williams, Zyzanski, and Wright (1992). They reported that there was an additive effect for life events and hassles on the risk of inpatient admission among 444 Navajo Indians. The dependent variable in this study was not a continuous measure of somatic or psychological symptoms as it was in most of the other studies. A relative risk model for predicting likelihood of admission, given high or low scores on life events and hassles measures, was used. This study indicated that daily hassle scores were associated with increased outpatient use, whereas life events were not related to use of health care services.

Although numerous studies have found significant effects for hassles on health outcomes, most have found limited support for uplifts (DeLongis et al., 1982; Jandorf et al., 1986; Kanner et al., 1981; Monroe, 1983; Wolf et al., 1989). In a study of 100 young women (mean age 35.8 years) with 77 of the participants available at the 5-year follow-up, Erlandsson (2008) found both hassles and uplifts to be fairly stable over a 5-year period and a balance was maintained between the two measures.

Although the life event measures have been challenged with regard to interdependence among the items, Hassles and Uplifts scales are not without problems. They have been particularly challenged in relation to the potential confounding of measures and health outcomes. Part of the argument concerns the question of whether day-to-day stressors can be validly measured without including a subjective component. This challenge strikes at the very core of the theoretical underpinnings of the Hassles and Uplifts Model, because saliency and the subjective nature of perceived threat are basic elements in defining day-to-day events as hassles.

Use and Testing of the Hassles and Uplift Model in Nursing Studies Across the Life Span

Empirical Studies of the Effects of Hassles and Uplifts on Health Outcomes

The Hassles and Uplifts Model has been tested in relation to a wide variety of health-related outcomes, in several cultures, and across the life span. A significant relationship has consistently been found between psychological symptoms and daily hassles whether the studies have used measures developed by Lazarus's group (DeLongis et al., 1982; Zarski, 1984) or others. Recent studies with the cognitively impaired (Elder et al., 2003), family caregivers (Hunt, 2003; Travis et al., 2007; Winslow, 2003), mothers of preterm infants (Reid & Bramwell, 2003), the hearing impaired (Knussen et al., 2005), and adolescent mothers (Sadler, Swartz, & Ryan-Krause, 2003) all supported the importance of assessing hassles.

In addition to predicting physical symptoms, the timing and changes in hassles and uplifts have been examined in relation to episodes of physical symptoms (Stone, Reed, & Neale, 1987) and the onset of common colds (Evans, Pitts, & Smith, 1988; Evans & Edgerton, 1991). In these studies, desirable events (uplifts) decreased and undesirable events (hassles) increased 3 or 4 days before the illness onset. These studies provide strong support for the role of micro-stressors on health outcomes because they used prospective designs with repeated measures analysis. They also suggested a role for uplifts in health outcomes, whereas earlier retrospective studies did not.

Other health-related outcomes that have been examined as dependent measures and found to be related to hassles or uplifts or both include episodes of hospitalization and outpatient visits (Williams et al., 1992), symptoms of irritable bowel syndrome (Dancey, Whitehouse, Painter, & Backhouse, 1995), quality of sleep (Weller & Avinir, 1993), perinatal mood disturbances (Monk, Leight, & Fang, 2008), and alcohol dependency (Boyd, Baliko, Cox, & Tavakoli, 2007). Dancey et al. (1995) used a prospective design to examine the relationship between daily symptoms of irritable bowel syndrome and hassles and uplifts. They found that total symptoms were associated with hassles in the following week; hassles in any week, however, were not associated with symptoms in the following week. There was no association between uplifts and irritable bowel symptoms. In contrast, Weller and Avinir (1993) found that hassles alone, uplifts alone, and a combined hassles and uplifts score were each correlated with quality of sleep in a sample of 41 people without sleeping disorders.

Hassles have also been found to be related to role changes and the number of health problems among parents and partners of individuals with traumatic brain injury (Leathem, Heath, & Woolley, 1996) and to be greater in Type A college students compared to Type B students (Margiotta, Davilla, & Hicks, 1990). Thus, there is significant empirical evidence that negative day-to-day events impact many aspects of personal health, whereas the role of positive day-to-day events remains unclear.

Effects of Hassles and Uplifts on Health Across the Age Continuum

Early studies examining the effects of hassles and uplifts on health outcomes were carried out with adults between the ages of 18 and 64 (DeLongis et al., 1982; Jandorf et al., 1986; Kanner et al., 1981; Monroe, 1983; Zarski, 1984). The hassles and uplifts measures used in these studies reflected items that were expected to be relevant to the working adult population. Theoretically, the Hassles and Uplifts Model is applicable for populations across the age continuum. Several studies were undertaken to examine whether or not hassles had an impact on health outcomes for both older and younger populations and, if so, whether the impact of hassles was the same or different for individuals at different developmental stages. Implicit in most of these studies is the assumption that the actual day-to-day events relevant to different age groups vary. Some of these studies will be reviewed.

Hassles and Older Adults

Two studies were implemented with the explicit purpose of comparing hassles and uplifts in older and younger adults. Folkman, Lazarus, Pimley, and Novacek (1987) used a retrospective, repeated measures longitudinal design with a revised version of the original Hassles and Uplifts scales. The sample consisted of 150 adults in their early forties and 141 adults in their late sixties. This study found a significant effect for age on the types of hassles endorsed by younger versus older adults. Younger adults reported significantly more hassles in the domains of work, finance, home maintenance, family, friends, and personal life, whereas older adults reported more hassles in the domains of environmental and social issues and health. The researchers concluded that these differences logically reflected differences in developmental tasks, with younger

adults concerned with work, home, and family and older adults concerned with health and the broader environmental and social issues. This study did not examine the effects of hassles on health outcomes, nor did it include examination of uplifts. Ewedemi and Linn (1987) examined the differences in hassles between younger and older adults who were outpatients at a Veterans Medical Center. This study used a descriptive cross-sectional design with 25 younger and 25 older adults with chronic disease who completed study measures on only one occasion. The hassles and uplifts measures for this study consisted of 40 of the original 117 hassles items and 40 of the 135 original uplifts. The authors indicated that these items were selected because they were applicable to men who were in the age ranges being studied. Subjects in the study were categorized as being in "good" or "poor" health depending on self-rating of their health on a 5-point scale. Study findings indicated that hassles were greater for those who rated their health as poor, but this did not differ by age group. The results became insignificant when 11 items (that were considered to confound health outcomes) were eliminated from the scale. This study did not find any associations between uplift scores and age or perceived health.

In contrast, Weinberger and colleagues (1987) implemented their study using a sample of 134 older adults with arthritis and a mean age of 66 years. These authors also modified the original Hassles and Uplifts scales based on responses from 44 pretest telephone interviews. Seventy-three items were retained for this study; the omitted items were related to work, sexual relationships, and raising children. The authors stated that these items were probably not relevant to an elderly population that was not working. In addition, this study examined the effects of life events on arthritis-specific functional status. Uplifts were excluded from the study because pretest data suggested respondents had a difficult time responding to the uplifts items. The authors stated that respondents were unwilling to estimate or were uncomfortable estimating the frequency of experiencing uplifts. The study found that hassles were better predictors of arthritis-specific functional status than life events, and that hassles were strongly related to health status. Thus, findings in these earlier studies with adults in their middle years were replicated in this study with older adults.

Similarly, several studies have been implemented with caregivers of family members with dementia and stroke (Kinney & Stephens, 1989a; Kinney, Stephens, Franks, & Norris, 1995). The samples in these studies have generally been late-middle-aged adults with average ages from 57 to 60 years. These studies used a scale specifically targeting the unique hassles that would be faced by caregivers of family members (Kinney & Stephens, 1989a) and found that hassles were associated with caregivers' well-being (Kinney & Stephens, 1989b). Uplifts were not directly associated with well-being, but when caregivers' uplifts outnumbered their hassles the net effect was lower levels of caregiver distress. In a more recent study, Elder and colleagues (2003) found that caring for the cognitively impaired client provided many uplifts for nurses and few hassles. However, the hassles that occurred were of high importance as they were the engagements with family members.

Hassles and Children and Adolescents

Studies have also been implemented to examine the effects of hassles on health outcomes among children and adolescents. Kanner and Feldman (1991) studied the effects of perceived control over daily hassles and uplifts in a sample of 140 sixth graders. This cross-sectional study used a 50-item Children's Hassles and Uplifts Scale that consisted of 25 items reflecting hassles and 25 items reflecting uplifts in areas such as school, family, or friends. Hassles and uplifts were rated with regard to whether they had occurred in the past month and also rated on a 3-point scale with regard to their relative effect. Results of this study indicated that the number of hassles and the number of uplifts were significantly related to depression scores for both boys and girls. In addition, perceived control over uplifts was associated with better functioning, and lower control over hassles was associated with poorer functioning, in which functioning reflected both depression scores and levels of restraint.

Several studies of "day-to-day" events have been completed with adolescents. Miller, Tobacyk, and Wilcox (1985) examined which of the 117 hassles items and 135 uplifts items from the original scale were most frequently endorsed by 38 high school students. Subjects in this convenience sample had a mean age of 17 years and were found to endorse hassles that seemed developmentally appropriate, such as troublesome thoughts about one's future, concerns about weight, misplacing or losing things, social obligations, and fear of rejection. In addition, a significant bivariate relationship was found between adolescent hassles scores and their self-rating of their physical and psychological health on 9-point semantic differential scales. Uplifts were not significantly related to either physical or psychological health.

Wagner et al. (1988) also studied the impact of negative daily events on psychological health. Their study of 58 adolescents with a mean age of 18 years measured daily negative events, major negative events, and psychological symptoms at three time points: (a) 1 month before high school graduation, (b) 2 weeks after starting college, and (c) 3 months after the semester began. There was a single measure of daily and major events for this study, the Adolescent Perceived Events Scale. Causal modeling analysis using LISREL confirmed significant path coefficients between major events and daily events and between daily events and psychological symptoms, with no significant direct path relationship between major events and symptoms. The study supported the role of daily events in psychological health for adolescents and the effect of major life events on psychological symptoms mediated by daily events.

A related study (Wolf et al., 1989) examined the effect of hassles, uplifts, and life events on the psychological well-being of freshman medical students. This young adult sample of 55 students had a mean age of 24 years. The students completed the Medical Education Hassles/Uplifts Scale and other scales at least six times during a 9-month period. As in other studies, hassles were a better predictor of both concurrent and subsequent negative mood when compared to life events. This study, however, found that life events contributed to subsequent positive moods. Uplifts were found to be unrelated to psychological well-being.

The results of studies of hassles across the life span confirm that although specific hassles differ depending on age and development, day-to-day micro-stressors that are relevant to the individuals have a negative effect on health outcomes. This was demonstrated when the Hassles Scale was a broad and general measure, such as the original Hassles and Uplifts scales (Kanner et al., 1981), or with investigator-developed scales that addressed specific populations, such as caregivers or medical students (Kinney & Stephens, 1989a; Wolf et al., 1989). Furthermore, the relative strength of hassles as a predictor of health state and the mediating effect of hassles have been supported in samples across the age continuum (Wagner et al., 1988; Weinberger et al., 1987).

Effects of Hassles and Uplifts
Across Different Cultural Groups

Research examining the effects of hassles and uplifts has been implemented in many countries throughout the world, and a few studies in the United States have used samples from diverse ethnic and racial groups. In England, several studies of hassles as predictors of specific illness symptoms, upper respiratory infections, and irritable bowel syndrome have been implemented (Dancey et al., 1995; Evans & Edgerton, 1991; Evans et al., 1988). Studies have also been conducted in New Zealand (Leathem et al., 1996), Canada (Ravindran, Griffiths, Merali, & Anisman, 1996), and Israel (Weller & Avinir, 1993). In the study by Weller and Avinir, the Hassles and Uplifts Scale was translated into Hebrew. In general, studies in different countries have found hassles to be related to the health outcome measures being studied.

The majority of studies examining the effects of hassles and uplifts on health outcomes have used samples composed of people that were predominantly White, well educated, and middle or upper middle class. Three exceptions are Williams et al.'s (1992) study with Navajo Indian subjects, Weinberger et al.'s (1987) study with older, Black women, and Ivancevich's (1986) study with hourly assembly-line employees. Both Williams et al. and Weinberger et al. used revised versions of the original Hassles and Uplifts scales (Kanner et al., 1981) to make the scale more culturally and developmentally appropriate to their samples. In the study with Navajo Indians, the authors deleted selected items and also added many items that they describe as culturally relevant (Williams et al., 1992). The tool used with older Black women omitted 44 of the original 117 items that were considered inappropriate for this population based on pretest telephone interviews (Weinberger et al., 1987). Ivancevich's study with assembly-line workers used the original tool developed by Kanner and colleagues (1981)

and found that hassles most frequently cited were health of a family member, too many things to do, trouble relaxing, misplacing or losing things, too many interruptions, and unchallenging work. Furthermore, Ivancevich reported that test-retest correlations for both the Uplifts and Hassles scales were similar to those found in earlier studies with more upper-middle-class samples. Recent cross-cultural hassles and uplift studies have included Mexican American caregivers (Kao, 2011), Singaporean nurses (Lim, Hepworth, & Bogossian, 2011), low-income Mexican Americans (Clark, Zimmer, & Sanchez, 2009), and Chinese American urban adolescents (Ozer & McDonald, 2006). More studies are needed before the role of day-to-day events in predicting health outcomes can be generalized across cultures and socioeconomic groups. Research to date, however, supports the applicability of the Hassles and Uplifts Model across diverse populations.

HASSLES AND UPLIFTS AND NURSING KNOWLEDGE

Overview of Studies

Nurse scientists have been particularly attracted to the Hassles and Uplifts Model as a possible explanation and predictor of health outcomes. Studies have examined the model as applied to such diverse health outcomes as perimenstrual symptoms (Woods, Most, & Longenecker, 1985), rheumatoid arthritis (Crosby, 1988), perceptions of health in adolescent females (De Maio-Esteves, 1990), and depression in female nursing students (Williams, Hagerty, Murphy-Weinberg, & Wan, 1995). In addition, hassles and uplifts have been examined in relationship to symptoms of genital herpes (Swanson, Dibble, & Chenitz, 1995), as a covariate in understanding perceived health among subjects quitting smoking (Macnee, 1991), and as a predictor of exercise behavior in perimenopausal women (M. S. Evans & Nies, 1997). Recent nursing research studies of hassles and uplifts include problems caring for people with cognitive impairment (Elder et al., 2003), medication confusion in older adults (Travis et al., 2007), psychological and social adaptation of middle-aged widows (Ungar & Florian, 2004), and hearing impairment in older adults (Knussen et al., 2005) and those using HIV medications (Beals, Wight, Aneshensel, Murphy, & Miller-Martinez, 2006).

The empirical use of the Hassles and Uplifts Model in nursing has centered on examination of common negative daily stressful events, or hassles, and the link between symptom expression and underlying illness state. Consistent with other empirical uses of the model, nurse researchers have focused mainly on examining the impact of hassles on health states and have not investigated uplifts as protective factors in health. Nursing studies, like those in other disciplines, have consistently found a significant relationship between a person's psychological perception of micro-stressors and the individual's subsequent perceptions of health or symptom expression or both.

Appropriateness and Use of the Model for Nursing

The process nature of the Hassles and Uplifts Model has made it particularly appropriate for nursing studies. One of the first nursing studies to use the Hassles and Uplift Model applied it to the examination of the experience of perimenstrual symptoms and the relationship of symptom level to stress (Woods et al.,1985). In that study, the Hassles and Uplifts Model was used as the conceptual basis for attempting to explain the influence of a women's psychosocial context on their experience of perimenstrual symptoms. Nursing studies using the Hassles and Uplift Model share a basic premise identified in Woods et al.'s study: *Individuals who perceive life as more stressful, experience and act on symptoms of illness more than those whose environment is individually perceived as less stressful.* Stress, coping, and the subsequent impact of these variables on health has historically been considered integral to the practice of nursing. From this perspective, the Hassles and Uplift Model is both relevant and appropriate for nursing studies.

Most of the nursing research using the Hassles and Uplifts Model as the conceptual basis of study is predicated on the assumption that daily, common, continuous stressor events, referred to as hassles, have more and different impact than major stress events on individual perceptions of health. Only Woods et al.'s (1985) study does not make this assumption, instead trying to contrast the impact of major stress events with the impact of daily hassles.

Implications of Hassles and Uplifts for Nursing Theory, Practice, and Research

The Hassles and Uplifts Model takes stress and coping theory beyond the linear perspective of inputs and outputs that are reflected in the physiological models of stress and coping (Selye, 1950) and life events theory (Holmes & Rahe, 1967). It is a well-developed and tested model, clearly grounded and conceptualized within the larger TTSC (Lazarus & Folkman, 1984). Relationships within the model are explicitly stated, and the concepts are theoretically and operationally defined. These relationships and concepts have received considerable testing and, at least for the hassles portion of the model, have been repeatedly supported in a wide range of studies in both nursing and other disciplines. The use of the model for developing and testing knowledge about the relationships between stress and health is evident given the large number of publications and studies based on the model.

The Hassles and Uplifts Model is very consistent with nursing's holistic view of persons and health and is congruent with most nursing theories. The model not only has use for theoretical knowledge development but also has been applied and tested in clinical nursing studies that have direct implications for practice. Research has supported the relationship of hassles to symptoms from rheumatoid arthritis, perimenstrual symptoms, genital herpes symptoms, and depression. These results suggest and assist the development of nursing practice models that address the need to direct nursing care toward understanding and perhaps modifying clients' perceptions and coping approaches to day-to-day events. Knowledge gained from studies using the Hassles and Uplifts Model suggests that a combination of increasing hassles with decreasing uplifts leads to the development of common illnesses such as the cold (Evans & Edgerton, 1991; Evans et al., 1988). These results suggest the possibility of assisting clients to identify high-risk periods in their lives and a need to increase their self-care in other ways to perhaps offset the potential effects of day-to-day stressors. Therefore, the Hassles and Uplifts Model, because of the level of theory it represents and the extensive testing it has received, has many implications for nursing practice that need to be explored and tested further.

Implications for future research using the Hassles and Uplifts Model are extensive. The model has significant potential to be used as a means for controlling statistically for the effects of day-to-day stresses and strains when researchers are seeking to explore other factors that impact health outcomes. The model has received only limited testing in diverse cultures; therefore, additional studies with different socioeconomic groups are also needed. Issues of measurement and study design need continued examination. Furthermore, although results of empirical studies have consistently supported the effects of day-to-day events (that are perceived as salient and threatening on health outcomes), findings regarding the effects of positively toned events are inconsistent and controversial. Lazarus and colleagues originally proposed equal and balancing effects for hassles and uplifts. Empirical studies, however, suggest that uplifts may act more as modifiers for the effects of hassles or may have only an interaction effect on health outcomes.

In summary, the Hassles and Uplifts Model is a well-tested model that is congruent with nursing's perspective of health and well being and has demonstrated utility for nursing practice. Future research is needed using samples from diverse cultures and socioeconomic backgrounds to test the possible modifier effect of uplifts on the effects of hassles.

REFERENCES

Amster, L., & Kraus, H. (1974). The relationship between life crises and mental deterioration in old age. *International Journal of Aging and Human Development, 5,* 51–55.

Antonovsky, A., & Kats, R. (1967). The life crisis history as a tool in epidemiological research. *Journal of Health and Social Behavior, 8,* 15–21.

Bakan, G., & Akyol, A. D. (2008). Theory-guided interventions for adaptation to heart failure in Turkey. *Journal of Advanced Nursing, 61*(6), 596–608.

Baldwin, C. W., Hibbein, J., Herr, S., Lohner, I., & Core, D. (2002). Self-care as defined by members of the Amish community utilizing the theory of modeling and role-modeling. *Multicultural Nursing and Health, 8,* 60–64.

Beals, K. P., Wight, R. G., Aneshensel, C. S., Murphy, D. A., & Miller-Martinez, D. (2006). The role of family caregivers in HIV medication adherence. *AIDS Care, 18*(6), 589–596.

Beck, C. T. (2008). Impact of birth trauma on breastfeeding. *Nursing Research. 57*(4), 228–36.

Benson, H., & Casey, A. (2008). *Stress management: Approaches for preventing and reducing stress.* (Harvard Medical School Special Health Report). Boston, MA: Harvard Health Publications.

Ben-Zur, H., & Michael, K. (2009). Social comparisons and well-being following widowhood and divorce. *Death Studies, 33*(3), 220–238.

Bettelheim, B. (1960). *The informed heart.* New York, NY: Free Press.

Black, N., Griffiths, J., & Pope, C. (1996). Development of a symptom severity index and a symptom impact index for stress incontinence in women. *Neurology & Urodynamics, 15*(6), 630–640.

Blegen, M. A., & Tripp-Reimer, T. (1997). Implications of nursing taxonomies for middle-range theory development. *Advances in Nursing Science, 19*(3), 37–49.

Bost, N., & Wallis, M. (2006). The effectiveness of a 15 minute weekly massage in reducing physical and psychological stress in nurses. *Australian Journal of Advanced Nursing, 23*(4), 28–33.

Boyd, M. R., Baliko, B., Cox, M. F., & Tavakoli, A. (2007). Stress, coping, and alcohol expectancies in rural African-American women. *Archives of Psychiatric Nursing, 21*(2), 70–79.

Bramston, P., & Fogarty, G. J. (1995). Measuring stress in the mildly intellectually handicapped: The factorial structure of the Subjective Stress Scale. *Research in Developmental Disabilities, 16*(2), 117–131.

Breznitz, S., & Goldberger, L. (1993). Stress research at a crossroads. In L. Goldberger & S. Breznitz (Eds.), *Handbook of stress: Theoretical and clinical aspects.* New York, NY: Free Press.

Brown, G. W., & Harris, T. O. (1978). *Social origins of depression.* New York, NY: Free Press.

Brown, G. W., & Harris, T. (1982). Fall off in the reporting of life events. *Social Psychiatry. 17,* 23–28.

Budd, K. S., Workman, D. E., Lemsky, C. M., & Quick, D. M. (1994). The Children's Headache Assessment Scale (CHAS): Factor structure and psychometric properties. *Journal of Behavioral Medicine, 17*(2), 159–179.

Byrne, C. P., Velamoor, V. R., Cernovsky, Z. Z., Cortese, L., & Losztyn, S. (1990). A comparison of borderline and schizophrenic patients for childhood life events and parent child relationships. *Canadian Journal of Psychiatry. 35*(7), 590–595.

Cannon, W. B. (1932). *The wisdom of the body.* New York, NY: Norton.

Cavendish, R., Luise, B., Home, K. et al. (2000). Opportunities for enhanced spirituality relevant to well adults. *International Journal of Nursing, 11*(4), 151–163.

Charles, S. T., Luong, G., Almeida, D. M., Ryff, C. D., Sturm, M., & Love, G. (2010). Fewer ups and downs: Daily stressors mediate age differences in negative affect. *Journal of Gerontology: Psychological Sciences, 65B*, 279–286.

Chilcote, R. L. (2007). Art therapy with child tsunami survivors in Sri Lanka. *Art Therapy, 24*(4), 156–162.

Chou, M. H., & Lin, M. F. (2006). Exploring the listening experiences during guided imagery and music therapy of outpatients with depression. *Journal of Nursing Research, 14*(2), 93–102.

Clark, L., Zimmer, V., & Sanchez, J. (2009). Cultural values and political economic contexts of diabetes among low-income Mexican Americans. *Transcultural Nursing, 20*(4), 382–394.

Cochrane, R., & Robertson, A. (1973). The life events inventory: A measure of the relative severity of psychosocial stressors. *Journal of Psychosomatic Research, 17*, 135–139.

Coddington, R. D. (1972a). The significance of life events as etiologic factors in the diseases of children. I. A survey of professional workers. *Journal of Psychosomatic Research, 16*, 7–18.

Coddington, R. D. (1972b). The significance of life events as etiologic factors in the diseases of children. II. A survey of a normal population. *Journal of Psychosomatic Research, 16*, 205–213.

Coddington, R. D., & Troxell, J. R. (1980). The effect of emotional factors on football injury rates: A pilot study. *Journal of Human Stress, 6*, 3–5.

Cohen, F., Horowitz, M. J., Lazarus, R., Moos, R., Robins, L., Rose, R., & Rutter, M. (1982). Panel report on psychosocial assets and modifiers of stress. In G. R. Elliott & C. Eisdorfer (Eds.), *Stress and human health*: Analysis and implications of research (pp. 147–184). New York, NY: Springer

Cohen, S., Kessler, R. C., & Gordon, L. U. (1995). *Measuring stress: A guide for health and social scientists*. New York, NY: Oxford University Press.

Cohen, S., Tyrrell, D. A., & Smith, A. P. (1991). Psychological stress in humans and susceptibility to the common cold. *New England Journal of Medicine, 325*, 606–612.

Cohen-Sandler, R., Berman, A. L., & King, R. A. (1982). Life stress and symptomatology: Determinants of suicidal behavior in children. *Journal of the American Academy of Child Psychiatry, 21*, 178–186.

Collins, E. G., White-Williams, C., & Jalowiec, A. (1996). Spouse stressors while awaiting transplantation. *Heart & Lung: Journal of Acute & Critical Care, 25*, 1–13.

Compas, B. E., Davis, G. E., Forsythe, C. J., & Wagner, B. M. (1987). Assessment of major and daily stressful events during adolescence: The Adolescent Perceived Event Scale. *Journal of Consulting and Clinical Psychology, 55*(4), 534–543.

Cossette, S., D'Aoust, L., Morin, M., Heppell, S., & Frasure-Smith, M. (2009). The systematic development of a nursing intervention aimed at increasing enrollment in cardiac rehabilitation for acute coronary syndrome patients. *Progress in Cardiovascular Nursing, 24*(3), 71–79.

Costa, P. T., Somerfield, M., & McCrae, R. R. (1996). Personality and coping: A reconceptualization. In M. Zeidner & N. S. Endler (Eds.), *Handbook of coping*. New York, NY: John Wiley.

Costantini, A. F., Braun, J. R., Davis, J., & Ivervolino, A. (1974). The life change inventory: A device for quantifying psychological magnitude of changes experienced by college students. *Psychological Reports, 34*, 991–1000.

Cox, T. (1978). *Stress*. Baltimore, MD: University Park Press.

Crandall, C. S., Preisler, J. J., & Aussprung, J. (1992). Measuring life event stress in the lives of college students: The Undergraduate Stress Questionnaire (USQ). *Journal of Behavioral Medicine, 15*(6), 627–662.

Cropley, M., & Steptoe, A. (2005). Social support, life events and physical symptoms: A prospective study of chronic and recent life stress in men and women. *Psychology, Health and Medicine, 10*, 317–325.

Crosby, L. J. (1988). Stress factors, emotional stress and rheumatoid arthritis disease activity. *Journal of Advanced Nursing, 13*(4), 452–461.

Dancey, C. P., Whitehouse, A., Painter, J., & Backhouse, S. (1995). The relationship between hassles, uplifts, and irritable bowel syndrome: A preliminary study. *Journal of Psychosomatic Research, 39*(7), 827–832.

DeLongis, A., Coyne, J. C., Dakof, G., Folkman, S., & Lazarus, R. S. (1982). Relationship of daily hassles, uplifts, and major life events to health status. *Health Psychology, 1*, 119–136.

DeLongis, A., Folkman, S., & Lazarus, R. S. (1988). The impact of daily stress on health and mood: Psychological and social resources as mediators. *Journal of Personality and Social Psychology, 54*(3), 486–495.

DeLongis, A., Holtzman, S, Puterman, E., & Lam, M. (2010). Dyadic coping: Support from the spouse in times of stress. In J. Davila & K. Sullivan (Eds.), *Social support processes in intimate relationships*. New York, NY: Oxford Press.

De Maio-Esteves, M. (1990). Mediators of daily stress and perceived health status in adolescent girls. *Nursing Research, 39*(6), 360–364.

Derogatis, L. R., & Coons, H. L. (1993). Self-report measures of stress. In L. Goldberger & S. Breznitz (Eds.), *Handbook of stress: Theoretical and clinical aspects.* New York, NY: Free Press.

DeSanto-Madeya, S. (2006). The meaning of living with spinal cord injury 5 to 10 years after the injury. *Western Journal of Nursing Research, 28,* 265–289.

Deutsch, L. J., & Erickson, M. T. (1989). Early life events as discriminators of socialized and undersocialized delinquents. *Journal of Abnormal Child Psychology, 17*(5), 541–551.

Dohrenwend, B. P., Link, B. G., Kern, R., Shrout, P. E., & Markowitz, J. (1990). Measuring life events: The problem of variability within event categories. *Stress Medicine, 6,* 179–187.

Dohrenwend, B. P., Raphael, K. G., Schwartz, S., Stueve, A., & Skodol, A. (1993). The structured event probe and narrative rating method for measuring stressful life events. In L. Goldberger & S. Breznitz (Eds.), *Handbook of stress: Theoretical and clinical aspects* (pp. 174–199). New York, NY: Free Press.

Dohrenwend, B. S., Krasnoff, L., Askenasy, A. R., & Dohrenwend, B. P. (1978). Exemplification of a method for scaling life events: The PERI Life Events Scale. *Journal of Health Social Behavior, 19,* 205–229.

Dohrenwend, B. S., Krasnoff, L., Askenasy, A. R., & Dohrenwend, B. P. (1982). The psychiatric epidemiology research interview life events scale. In L. Goldberger & S. Breznitz (Eds.), *Handbook of stress: Theoretical and clinical aspects.* New York, NY: Free Press.

Dykema, J., Bergbower, K., & Peterson, C. (1995). Pessimistic explanatory style, stress and illness. *Journal of Social and Clinical Psychology, 14*(4), 357–371.

Eilert-Petersson, E., & Olsson, H. (2003). Humour and slimming related to the Neuman Systems Model: A study of slimming women in Sweden. *Theoria Journal of Nursing Theory, 12*(3), 4–18.

Elder, R., Wollin, J., Härtel, C., Spencer, N., & Sanderson, W. (2003). Hassles and uplifts associated with caring for people with cognitive impairment in community settings. *International Journal of Mental Health Nursing, 12*(4), 271–278.

Elliott, G. R., & Eisdorfer, C. (1982). *Stress and human health.* New York, NY: Springer.

Erickson, H., Tomlin, E., & Swain, M. (1983). *Modeling and role-modeling: A theory and paradigm for nursing.* Englewood Cliffs, NJ: Prentice-Hall.

Eriksen, H. R., & Ursin, H. (2005). Stress—it is all in the brain. In B. B. Arnetz & R. Ekman (Eds.), *Stress in health and disease* (pp. 46–68). Weinheim, Germany: Wiley-VCH.

Erlandsson, L.-K. (2008). Stability in women's experiences of hassles and uplifts: A five-year follow-up survey. *Scandinavian Journal of Occupational Therapy, 15,* 95-104.

Evans, M. S., & Nies, M. A. (1997). The effects of daily hassles on exercise participation in perimenopausal women. *Public Health Nursing, 14*(2), 129–133.

Evans, P. D., & Edgerton, N. (1991). Life-events and mood as predictors of the common cold. *British Journal of Medical Psychology, 64,* 35–44.

Evans, P. D., Pitts, M. K., & Smith, K. (1988). Minor infection, minor life events and the four day desirability dip. *Journal of Psychosomatic Research, 32*(4/5), 533–539.

Ewedemi, F., & Linn, M. W. (1987). Health and hassles in older and younger men. *Journal of Clinical Psychology, 43*(4), 347–353.

Figley, C. R., & McCubbin, H. I. (1983). *Stress and the family, Volume II: Coping with catastrophe.* New York, NY: Brunner/Mazel.

Folkman, S., Lazarus, R.S., Pimley, S., & Novacek, J. (1987). Age differences in stress and coping processes. *Psychology and Aging, 2*(2), 171–184.

Frost, M. H. (1993). Commentary on stressors and health outcomes: Implications for nursing research, theory, practice and policy agendas. In J. S. Barnfather & B. L. Lyon (Eds.), *Stress and coping: State of the science and implications for nursing theory, research, and practice* (pp. 43–64). Indianapolis, IN: Sigma Theta Tau Center Nursing Press.

Frost, M. H., Orth, K., & Werner, J. (2000). Stressors and chronic conditions. In J. S. Werner & M. H. Frost (Eds.), *Stress and coping: State of the science and implications for nursing theory, research and practice,* Volume II. Glenview, IL: Midwest Nursing Research Society Press.

Funch, D. P., & Marshall, J. R. (1984). Measuring life stress: Factors affecting fall-off in the reporting of life events. *Journal of Health and Social Behavior, 15,* 453–464.

Gadzella, B. M. (1994). Student-life stress inventory: Identification of and reactions to stressors. *Psychological Reports, 74,* 395–402.

Garcia, C. (2010). Conceptualization and measurement of coping during adolescence: A review of the literature. *Journal of Nursing Scholarship, 42*(2), 166–185.

Gerstle, D. S., All, A. C., & Wallace, D. C. (2001). Quality of life and chronic nonmalignant pain. *Pain Management Nursing, 2*(3), 98–109.

Gibbons, C., Dempster, M., & Moutray, M. (2009). Index of sources of stress in nursing students: a confirmatory factor analysis. *Journal of Advanced Nursing, 65*(5), 1095–1102.

Glen, S., Simpson, A., Drinnan, D., McGuinness, D., & Sandberg, S. (1993). Testing the reliability of a new measure of life events and experiences in childhood: The Psychosocial Assessment of Childhood Experiences (PACE). *European Child and Adolescent Psychiatry, 2*(2), 98–110.

Glidden, L. M. (1993). What we do not know about families with children who have developmental disabilities: Questionnaire on resources and stress as a case study. *American Journal of Mental Retardation, 97*(5), 481–495.

Goodman, L., Corcoran, C., Turner, K., Yuan, N., & Green, B. (1998). Assessing traumatic event exposure: General issues and preliminary findings for the Stressful Life Events Screening Questionnaire. *Journal of Traumatic Stress, 11*(3), 521–542.

Gupta, M. A., & Gupta, A. K. (1995). The Psoriasis Life Stress Inventory: A preliminary index of psoriasis-related stress. *Acta Dermato-Venereologica, 75*(3), 240–243.

Hammoudeh, A. J., Alhaddad, I.A. (2009). Triggers and the onset of acute myocardial infarction. *Cardiology in Review, 17*(6), 270–274.

Hawkins, N. G., Davies, R., & Holmes, T. H. (1957). Evidence of psychosocial factors in the development of pulmonary tuberculosis. *American Review of Tuberculosis and Pulmonary Diseases, 75,* 768–780.

Henderson, S., Byrne, D. G., & Duncan-Jones, P. (1981). *Neurosis and the social environment.* New York, NY: Academic Press.

Herschbach, P., Duran, G., Waadt, S., Zettler, A., Amm, C., & Marten-Mittag, B. (1997). Psychometric properties of the Questionnaire on Stress in patients with diabetes—Revised (QSD-R). *Health Psychology, 16*(2), 171–174.

Hinds, P. S. (2000). Fostering coping by adolescents with newly diagnosed cancer. *Seminars in Oncology Nursing, 16*(4), 317–336.

Hinkle, L. E. (1973). The concept of "stress" in the biological and social sciences. *Science, Medicine, and Man, 1,* 31–48.

Hobfoll, S. E., Freedy, J. R., Green, B., & Solomon, S. (1996). Coping in reaction to extreme stress: The roles of resource loss and resource availability. In M. Zeidner & N. S. Endler (Eds.), *Handbook of coping.* New York, NY: John Wiley.

Holmes, T. H. (1979). Development and application of a quantitative measure of life change magnitude. In J. E. Barrett, R. M. Rose, & G. I. Klerman (Eds.), *Stress and mental disorder.* New York, NY: Raven Press.

Holmes, T. H., & Masuda. M. (1974). Life change and illness susceptibility. In B. S. Dohrenwend & B. P. Dohrenwend (Eds.), *Stressful life events:*

Their nature and effects (pp. 45–72). New York, NY: John Wiley.

Holmes, T. H., & Rahe, R. (1967). The Social Readjustment Rating Scale. *Journal of Psychosomatic Research, 12,* 213–218.

Horowitz, M. (1979). *Impact of Event Scale (IES).* San Francisco: University of California Press.

Horowitz, M. J., Schaefer, C., Hiroto, D., Wilner. N., & Levin, B. (1977). Life event questionnaires for measuring presumptive stress. *Psychosomatic Medicine, 39,* 413–431.

Hunt, C. K. (2003). Concepts in caregiver research. *Journal of Nursing Scholarship, 35*(1), 27–32.

Hurst, M. W., Jenkins, C. D., & Rose, R. M. (1978). The assessment of life change stress: A comparative and methodological inquiry. *Psychosomatic Medicine, 40,* 126–141.

Hymovich, D. (1983). The Chronicity Impact and Coping Instrument: Parent questionnaire. *Nursing Research, 32*(5), 275–281.

Ivancevich, J. M. (1986). Life events and hassles as predictors of health, symptoms, job performance, and absenteeism. *Journal of Occupational Behavior, 7,* 39–51.

Jandorf, L., Deblinger, E., Neale, J. M., & Stone, A. A. (1986). Daily versus major life events as predictors of symptom frequency: A replication study. *Journal of General Psychology, 113*(3), 205–218.

Janis, I. L. (1951). *Air war and emotional stress.* New York, NY: McGraw-Hill.

Jenkins, R., & Elliott, P. (2004). Stressors, burnout and social support: Nurses in acute mental health settings. *Journal of Advanced Nursing, 48*(6), 622–631.

Jirovec, M. M.., Jenkins, J., Isenberg, M., & Baiardi, J. (1999). Urine control theory derived from Roy's conceptual framework. *Nursing Science Quarterly, 2*(3), 251–255.

Johannisson, K. (2006). Modern fatigue: A historical perspective. In B. B. Arnetz & R. Ekman (Eds.), *Stress in health and disease* (pp. 1–19). Weinheim, Germany: Wiley-YCH.

Johnson, D. E. (1980). The behavioral system model for nursing. In J. P. Riehl & C. Roy (Eds.), *Conceptual models for nursing practice* (2nd ed.). New York, NY: Appleton-Century-Crofts.

Johnson, J. H., & McCutcheon, S. M. (1980). Assessing life stress in older children and adolescents: Preliminary findings with the life events checklist. In I. B. Sarason & C. C. Spielberger (Eds.), *Stress and anxiety* (Vol. 7, pp. 111–125). Washington, DC: Hemisphere.

Jopp, D., & Schmitt, M. (2010). Dealing with negative life events: Differential effects of personal resources, coping strategies, and control beliefs. *European Journal of Ageing, 7*(3), 167–180.

Kanner, A. D., Coyne, J., Schaefer, C., & Lazarus, R. (1981). Comparison of two modes of stress measurements: Daily hassles and uplifts versus major life events. *Journal of Behavioral Medicine, 4,* 1– 39.

Kanner, A. D., & Feldman, S. S. (1991). Control over uplifts and hassles and its relationship to adaptational outcomes. *Journal of Behavioral Medicine, 14*(2), 187–201.

Kao, H.-F. S. (2011). Medication administration hassles for Mexican American family caregivers of older adults. *Nursing & Health Sciences, 13*(2), 133–140.

Kessler, R. C., & Wethington, E. (1991). The reliability of life event reports in a community survey. *Psychological Medicine, 21,* 723–738.

Kidney, W. C. (1993). *Webster's 21st century dictionary.* Nashville, TN: T. Nelson.

Kinney, J. M., & Stephens, M. A. P. (1989a). Caregiving hassles scale: Assessing the daily hassles of family members with dementia. *The Gerontologist, 29*(3), 328–332.

Kinney, J. M., & Stephens, M. A. P. (1989b). Hassles and uplifts of giving care to a family member with dementia. *Psychology and Aging, 4*(4), 402–408.

Kinney, J. M., Stephens, M. A. P., Franks, M. M., & Norris, V. K. (1995). Stresses and satisfactions of family care givers to older stroke patients. *Journal of Applied Gerontology, 14,* 3–21.

Knussen, C., Tolson, D., Swan, I. R. C., Stott, D. J., & Brogan, C. A. (2005). Stress proliferation in caregivers: The relationships between caregiving stressors and deterioration in family relationships. *Psychology and Health, 20*(2), 207–221.

Lamb, S. E., Hansen, Z., Lall, R., Castelnuovo, E., Withers, E. J., Nichols, V., & Underwood, M. R. (on behalf of the Back Skills Training Trial investigators). (2010). Group cognitive behavioural treatment for low-back pain in primary care: A randomised controlled trial and cost-effectiveness analysis. *Lancet, 375*(9718), 916–923.

Lange, A., Kooiman, K., Huberts, L., & van Oostendorp, E. (1995). Childhood unwanted sexual events and degree of psychopathology of psychiatric patients: Research with a new anamnestic questionnaire (CHUSE). *Acta Psychiatrica Scandinavia, 92*(6), 441–446.

Lazarus, R. S. (1966). *Psychological stress and the coping process.* New York, NY: McGraw-Hill.

Lazarus, R. S. (1993). From Psychological stress to the emotions: A history of changing outlooks. *Annual Review of Psychology, 44,* 1-21.

Lazarus, R. S., & Folkman, S. (1984). *Stress, appraisal, and coping.* New York, NY: Springer.

Leathem, J., Heath, E., & Woolley, C. (1996). Relatives' perceptions of role change, social support and stress after traumatic brain injury. *Brain Injury, 10,* 27–38.

Lepore, S. J., & Evans, G. W. (1996). Coping with multiple stressors in the environment. In M. Zeidner & N. S. Endler (Eds.), *Handbook of coping.* New York, NY: John Wiley.

Levenstein, S., Prantera, C., Varvo, V., Scribano, M. L., Berto, E., Luzi, C., & Andreoli, A. (1993). Development of the Perceived Stress Questionnaire: A new tool for psychosomatic research. *Journal of Psychosomatic Research, 37,* 19–32.

Levine, S., & Scotch, N. A. (1970). *Social stress.* Chicago, IL: Aldine.

Lewin, K. A. (1935). *A dynamic theory of personality.* New York, NY: McGraw-Hill

Li Y, Shi J, & Zheng X. (2002). The theory of modeling and role-modeling and systematic holistic nursing care [Chinese]. *Chinese Nursing Research,16*(4). 189–190.

Lietzen, R., Virtanen, P., Kivimaki, M., Sillanmaki, L., Vahtera, J., & Koskenvuo, M. (2011). Stressful life events and the onset of asthma. *European Respiratory Journal, 37*(6), 1360–1365.

Lim, J., Hepworth, J., & Bogossian, F. (2011). A qualitative analysis of stress, uplifts and coping in the personal and professional lives of Singaporean nurses. *Journal of Advanced Nursing, 67*(5), 1022–1033.

Lombardo, S. L., & Roof, M. (2005). Clinicians' forum. A case study applying the modeling and role-modeling theory to morbid obesity. *Home Healthcare Nurse, 23*(7), 425–428.

Lyon, B. L., & Werner, J. S. (1987). Stress. *Annual Review of Nursing Research, 5,* 3–22.

Macnee, C. L. (1991). Perceived well-being of persons quitting smoking. *Nursing Research, 40*(4), 200–203.

Madu, S. N., & DeJong, E. S. (2002). Changing stress levels through gaining information on stress. *Curationis, 25*(1), 28–34.

Margiotta, E. W., Davilla, D. A., & Hicks, R. A. (1990). Type A-B behavior and the self-report of daily hassles and uplifts. *Perceptual and Motor Skills, 79*(3), 777–778.

Mason, J. W. (1975). A historical view of the stress field: Part I. *Journal of Human Stress, 1,* 6–12.

McCain, N. L., Munjas, B. A., Munro, C. L., Elswick, R. K., Jr., Robins, J. L. W., Ferreira-Gonzalez, A., . . . Garrett, C.T., et al. (2003). Effects of stress management on PNI-based outcomes in persons with HIV disease. *Research in Nursing & Health, 26*(2), 102–117.

McCubbin, M. (2002, July). Family stress, perceived social support and coping following the diagnosis of a child's congenital heart disease. *Journal of Advanced Nursing, 39*(2), 190–198.

McCubbin, H. I., & Figley, C. R. (1983). *Stress and the family, Volume I: Coping with normative transitions.* New York, NY: Brunner/Mazel.

McCubbin, H. I., & Patterson, J. M. (1983). The family stress process: The Double ABCX Model of Adjustment and Adaptation. *Marriage and Family Review, 6,* 7–35.

McCubbin, H. I., Patterson, J., Bauman, E., & Harris, L. (1981). *Adolescent-Family Inventory of Life Events and Changes (A-FILE).* Madison, WI: Family Stress, Coping and Health Project.

McCubbin, H. I., Patterson, J., & Wilson, L. (1980). *Family Inventory of Life Events and Changes (FILE).* Madison, WI: Family Stress, Coping and Health Project.

Mechanic, D. (1968). *Medical sociology.* New York, NY: Free Press.

Meeks, S., Shah, S., & Ramsey, S. (2009). The Pleasant Events Scale—nursing home version: A useful tool for behavioral interventions in long-term care. *Aging and Mental Health, 13,* 445–455.

Miller, M. J., Tobacyk, J. J., & Wilcox, C. T. (1985). Daily hassles and uplifts as perceived by adolescents. *Psychological Reports, 56,* 221–222.

Miller, T. W. (1981). Life events scaling: Clinical methodological issues. *Nursing Research, 30*(5), 316–320.

Mitchell, A. M., Wesner, S., Garand, L., Gale, D. D., Havill, A., & Brownson, L. (2007). A support group intervention for children bereaved by parental suicide. *Journal of Child & Adolescent Psychiatric Nursing, 20*(1), 3–13.

Monk, C., Leight, K. L., & Fang, Y. (2008). The relationship between women's attachment style and perinatal mood disturbance: Implications for screening and treatment. *Archives of Women's Mental Health, 11*(2), 117–129.

Monroe, S. M. (1983). Major and minor life events as predictors of psychological distress: Further issues and findings. *Journal of Behavioral Medicine, 6*(2), 189–205.

Murphy, S. P., Powers, M. J., & Jalowiec, A. (1985). Psychometric evaluation of the Hemodialysis Stressor Scale. *Nursing Research, 34*(6), 368–371.

Murrell, S. A., Norris, F. H., & Hutchins, G. M. (1984). Distribution and desirability of life events in older adults: Population and policy implications. *Journal of Community Psychology, 12,* 301–311.

Neufeldt, V., & Guralnik, D. B. (1996). *Webster's new world college dictionary.* New York, NY: Macmillan.

Neuman, B. (1989). The Neuman systems model: Applications in nursing education and practice (2nd ed.). Norwalk, CT: Appleton-Lange.

Norbeck, J. S. (1984). Modification of life event questionnaires for use with female respondents. *Research in Nursing and Health, 7,* 61–71.

Norris, F. H., & Hamblen, J. L. (2004). Standardized self-report measures of civilian trauma and PTSD. In J. P. Wilson, T. M. Keane, & T. Martin (Eds.), *Assessing psychological trauma and PTSD* (pp. 63–102). New York, NY: Guilford.

Ozer, E.J., & McDonald, K. L. (2006). Exposure to violence and mental health among Chinese American urban adolescents. *Journal of Adolescent Health, 39*(1), 73–79.

Paterson, R. J., & Neufeld, R. W. (1989). The stress response and parameters of stressful situations. In R. W. Neufeld (Ed.), *Advances in the investigation of psychological stress.* New York, NY: John Wiley.

Paykel, E. S. (1983). Methodological aspects of life event research. *Journal of Psychosomatic Research, 27,* 341–352.

Paykel, E. S. (1997). Interview for recent life events. *Psychological Medicine, 27,* 301–310.

Perry R. N. B. (2009). Role modeling excellence in clinical nursing practice. *Nurse Education in Practice, 9*(1), 36–44.

Rahe, R. H. (1968). Life-change measurement as a predictor of illness. *Proceedings of Research in Social Medicine, 61,* 1124–1126.

Rahe, R. H. (1972). Subjects' recent life changes and their near-future illness reports. *Annals of Clinical Research, 4,* 250–265.

Rahe, R. H. (1975). Epidemiological studies of life change and illness. *International Journal of Psychiatry in Medicine, 6,* 133–146.

Rahe, R. H. (1977). Life change measurement clarification. *Psychosomatic Medicine. 40,* 95–98.

Ravindran, A. V., Griffiths, J., Merali, Z., & Anisman, H. (1996). Primary dysthymia: A study of several psychosocial, endocrine and immune correlates. *Journal of Affective Disorders, 40,* 73–84.

Ray, S. L. (2009). The experience of contemporary peacekeepers healing from trauma. *Nursing Inquiry, 16*(1), 53–63.

Reid, T., & Bramwell, R. (2003). Using the parental stressor scale: NICU with a British sample of mothers of moderate risk preterm infants. *Journal of Reproductive & Infant Psychology, 21*(4), 279–291.

Reynolds, F., Lim, K. H., & Prior, S. (2008). Narratives of therapeutic art-making in the context of marital breakdown: Older women reflect on a significant mid-life experience. *Counselling Psychology Quarterly, 21*(3), 203–214.

Roosa, M. W., Sandler, I. N., Gehring, M., Beals, J., & Cappo, L. (1988). The children of alcoholics life-events schedule: A stress scale for children of alcohol abusing parents. *Journal of Studies on Alcohol, 49*(5), 422–429.

Roy, C. (1984). *Introduction to nursing: An adaptation model* (2nd ed.). Englewood Cliffs, NJ: Prentice Hall.

Rutter, M. (1989). Pathways from childhood to adult life. *Journal of Child Psychology and Psychiatry, 30,* 23–51.

Sadler, L. S., Swartz, M. K., & Ryan-Krause, P. (2003). Supporting adolescent mothers and their children through a high school–based child care center and parent support program. *Journal of Pediatric Health Care, 17*(3), 109–117.

Sandler, I. N., Nolichuk, S., Brauer, S. L., & Fogas, B. (1986). Significant events of children of divorce: Toward the assessment of a risky situation. In S. M. Averback & A. Stolberg (Eds.), *Crisis intervention with children and families* (pp. 65–87). New York, NY: Hemisphere.

Sarason, I. G., Johnson, J. H., & Siegel, J. M. (1978). Assessing the impact of life changes: Development of Life Experiences Survey. *Journal of Consulting and Clinical Psychology, 46,* 932–946.

Schmelz, J. O., Bridges, E. J., Duong, D. N., & Ley, C. (2003). Care of the critically ill patient in a military unique environment: A program of research. *Critical Care Nursing Clinics of North America, 15,* 171–181.

Scollan-Koliopoulos, M., & Koliopoulos, J. S. (2010). Evaluation and management of apparent life-threatening events in infants. *Pediatric Nursing, 36*(2), 77–78.

Scott, D. W., Oberst, M., & Dropkin, M. (1980). A stress coping model. *Advances in Nursing Science, 3,* 9–23.

Selye, H. (1950). Forty years of stress research: Principal remaining problems and misconceptions. *Canadian Medical Association Journal, 115,* 53–55.

Selye, H. (1956). *The stress of life.* New York, NY: McGraw-Hill.

Selye, H. (1993). History of the stress concept. In L. Goldberger & S. Breznitz (Eds.), *Handbook of stress: Theoretical and clinical aspects.* New York, NY: Free Press.

Selye, H. (1998). A syndrome produced by diverse nocuous agents. *The Journal of Neuropsychiatry and Clinical Neurosciences, 10*(2), 230–231.

Skalski, C., DiGerolamo, L., & Gigliotti, E. (2006). Stressors in five client populations—Neuman's systems model. *Journal of Advanced Nursing, 56*(1), 69–78.

Stokes, S. A., & Gordon, S. E. (1988). Development of an instrument to measure stress in the older adult. *Nursing Research, 37,* 16–19.

Stokes, S. A. & Gordon, S. E. (2003). Common stressors experienced by the well elderly: Clinical implications. *Journal of Gerontological Nursing, 29*(5), 25–29.

Stone, A. A., Reed, B. R., & Neale, J. M. (1987). Changes in daily event frequency precede episodes of physical symptoms. *Journal of Human Stress, 13,* 70–74.

Stowell, J. R., Hedges, D. W., Ghambaryan, A., Key, C., Bloch, G. J. (2009). Validation of the Symptoms of Illness Checklist (SIC) as a tool for health psychology research. *Journal of Health Psychology, 14,* 68–77.

Swanson, J. M., Dibble, S. L., & Chenitz, W. C. (1995). Clinical features and psychosocial factors in young adults with genital herpes. *Image: Journal of Nursing Scholarship, 27,* 16–22.

Swearingen, E. M., & Cohen, L. H. (1985). Life events and psychological distress: A prospective study of young adolescents. *Developmental Psychology, 21,* 1045–1054.

Tolor, A., Murphy, V., Wilson, L. T., & Clayton, J. (1983). The High School Readjustment Scale: An attempt to quantify stressful events in young people. *Research Communication in Psychology, Psychiatry, and Behavior, 8,* 85–111.

Towbes, L. C, Cohen, L. H., & Glyshaw, K. (1989). Instrumentality as a life-stress moderator for early versus middle adolescents. *Journal of Personality and Social Psychology, 57,* 109–119.

Travis, S. S., McAuley, W. J., Dmochowski, J., Bernard, M. A., Hsueh-Fen, S., Kao, H.-F. N., & Greene, R. (2007). Factors associated with medication hassles experienced by family caregivers of older adults. *Patient Education and Counseling, 66*(1), 51–57.

Turan, T., Başbakkal, Z., & Ozbek, S. (2008). Effect of nursing interventions on stressors of parents of premature infants in neonatal intensive care unit. *Journal of Clinical Nursing, 17,* 2856–2866.

Turner, R. J., & Wheaton, B. (1995). Checklist measurement of stressful life events. In S. Cohen, R. C. Kessler, & L. U. Gordon (Eds.), *Measuring stress: A guide for health and social scientists.* New York, NY: Oxford University Press.

Twisk, J. W., Snel, J., de Vente, W., Kemper, H. C., & van Mechelen W. (2000). Positive and negative life events: The relationship with coronary heart disease risk factors in young adults. *Journal of Psychosomatic Research, 49*(1), 35–42.

Ungar, L., & Floridan, V. (2004). What helps middle-aged widows with their psychological and social adaptation several years after their loss? *Death Studies, 28*(7), 621–641.

Unger, W. S., Gould, R. A., & Babich, M. (1998). The development of a scale to assess war-time atrocities: The War Events Scale. *Journal of Traumatic Stress, 11*(2), 375–383.

Van Pelt, D. C., Schultz, R., Chelluri, L., & Pinsky, M. R. (2010). Patient-specific, time-varying predictors of post-ICU informal caregiver burden: The caregiver outcomes after ICU discharge project. *CHEST, 137*(1), 88–94.

Volicer, B. J., & Bohannon, M. W. (1975). A hospital stress rating scale. *Nursing Research, 24*(5), 352–359.

Wagner, B. M., Compas, B. E., & Howell, D. C. (1988). Daily and major life events: A test of an integrative model of psychosocial stress. *American Journal of Community Psychology, 16*(2), 189–205.

Weinberger, M., Hiner, S. L., & Tierney, W. M. (1987). In support of hassles as a measure of stress in predicting health outcomes. *Journal of Behavioral Medicine, 10,* 19–31.

Weisaeth, L. (1993). Disasters: Psychological and psychiatric aspects. In L. Goldberger & S. Breznitz (Eds.), *Handbook of stress: Theoretical and clinical aspects.* New York, NY: Free Press.

Weisaeth, L. (2005). Stress at the societal and organizational level. In B. B. Arnetz & R. Ekman (Eds.), *Stress in health and disease* (pp. 69–90). Weinheim, Germany: Wiley-VCH.

Weitzel , M. L., & McCahon, C. P. (2008, March). Stressors and supports for baccalaureate nursing students completing an accelerated program. *Journal of Professional Nursing, 24*(2), 85–89.

Weller, L., & Avinir, O. (1993). Hassles, uplifts, and quality of sleep. *Perceptual and Motor Skills, 76,* 571–576.

Werner, J. S. (1993). Stressors and health outcomes: Synthesis of nursing research, 1980–1990. In J. S. Barnfather & B. L. Lyon (Eds.), *Stress and coping: State of the science and implications for nursing theory, research, and practice* (pp. 11–41). Indianapolis, IN: Sigma Theta Tau Center Nursing Press.

Werner, J. S. (1996). Stress: Nursing assessment and role in management. In S. M. Lewis, I. Collier, & M. Heitkemper (Eds.), *Medical surgical nursing: Assessment and management of clinical problems.* St. Louis, MO: C. V. Mosby.

Werner, J. S., Frost, M. H., & Orth, K. (2000). Stressors and health outcomes: Synthesis of nursing research, 1991–1995. In J. S. Werner & M. H. Frost (Eds.), *Stress and coping: State of the science and implications for nursing theory, research and practice, Volume II.* Glenview, IL: Midwest Nursing Research Society Press.

Werner, J. S., & O'Neill, S. E. (1992). Stress: Nursing assessment and role in management. In S. M. Lewis & I. Collier (Eds.), *Medical-surgical nursing: Assessment and management of clinical problems.* St. Louis, MO: C. V. Mosby.

Williams, R. A., Hagerty, B. M., Murphy-Weinberg, V., & Wan, J.-Y. (1995). Symptoms of depression among female nursing students. *Archives of Psychiatric Nursing, 9*(5), 269–278.

Williams, R., Zyzanski, S., & Wright, A. (1992). Life events and daily hassles and uplifts as predictors of hospitalization and outpatient visitation. *Social Science and Medicine, 34,* 63–68.

Winslow, B. W. (2003). Family caregivers' experiences with community services: A qualitative analysis. *Public Health Nursing, 20*(5), 341–348.

Wittchen, H., Essau, C. A., Hecht, H., Teder, W., & Pfister, H. (1989). Reliability of life event assessments: Test-retest reliability and fall-off effects of the Munich Interview for the Assessment of Life Events and Conditions. *Journal of Affective Disorders, 16,* 77–91.

Wolf, T. M., Elston, R. C., & Kissling, G. E. (1989, Spring). Relationship of hassles, uplifts, and life events to psychological well-being of freshman medical students. *Behavioral Medicine, 15*(1), 37–45.

Wolff, H. G., Wolff, S. G., & Hare, C. (Eds.). (1950). *Life stress and bodily disease.* Baltimore, MD: Williams & Wilkins.

Woods, N. F., Most, A., & Longenecker, G. D. (1985). Major life events, daily stressors, and perimenstrual symptoms. *Nursing Research, 34*(5), 263–267.

Yarcheski, T. J., Mahon, N. E., Yarcheski, A., Hanks, M. M. (2010). Perceived stress and wellness in early adolescents using the Neuman Systems Model. *Journal of School Nursing, 26*(3), 230–237.

Yeaworth, R., York, J., Hussey, M., Ingle, M., & Goodwin, T. (1980). The development of an adolescent life changes event scale. *Adolescence, 15,* 91–97.

Yeh, C. H. (2001). Adaptation in children with cancer: Research with Roy's model. *Nursing Science Quarterly, 14*(2), 141–148.

Zarski, J. J. (1984). Hassles and health: A replication. *Health Psychology, 3*(3), 243–251.

Zautra, A. J., & Reich, J. W. (1983). Life events and perceptions of life quality: Developments in a two-factor approach. *Journal of Community Psychology, 1,* 121–132.

Zhan, L. (2000). Cognitive adaptation and self-consistency in hearing-impaired older persons: Testing Roy's adaptation model. *Nursing science quarterly, 13*(2), 158–165.

7

STRESS AND BEHAVIOR

Coping via Information Technology

LINDA S. WEGLICKI AND NEVEEN FARAG AWAD

More than half a century has passed since Hans Selye (1956) first introduced the "general adaptation syndrome" and the concept of *stress*, a term referring to the "physiological reactions brought about by a broad range of environmental stimuli." Literally thousands of studies on the negative physical and mental health consequences of major and minor life events have been conducted subsequently. Since the late 1970s, stress theory has been elaborated to incorporate factors which moderate or buffer the effects of stress on physical and mental health. Each of these moderating factors—coping resources, coping strategies, and social support—now has its own thriving science. The emergence of the ability to adapt to stress and adversity is a central facet of human development. Successful adaptation to stress includes the ways in which individuals manage their emotions, think constructively, regulate and direct their behavior, control their autonomic arousal, and act on the social and nonsocial environments to alter or decrease sources of stress. These processes have all been included to varying degrees within the construct of coping (e.g., Compas, Conner-Smith, Saltzman, Thomsen, & Wadsworth, 2001).

Psychological Stress Theory (PST) (Lazarus, 1966; Lazarus & Folkman, 1984), a framework for studying psychological stress, holds that stress is contextual, meaning that it involves a transaction between the person and the environment, and it is a process, meaning that it changes over time.

Psychological stress, therefore, is a relationship between the person and the environment that is appraised by the person as taxing or exceeding his or her resources and endangering his or her well-being (Lazarus & Folkman, 1984, p. 21). (See Chapter 9 of this text for more details on this framework.)

Stress theory has been elaborated on to include factors that moderate or buffer the effects of stress on predominately mental and, to a lesser degree, physical health. Social support has been shown to buffer the relationship between life stress and psychological distress and physical health outcomes (see Chapter 14 of this text). However, little attention has been paid to the many personal variables that are associated with the capacity to effectively utilize information technology (e.g., social networks, e-health applications) as a form of social support to manage life stress(es).

With the advent of information systems (IS) and computer-mediated communication (CMC), individuals of all ages have access to an ever-widening network of supportive relationships through real-time online interaction. Whereas little research has addressed how people use network resources for social support and coping, preliminary research suggests that the interaction within these networks exhibits a variety of social support messages and behaviors (Sullivan, 1997), and they appear to be an outlet for older adult friendships (Furlong, 1989).

Computer information technology (CIT) and computer-mediated communications, including information systems, computerized behavioral programs (CBPs), social networks (SN), and e-health applications that help individuals improve or alter lifestyle behaviors, have the potential to play a very important role in stress, coping, social support, and physical and mental health outcomes. To be effective, however, as a coping strategy or a form of social support, CIT applications *must* build upon theoretical frameworks of technology acceptance, behavior, and stress adaptation. To date, an integrative theory that focuses on the constructs that affect the promotion of effective healthy coping behaviors when using CIT systems has not been espoused. The integration of stress and behavioral theory with information systems theory will aid nurses, nurse scientists, and health care practitioners to design and test theoretically driven studies that include real-time, state-of-the-art CIT applications to promote successful coping and healthy responses to stress.

The purpose of this chapter is to present a theoretical model, the Theory of Behavior and Stress: Coping via Information Technology (BS-CIT) that integrates and extends the Theory of Planned Behavior (TPB) (Ajzen, 1991), major concepts within the Stress and Coping Theory (SCT) (Lazarus & Cohen, 1977), and the Technology Acceptance Model (TAM) (Davis, 1989, 1993) into a novel framework for assessing the use of information technologies to mitigate stress and its effects, resulting in positive health outcomes. Theoretical model variables include factors that directly and indirectly affect intention to use, actual use, and the impact of technology-based, stress-reducing health interventions. (See Figure 7.1.)

The integration and extension of the TPB, TAM, and actual technology use (i.e., use of social networks) to promote coping with stress and health is appropriate at this time for a number of reasons: (1) both the TAM and TPB are the preferred frameworks relative to their major constructs of interest (technology acceptance and health behavior change, respectively); (2) the Theory of Behavior and Stress: Coping via Information Technology (BS-CIT) is a logical extension and integration as the TAM builds on elements of the TPB; (3) it is well recognized that there is a growing percentage of the population (including children and

adults of all ages) who embrace and use new and emerging forms of information technology; (4) the body of research using, supporting, and evaluating the efficacy and predictability of both the TPB and TAM is rich and therefore sufficient to make suggestions for refinement and revisions that advance their usefulness; and (5) there is a lack of theory surrounding how information technology can be used to affect stress, coping, and health behaviors.

This chapter is organized in three sections. Section 1 provides a brief overview of Stress and Coping Theory (SCT), the Theory of Planned Behavior (TPB), and the Technology Acceptance Model (TAM), respectively, which were used to derive the integrated Theory of Behavior and Stress: Coping via Information Technology (BS-CIT). Each foundational model and its major constructs are briefly described. Section 2 presents a review of the literature regarding the application of TAM to stress and coping and health behaviors. Finally, section 3 describes the derived BS-CIT model in detail, including the proposed theoretical assumptions, the major integrated model constructs, mediating factors, and their anticipated effects on technology use and health outcomes including healthy behaviors, stress adaptation, and coping.

Section 1. Stress and Coping Theory (SCT) and Lazarus's Psychological Stress Theory (PST)

Criticisms of Selye's general adaptation syndrome indicate that he did not specify mechanisms that may explain the cognitive transformation of "objective" noxious events into the subjective experience of being distressed, and he did not take into account coping mechanisms as important mediators of the stress–outcome relationship. Coupled with this argument is that the stress experienced by humans is almost always the result of cognitive mediation (Arnold 1960; Janis, 1958; Lazarus, 1966, 1982), which has led to more than 50 years of work on the development of psychological and transactional stress theories (e.g., Lazarus, 1966, 1991, 1998, 2000a, 2000b; Lazarus & Folkman, 1984; Lazarus & Launier, 1978).

Agreeing on a common definition of stress is difficult, even today. However, most theorists,

Figure 7.1 Theory of Behavior and Stress: Coping via Information Technology (BS-CIT)

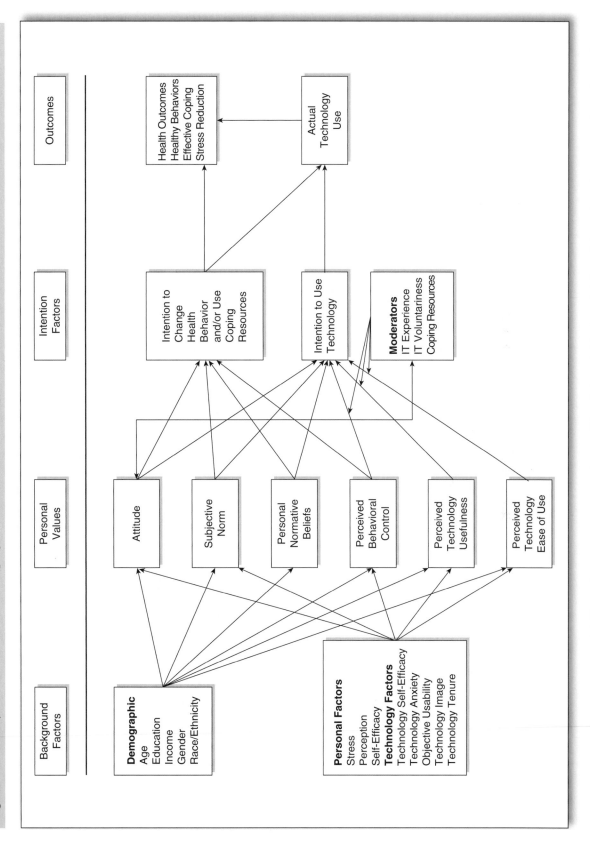

psychologists, and sociologists do agree that there is no singly acceptable definition of stress because it is a highly subjective phenomenon. It is well recognized that what is stressful for one person may be pleasurable or have little effect on others, resulting in wide variation in stress response. Central concepts to PST include appraisal (i.e., individuals' evaluation of the significance of what is happening for their well-being) and coping (i.e., individuals' efforts in thought and action to manage specific demands) (Lazarus, 1993).

Lazarus and Folkman (1984) identified two types of stress appraisal: primary (whether or not what is happening is relevant to one's values, goal commitments, beliefs, and situational intentions) and secondary (what can be done about a troubled person–environment interaction). Coping (as in process) is viewed as *"constantly changing cognitive and behavioral efforts to manage specific external and/or internal demands that are appraised as taxing or exceeding resources of the person"* (Lazarus & Folkman, 1984, p. 141). PST, as evolved by Lazarus and others, was modified to include the conjoining of stress and emotion and emotional states to social and physical conditions and what Lazarus describes as the transactional theory of emotion and coping (Lazarus & Folkman, 1987) and cognitive-motivational-relational theory of emotions (Lazarus, 1991, 2000b). PST and derivative theories of stress continue to guide studies focused on a wide variety of health conditions such as anxiety and depression, caregiving stress, the immune system, inflammation and aging, insomnia, and sleep deprivation.

The Theory of Planned Behavior (TPB)

The Theory of Planned Behavior (Ajzen, 1985, 1991), an extension of the Theory of Reasoned Action (TRA) (Ajzen & Fishbein, 1980), is a mid-level theory developed to explain and predict human behavior; it examines how "processing of available information mediates the effects of biological and environmental factors on behavior" (Ajzen, 1985, p. 179). The TPB hypothesized that attitude, subjective norms, and perceived behavioral control predict intention; and intention along with perceived behavioral control predicts and/or explains actual behavior. Intention, a central factor in performing a behavior, is assumed to capture the motivational factors that influence a

behavior. With regard to prediction of behavior, many studies have substantiated the predictive validity of behavioral intentions (Albarracín, Johnson, Fishbein, & Muellerleile, 2001; Blue, 1995; Godin & Kok, 1996). The TPB (Ajzen & Madden, 1986; Ajzen, 1988, 1991) is one of the most widely used health behavior theories used to understand both the determinants of health behaviors and the process of health behavior change (Ajzen, 2005; Armitage & Conner, 2001; Noar & Zimmerman, 2005).

Technology Acceptance Model (TAM)

Internet users, especially the young, spend a lot of time on the Internet to interact with others in order to communicate in social networking (e.g., MySpace, Facebook, or various blogs). To make efficient use of these new opportunities, the principles of user acceptance, behaviors, and adoptions must be analyzed. In this respect, existing user acceptance models may be adapted to extract recommendations, for example, for practitioners to build new models of how technology is used to aid in behavioral changes, and health behavioral changes more specifically. Understanding the conditions under which information systems are or are not accepted and used in health care and health promotion is important (Fogg, 2002). Among the different proposed models, the Technology Acceptance Model (TAM) (Davis, 1989; Davis, Bagozzi, & Warshaw, 1989) offers a powerful and parsimonious explanation for user acceptance and usage behavior. The TAM represents how individuals come to use and accept a given technology. TAM builds on Fishbein and Ajzen's (1975) Theory of Reasoned Action and Theory of Planned Behavior (Ajzen, 1985) in order to explain why individuals either accept or reject new technological systems.

Many applications and replications have established the robustness of TAM (Adams, Nelson, & Todd, 1992; Chin & Todd, 1995; Davis, 1989, 1993; Davis et al., 1989; Davis & Venkatesh, 1996; Gefen and Straub, 1997; Igbaria, Zinatelli, Cragg, & Cavaye, 1997; Mathieson, 1991; M. Morris & Dillon, 1997; Segars & Grover, 1993; Subramanian, 1994; Szajna, 1994, 1996; Taylor & Todd 1995b; Venkatesh, 1999; Venkatesh & Davis, 1996). Overall, the TAM has been empirically shown to successfully predict about 40% of a system's use (Ajzen & Fishbein, 1980; Hu, Chau,

Liu Sheng, & Tam, 1999). However, Legris, Ingham, and Collerette (2003) argue that while the TAM is a useful model for exploring information systems, it must be integrated into a broader and more innovative model that includes variables related to human and social change processes (such as relationships of people with technological interventions and their health behaviors); we attempt to address such integration through the introduction of the model of Behavior and Stress: Coping via Information Technology (BS-CIT).

There have been a number of proposed extensions to the TAM, further supporting its use as the predominant model of technology acceptance. For example, Gefen and Straub (2000) proposed that perceived usefulness (PU) and perceived ease of use (PEOU) directly affect intention to use and ignore the influence of the mediating variable, attitude toward using. Building on this, Venkatesh and Davis (2000) proposed a second version of the TAM, referred to as TAM2, which incorporates additional constructs, including subjective norms; we build on TAM2 and the TPB in our integrative model.

Section 2. TAM Applied to Health Care

The health care context remains an area of relatively minimal domain-specific examination of the technology acceptance model (TAM). The ability to understand the use and acceptance of technology in health care will facilitate implementation efforts and advancement of the use of new technologies to promote healthy behaviors (Al-Gahtani & King, 1999; Davis, 1989) and healthy responses to stress. Prior literature has examined TAM in the health care setting, primarily related to physicians' telemedicine technology (Chau & Hu, 2002a, 2002b; Hu et al., 1999). Few studies have applied TAM within nursing practice. The TAM was applied to examine public health nurses' intention toward web-based learning (Chen, Yang, Tang, & Huang, 2007) and nurses' intention of adopting an electronic logistics information system in Taiwan (Tung, Chang, & Chou, 2008). Limited studies have been conducted on the use of TAM in influencing health behaviors. Wilson and Lankton (2004) applied the TAM to e-health acceptance among a group

of middle-aged to elderly female medical patients; the results confirmed the significance of the main TAM constructs (PEOU and PU) on e-health acceptance. However, the results did not find support for the effect of intrinsic motivation on behavioral intentions; thus, the authors underscored the need for further model development in the context of acceptance of e-health technologies. According to Kukafka, Johnson, Linfante, and Allegrante (2003), interventions designed to improve the success of information technology (IT) have omitted two fundamental propositions: (1) IT usage is influenced by multiple factors and (2) interventions must be multidimensional. Kukafka and colleagues emphasized the need to move beyond the current dominant approach that employs a single model to examine factors associated with IT acceptance and subsequent positive use behavior. In addition, few of the prior studies included background factors, such as age, education, and online tenure, which have been shown to be relevant in the application of TAM (e.g., Gefen & Straub, 2002).

Thus, in presenting our model, we synthesized elements from the TPB, TAM, and TAM2, therefore following the recommendations of Kukafka et al. (2003). The mixed results across various prior studies underline the need for a rigorous and robust examination of the predictors of technology use in health care, and the introduction of a health behavior information technology model—it is this gap in the current literature that we aim to fill by proposing this integrated theory.

In addition, we aim to examine health behavior in the context of stress and coping as well as technology acceptance. Individuals cope with disruptions by using two key sub-processes that continuously influence each other (Lazarus, 1966; Lazarus & Folkman, 1984). First, individuals evaluate the potential consequences of an event (appraisal). They assess the nature of the particular event and its personal importance and relevance (primary appraisal). Second, individuals perform different actions to deal with the situation at hand (coping efforts). They rely on a combination of cognitive and behavioral efforts, both of which have been categorized as either problem- or emotion-focused (Folkman, 1992; Lazarus & Folkman, 1984). Problem-focused coping aims at managing the disruptive issue itself. It is oriented toward dealing with the specific aspects of the situation by changing the environment (e.g., altering or alleviating environmental pressures, barriers, resources, or procedures) or changing one's self (e.g., developing new standards of behavior, shifting levels of aspiration, finding new channels of gratification, and learning new skills or procedures) (Lazarus & Folkman, 1984).

Emotion-focused coping changes one's perception of the situation, but it does not alter the situation itself. It aims at regulating personal emotions and tensions, restoring or maintaining a sense of stability, and reducing emotional distress . The specific combination of problem- and emotion-focused coping efforts depends upon one's appraisals of a given situation (Lazarus & Folkman, 1984). The Theory of BS-CIT seeks to combine research on technology acceptance, health behavior, and stress and coping. This is accomplished by applying coping mechanisms (resources) as a moderating variable to the acceptance factors (personal values and intentions factors) and health outcome variables in the model.

Section 3. Behavior and Stress: Coping via Information Technology (BS-CIT)

The Theory of Behavior and Stress: Coping via Information Technology is a model designed to explore the use of IT and its impact on promoting health behaviors (e.g., activities undertaken to cope with stress and/or stressors) and effective coping and stress-reduction outcomes. The BS-CIT (Figure 7.1) proposes that background factors have an indirect effect on actual use of technology applications designed to influence health behaviors to reduce stress. The background factors (i.e., demographic, personal, and technology) directly affect personal values (i.e., attitude, subjective norm, personal normative beliefs, perceived behavioral control, perceived technology usefulness, and perceived technology ease of use). Personal values (technology- and nontechnology-related) directly affect intention factors (i.e., intention to change health behavior, intention to use coping resources, intention to use technology), and intention factors directly influence actual technology use and/or health outcomes. Moderating factors, including IT

experience and voluntariness, and coping resources were added to the model and are expected to moderate the relationship between technology-related personal values (e.g., perceived behavioral control, perceived technology usefulness, and perceived technology ease of use) and intention to use technology.

Research suggests that it is important to understand the antecedents of the key TAM constructs, perceived ease of use (PEOU) and perceived usefulness (PU) (Venkatesh & Davis, 1996), by examining the actual behavioral experience that may shape the evolution of beliefs such as PEOU (Doll & Ajzen, 1992; Davis et al., 1989; Fazio & Zanna, 1978a, 1978b, 1981; Venkatesh & Davis, 1996). Aligned with Venkatesh (2000), we integrate experience-based items, such as technology tenure, as factors affecting PEOU. We also extend Venkatesh's (2000) work by examining whether these factors also affect PU and other personal value constructs, such as subjective norms and attitudes that stem from the TPB (Ajzen, 1985). Thus, in extending and integrating the TPB and TAM for use in health behaviors, we examine antecedents of PEOU in the context of health outcomes (e.g., reduction in stress, effective coping) and include self-efficacy, perceived behavioral control, and emotion (technology anxiety). Self-efficacy has been shown to be a strong determinant of PEOU (Compeau & Higgins, 1995a, 1995b).

In accordance with Venkatesh (2000), emotion is conceptualized as computer anxiety. Control is an important factor, both in terms of technology acceptance and in terms of health behaviors and coping. Despite being a widely used construct in nursing and psychology, there is no single clear definition of the construct of control. While various researchers label and define control constructs differently (e.g., see locus of control [Rotter, 1966], health locus of control [B. S. Wallston & Wallston, 1981; K. A. Wallston, Wallston, & DeVellis, 1978], and personal control [Rodin, 1990]), in general, control is "one's perception of one's ability to alter a situation, response, or outcome" (Ruiz-Bueno, 2000, p. 461). According to Armitage and Conner (2001), "self-efficacy is more concerned with cognitive perceptions of control based on internal control factors, whereas perceived behavioral control (PBC) also reflects more general, external factors" (p. 476). This distinction between the concepts identifies the need to examine self-efficacy as well as PBC in relation to stress and coping in order to more fully understand their impact on behaviors, as we have in the BS-CIT model.

PEOU has been shown to be a determinant of attitude consistent with TPB (see Davis et al., 1989; Taylor & Todd, 1995a, 1995b), while internal and external control has been shown to relate to PBC in the TPB. In the BS-CIT model, we relate internal control (self-efficacy) to PEOU, thus departing from the basic framework of TPB and toward an updated framework, similarly used in prior work (Oliver & Bearden, 1985; Venkatesh, 2000; Venkatesh & Davis, 1996). Aligned with other prior literature, in the BS-CIT model we include both internal (self-efficacy) (de Vries, Dijkstra, & Kuhlman, 1988; McCaul, O'Neill, & Glasgow, 1988; Ronis & Kaiser, 1989; Terry, 1993; Wurtele, 1988) and external control (perceived behavioral control) (Kimieck, 1992; Schifter & Ajzen, 1985). In addition to prior literature, it will also include moderators for stress and coping.

BS-CIT Theory Assumptions

BS-CIT assumptions are presented in order to specify the type of context that is best suited for the applications of the model. The following assumptions show the unique contribution of the chapter in addressing a gap in the literature, and reflect behavioral science and information technology use perspectives:

1. Individuals engage in health-related behaviors that they are willing to change to promote quality of life.

2. Degree of willingness to change health behaviors varies according to background and personal value factors.

3. Degree of willingness to use information systems in response to stress/stressors varies according to background and personal value and technology factors.

4. Background factors directly influence personal values.

5. Background factors indirectly influence intentions and health practices and behaviors.

6. Background factors indirectly influence intentions and actual technology usage.

7. Background factors interact with coping mechanisms to influence personal values and indirectly influence health practice and behaviors.

8. Personal values directly influence intention behaviors and indirectly influence actual behavior, stress, and healthy coping outcomes.

9. Intention factors directly influence actual behaviors.

10. Moderating factors important to the relationship between personal value factors and intention factors will indirectly influence outcomes including actual technology use and health behavior changes; these include factors of stress and coping.

11. Within Stress and Coping Theory, contextual information is critical for a full appreciation of life events effects (stress).

The above assumptions emphasize the role of the individual in shaping, maintaining, or changing/adapting health behaviors by using information systems for modifying or adapting health behaviors (e.g., using IT technology to cope with stress/stressors) that can lead to an improved quality of life.

Background Factors for BS-CIT

Background factors of interest include demographic (i.e., age, education, income, gender, and race/ethnicity), personal (i.e., stress perception, stress appraisal, perceived behavioral control, and self-efficacy), and technologic (computer anxiety, objective usability, perceived enjoyment, technology experience, and user acceptance) factors and their indirect effects on intention to change health behavior, intention to use coping resources, intention to use technology, actual technology use, and health outcomes. Each of the constructs under demographic and personal background factors in the BS-CIT model will be described relative to health behaviors, stress, and to information technology use. Constructs of interest under technology factors will be described relative to information technology use.

Demographic Factors

Socio-demographic background characteristics such as age, gender, race/ethnicity, and culture have been identified as having powerful influences on an individual's ability to achieve and impact health outcomes (U.S. Department of Health & Human Services [USDHHS], 2010; http://www.healthypeople.gov/2020/about/DisparitiesAbout.aspx). However, the relationship between socioeconomic and demographic factors and health behaviors/outcomes is not well established. With respect to background factors and information technology use, researchers have found that computer and Internet use, and, thus information systems, are related to age, gender, education, income, technology tenure, and race (Awad & Krishnan, 2006; Hoffman, Kalsbeek, & Novak, 1996) and that the demographics of use have remained fairly consistent since 2002 (Rainie, 2005).

However, the degree to which such factors impact the use of information systems for coping with stress and fostering health has gone unexplored. Therefore, constructs under demographic background (i.e., age, education, gender, income, and race/ethnicity) are included in the BS-CIT organizing framework in order to sufficiently determine the predictive accuracy of the theory, including all internal and external factors important to determine a given behavior (Ajzen, 1991). We briefly discuss each of these factors individually.

Age. Numerous reasons for the age differences in life span have been debated over the years. Some of the most commonly cited reasons include genetic makeup, nutrition, sanitation, education, the interactions between genes and the environment (Duff et al., 2006; Westendorp, 2006), medical and technological advances and decreases in the proportion of the community-dwelling population (Crimmins, Ingegneri, & Saito, 1997), and lifestyle behaviors (Duff et al., 2006) that often result in increased rates of disease and disability such as obesity (Olshansky et al., 2005; Preston, 2005), and the numerous health consequences associated with smoking (Office of the Surgeon General, 2010). From a theory-based perspective, it is important to more fully understand the relationship between age and lifestyle behaviors.

Age has been shown to moderate all of the key relationships in the TAM (Venkatesh & Bala, 2008). Age was identified as one of four key moderating variables for the TAM in addition to experience, voluntariness, and gender (Venkatesh, Morris, Davis, & Davis, 2003). Both gender and age differences have been reported in technology acceptance contexts (Morris & Venkatesh, 2000; Venkatesh & Morris, 2000; Venkatesh et al., 2003). Levy (1988) suggests that studies of gender differences can be misleading without reference to age. Accordingly, Venkatesh et al. (2003) illustrated that the TAM is moderated by gender and age. As a first step in understanding this complex relationship, age, as a background factor, is expected to have an indirect effect on influencing health outcomes that may be impacted by CIT designed to cope with stressful situations.

Education. Education is often identified when addressing causes of health disparities in the United States; it is generally recognized that individuals and populations with the unhealthiest behaviors have the least education and lowest incomes (Robert Wood Johnson Foundation [RWJF] Commission to Build a Healthier America, 2009; USDHHS, 2000, http://www.healthypeople.gov/2010/About/). Higher levels of education are generally associated with beliefs in health prevention and the ability to understand health-related information necessary to practice health-promoting behaviors (RWJF Commission to Build a Healthier America, 2009). In addition, lower levels of education have been associated with higher tobacco use rates, higher rates and percentages of overweight/obesity, lower rates of successful smoking cessation (American Cancer Society [ACS], 2006; Office of the Surgeon General, 2010) and weight loss (Molarius, Seidell, Sans, Tuomilehto, & Kuulasmaa, 2000), and more difficulty in dealing with stress-related events (Grzuwacz, Almeida, Neupert, & Ettner, 2004). Education has been identified as a factor in one's ability to process information (Schmidt & Spreng, 1996).

Along this same vein, previous research indicates that individuals with more advanced education gather information from a greater number of sources (including both technology-mediated sources and offline sources such magazines, friends, store visits, etc.) (Klein & Ford, 2003). As education and income are viewed as being intrinsically related and therefore often serve as proxy measures for one another, both are included as personal background factors. We expect that education will be associated with information processing and will affect an individual's attitude toward, and use of, a health technology intervention to promote healthy behaviors and outcomes such as successful coping.

Income. Differences in socioeconomic status (SES) have consistently been associated with health disparities; as with education, income inequities have been associated with differences in disease and death including heart disease, chronic respiratory disorders, diabetes, obesity, cancers, and others (ACS, 2006; CDC, 2004, 2006). Those with lower incomes generally have less access to medical care and are less likely to engage in health-promoting behaviors such as exercise, eating healthy foods, avoiding tobacco use, and following recommended cancer screening; this behavior pattern often leads to increased stress (RWJF Commission to Build a Healthier America, 2009) and shorter life spans.

From the technology perspective, income has not been shown to have a significant impact on time spent in online social networks, such as Facebook (Ellison, Steinfeld, & Lampe, 2007). The main area where income has an affect is in regard to stress and health disparities. Thus, we expect income/SES will directly affect an individual's personal values and therefore indirectly affect actual use of a health-directed (or stress reduction) technology intervention.

Gender. It is well known that gender differences exist in rates of unhealthy and high-risk behaviors and resulting morbidity and mortality. For example, cigarette smoking, the single largest preventable cause of disease and premature death in the United States, is higher among adult men (22.3%) than adult women (17.4%) (American Thoracic Society, 2010), resulting in more than 443,000 U.S. deaths per year (Office of the Surgeon General, 2010). This and other examples of gender-based health disparities can be modified by changing health behaviors and adopting healthier lifestyles. While it is not currently known if participation in creative intervention programs—such as programs using information technology—can effectively modify and alter lifestyle behaviors or reduce the stress associated with those behaviors, it is this question we attempt to address with the BS-CIT Model. Research suggests that technology use is related to gender. For example, men are more likely than women to use the Internet (Fox & Jones, 2009). However, more women (64%) than men (57%) use the Internet for

health information (Fox & Jones, 2009). Davis's original TAM (1989) as well as subsequent work using the model make no reference to gender influences in IT acceptance models or IT diffusion processes. Gefen and Straub (1997) suggested, based on their exploratory study of gender differences in the perception of e-mail, that gender "has a measurable, indirect effect on e-mail usage" (p. 397). Gender differences have also been found to impact perception of a technology's usefulness as well as technology use anxiety (Gilroy & Desai, 1986). According to gender schema theory, such differences stem from socialization processes reinforced from birth rather than biological differences (Bem, 1981; Bem & Allen, 1974; Kirchmeyer, 1997; Lubinski, Tellegen, & Butcher, 1983; Motowidlo, 1982). Thus, we expect that gender will have a direct effect on personal values and therefore an indirect effect on actual use of a technology-based health/stress-reduction intervention.

Race/Ethnicity/Culture. Race, ethnicity, and cultural factors have historically been viewed as critical factors in determining health status, healthy behaviors, health-seeking behaviors, and the quality of care one receives (CDC, 2004; Williams, 1994). While it is well known that minority groups are disproportionately represented in low socioeconomic strata in the United States, less recognized is that at most levels of SES, morbidity and mortality rates are higher for Blacks than for Whites (Office of Behavioral and Social Science Research [OBSSR], n.d.). Evidence suggests that the reasons for these disparities are complex (RWJF Commission to Build a Healthier America, 2009; USDHHS, 2010). In addition, minority groups have higher rates of infant mortality, heart disease, death from certain cancers (e.g., prostate and breast), and HIV/AIDS and are more likely to die from diabetes and have higher rates of hypertension and obesity than White non-Hispanics (CDC, 2006).

Despite the Healthy People 2010 objectives and forecasts, Levine et al. (2001) found no "sustained decrease in black-white disparities" in life expectancy or age-adjusted mortality, based on historical and estimated data from the National Center for Health Statistics and U.S. Census Bureau since the mid 1940s. If ethnic group differences in health are not simply attributable to socioeconomic status, then research is needed to understand race/ethnicity and health behaviors and the role of technology-based health interventions in this relationship. A clear understanding of the impact of the ethnicity on information systems usage does not exist. Nor has technology use been studied in relation to stress and coping; as such we propose to examine this relationship within BS-CIT. We expect that race/ethnicity will have a direct effect on personal values and an indirect effect on actual use of technology-based health interventions.

Personal Factors

Personal factors including stress perception, stress appraisal, and self efficacy are generally considered modifiable and have been shown to have a direct effect on health values and an indirect effect on health and healthy behaviors. The impact of personal factors on personal values, intention factors, and actual technology use and its influence on health outcomes (e.g., stress reduction, effective coping, and healthy behaviors) are described below.

Stress Perception. Within the transactional model of stress and coping, stressors are demands of an individual's internal or external environment that upset balance, thereby affecting physical and psychological well-being and requiring action to restore balance (Lazarus & Cohen, 1977). The individual's perception of stress is dependent on the meaning of the stimulus within the person–environment transaction that is evaluated within processes of the individual's coping ability (e.g., resources and options) (Antonovsky, 1979; Cohen, 1984; Lazarus, 1996).

Coping efforts are aimed at regulating the stress/stressor which is mediated via primary and secondary appraisal processes in order to improve functional status, emotional well-being, and healthy behaviors. They can change over time due to coping effectiveness, altered requirements, or improvements in personal abilities. According to Ajzen (1991), one's beliefs and evaluations of those beliefs (perception of stress) affect attitude toward the behavior. Thus, we expect that stress perception will have a direct effect on personal values and therefore an indirect effect on actual use of technology-based health and coping interventions, resulting in positive health outcomes.

Behavioral Self-Efficacy (BSE). Self-efficacy (SE), first identified in Bandura's Social Cognitive Theory (SCT), is one of the most powerful predictors of health behavior (Bandura, 1997). According to Bandura, those with a strong sense of SE are believed to develop strong intentions to act, to expend more effort to achieve their goals, and to persist longer when faced with barriers, obstacles, and stress (Bandura, 1988). Perceived SE (also called self-determination) is therefore believed to play a central role in the determination of health behavior. Self-efficacy has also been viewed as a "notion conceptually related to perceived behavioral control (PBC)" (Godin & Kok, 1996, p. 88). Ajzen (1991) argued that self-efficacy and PBC constructs were synonymous. Others have argued against using the terms interchangeably (Bandura, 1992; de Vries et al., 1988; Terry, 1993) and have reported differences in direct versus indirect effects of the two constructs on behavior (Dzewaltowski, Noble, & Shaw, 1990) and intentions (White, Terry, & Hogg, 1994). Several researchers reported SE predicted intentions, while PBC predicted behavior (Terry & O'Leary, 1995; White et al., 1994). These studies provide support for distinction between the two constructs, SE and PBC, and the need to study their individual effects on behavior. Research underscores the influential role of perceived control in stress reactions (Lazarus & Folkman, 1984). Being able to exercise control over stressors can diminish stress (stress reduction) by instilling and strengthening beliefs about one's coping efficacy. According to Bandura (1988), cognitive changes serve as proximal determinants of stress reaction and level of stress during encounters with stressors. Therefore, we include the addition of the construct of behavioral self-efficacy and expect that it will have a direct effect on personal values and an indirect effect on use of technology-based interventions.

Technology Factors

Access. Access to health information continues to be revolutionized by advances in IT, particularly health information via the World Wide Web and the Internet. Estimates suggest that more than half (Horringan & Rainie, 2002) and as much as 80% of adults (Taylor, 2003) with Internet access use it for health care purposes (Baker, Todd, Wagner, & Bundorf, 2003). According to the Pew Report Health Information Online (Fox, 2005),

95 million American adults (18+) use the Internet to find health information. The Internet can be a powerful tool by which individuals obtain health-promoting information about an illness, treatment options, and programs designed to promote sustainable personal healthy behaviors. Individuals can select information that is most relevant to their needs and lifestyle. The percentage of those interested in health information varies by age and gender (race, ethnicity, and cultural influence were not reported). Therefore, the BS-CIT encompasses attention to the development of age-related health behavior interventions designed to promote healthy behavioral change and a healthy lifestyle.

Technology Self-Efficacy. Internal control is conceptualized as technology self-efficacy in the context of technology acceptance. Internal control represents one's belief about her or his ability to perform a specific task using a computer (Compeau & Higgins, 1995a, 1995b; Venkatesh, 2000). Prior experimental evidence supporting the causal flow from computer self-efficacy to system-specific PEOU has been established (Venkatesh & Davis, 1996). In this chapter we expand the construct of computer self-efficacy to technology self-efficacy. Thus, we expect that technology self-efficacy will affect PEOU (Venkatesh & Davis, 1996). It is clear that self-efficacy is an important construct of influence for both health behaviors as well as technology, thus one of the unique contributions of the BS-CIT Model is the inclusion of efficacy as two unique background factors (technology self-efficacy and self-efficacy), each of which has a direct effect on personal values and an indirect effect on use of technology-based health applications.

Technology Anxiety. Technology anxiety is defined as an individual's apprehension, or even fear, when she or he is faced with the possibility of using technology (Simonson, Maaurer, Montag-Torard, & Whitaker, 1987). Technology anxiety, like technology self-efficacy, relates to users' general perceptions about technology use. While technology self-efficacy relates to judgments about ability, technology anxiety is a negative affective reaction toward technology use. Researchers have used the construct of technology anxiety to capture the emotional aspect of technology usage (Venkatesh, 2000) and found stress related to

system use had a negative influence on the PEOU of a new system. Technology anxiety has also been shown to have a significant impact on attitudes (Howard & Smith, 1986; Igbaria & Chakrabarti, 1990; Igbaria & Parasuraman, 1989; Morrow, Prell, & McElroy, 1986; Parasuraman & Igbaria 1990), intention (Elasmar & Carter, 1996), behavior (Compeau & Higgins, 1995a; Scott & Rockwell, 1997; Todman & Monaghan, 1994), learning (Liebert & Morris, 1967; Martocchio, 1994; Morris Davis, & Hutchings, 1981), performance (Anderson, 1996; Heinssen, Glass, & Knight, 1987), and perceived ease of use (Venkatesh, 2000). Thus, we include technology anxiety as a determinant of personal values and expect it to have an indirect effect on use of technology-based health and stress and coping interventions.

Objective Usability. Objective usability assesses the usability of the system over time; it is a construct that allows for a comparison of systems based on the actual level (rather than perceived level) of effort required to complete specific tasks (Venkatesh, 2000). Objective usability was first defined and operationalized in conjunction with the TAM (Venkatesh & Davis, 1996) and is consistent with the conceptualization of objective usability in human-computer interaction research (Card, Moran, & Newell, 1983). The idea behind objective usability is that direct behavioral experience can shape system-specific PEOU over time (Doll & Ajzen, 1992; Fazio & Zanna, 1978a, 1978b, 1981).

For example, an individual may exhibit low computer self-efficacy, high computer anxiety, and high stress initially; however, with increasing direct experience with the target system, she or he is expected to cope with the system partly depending on the extent to which the system is easy to use from an objective standpoint. Therefore, because most responses to stress and adaptive coping resulting in healthy outcomes may involve multiple resources for the change to occur and be sustainable, we expect that objective usability will directly affect personal values relative to the technology over time, and thus will indirectly affect use of technology-based health interventions.

Technology Image. Technology image was initially defined by Moore and Benbasat, (1991) as "the degree to which use of an innovation is perceived to enhance one's image or one's status or social symbol" (p. 137). In this case, the innovation that we are examining is technology-based health information as accessed through social network sites. Individuals have been shown to respond to social norms to establish or maintain a favorable image within a reference group, such as their peer group or colleague cohort (Kelman, 1958). In addition, individuals often turn to social network sites for stress and coping, but still work to balance their ability to cope with their desire to maintain a positive image (Ellison et al., 2007). Thus, we expect that image will have a direct effect on personal values, and therefore an indirect effect on the use of a technology-based health intervention.

Technology Tenure. Experience within a given technological medium, for example the online medium, has been shown to affect behavior. For example, Brucks (1985) found that online novices search the least out of all users, as they do not understand the nuances of the online environment and therefore they oversimplify. In a similar vein, higher general knowledge of a domain has been shown to affect consumer behavior by enabling users to assimilate greater amounts of domain-specific information (Punj & Staelin, 1983). Thus, we expect that technology tenure will have a direct effect on personal values and an indirect effect on actual use of a technology-based health intervention. However, little to no research has explored technology tenure and its impact on stress and coping. As technological mediums are constantly changing and emerging, we believe this to be an important variable within the model.

Personal Values

Personal value factors are the elements that contribute to people adopting technology in order to change their health behaviors, use coping resources, and use technology. BS-CIT personal value constructs were adapted from the TPB, the TAM, as well as various extensions of the two models. As within these theories, these constructs are believed to have a direct effect on intention to change health behavior and intention to accept a technology-based intervention. However, within the BS-CIT, personal values and intentions are moderated by technology factors (e.g., experience and voluntariness) described below.

Attitude. Within the TPB, attitude is conceptualized as a multidimensional construct consisting of cognition, affect, and cognitive responses (Ajzen, 1985). The cognition portion of attitude reflects an individual's information about and perceptions of a particular attitude (e.g., attitude object is smoking cessation behavior); affective responses are feelings toward the object; and cognitive responses are concerned with behavioral inclinations and commitments (Ajzen, 2001). Attitude toward a behavior is an expression of a person's positive or negative evaluation of performing a behavior. Recent work suggests that people often hold dual attitudes toward objects, such as "one attitude of implicit or habitual, the other explicit" (Ajzen, 2001, p. 39); an in-depth discussion of dual attitudes can be found in Wilson, Lindsey, & Schooler (2000). Attitude is therefore believed to be a product resulting from behavioral beliefs as well as the outcome evaluation of performing the behavior. In the BS-CIT, attitude is expected to directly affect intention to change a health behavior as well as intention to use technology-based interventions and indirectly affect actual behavior change.

Subjective Norm. Consistent with the TRA, subjective norm is defined as a "person's perception that most people who are important to him think he should or should not perform the behavior in question" (Fishbein & Ajzen, 1975, p. 302). Venkatesh and Davis (2000) extended the TAM to include the construct of subjective norm. Subjective norm is included as a direct determinant of intention to use technology (Venkatesh & Davis, 2000). We theorize that subjective norm directly affects intention to change health behavior and intention to use technology and indirectly affects actual use and actual health behavioral change.

Personal Normative Beliefs. The construct and conceptualization of personal normative beliefs (PNB) have undergone revision since first operationalized by Fishbein (1967). Schwartz and Tessler (1972) argued for the inclusion of the construct and emphasized PNB to be the moral obligation to perform an act, which according to Ajzen (1985) is influenced by the likelihood that important others would approve or disapprove of a particular behavior. Both Schwartz and Tessler (1972) and Ajzen and Fishbein (1969) found that PNBs made consistent and substantial contributions to the explanation of variance in intentions. Schwartz and Tessler (1972) amended the operationalization of the PNB construct, which resulted in an independent impact of PNB on intention. Personal normative beliefs and attitude toward the act/behavior have been shown to be predictors of intentions. Social support may also be necessary (Schwartz & Tessler, 1972), but the literature remains in debate regarding the relative significance of social support in comparison to attitude and personal normative beliefs. To address this debate, we include social support in the BS-CIT model. Within BS-CIT, we theorize that personal normative beliefs directly affect intention to change health behavior and intention to use technology and indirectly affect actual use and actual health behavioral change.

Perceived Behavioral Control. Perceived behavioral control (PBC) reflects a person's beliefs as to how easy or difficult it will be to perform the behavior. In the TPB, important beliefs determine the intention and actions of a person (Ajzen, 1991) and are antecedents to PBC. Control beliefs may be influenced by past behavior and also by information about the behavior received from family, friends, the media, and other sources that impact the perceived difficulty in performing the specific behavior (e.g., smoking, overeating, poor food choices). Control beliefs reflect a balance between the resources and opportunities a person believes they possess, along with barriers that impede the behavior or deal with stress/stressors. PBC has an indirect effect on the behavior depending on the type of behavior and the nature of the situation (Armitage & Conner, 2001; Blue, 1995). Perceived control is a robust predictor of a person's behavior, motivation, performance, and emotion (Skinner, 1995) and can predict success or failure in very diverse domains, ranging from changing one's health behaviors (e.g., successfully quitting smoking or effectively using coping resources) to ability to use various types of information technology (e.g., cell phones, personal assistants [PDAs], computers, and electronic games). Ajzen (1991) argued that the addition of PBC and ability to measure it improves the predictive accuracy when behaviors not under volitional control (e.g., unexpected and multiple stressors,

addictive behaviors such as smoking and drug use) are studied. We therefore theorize that PBC directly affects intention to change health behavior, use coping resources, and intention to use technology, and indirectly affects actual use and health outcomes.

Perceived Technology Usefulness. TAM highlights two important antecedent dimensions of IT use. The first dimension, perceived usefulness (PU), is the degree to which "people tend to use or not use an application to the extent they believe it will help them perform" (Davis, 1989, p. 320) or is useful in dealing with stressful situations. PU was found to have a significant influence upon system utilization because of a user's belief in the existence of a use–performance relationship. Davis argues that the theoretical foundations for PU, as a predictor of usage behavior, are derived from several diverse research streams, including self-efficacy theory, cost-benefit paradigm, and adoption of innovations research. Hu et al. (1999) utilized TAM in medical-related research and confirmed that PU is an important factor that impacts the adoption of telemedicine technology by physicians for the completion of work-related tasks. We theorize that perceived technology usefulness directly affects intention to use technology, intention to change health behavior, intention to use coping resources, and indirectly affects actual technology use and health outcomes.

Perceived Technology Ease of Use. The second antecedent dimension to IT use, perceived ease of use (PEOU), is defined as "the degree to which a person believes that using a particular system would be free of effort" (Davis, 1989, p. 320) and cognitive burden (Davis, 1989; Davis & Venkatesh, 1996, 2004; Lederer, Manupin, Sena, & Zhuang, 2000; Szajna, 1996). Research shows that individuals are more likely to interact with new technologies if they perceive that relatively little cognitive effort will be expended during the interaction (Adams et al., 1992). PEOU represents an intrinsically motivating aspect of human–computer interactions (Davis, 1989) that changes over time as the user gradually learns the process (Davis & Venkatesh, 2004). PEOU is posited to influence behavioral intentions to use IT through two causal pathways: a direct effect as well as an indirect effect through perceived usefulness. The latter relationship is supported by the notion that to the extent the lower cognitive burden imposed by a technology frees up attention resources to focus on other matters, it serves the instrumental ends of a user (Davis et al., 1989). Thus, we theorize that perceived technology ease of use directly affects intention to use technology, intention to change health behavior and use coping resources, and indirectly affects actual technology use and intention to change health behavior and use coping resources through PU. In addition, perceived technology ease of use indirectly affects actual use and health outcomes.

Moderating Factors

Several factors have been previously presented as moderating factors of the TAM, including technology experience and voluntariness (Venkatesh & Davis, 2000). Likewise, coping resources have been identified as a key moderating factor important in both SRT as well as the TPB. For purposes of this chapter, coping resources will be described as social support. These constructs modify the relationship between the personal value factors (e.g., perceived behavioral control, perceived technology usefulness, perceived technology ease of use, and attitude) and the intention factors in the BS-CIT model.

Technology Experience. Over repeated interactions with a given information system, the impact of various factors on use, such as PEOU and subjective norm, on PU and intention to use, can change over time (Karahanna, Straub, & Chervany, 1999). Karahanna et al. (1999) found that the personal values factor of attitude was more important with increasing experience, while subjective norm became less important with increased experience. In addition, Davis et al. (1989) and Szajna (1996) provided empirical evidence that PEOU becomes decreasingly significant with increased experience. In addition, PU, attitude toward behavior, and PBC were all found to be more salient with increasing experience, whereas subjective norm was found to be less salient with increasing experience (Taylor & Todd, 1995a, 1995b). We include all three linkages between PEOU and PU in accordance with the original TAM (Davis et al., 1989). However, because health technology interventions generally occur over time or are used repeatedly over time, we incorporate Szajna's (1996) revision

suggesting that pre-implementation (e.g., brief introduction to information system), both PU and PEOU, directly affects intention to use technology. Moreover, regarding post-implementation (i.e., after the system has been used more than once), we theorize that PU will directly impact intention to use technology, whereas PEOU will indirectly affect intention to use technology through PU. Thus, the BS-CIT model includes experience as a moderating variable between the background factors and the personal values factors, as well as between some of the personal value factors.

IT Voluntariness. Voluntariness is defined as "the extent to which potential adopters perceive their adoption decision to be non-mandated" (Agarwal & Prasad, 1997, p. 564). Perceived voluntariness was first proposed as influential in the context of acceptance behavior by Moore and Benbasat (1991) and was confirmed as a significant moderating variable in regard to technology acceptance, along with experience, gender, and age, by Venkatesh et al. (2003). They found that in settings where the use of the technology was mandatory, constructs related to social influence were significant, whereas in voluntary settings constructs related to social influence were not significant (Venkatesh et al., 2003). Thus, voluntariness is included as a moderating variable between the personal value factors and the intention factors in the BS-CIT model.

Coping Resources (Social Support)

Social support has been positively linked to healthy behaviors (e.g., Watkins & Kligman, 1993; Weinert & Burman, 1994) and moderation of life stress (Cobb, 1976); lack of social support has been equated with increased illness and decreased participation in healthy activities (Svanborg, 1990). The association between social support and stress has a long-standing history among theorists. Empirical investigations from these theories revealed the relationship between the two constructs is complex; this is due to both positive and negative effects of social support within the stress-response process. For example, social support has been found to assist individuals to cope with stress; on the other hand, social support has been found to be a source of stress. However, in general, social support is believed to aid individuals in coping with stress (Antonucci & Akiyama, 1987; 2000). Having support systems becomes increasingly important for older adults whose personal and support resources often diminish with aging. In addition, personal well-being was found to be related to the quality of the support relationships (Beckerman & Northrop, 1996). Dean (1992) suggested that age, rather than having direct influence, is significantly related to social and psychosocial variables that directly impact behavior and health. Within the BS-CIT, social support is expected to directly affect intention to change health behavior and intention to use technology, and indirectly affect the actual use of technology-based interventions designed to modify or change health-promoting behaviors.

Intention Factors

Intentions, a central factor in performing a behavior (Ajzen, 1985, 1991), are assumed to capture the motivational factors that influence a behavior—or indications of how hard or how much effort a person is willing to try or exert in performing a health behavior or using coping resources to reduce stress.

Intention to Change Health Behavior. Since the introduction of the TPB in the 1980s, there has been increasing attention to the relationship between intentions and behavior. A number of studies have substantiated the predictive validity of behavioral intentions (e.g., Albarracín et al., 2001; Godin, Valois, Lepage, & Desharnais, 1992; Sheeran & Orbell, 1998). According to Ajzen (2005), when attitude toward a behavior, subjective norm, and perception of behavioral control are combined, this leads to behavioral intention. Generally, the more favorable one's attitude, subjective norm, and PBC, the greater the likelihood of the person's intention to perform a given behavior. Within the BS-CIT framework, intention to change health behavior is therefore an antecedent to health behavior change(s). Studies on implementation and intention show that helping people to make plans to behave in a certain way can improve the intention–behavior link. However, according to Goh (2006), intentions may be overruled by habits. Behaviors become habitual when performed frequently and when performed in a stable environment. Under conditions where habits conflict with intentions, intentions become poor predictors of behavior. It is possible, however, to break bad habits by replacing a habitual sequence with an alternatively more healthful sequence, which can be supported by e-health applications and interventions. Thus overall, we expect intention to change health behavior to be a significant predictor of participating in a technology health intervention in the absence of conflicting habits.

Intention to Use Coping Resources. After individuals determine (appraise) a situation as irrelevant, benign-positive, or stressful (and further as harm or loss, threat, or challenging) they next appraise coping resources to manage the stress/stressor. Individuals draw upon three kinds of coping: problem-focused (planful problem solving), emotion-focused (used to regulate negative emotion), and meaning-focused (regulates positive emotions) (Folkman, 2010). According to Folkman (2010), the three types of coping represent a "dynamic system of processes that are highly interactive" (p. 902). Coping resources vary individually, at a point in time, and from stressor to stressor. For example, a newly diagnosed cancer patient may benefit from personal social support provided directly from a family member or friend initially following diagnosis in order seek emotional support and/or distance themselves from the diagnosis (a coping resource aiding emotion-focused coping). Later that same individual may turn to various forms of information technology (such as the Internet or social networks) or health care professionals for information to aid in treatment decision making (a coping resource for problem-solving coping). Little research has examined the factors individuals use in selecting coping resources for different stressful situations; nor is there research examining actual intention to use coping resources (either singularly or collectively). Therefore, in order to fill this gap, intention to use coping resources following appraisal of stress/stressor and various coping resources will be examined in the BS-CIT model.

Intention to Use Technology. Intention to use technology measures how users intend to use a system. According to TAM it is the function of PU and PEOU. Intention to use technology can be used to measure users' attitude of acceptance or rejection of a system (Gefen & Straub, 1997;

Legris et al., 2003; Venkatesh, 2000; Venkatesh & Davis, 2000). As previously identified, the TAM has been shown to be robust and parsimonious and typically explains 40% of usage intentions and 30% of usage behavior (Hu et al., 1999; Venkatesh & Davis, 2000). Other studies compared the benefits of TAM and TPB in different research scenarios and urged more theoretical models (Mathieson, 1991). Taylor and Todd (1995a, 1995b) integrated TAM and TPB and established a decomposed TPB. The decomposed model incorporated additional factors such as the personal value factor, perceived behavioral control, and experience; these were shown to be important determinants of behavior. The decomposed TPB elaborated TAM and provided a more complete understanding of usage.

The BS-CIT model further decomposes and integrates TPB and TAM specific to the context of adoption of technology-based health interventions. There is limited research examining intention to use technology relative to stress and coping. Two studies were found that examined teenagers' intention to use online social networks (Baker & White, 2010; Livingston, 2008) for stress and coping (Livingston, 2008) and to test the validity of an extended theory of planned behavior model, incorporating the additions of group norm and self-esteem influences, to predict frequent social networking skills (SNS) use (Baker & White, 2010). Given the limited work in this area, we propose inclusion of intention to use the technology-based health intervention, intention to change health behaviors, and to use coping resources as antecedents of actual technology usage and health outcomes.

Actual Technology Use

Few studies have captured the actual usage of information systems and technology (Devaraj & Kohli, 2003). The comparability of self-reported usage and objective or actual usage remains a controversial point in IS research (Straub, Limayem, & Karahanna-Evaristo, 1995; Venkatesh & Davis, 2000). The actual usage of an information system is represented by the total number of times a person accesses a technology-based coping and/or health intervention, the time the user spends using the intervention, and depth of usage of the user. The BS-CIT model theorizes a direct link from actual technology usage to actual coping and positive health outcomes.

Health Outcomes

According to Glanz, Rimer, and Lewis (2002), in the broadest sense, "health behaviors are the actions of individuals, groups, and organizations . . . to improve coping skills, and enhance quality of life" (p. 10). Gochman (1982) further defined health behavior as "personal attributes such as beliefs, expectations, motives, values, perceptions, and other cognitive elements; personality characteristics; . . . and overt behavior patterns, actions, and habits that relate to health maintenance, to health restoration, and to health improvement" (p. 169). In other words, health behaviors are the actions expressed by individuals to protect, maintain, or promote their health status. Behavioral factors such as cigarette smoking, diet and activity patterns, sexual behavior, and behaviors related to avoidable injuries (e.g., bicycle helmet and seat belt use) are among the most important factors contributing to morbidity and mortality (McGinnis & Foege, 1993). Health behaviors are the central focus of health education (Glanz et al., 2002), whether designed to promote individual or social change toward optimal health. Therefore, we expect that current heath behaviors, as a central construct in health education programs, applied using the BS-CIT model will have a direct effect on personal values, and therefore an indirect effect on use of the technology-based stress-reducing intervention(s) and positive health outcomes (e.g., healthy behaviors, stress reduction, effective coping).

The use of coping strategies leading to effective coping results in stress reduction, improved physical functioning and psychological well-being, and healthy outcomes—the desired health outcomes of the proposed BS-CIT model. In contrast and undesired is ineffective coping, which leads to poor health outcomes (e.g., burnout, anxiety and depression, denial, altered sleep and insomnia, and higher morbidity and mortality—leading to poor quality of life and personal well-being) and a number of unhealthy behaviors such as personal isolation, and substance use and abuse (e.g., drugs, alcohol, food).

UNIQUENESS OF THE BS-CIT MODEL

The BS-CIT model offers several unique contributions to nursing theory and practice. From a theoretical perspective, it is the first model to combine elements from the technology acceptance literature and from the health behavior and stress and coping literature in order to address the context of using technology to promote health. In addition, the stages of the model, moving from background factors, to personal factors, to intention factors, and finally to outcomes, offers a unique progression in examining the phenomenon of using technology to impact health and promote healthy outcomes. From an application perspective, minimal research exists that truly develops a theory behind what elements are significant predictors of the use of technology to impact health behavior, which is what we attempt to address through the use of the BS-CIT model. Within the BS-CIT model, we believe it is important to assess the impact of technology-based health interventions over time, and therefore we include technology experience as a moderating factor. Furthermore, we propose that the relative impact of the personal value factors will change across subsequent uses of stress and coping and health-promoting interventions. This is not a static model. Further research is necessary to test the application of this model over time. We expect that over time, different background and value factors will become less important in comparison to other factors as individuals move through the process of modifying and changing their health behaviors and/or coping with stress through their participation in information systems interventions.

Future Work

This chapter presents an important first step in the development of a theoretical model, Theory of Behavior and Stress: Coping via Information Technology (BS-CIT), to guide the development, implementation, and testing of technology-based health interventions designed to foster healthier lifestyles among individuals in a society who are increasingly relying on advancing technology and information systems. The proposed model will benefit from future work that aims to test and extend the proposed framework. Future work using the BS-CIT model should include (1) development and testing of study measures that tap all the proposed model constructs, (2) testing of the BS-CIT with diverse health behaviors and stressful events,

(3) testing of the BS-CIT in diverse racial/ethnic populations across the age continuum, and (4) testing the effects of the BS-CIT with diverse technology systems. In the long run, we believe the BS-CIT can aid nurses and health care providers and clinicians, researchers, and practitioners in developing health-promoting programs and interventions that are based on constructs that have been shown to influence stress and coping, health behavior, as well as information systems use. We believe the BS-CIT model can maximize information systems to promote health, healthy behaviors, and cope with stress across the age continuum, resulting in a healthier American society.

References

Adams, D. A., Nelson, R. R., & Todd, P. A. (1992). Perceived usefulness, ease of use and usage of information technology: A replication. *MIS Quarterly, 16*(2), 227–250.

Agarwal, R., & Prasad, J. A. (1997). The role of innovation characteristics and perceived voluntariness in the acceptance of information technologies. *Decision Sciences, 28*(3), 557–582.

Ajzen, I. (1985). From intention to action: A theory of planned behavior. In J. Kuhl & J. Beckman (Eds.), *Action control: From cognition to behavior* (pp. 11–39). New York, NY: Springer Verlag.

Ajzen, I. (1988). *Attitudes, personality, and behavior.* Chicago, IL: Dorsey Press.

Ajzen, I. (1991). The Theory of Planned Behavior. *Organizational Behavior and Human Decision Processes, 50,* 179–211.

Ajzen, I. (2001). Nature and operation of attitudes. *Annual Review of Psychology, 52,* 27–58.

Ajzen, I. (2005). Understanding health-related lifestyle behaviors. Background paper for Session on Lifestyles, Health, and Mortality. In *Proceedings of the World Congress of the International Forum for Social Sciences and Health (IFSSH)*: Health Challenges of the Third Millennium, Yeditepe University.

Ajzen, I., & Fishbein, M. (1969). The prediction of behavioral intentions in a choice situation. *Journal of Experimental Social Psychology, 5,* 400–416.

Ajzen, I., & Fishbein, M. (1980). *Understanding attitudes and predicting social behavior.* Englewood Cliffs, NJ: Prentice-Hall.

Ajzen, I., & Madden, T. (1986). Prediction of goal-directed behavior: Attitudes, intentions, and perceived behavioral control. *Journal of Experimental Social Psychology, 22,* 453–474.

Albarracín, D., Johnson, B. T., Fishbein, M., & Muellerleile, P. A. (2001). Theories of reasoned action and planned behavior as models of condom use: A meta-analysis. *Psychological Bulletin, 127,* 142–161.

Al-Gahtani, S. S., & King, M. (1999). Attitudes, satisfaction and usage: Factors contributing to each in the acceptance of information technology. *Behavior and Information Technology, 18*(4), 277–297.

American Cancer Society (ACS). (2006). *Cancer prevention and early detection facts and figures, 2006.* Atlanta, GA: American Cancer Society.

American Thoracic Society. (2010). *Smoking cessation.* Retrieved January 3, 2011, from http://www.thoracic.org/clinical/best-of-the-web/pages/patient-education/smoking-cessation.php

Anderson, A. A. (1996). Predictors of computer anxiety and performance in information systems. *Computers in Human Behavior, 12*(1), 61–77.

Antonucci, T. C., & Akiyama, H. (1987). Social networks in adult life and a preliminary examination of the convoy model. *Journal of Gerontology, 42*(5), 519–527.

Antonucci, T. C., Lansford, J. E., & Ajrovich, K. J. (2000). Social support. In G. Fink (Ed.), *Encyclopedia of stress* (Vol. 3, pp. 479–483). San Diego, CA: Academic Press.

Antonovsky, A. (1979): *Health, stress and coping.* San Francisco, CA: Jossey-Bass.

Armitage, C. J., & Conner, M. (2001). Efficacy of the theory of planned behavior: A meta-analytic review. *British Journal of Social Psychology, 40,* 471–499.

Arnold, M. B. (1960). *Emotion and personality.* New York, NY: Columbia University Press.

Awad, N. F., & Krishnan, M. S. (2006). The personalisation privacy paradox: An empirical evaluation of information transparency and the willingness to be profiled online for personalisation. *MIS Quarterly, 30*(1), 13–28.

Baker, L., Todd, H., Wagner, S., & Bundorf, M. K. (2003, May). Use of the Internet and e-mail for health care information: Results from a national survey. *Journal of the American Medical Association, 289,* 2400–2406.

Baker, R. K., & White, M. (2010). Predicting adolescents' use of social networking sites from an extended theory of planned behaviour perspective. *Computers in Human Behavior, 26,* 1591–1597.

Bandura, A. (1988). Perceived self-efficacy: Exercise of control through self-belief. In J. P. Dauwalder, M. Perez, & V. Hobbi (Eds.), *Annual series of European research in behavior therapy* (Vol. 2, pp. 27–59). Lisse, Netherlands: Swets & Zietlinger.

Bandura, A. (1992). On rectifying the comparative anatomy of perceived control: Comments on 'Cognates of Personal Control.' *Applied and Preventive Psychology, 1,* 121–126.

Bandura, A. (1997). *Self-efficacy: The exercise of control.* New York, NY: W. H. Freeman.

Beckerman, A., & Northrop, C. (1996). Hope, chronic illness and the elderly. *Journal of Gerontological Nursing, 22,* 19–25.

Bem, D. J., & Allen, A. (1974). On predicting some of the people some of the time: The search for cross-situational consistencies in behavior. *Psychological Review, 81,* 506–520.

Bem, S. L. (1981). The BSRI and gender schema theory: A reply to Spence and Helmreich. *Psychological Review, 88,* 369–371.

Blue, C. L. (1995). The predictive capacity of the theory of reasoned action and the theory of planned behavior in exercise research: An integrated literature review. *Research in Nursing & Health, 18,* 105–121.

Brucks, M. (1985). The effects of product class knowledge on information search behavior. *Journal of Consumer Research, 21*(1), 1–16.

Card, S., Moran, T. P., & Newell, A. (1983). *The psychology of human-computer interaction.* Hillsdale, NJ: Lawrence Erlbaum Associates.

Centers for Disease Control and Prevention (CDC). (2004). *The burden of chronic diseases and their risk factors. National and state perspectives.* Atlanta, GA: U.S. Department of Health and Human Services. Available from http://www.cdc.gov/nccdphp/burdenbook2004/pdf/burden_book2004.pdf

Centers for Disease Control and Prevention (CDC). (2006). *Chartbook on trends in the health of Americans, 2006.* National Center for Health Statistics, United States. Hyattsville, MD: U.S. Government Printing Office.

Chau, P. Y. K., & Hu, P. J. (2002a). Examining a model of information technology acceptance by individual professionals: An exploratory study. *Journal of Management Information Systems, 18*(4), 191–229.

Chau, P. Y. K., & Hu, P. J. (2002b). Investigating healthcare professionals' decisions to accept telemedicine technology: An empirical test of competing theories. *Information and Management, 39,* 297–311.

Chen, I. J., Yang, K. F., Tang, F. I., Huang, C. H., & Yu, S. (2007). Applying the technology acceptance model to explore public health nurses' intentions towards web-based learning: A cross-sectional questionnaire survey. *International Journal of Nursing Studies, 45*(6), 869–878.

Chin, W. W., & Todd, P. A. (1995). On the use, usefulness, and ease of use of structural equation modeling in MIS research: A note of caution. *MIS Quarterly, 19,* 237–246.

Cobb, S. (1976). Presented as part of the presidential address at the Community Health and Psychiatry Program in Medicine at Brown University before the Society at its Annual Meeting, March 27, 1976. In *Toward an integrated medicine: Classics from psychosomatic medicine, 1958–1979,* Chapter 18: Social support as a moderator of life stress, (pp. 377–398). Washington, DC: Psychological Press Inc.

Cohen, F. (1984). Coping. In J. D. Matarazzo, C. M. Weiss, J. A. Herd, N. E. Miller, & S. M. Weiss (Eds.), *Behavioral health: A handbook of health enhancement and disease prevention.* New York, NY: Wiley.

Compas, B. E., Connor-Smith, J. K., Saltzman, H., Thomsen, A. H., & Wadsworth, M. E. (2001). Coping with stress during childhood and adolescence: Progress, problems, and potential in theory and research. *Psychological Bulletin, 127,* 87–127.

Compeau, D. R., & Higgins, C. A. (1995a). Application of social cognitive theory to training for computer skills. *Information Systems Research, 6*(2), 118–143.

Compeau, D. R., & Higgins, C. A. (1995b). Computer self-efficacy: Development of a measure and initial test. *MIS Quarterly, 19*(2), 189–211.

Crimmins, E. M., Ingegneri, D., & Saito, Y. (1997). Trends in disability-free life expectancy in the United States: 1970–90. *Population and Development Review, 23*(3), 555–572. Retrieved November 15, 2006, from http://proxy.lib.wayne.edu:3245/itx/printdoc.do?prodId=ITOF&userGroupName=1om

Davis, F. D. (1989). Perceived usefulness, perceived ease of use, and user acceptance of information technology. *MIS Quarterly, 13*(3), 319–340.

Davis, F. D. (1993). User acceptance of information technology: System characteristics, user perceptions and behavioral impacts. *International Journal of Man-Machine Studies, 38*(3), 475–487.

Davis, F. D., Bagozzi, R. P., & Warshaw, P. R. (1989, August). User acceptance of computer technology: A comparison of two theoretical models. *Management Science, 35(8),* 982–1003.

Davis, F. D., & Venkatesh, V. (1996). A critical assessment of potential measurement biases in the technology acceptance model: Three experiments. *International Journal of Human Computer Studies, 45,* 19–45.

Davis, F. D., & Venkatesh, V. (2004). Toward preprototype user acceptance testing of new information systems: Implications for software project management. *IEEE Transactions on Engineering Management, 51*(1), 31–46.

Dean, K. (1992). Health-related behaviors: Concept and methods. In M. G. Ory, I. L. P. Abeles, & P. D. Lipman (Eds.), *Aging, health, and behavior* (pp. 27–56). Newbury Park, CA: Sage.

Devaraj, S., & Kohli, R. (2003). Performance impacts of information technology: Is actual usage the missing link? *Management Science, 49*(3), 273–289.

de Vries, H., Dijkstra, M., & Kuhlman, P. (1988). Self-efficacy: The third factor besides attitude and subjective norm as predictor of behavioral intentions. *Health Education Research, 3,* 273–282.

Doll, J., & Ajzen, I. (1992). Accessibility and stability of predictors in the theory of planned behavior. *Journal of Personality and Social Psychology, 63,* 754–765.

Duff, G. W., Libby, P., Ordovas, J. M., & Reilly, P. R. (2006). The future of living well to 100. *American Journal of Clinical Nutrition, 83*(Suppl), 488S–490S.

Dzewaltowski, D. A., Noble, J. M., & Shaw, J. M. (1990). Physical activity participation—Social cognitive theory versus the theories of reasoned action and planned behavior. *Journal of Sport and Exercise Psychology, 12,* 399–405.

Elasmar, M. G., & Carter, M. E. (1996). Use of e-mail by college students and implications for curriculum. *Journal of Mass Communication Educator, 51*(2), 46–54.

Ellison, N. B., Steinfeld, C., & Lampe, C. (2007). The benefits of Facebook "Friends": Social capital and college students' use of online social network sites. *Journal of Computer-Mediated Communication, 12*(4), article 1.

Fazio, R. H., & Zanna, M. (1978a). Attitudinal qualities relating to the strength of the attitude-perception and attitude-behavior relationship. *Journal of Experimental Social Psychology, 14,* 398–408.

Fazio, R. H., & Zanna, M. (1978b). On the predictive validity of attitudes: The roles of direct experience and confidence. *Journal of Personality, 46,* 228–243.

Fazio, R. H., & Zanna, M. (1981). Direct experience and attitude-behavior consistency. In L. Berkowitz (Ed.), *Advances in experimental social psychology* (pp. 161–202). San Diego, CA: Academic Press.

Fishbein, M. (1967). Attitude and the predication of behavior. In M. Fishbein (Ed.), *Readings in attitude theory and measurement.* New York, NY: John Wiley.

Fishbein, M., & Ajzen, I. (1975). *Belief, attitude, intention, and behavior: An introduction to theory and research.* Reading, MA: Addison-Wesley Publishing.

Fogg, B. J. (2002). *Persuasive computers using technology to change what we think and do.* San Francisco, CA: Morgan Kaufman Publishers.

Folkman, S. (1992). Making the case for coping. In B.N. Carpenter (Ed.). *Personal coping: Theory, research, and application.* Westport, CT: Praeger/Greenwood.

Folkman, S. (2010). Stress, coping, and hope. *Psycho-Oncology, 19,* 901–908.

Fox, S. (2005). *Health information online.* Washington: DC: Pew Internet & American Life Project.

Fox, S., & Jones, S. (2009). *The Pew Report: The social life of health information.* Retrieved November 20, 2010, from http://www.pewinternet.org/Reports/2009/8-The-Social-Life-of-Health-Information/02-A-Shifting-Landscape/2-61-of-adults-in-the-US-gather-health-information-online.aspx?q=Internet%20use%20by%20gender

Furlong, M. S. (1989). An electronic communication for older adults: The SeniorNet Network. *Journal of Communication, 39*(3), 145–153.

Gefan, D., & Straub, D. W. (1997). Gender differences in the perception and use of e-mail: An extension to the technology acceptance model. *MIS Quarterly, 21*(4), 389–400.

Gefen, D., & Straub, D. (2000). The relative importance of perceived ease of use in IS adoption: A study of e-commerce adoption. *Journal of the Association for Information Systems, 8*(1), 1–28.

Gefan, D., & Straub, D. W. (2002). Nurturing clients' trust to encourage engagement success during the customization of ERP systems. *Omega: The International Journal of Management Science, 30*(4), 287–299.

Gilroy, D. F., & Desai, H. B. (1986). Computer anxiety: Sex, race, and age. *International Journal of Man-Machine Studies, 25,* 711–719.

Glanz, K., Rimer, B. K., & Lewis, F. M. (2002). *Health behavior and health education: Theory, research, and practice.* San Francisco, CA: Jossey-Bass.

Gochman, D. S. (1982). Labels, systems, and motives: Some perspectives on future research. *Health Education Quarterly, 9,* 167–174.

Godin, G., & Kok, G. (1996). The theory of planned behavior: A review of its applications to health-related behaviors. *The American Journal of Health Promotion, 11*(2), 87–98.

Godin, G., Valois, P., Lepage, L., & Desharnais, R. (1992). Predictors of smoking behavior: An application of Ajzen's theory of planned behavior. *British Journal of Addiction, 87,* 1335–1343.

Goh, Y. I. (2006). A critical review of the effectiveness of a multimedia program to prevent fetal alcohol syndrome. *Health Promotion Practice, 7*(X), 1–5.

Grzuwacz, J. G., Almeida, D. M., Neupert, S. D., & Ettner, S. L. (2004). Socioeconomic status and health: A micro-level analysis of exposure and vulnerability to daily stress. *Journal of Health and Social Behavior, 45*(1). Available online: http://hsb.sagepub.com/content/45/1/1

Heinssen, R. K. J., Glass, C. R., & Knight, L. A. (1987). Assessing computer anxiety: Development and validation of the computer anxiety rating scale. *Computers in Human Behavior, 3*(1), 49–59.

Hoffman, D. L., Kalsbeek, W. D., & Novak, T. P. (1996). Internet and Web use in the U.S.: Baselines for commercial development. Special Section on "Internet in the Home." *Communications of the ACM, 39*(12), 36–46.

Horrigan, J., & Rainie, L. (2002). *Getting serious online: As Americans gain experience, they use the Web more at work, write emails with more significant content, perform more online transactions, and pursue more serious activities.* Washington, DC: Pew Internet & American Life Project. Retrieved from http://www.pewinternet.org

Howard, G. S., & Smith, R. D. (1986). Computer anxiety in management: Myth or reality? *Communications of the ACM, 29*(7), 611–615.

Hu, P. J., Chau, P. Y. K., Liu Sheng, O. R., & Tam, K. Y. (1999). Examining the technology acceptance model using physician acceptance of telemedicine technology. *Journal of Management Information Systems, 16*(2), 91–112.

Igbaria, M., & Chakrabarti, A. (1990). Computer anxiety and attitudes toward microcomputer use. *Behavior and Information Technology, 9*(3), 229–241.

Igbaria, M., & Parasuraman, S. (1989). A path analytic study of individual characteristics, computer anxiety, and attitudes toward microcomputers. *Journal of Management, 15*(3), 373–388.

Igbaria, M., Zinatelli, N., Cragg, P., & Cavaye, A. L. M. (1997). Personal computing acceptance factors in small firms: A structural equation model. *MIS Quarterly, 21*(3), 279–305.

Janis, I. L. (1958). *Psychological stress: Psychoanalytic and behavioral studies of surgical patients.* New York, NY: John Wiley.

Karahanna, E., Straub, D. W., & Chervany, M. L. (1999). Information technology adoption across time: A cross-sectional comparison of pre-adoption and post-adoption beliefs. *MIS Quarterly, 23*(2), 183–213.

Kelman, H. C. (1958). Compliance, identification, and internalization: Three processes of attitude change. *Journal of Conflict Resolution, 2,* 51–60.

Kimieck, J. (1992). Predicting vigorous physical activity of corporate employees: Comparing the theories of reasoned action and planned behavior. *Journal of Sport and Exercise Psychology, 14*(2), 192–206.

Kirchmeyer, C. (1997). Relational demography and career success: A longitudinal study of mid-career managers. *Proceedings of the Academy of Management Meeting.*

Klein, L. R., & Ford, G. T. (2003). Consumer search for information in the digital age: An empirical study of prepurchase search for automobiles. *Journal of Interactive Marketing, 17*(3), 29–49.

Kukafka, R., Johnson, S. B., Linfante, A., & Allegrante, J. P. (2003). Grounding a new information technology implementation framework in behavioral science: A systematic analysis of the literature in IT use. *Journal of Biomedical Informatics, 36*(3), 218–227.

Lazarus, R.S. (1966). *Psychological stress and the coping process.* New York, NY: McGraw-Hill.

Lazarus, R.S. (1991). *Emotion and adaptation.* New York, NY: Oxford University Press.

Lazarus, R.S. (1993). From psychological stress to the emotions: A history of changing outlooks. *Annual Review of Psychology, 44,* 1–21.

Lazarus, R. S. (1998). *Fifty years of research and theory by R. S. Lazarus: An analysis of history and perennial issues.* Mahwah, NJ: Lawrence Erlbaum.

Lazarus, R. S. (2000a). Toward better research on stress and coping. *American Psychologist, 55*(6), 665–673.

Lazarus, R. S. (2000b). Evolution of a model of stress, coping, and discrete emotions. In V. H. Rice (Ed.), *Handbook of stress, coping, and health: Implications for nursing research, theory, and practice* (pp. 195–222). Thousand Oaks, CA: Sage.

Lazarus, R. S., & Cohen, J. B. (1977). Environmental stress. In I. Altman and J. F. Wohlwill (Eds), *Human behavior and environment* (Volume 2). New York, NY: Plenum.

Lazarus, R. S., & Folkman, S. (1984). *Stress, appraisal, and coping.* New York, NY: Springer.

Lazarus, R. S., & Folkman, S. (1987). Transactional theory and research on emotions and coping. *European Journal of Personality, 1,* 141–169.

Lazarus, R. S., & Launier, R. (1978). Stress related transactions between person and environment. In L. A. Pervin & M. Lewis (Eds.), *Perspectives in interactional psychology* (pp. 287–327). New York, NY: Plenum.

Lederer, A. L., Manupin, D. J., Sena, M. P., & Zhuang, Y. (2000). The technology acceptance model and the world wide web. *Decision Support Systems, 29,* 269–282.

Legris, P., Ingham, J., & Collerette, P. (2003). Why do people use information technology? A critical review of the technology acceptance model. *Information & Management, 40,* 191–204.

Levin, R. S., Foster, J. E., Fullilove, R. E., Fulllilove, M. T., Briggs, N. C., Hull, P. C., et al. (2001, September–October). Black-white inequalities in mortality and life expectancy, 1933–1999: Implications for Healthy People 2010. *Public Health Reports, 116,* 474–483.

Levy, F. (1988). Incomes, families, and living standards. In R. E. Litan et al. (Eds.), *American living standards: Threats and challenges.* Washington, DC: Brookings Institute.

Liebert, R. M., & Morris, L. W. (1967). Cognitive and emotional components of test anxiety: A distinction and some initial data. *Psychological Reports, 20,* 975–978.

Livingston, S. (2008). Taking risky opportunities in youthful content creation: Teenagers' use of social networking sites for intimacy, privacy and self-expression. *New Media & Society, 10*(3), 393–411.

Lubinski, D., Tellegen, A., & Butcher, J. A. (1983). Masculinity, femininity, and androgyny viewed and assessed as distinct concepts. *Journal of Personality and Social Psychology, 44,* 428–439.

Martocchio, J. J. (1994). Effects of conceptions of ability on anxiety, self-efficacy, and learning in training. *Journal of Applied Psychology, 79,* 819–825.

Mathieson, K. (1991). Predicting user intentions: Comparing the technology acceptance model with the theory of planned behavior. *Information Systems Research, 1991, 2,* 173–191.

McCaul, K. D., O'Neill, H. K., & Glasgow, R. E. (1988). Predicting the performance of dental hygiene behaviors: An examination of the Fishbein and Ajzen model and self-efficacy expectations. *Journal of Applied Social Psychology, 18,* 114–128.

McGinnis, M. J., & Foege, W. H. (1993). Actual causes of death in the United States. *Journal of the American Medical Association, 270,* 2207–2212.

Molarius, A., Seidell, J. C., Sans, S., Tuomilehto, J., & Kuulasmaa, K. (2000). Educational level, relative body weight, and changes in over 10 years: An international perspective from the WHO MONICA Project. *American Journal of Public Health, 90,* 1260–1268.

Moore, G. C., & Benbasat, I. (1991). Development of an instrument to measure the perceptions of adopting an information technology innovation. *Information Systems Research, 2*(3), 192–222.

Morris, L. W., Davis, M. A., & Hutchings, C. H. (1981). Cognitive and emotional components of anxiety: Literature review and a revised worry-emotionality scale. *Journal of Educational Psychology, 73,* 541–555.

Morris, M., & Dillon, A. (1997). How user perceptions influence software use. *IEEE Software, 14*(4), 58–65.

Morris, M. G., & Venkatesh, V. (2000). Age differences in technology adoption decisions: Implications for a changing workforce. *Personnel Psychology, 53,* 375–403.

Morrow, P. C., Prell, E. R., & McElroy, J. C. (1986). Attitudinal and behavioral correlates of computer anxiety. *Psychological Reports, 59,* 1199–1204.

Motowidlo, S. J. (1982). Relationship between self-rated performance and pay satisfaction among sales representatives. *Journal of Applied Psychology, 67,* 209–213.

Noar, S. M., & Zimmerman, R. S. (2005). Health behavior theory and cumulative knowledge regarding health behaviors: Moving in the right direction? *Health Education Research, 20*(3), 275–290.

Office of Behavioral and Social Science Research (OBSSR). (n.d.). *Office of Behavioral and Social Science Research strategic plan, FY 2002–2006.* National Institutes of Health, 77. Retrieved January 15, 2007, from http://obssr.od.nih.gov/about_obssr/strategic_planning/health_disparities/healthdisp.aspx

Office of the Surgeon General (Ed.). (2010). *How tobacco smoke causes disease: The biology and behavioral basis for smoking-attributable disease: A report of the Surgeon General.* Atlanta, GA: U.S. Department of Health & Human Services, Centers for Disease Control and Prevention, National Center for Chronic Disease Prevention and Health Promotion, Office on Smoking and Health.

Oliver, R. L., & Bearden W. O. (1985). Crossover effects in the theory of reasoned action: A moderating influence attempt. *Journal of Consumer Research, 12,* 324–340.

Olshansky, S. J., Passaro, D. J., Hershow, R. C., Layden, J., Carnes, B. A., Brody, J., et al. (2005). A potential decline in life expectancy in the United States in the 21st century. *New England Journal of Medicine, 352*(11), 1138–1145.

Parasuraman, S., & Igbaria, M. (1990). An examination of gender differences in the determinants of computer anxiety and attitudes toward microcomputers among managers. *International Journal of Man-Machine Studies, 32*(3), 327–340.

Preston, S. H. (2005). Deadweight?—The influence of obesity on longevity. *New England Journal of Medicine, 352*(11), 1135–1137.

Punj, G. N., & Staelin, R. (1983). A model of consumer information search behavior for new automobiles. *Journal of Consumer Research, 9*(4), 366–380.

Rainie, L. (2005, November 11). Search engine use shoots up in the past year and edges towards email as the primary Internet application. Washington, DC: PEW Internet & American Life Project.

Robert Wood Johnson Foundation (RWJF) Commission to Build a Healthier America. (2009). *Beyond health care: New directions to a healthier America.* Retrieved January 3, 2011, from http://www.commissiononhealth.org

Rodin, J. (1990). Control by any other name: Definitions, concepts, and processes. In J. Rodin, C. Schooler, & K. W. Schaie (Eds.), *Self-directedness: Cause and effects throughout the life course* (pp. 1–15). Mahwah, NJ: Erlbaum Publishers.

Ronis, D. L., & Kaiser, M. K. (1989). Correlates of breast self-examination in a sample of college women: Analyses of linear structural relations. *Journal of Applied Social Psychology, 19*(13), 1068–1084.

Rotter, J. B. (1966). Generalized expectancies for internal versus external control of reinforcement. *Psychological Monographs, 80*(1, Whole No. 609), 1–28.

Ruiz-Bueno, J. B. (2000). Locus of control, perceived control, and learned helplessness. In V. H. Rice (Ed.), *Handbook of stress, coping, and health: Implications for nursing research, theory, and practice* (pp. 461–482). Thousand Oaks, CA: Sage.

Schifter, D. E., & Ajzen, I. (1985). Intention, perceived behavioral control and weight loss: An application of the theory of planned behavior. *Journal of Personality and Social Psychology, 49,* 843–851.

Schmidt, J. B., & Spreng, R. A. (1996, Summer). A proposed model of consumer information search. *Journal of the Academy of Marketing Science, 24*(3), 246–256.

Schwartz, S., & Tessler, R. (1972). A test of a model for reducing measured attitude-behavior discrepancies. *Journal of Personality and Social Psychology, 24,* 225–236.

Scott, C. R., & Rockwell, S. C. (1997). The effect of communication, writing, and technology apprehension on likelihood to use new communication technologies. *Communication Education, 46,* 44–62.

Segars, A. H., & Grover, V. (1993). Re-examining perceived ease of use and usefulness: A confirmatory factor analysis. *MIS Quarterly,* *18*(4), 517–525.

Selye, H. (1956). *The stress of life.* New York, NY: McGraw-Hill.

Sheeran, P., & Orbell, S. (1998). Do intentions predict condom use? Meta-analysis and examination of six moderating variables. *British Journal of Social Psychology, 37,* 231–250.

Simonson, M. R., Maaurer, M., Montag-Torard, M., & Whitaker, M. (1987). Development of a standardized test of computer literacy and a computer anxiety index. *Journal of Educational Computing Research, 3,* 231–247.

Skinner, E. A. (1995). *Perceived control, motivation, and coping, (Individual Differences and Development,* Volume 8). Thousand Oaks, CA: Sage.

Straub, D. M., Limayem, E., & Karahanna-Evaristo, E. (1995). Measuring system usage: Implications for IS theory testing. *Management Science, 41,* 1328–1342.

Subramanian, G. H. (1994). A replication of perceived usefulness and perceived ease of use measurement. *Decision Sciences, 25*(6), 863–874.

Sullivan C.F. (1997, April). *Cancer support groups in cyberspace: Are there gender differences in message functions?* Paper presented at the Central States Communication Association annual meeting convention, St. Louis, MO.

Svanborg, A. (1990, October). Aging, health and vitality: Results from the Gothberg longitudinal study. Paper presented at the 19th Annual Scientific and Educational Meeting of the Canadian Association of Gerontology. Victoria, British Columbia.

Szajna, B. (1994). Software evaluation and choice: Predictive validation of the technology acceptance instrument. *MIS Quarterly, 18,* 319–324.

Szajna, B. (1996). Empirical evaluation of the revised technology acceptance model. *Management Science, 42,* 85–92.

Taylor, H. (2003, August 11). *Cyberchondriacs update.* Harris Poll No. 44.

Taylor, S., & Todd, P. A. (1995a). Understanding information technology usage: A test of competing models. *Information Systems Research, 6,* 144–176.

Taylor, S., & Todd, P. A. (1995b). Assessing IT usage: The role of prior experience. *MIS Quarterly, 19*(4), 561–570.

Terry, D. J. (1993). Self-efficacy expectancies and the theory of reasoned action. In D. J. Terry, C. Gallois, & M. McCamish (Eds.), *The theory of reasoned action: Its application to AIDs-preventive behavior* (pp. 135–151). Oxford, England: Pergamon.

Terry, D. J., & O'Leary, J. E. (1995). The theory of planned behavior: The effects of perceived behavioral control and self-efficacy. *British Journal of Social Psychology, 34,* 199–220.

Todman, J., & Monaghan, E. (1994). Qualitative differences in computer experience, computer anxiety, and students' use of computers: A path model. *Computers in Human Behavior, 10*(4), 529–539.

Tung, F. C., Chang, S. C., & Chou, C. M. (2008). An extension of trust and TAM model with IDT in the adoption of the electronic logistics information system in HIS in the medical industry. *International Journal of Medical Informatics, 77*(5), 324–335.

U.S. Department of Health & Human Services (USDHHS). (2000). Healthy people 2010: About healthy people. Retrieved August 25, 2011, from http://www.healthypeople.gov/2010/About/

U.S. Department of Health & Human Services (USDHHS). (2010). Healthy people 2020. Retrieved January 20, 2010, from http://www.healthypeople.gov/2020/about/DisparitiesAbout.aspx

Venkatesh, V. (1999). Creation of favorable user perceptions: Exploring the role of intrinsic motivation. *MIS Quarterly, 23*(2), 239–260.

Venkatesh, V. (2000). Determinant of perceived ease of use: Integrating control, intrinsic motivation, and emotion into the technology acceptance model. *Information Systems Research, 11,* 342–365.

Venkatesh, V., & Bala, H. (2008). Technology Acceptance Model 3 and a research agenda on interventions. *Decision Sciences, 39*(2), 273–315.

Venkatesh, V., & Davis, F. D. (1996). A model of the perceived ease of use development and test. *Decision Sciences, 27*(3), 451–481.

Venkatesh, V., & Davis, F. D. (2000). A theoretical extension of the technology acceptance model: Four longitudinal field studies. *Management Science, 46,* 186–204.

Venkatesh, V., & Davis, R. D. (2004). Toward preprototype user acceptance testing of new information systems: Implications for software project management. *IEEE Transactions on Engineering Management, 51*(1), 31–46.

Venkatesh, V., & Morris, M. G. (2000). Why don't men ever stop to ask for directions? Gender, social influence, and their role in technology acceptance and usage behavior. *MIS Quarterly, 24,* 115–139.

Venkatesh, V., Morris, M. G., Davis, G. B., & Davis, F. D. (2003). User acceptance of information technology: Toward a unified view. *MIS Quarterly, 27*(3), 425–478.

Wallston, B.S., & Wallston, K.A. (1981). Health locus of control. In H. Lefcourt (Ed.), *Research with the Locus of Control Construct* (Vol. 1). New York, NY: Academic Press.

Wallston, K. A., Wallston, B. S., & DeVellis, R. (1978). Development of the multidimensional health locus of control (MHLC) scales. *Health Education Monographs, 6,* 160–170.

Watkins, A.J., & Kligman, E. W. (1993). Attendance patterns of older adults in a health promotion program. *Public Health Reports, 106*(1), 86–90.

Weinert, C., & Burman, M. E. (1994). Rural health and health-seeking behaviors. *Annual Review Nursing Research, 12,* 65–92.

Westendorp, R. G. J. (2006). What is healthy aging in the 21st century? *American Journal of Clinical Nutrition, 83*(2), 404S–409S.

White, K. M., Terry, D. J., & Hogg, M. A. (1994). Safer sex behavior: The role of attitudes, norms, and control factors. *Journal of Applied Social Psychology, 21,* 213–228.

Williams, D. (1994). The concept of race in health services research: 1966–1990. *Health Services Research, 29*(3), 261–274.

Wilson, E. V., & Lankton, N. K. (2004, July–August). Modeling patients' acceptance of provider-delivered e-health. *Journal of American Medical Information Association, 11*(4), 241–248.

Wilson, T. D., Lindsey, S., & Schooler, T. Y. (2000). A model of dual attitudes. *Psychological Review, 107*(1), 101–126.

Wurtele, S. K. (1988). Increasing women's calcium intake: The role of health beliefs, intentions and health value. *Journal of Applied Social Psychology, 18*(8), 627–639.

PART IV

INTERACTIONAL AND TRANSACTIONAL MODELS

8

SALUTOGENESIS

Origins of Health and Sense of Coherence

MARTHA E. HORSBURGH AND ALANA L. FERGUSON

Recalling an event that occurred toward the end of his incarceration in the concentration camps of Nazi Germany, Victor Frankl (1959) wrote,

> Not only our experiences, but all we have done, whatever great thoughts we may have had, and all we have suffered, all this is not lost, though it is past; we have brought it into being. Having been is also a kind of being, and perhaps the surest kind. Then I spoke of the many opportunities of giving life a meaning. I told my comrades (who lay motionless, although occasionally a sigh could be heard) that human life, under any circumstances, never ceases to have a meaning, and that this infinite meaning of life includes suffering and dying, privation and death. I asked the poor creatures who listened to me attentively in the darkness of the hut to face up to the seriousness of our position. They must not lose hope but should keep their courage in the certainty that the hopelessness of our struggle did not detract from its dignity and its meaning. (p. 104)

Frankl and many others lost family members and friends to World War II concentration camps, were stripped of their possessions, and suffered from hunger, cold, and brutality. The threat of extermination faced them every hour of every day. Scarred forever by this horrific adversity, Frankl was especially haunted by the nature of survival. He witnessed some apparently strong individuals falter and fail, while others who might have seemed weaker were in fact able to live on. Beyond the question of how he himself had survived, Frankl was troubled by how and why others had done so. This same question stimulated medical sociologist Aaron Antonovsky's life's work—the scientific search for factors that facilitate human health and well-being in the face of pathogens, stresses, and strains that are endemic in the human condition. He named this concept *salutogenesis*, the origins of health, and "good beginnings" (Antonovsky, 1979).

DEVELOPMENT OF THE SALUTOGENIC MODEL

Born in Brooklyn in 1923, Aaron Antonovsky studied history and economics as an undergraduate. He served in the U.S. Army during World War II and later studied at Yale University, receiving both master's and doctoral degrees in sociology. He emigrated with his wife to Israel in 1960 and served as professor and chair of the Department of Sociology of Health, Faculty of Health Services, Ben-Gurion University, Beersheba (Antonovsky, 1987).

Influenced by Hans Selye's (1956) work on the "generalized adaptation syndrome," René Dubos's (1960, 1968) contributions on psychosocial and cultural influences on human adaptation, and the work of many other scientists of his time, Antonovsky (1972) published the first of his formulations in the area of individual stress, coping, and health. Antonovsky argued that it was time to move beyond consideration of individual diseases and their unique etiologies to search for common phenomena that enhance individuals' abilities to adapt to threats in general. He put forward three key positions. First, serious consideration should be given to a common etiology of disease. Second, health should be measured using a "breakdown" continuum, with "no breakdown" at one extreme and "life-threatening breakdown" at the other. Finally, he maintained that persons use "generalized resistance resources" (GRR) to resolve tensions that occur from a variety of internal and external stressors and demands.

In his book *Health, Stress and Coping* (1979), Antonovsky developed the perspective associated with salutogenesis. Research with menopausal women suggested to him that cultural stability exerted positive benefits for individual health. Additional work with a sub-sample of these women, who were concentration camp survivors of World War II, led Antonovsky to ask what he called "the revolutionary question and the origin of my concern," namely, how these beleaguered individuals managed to remain reasonably healthy. He argued that salutogenesis could add an important new facet to *pathogenesis,* the traditional medical model. He therefore advocated allocation of resources to study the origins of health.

Analyzing American epidemiological data, Antonovsky (1979) concluded that at any one time, "at least one third and quite possibly a majority of the population of any modern industrial society is characterized by some morbid condition" (p. 15). He noted that pathogenesis, which focuses on individual diseases, categorizes persons in an artificially dichotomous way, as either "non-patients" or "patients." Non-patients are further classified as "healthy" or "sick" (self-diagnosed or diagnosed by another layperson), whereas patients are further classified as "diseased," with clear or unclear medical diagnosis, or "not diseased," displaying hypochondriac and malingerer tendencies. The central question of pathogenesis—"Why do people get this or that disease?"—reinforces the categorization of individuals in this manner.

In contrast to the pathogenic approach, Antonovsky (1979) argued that it is only when we ask why people stay healthy that we begin to

search for factors that can promote health despite the "ubiquity of pathogens—microbiological, chemical, physical, psychological, social, and cultural" (p. 13). The central question of salutogenesis thus offers three distinct advantages: It focuses attention on the common denominators of health, including individuals' subjective interpretations; it embraces the notion of multiple causation and encourages a broad approach consistent with the field of health promotion; and it seeks to describe and explain factors that move individuals toward the healthy end of a health continuum. Health and illness are no longer viewed as dichotomies. Rather, a multidimensional health–illness continuum is posited, with "two poles that are useful only as heuristic devices and are never found in reality: absolute health and absolute illness" (p. 37).

This health–illness continuum, or "ease/dis-ease continuum" (Antonovsky, 1979, p. 65), is composed of two subjective dimensions as perceived by the individual and two objective dimensions as perceived by the health professional. The former includes four pain categories ranging from "none" to "severe" and four categories of functional limitations ranging from "none" to "severely limiting." The latter includes six prognostic implications ranging from "not acute or chronic" to "serious, acute, and life-threatening" and four action implications ranging from "no particular health-related action needed" to "active therapeutic intervention required" (p. 65). This offers the possibility of 384 individual combinations that may be used to describe an individual's location on the ease/dis-ease continuum. This mapping of ease/dis-ease profiles, and the search for factors that place an individual somewhere on the continuum, culminated in the development of the salutogenic model.

Antonovsky unexpectedly passed away in 1994. At the time of his death, the salutogenic model was just starting to be recognized as a strong theoretical base, especially for health promotion and public health interventions (Lindström & Eriksson, 2006). Lindström and Eriksson have perhaps produced the seminal articles since Antonovsky's passing, particularly through their systematic reviews of more than 200 articles using the salutogenic model.

The next sections of this chapter explain the concepts of the salutogenic model and relationships proposed among them, appraise the empirical support for the model, and review its practical applications 30 years after its introduction by Antonovsky and 10 years after the first version of this book chapter (Horsburgh, 2000). Over the past 10 years, much additional research in this area has been accomplished, particularly evaluations of the model's concepts and relationships. The future of this model is to rely upon practical applications through health promotion interventions, strategies, and policies.

THE SALUTOGENIC MODEL: CONCEPTS AND RELATIONSHIPS

The major substantive elements of the salutogenic model were elucidated by Antonovsky in 1979 (see Figure 8.1) and further refined in his subsequent book, *Unraveling the Mystery of Health: How People Manage Stress and Stay Well* (1987). The model seeks to describe the process of staying healthy despite exposure to stress. It is a cognitive model of human responses to stress that influences health over time, as well as within a sociocultural and historical context. The following are the main conceptual elements of the salutogenic model: (a) stressors; (b) tension, tension management, and stress; (c) generalized resistance resources–resistance deficits; (d) sense of coherence; and (e) individual placement on the health ease/dis-ease continuum, the outcome of interest. Each of these is briefly described, followed by a discussion of the relationships purported among them.

Stressors

Stressors are viewed within the salutogenic model (Antonovsky, 1979, 1987) as endemic to the human condition. Indeed, Antonovsky suggests that human existence is characterized by moderate to severe levels of stressors. In 1979, he differentiated stressors from other stimuli, noting that stressors upset the individual's homeostasis and present "demands to which there are no readily available or automatic responses" (p. 72). Stressors are viewed as human and environmental, occurring from within the individual or from without, and imposed or freely chosen or both. Stressors, when recognized as such by the individual, engender a state of "tension."

Tension, Tension Management, and Stress

Tension, tension management, and stress are differentiated within the salutogenic model (Antonovsky, 1979, 1987). A state of tension is viewed as the response to a stressor and is both an emotional and physiological phenomenon— "the recognition in the brain that some need one has is unfulfilled, that a demand on one has to be met, that one must do something if one is to realize a goal" (1987, p. 130). Outcomes associated with tension can be salutary, neutral, or negative with respect to health. The nature of the outcome depends on the ability of the individual to manage tension. Tension management is defined as "the rapidity and completeness with which problems are resolved and tension dissipated" (1979, p. 96). If tension management is effective, stress does not ensue and the impact on health may be neutral or even salutary. If tension is not managed effectively, the individual enters a state of stress. The ability of the individual to manage tension, and avoid or manage stress or both, is influenced by factors known as generalized resistance resources.

Generalized Resistance Resources–Resistance Deficits

In 1979, Antonovsky defined a *generalized resistance resource* (GRR) as "any characteristic of the person, group, or environment that can facilitate effective tension management" (p. 99). Later, GRRs were defined as "phenomena that provide one with sets of life experiences characterized by consistency, participation in shaping outcome, and an underload-overload balance" (Antonovsky, 1987, p. 19). GRRs include (a) material resources, such as money, shelter, and food; (b) knowledge and intelligence—a means to know the real world and to acquire skills; (c) ego identity—a sense of inner self that is integrated but flexible; (d) a coping strategy that is rational, flexible, and farsighted; (e) social supports—ties or deep interpersonal roots and commitment; (f) commitment and cohesion with one's cultural roots; (g) cultural stability; (h) ritualistic activities and answers provided by one's culture that anthropology labels collectively as magic (e.g., ceremony for crop failure and ceremony for accession of leaders); (i) religion and philosophy—a stable set of answers to life's perplexities; (j) preventive health orientation; (k) genetic and constitutional GRRs; and (l) an individual's state of health (Antonovsky, 1979, 1987). (See Figure 8.1.)

It is important to briefly discuss the GRR coping strategy. Antonovsky (1979, 1987) distinguishes

Figure 8.1 The Salutogenic Model

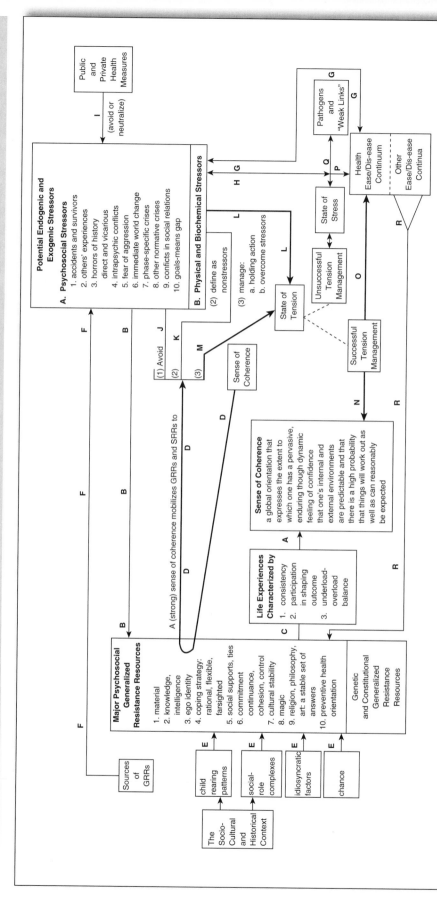

A, life experiences shape the sense of coherence; B, stressors affect the generalized resistance resources (GRRs); C, by definition, a GRR provides one with sets of meaningful, coherent life experiences; D, a strong sense of coherence mobilizes the GRRs and specific resistance resources (SRRs) at one's disposal; E, child-rearing patterns, social role complexes, idiosyncratic factors, and chance build up GRRs; F, the sources of GRRs also create stressors; G, traumatic physical and biochemical stressors affect health status directly, and health status affects the extent of exposure to psychosocial stressors; H, physical and biochemical stressors interact with endogenic pathogens and "weak links" and with stress to affect health status; I, public and private health measures avoid or neutralize stressors; J, a strong sense of coherence, mobilizing GRRs and SRRs, avoids stressors; K, a strong sense of coherence, mobilizing GRRs and SRRs, defines stimuli as nonstressors; L, ubiquitous stressors create a state of tension; M, the mobilized GRRs (and SRRs) interact with the state of tension and manage a holding action and the overcoming of stressors; N, successful tension management strengthens the sense of coherence; O, successful tension management maintains one's place on the health ease/dis-ease continuum; P, interaction between the state of stress and pathogens and weak links negatively affects health status; Q, stress is a general precursor that interacts with the existing potential endogenic and exogenic pathogens and weak links; R, good health status facilitates the acquisition of other GRRs. Note that A, C–E, and L–O represent the core of the salutogenic model. Reproduced with permission from Antonovsky (1979, pp. 184–185).

183

coping strategies from coping behaviors that individuals may employ to deal with stress. The former refers to an "overall plan of action for overcoming stressors" (1979, p. 112), a plan that is rational, flexible, and farsighted—*rational* in that it is fairly accurate and objective; *flexible* in that there is a willingness to consider and use alternative strategies; and *farsighted* in that the individual anticipates the response of the environment to his or her action plan. Antonovsky uses the latter term, coping behaviors or "coping," in a generic way to indicate actions taken by individuals to deal with stress. Used in this broad way, coping is not depicted within the salutogenic model.

To enhance the parsimony of the salutogenic model, Antonovsky (1987) merged GRRs and his earlier notions of stressors (discussed previously) into one concept, generalized resistance resources–resistance deficits (GRR–RDs). He ranked each GRR on a continuum: The higher a person is on the continuum, the more likely he or she is to have consistent, balanced life experiences and high participation in decision making. Conversely, the lower the person is on the continuum, the more likely he or she will have inconsistent, poorly balanced life experiences with low participation in decision making. In the first instance, the GRR–RDs are viewed as GRRs (e.g., high material resources and good state of health). In the second instance, they are viewed as generalized resistance deficits (GRDs) (e.g., low material resources and poor state of health). Both GRRs and GRDs contribute to the development of one's *sense of coherence*, a central concept of the salutogenic model.

The Sense of Coherence

Antonovsky (1979) introduced a central concept of the model of salutogenesis—the sense of coherence (SOC). Sense of coherence is an abstract phenomenon descriptive of individuals. It is an enduring view of the world, and "a crucial element in the basic personality structure of an individual and in the ambiance of a subculture, culture, or historical period" (p. 124). From birth, the salutogenic model (Antonovsky, 1979, 1987) views individuals as constantly in situations of challenge, response, tension, stress, and resolution. The more these experiences are characterized by "consistency, participation in

shaping outcome, and an underload-overload balance of stimuli" (1979, p. 187), the more an individual will begin to view the world as coherent and predictable. Childhood and adolescence are viewed as crucial points in the development of a person's SOC. By young adulthood, individuals are viewed as having acquired a tentative SOC that then becomes relatively stable throughout adulthood.

Antonovsky (1987) defined SOC as follows:

> A global orientation that expresses the extent to which one has a pervasive, enduring though dynamic feeling of confidence that (1) the stimuli deriving from one's internal and external environments in the course of living are structured, predictable, and explicable; (2) the resources are available to one to meet the demands posed by these stimuli; and (3) these demands are challenges, worthy of investment and engagement. (p. 19)

The SOC is an individual disposition characterized by the degree to which individuals expect their world to be comprehensible, manageable, and meaningful. *Comprehensibility* refers to the extent to which stimuli make cognitive sense and are relatively orderly, consistent, structured, and clear. *Manageability* is the perception that resources are at one's disposal that are adequate to meet the demands posed, whereas *meaningfulness* refers to the extent to which "one feels that life makes sense emotionally" (p. 18), that at least some of the demands posed by life are worth engagement, and these are viewed as challenges rather than burdens.

Although the three components of SOC are viewed as highly related to one another, they are discussed in terms of relative importance. Meaningfulness is viewed as the motivational component of the SOC, and it is the most central of the three components. Antonovsky (1987) stresses that a meaningful commitment must underlie the effort to comprehend and manage over the long term. Comprehensibility is viewed as second in importance because manageability is largely dependent on how one perceives stimuli. Antonovsky emphasizes, however, that this does not mean that manageability is unimportant. If people do not believe that they can manage, they are less likely to find meaning or to strive to comprehend. Antonovsky noted that it is SOC viewed as a whole that is the major determinant of an individual's placement on the health ease/dis-ease continuum.

Individual Placement on the Health Ease/Dis-Ease Continuum

As described earlier, an individual's placement on the health ease/dis-ease continuum ("breakdown" continuum is another term used to refer to this concept) is indicated by pain, functional limitation, prognostic implications, and action implications. It is both an objective and subjective phenomenon, and it embraces the notion of multicausality.

Relationships Among the Concepts of the Salutogenic Model

The salutogenic model proposes a recursive relationship between SOC and GRR–RDs. These factors help to shape the SOC, while a strong SOC helps to mobilize GRRs for the purpose of tension management. Poorly managed stressors lead to a state of tension, and poorly managed tension leads to stress and negative placement on the health ease/disease continuum. In both situations, in which GRRs or GRDs are chronic and built into the life situation of the person, they are viewed as the primary determinants of the strength of an individual's SOC (Antonovsky, 1987, p. 29).

Returning to the original question of why individuals undergoing high stress nevertheless stay healthy, the salutogenic model presents SOC as a "very major determinant of maintaining one's position on the health ease/dis-ease continuum and of movement toward the healthy end" (Antonovsky, 1987, p. 15). Antonovsky poses both cognitive and physiologic mechanisms through which the SOC exerts salutary benefits. In explaining cognitive mechanisms, Antonovsky used the work of Lazarus and Folkman (1984) regarding cognitive appraisals. He drew on research conducted in the basic sciences that pointed to physiological mechanisms linking chronic stress with immune suppression.

Antonovsky (1987) wrote that a strong SOC mobilizes persons' abilities to use resources toward both avoiding and managing stress. Upon initial confrontation with stimuli, a person with a strong SOC is more likely to define those stimuli as nonstressors. Even if the stimulus is initially appraised as a stressor, the person with a strong SOC is likely to view the stressor as having low relevance (less danger) and to feel less or shorter-lived tension. When an individual with a strong SOC perceives that he or she is confronted with a formidable stressor, the individual is more likely to feel a sense of engagement, commitment, and willingness to cope. Furthermore, he or she is likely to have developed a rich repertoire of GRRs on which to draw to deal with the stressor, both the behavioral aspects (coping) and the emotive aspects (emotional regulation). Tension is resolved relatively quickly and does not become stress, or stress is resolved relatively quickly. Finally, the person with a strong SOC is better able to judge the efficacy of his or her behaviors to manage tension and cope with stress and is more likely to discern the need for, and make use of, alternative actions.

LEVEL OF DEVELOPMENT OF THE SALUTOGENIC MODEL

The salutogenic model has relatively broad but clearly demarcated boundaries. It is purported to transcend culture and historical period. It is a cognitive model, however, and as such does not apply to individuals who lack the ability to perceive stressors (e.g., infants). The model has been developed and applied to children, adolescents, and across cultures. Investigators have recognized the importance of examining the development of SOC in childhood and adolescence because these periods of human growth and development are viewed as integral to promoting the development of a strong SOC in adulthood (Honkinen et al., 2009; Moons & Norekvål, 2006). Cross-cultural application of the model is imperative to understand if individuals of various cultures develop SOC in similar ways, as Antonovsky (1987) hypothesized.

The salutogenic model is highly abstract and encompasses a relatively large number of concepts (e.g., sense of coherence, ease/dis-ease continuum, and the GRR–RDs). Direction is provided, however, for operationalization of some of the main model concepts (e.g., sense of coherence, ease/dis-ease continuum).

Measurement: The Orientation to Life Questionnaire

A 29-item Sense of Coherence Questionnaire (SOC-29) was developed by Antonovsky (1987) to measure an individual's sense of coherence. A shorter version, the 13-item SOC-13, is composed of a subset of items from the SOC-29. Published as an appendix in Antonovsky's 1987 book, the measures were based on the theoretical definition of SOC and its three subconstructs—comprehensibility, manageability, and meaningfulness. Both the SOC-29 and SOC-13 are 7-point, semantic differential scales. Scores on the SOC-29 may range from 29 to 203, and those on the SOC-13 from 13 to 91. The SOC-29 has 11 comprehensibility, 10 manageability, and 8 meaningfulness items. The SOC-13 is composed of 5 comprehensibility, 4 manageability, and 4 meaningfulness items. To minimize response bias, almost half of the items have negatively worded stems that are reverse coded so that a higher score indicates a stronger SOC.

There is strong empirical support across cultures and developmental stages for the reliability of both the SOC-29 and SOC-13. Indeed the shorter, 13-item measure is as satisfactory as the longer version, and should generally be considered for use first in consideration of efficient use of participants' time and energy (Eriksson & Lindström, 2005). The SOC-29, SOC-13, or both, have been examined in inclusive samples, ranging from 20 to 20,000 participants and published in 33 languages (Eriksson & Lindström, 2005). More than half of the respondents have been women and include adults of all ages.

The first iteration of this book chapter (Horsburgh, 2000) noted only a few studies examining the two SOC measures in adolescents and children. This gap has been addressed over the past 10 years. Recent studies have included children and youth ranging from age 8 to 18 (Ristkari et al., 2009; Myrin & Lagerström, 2008). The SOC-13 has been used to assess children and adolescent's SOC in relation to perceived health, well-being, psychosocial factors, and psychological problems (Bronikowski & Bronikowska, 2009; Honkinen et al., 2009; Honkinen, Suominen, Välimaa, Helenius, & Rautava, 2005; Myrin & Lagerström, 2008).

Both measures have been investigated with healthy, community-based and clinical samples.

An abundance of recent literature examined SOC in specific clinical groups, including breast cancer survivors (Gibson, 2003) and professional groups (i.e., physicians) (Rabin, Matalon, Maoz, & Shiber, 2005). Despite diagnosed illness, adult clinical participants have reported a strong SOC (Ekman, Fagerberg, & Lundman, 2002; Gustavsson-Lilius, Julkunen, Keskivaara, & Hietanen, 2007; Schmitt et al., 2008). This finding is consistent with Antonovsky's (1979) view that SOC is fairly stable in adulthood in both clinical and community-based populations.

Normative data recently reported for the SOC-29 (Eriksson & Lindström, 2005) is consistent with findings reported by Antonovsky (1987, 1993). Antonovsky (1987) originally reported means ranging from 132.4 ($SD = 22.0$) to 160.4 ($SD = 16.7$) for the SOC-29 using Israeli and American samples. Recently reported data based on a review of 124 studies using the SOC-29 demonstrated similar means ranging from 100.50 ($SD = 28.50$) to 164.50 ($SD = 17.10$) (Eriksson & Lindström, 2005).

Normative data for the SOC-13 were not reported by Antonovsky in 1987. In 1993, he reported data from nine individual studies of Western, Judeo-Christian populations, and means ranged from 55 ($SD = .7$) to 68.7 ($SD = 10.0$). Again, these data are consistent with means recently reported. A review of 127 studies using the SOC-13 reported means ranging from 35.39 ($SD = .10$) to 77.60 ($SD = 13.80$) (Eriksson & Lindström, 2005).

Other shorter versions of the SOC-29 and SOC-13 have been developed and tested; however results of reliability and/or validity testing have been unsatisfactory (Eriksson & Lindström, 2005; Feldt et al., 2007; Olsson, Gassne, & Hansson, 2009). Of particular concern is the SOC-3 which had low reliability and demonstrated low correlations with both the SOC-13 and SOC-29 (Olsson et al., 2009). Most contemporary investigators are opting to use the SOC-13 as it has been shown to be as reliable and valid as the SOC-29 (Feldt et al., 2007).

Reliability

Evidence supports the reliability of both the SOC-29 and SOC-13 (Feldt et al., 2007). Eriksson and Lindström (2005) reported Cronbach's alpha internal consistency coefficients that ranged from

0.70 to 0.95 from 124 studies using the SOC-29, and from 0.70 to 0.92 from 127 studies using the SOC-13. Test-retest reliability of both scales has been reported and overall scores are satisfactory (Eriksson & Lindström, 2005).

Validity and Stability

The SOC is an abstract construct. Antonovsky (1993) stressed that there is no "gold standard" against which to compare the SOC construct. A large number of empirical studies, however, have examined whether the SOC-29 and the SOC-13 measure what they purport to measure. Recent literature reported significant support for content, criterion, and predictive validity of both measures (Bengtsson-Tops & Hansson, 2001; Eriksson & Lindström, 2005; Wainwright et al., 2007). Overall the SOC-13 and SOC-29 were found to be valid tools to measure factors which affect health, health potential, well-being, and movement toward greater health (Becker, Glascoff, & Felts, 2010; Ing & Reutter, 2003).

An area worth noting is the high bivariate correlations (average correlation = 0.88) among the three SOC factors—comprehensibility, manageability, and meaningfulness. This inhibits the ability to use the factors as separate indicators (C. G. Richardson, Ratner, & Zumbo, 2007). Individual items were selected by Antonovsky and colleagues on the basis that each "referred cleanly to one and only one of the three SOC components" (Antonovsky, 1993, p. 727). This approach might be expected to produce a measure with three identifiable subscales. However, factor analyses carried out by Antonovsky (1993) and others (Hawley, Wolfe, & Cathey, 1992; Hittner, 2007; Sandell, Blomberg, & Lazar, 1998) have failed to demonstrate support for individual subscales. Eriksson and Lindström (2005) explain that the SOC is a multidimensional concept—and to be used as Antonovsky intended, "a measurement of the whole" (p. 462). Therefore, use of the total SOC score is recommended, and the use of individual subscale scores is discouraged (Feldt et al., 2007).

Perhaps the only enduring shortcoming of the SOC-13 and SOC-29 is a relatively low explained variance in respondents' scores accounted for by the factor solutions. Eriksson and Lindström's (2005) systematic review reported approximately 50% of the variance explained, with the remaining variance unexplained.

Despite the outstanding concern of unexplained variance, researchers report Antonovsky's measures of SOC to be "psychometrically comparatively sound," reliable, valid, feasible, and cross-culturally valid (Eriksson & Lindström, 2005; Harri, 1998; Myrin & Lagerström, 2008). It has been proposed there is no need to further validate the SOC-13 or SOC-29. Rather, investigators are urged to implement the construct and the model into clinical practice and policy (Becker et al., 2010; Eriksson & Lindström, 2005).

LOGICAL AND EMPIRICAL ADEQUACY OF THE SALUTOGENIC MODEL

The structure of the salutogenic model (Antonovsky, 1979, 1987) appears to meet criteria proposed by Walker and Avant (1995) for logical adequacy of a model or theory. The salutogenic model appears logical and has been used in a variety of health-related disciplines including nursing, medicine, psychology, psychiatry, sociology, community health and epidemiology, and public health to generate relatively precise research questions and testable hypotheses. The content of the model intuitively "makes sense" and is consistent with, or draws on, related theory and research of other highly regarded scientists and social scientists of this time period.

The salutogenic model has been examined and used to the greatest extent by psychologists and public health researchers, and to a lesser extent by nurse researchers. Published empirical findings from psychological research and other, allied health disciplines, differ from work reported by nurse researchers in the following ways: (a) samples have often been drawn from community-based populations, (b) research designs have featured more control and internal validity (longitudinal designs were more common), and (c) measurement and theoretical issues have received more attention. These differences will be illustrated through select allied health examples of empirical examinations of the salutogenic model and specifically the SOC construct.

Allied health researchers have primarily drawn samples from community-based populations to evaluate the SOC construct. Sampling within the general, community-based population is meaningful to capture a stratified representative of the population. For example, neurobiologists Myrin and Lagerström (2008) designed a cross-sectional study with students from six schools in different socioeconomic areas in Stockholm, Sweden (n = 196 girls and n = 187 boys). Multivariate analyses significantly associated the following variables with a low SOC: life dissatisfaction, depression, worries about family, poor psychosomatic health, and being female.

Family medicine researchers Honkinen et al. (2009) conducted a longitudinal, 15-year follow-up study with parents and their children. This study examined psychological and psychopathological symptoms in childhood and whether they predicted a poor SOC in late adolescence. Measurement points were at birth and at ages 3, 12, 15, and 18. A total of 1,086 families were enrolled in the study when their children were 3 years of age. By the end of the study period, 787 parents and 792 adolescents remained in the study. Honkinen et al. (2009) reported that symptoms such as destructive behavior at age three (p = .004), attention problems and aggression at age 12 (p < .001), and anxiety and depression at age 15 (p < .001) all correlated with a lower SOC at age 18 (Honkinen et al., 2009). Consistent with the salutogenic model, negative relationships were supported between SOC, distress, and psychological symptomatology in a community-based sample.

From psychology and psychiatry, Schmitt et al. (2008) carried out a comparative study between cancer patient families (n = 214) and a healthy family control group (n = 170). Through multivariate analysis, with control of potential confounding factors, factors associated with family functioning, including SOC, were evaluated. No statistically significant differences were reported between the clinical sample and the control group for SOC.

Longitudinal designs have been more common with psychologists seeking to validate the SOC construct. For example, Finnish psychologists Vastamäki, Moser, and Ingmar Paul (2009) collected longitudinal data with the SOC-13 questionnaire. Participants (n = 74) were involved in a short-term and long-term unemployment intervention program. Vastamäki et al. (2009) reported significant changes in SOC, correlated to periods of employment and unemployment measured at baseline (T1) and 6 months post-intervention follow-up (T2).

Binary correlations showed that an individual's SOC was significantly strengthened at T2; the mean SOC score increased 3.83 points (p < .01) after the intervention. Limitations of this study are a lack of a control group and a smaller sample size; however, Vastamäki et al. (2009) were able to demonstrate considerable validity through normed comparison contrasts, secondary source contrasts, and nonequivalent dependent variables. Furthermore, their longitudinal design provided an understanding of how the SOC may develop in response to changes in adults' employment status.

Finally, measurement and theoretical issues of the SOC construct have received the most attention from psychologists and allied health researchers in the salutogenesis literature. Specifically, concerns around the variance of the SOC measure and the stability of the SOC construct have been emphasized.

Psychometric work led by psychologists has evaluated the distinctiveness of the SOC measure from other basic personality traits, such as extroversion and neuroticism. For example, psychologists Boscaglia and Clarke (2007) reported that SOC contributes uniquely to perceived health, over and above neuroticism, yet further longitudinal work is required to explore the clinical significance of these findings.

Systematic reviews and recent publications with inclusive samples have demonstrated that SOC is not as stable as Antonovsky initially anticipated (Eriksson & Lindström, 2005; B. Nilsson, Holmgren, Stegmayr, & Westman, 2003). Antonovsky initially anticipated SOC to stabilize around the age of 30 (Wolff & Ratner, 1999). The SOC appears to develop continually over most of the life-span, stabilizing late in adulthood (K. W. Nilsson, Leppert, Simonsson, & Starrin, 2010; Richardson et al., 2007). K. W. Nilsson et al. (2010) reported SOC did not stabilize until around age 70 in their random sample of 43,598 adult participants aged 18 to 85.

Researchers have found that psychological changes and significant negative life events can lower SOC, even in adulthood (Schnyder, Büchi, Sensky, & Klaghofer, 2000). Further, findings suggest that SOC is a stable construct for those with an initially high SOC and for those who have a stable life situation (B. Nilsson et al., 2003; Richardson & Ratner, 2005; Vastamäki et al., 2009). Individuals with an initially lower SOC appear to be especially susceptible to catastrophic life changes, such as a severe accident or financial challenges, which result in an even lower SOC score (Richardson & Ratner, 2005; Vastamäki et al., 2009). This aligns with Antonovsky's (1987) model which describes a person with a low SOC as more likely to become anxious and threatened in stressful situations.

Gender differences between SOC scores have also been recently reported. Numerous studies reported higher SOC scores in males (Hittner, 2007; K. W. Nilsson et al., 2010; Surtees, Wainwright, Luben, Khaw, & Day, 2003). Differences between men and women were usually smaller in adulthood (Eriksson & Lindström, 2005). Men have had scores ranging from 1 to 3 points higher than women in adulthood (K. W. Nilsson et al., 2010), while boys' SOC scores have been reported as many as 7 points higher than girls in childhood or adolescence (Myrin & Lagerström, 2008). Though these differences have statistical significance, 1 to 3 points are likely of little or no clinical significance.

Cross-cultural comparisons have not been measured to the extent of SOC development across age and gender. Even though 32 countries have applied the SOC questionnaires, there are few studies that have examined cultural stability and cross-cultural validation of the SOC construct. Bowman (1996, 1997) reported support for Antonovsky's (1987) expectation that cultural paths to the development of SOC will differ, yet similar levels of SOC will be attained with maturation. Bowman (1996) applied a correlational study design to compare a Native American sample (n = 81) and an Anglo-American sample (n = 105) and reported that these two different cultures can develop a similar level of SOC. Despite reporting significant differences in background information (socio-economic status and family of origin size), the mean SOC score for the Native American sample was 134.38 (SD = 24.64) and the mean score for the Anglo-American sample was 134.48 (SD = 21.61) (Bowman, 1996). A limitation of this study is that the mean age of the Native American sample was approximately 10 years older than the Anglo-American sample. Further longitudinal, cross-cultural comparisons would be beneficial. Particularly meaningful would be to cross-culturally compare the stability of SOC during negative life events in adulthood.

In summary, allied health research has evaluated the salutogenic model with an emphasis on community-based, healthy populations. Psychologists, in particular, have applied rigorous methods, including longitudinal designs and the use of controls. Further, psychological studies have most often identified concerns around the variance and stability of the SOC construct. SOC uniquely explains objective and subjective health, apart from variables such as neuroticism and extroversion, yet we do not have a strong empirical understanding of what this contribution entails. Further, SOC is not as stable as Antonovsky (1979) originally hypothesized. Psychologists have identified a gap in longitudinal, multivariate studies which take additional variables into account, such as neuroticism and significant negative life events in adulthood. These studies are needed to contribute an understanding of unaccounted for variance of the SOC measure and (in)stability of the SOC construct over the life span (Boscaglia & Clarke, 2007; Evans, Marsh, & Weigel, 2010).

EMPIRICAL ADEQUACY OF THE SALUTOGENIC MODEL IN NURSING RESEARCH

The empirical evidence garnered through nursing research is supportive of the salutogenic model, with some limitations; results are generally consistent with those of psychologists and other health-related disciplines previously reported. In general, nursing studies have primarily examined the model in clinical samples using descriptive, cross-sectional designs. Selected, recent nursing literature is evaluated in this section, documenting the empirical adequacy and relationships among concepts of the salutogenic model: GRR–RDs and SOC; SOC and symptoms and distress; SOC and tension management and coping behaviors; and SOC and subjective and objective health and well-being.

Generalized Resistance Resources and Deficits and the Sense of Coherence

The salutogenic model proposes that a strong SOC develops through successful applications of GRR–RDs over the life span. The relationship between GRR–RDs and the SOC is described as reciprocal and dynamic: Exposure to moderately stressful life events can enhance the development of GRR–RDs, thereby building SOC (Moons & Norekvål, 2006). Further, an initially strong SOC can trigger successful applications of GRR–RDs over time for effective problem solving and coping (Moons & Norekvål, 2006).

Nurse researchers have examined GRR–RDs, including spirituality, religion, social supports, material resources, income, and education. There are gaps in the evidence for some of Antonovsky's GRR–RDs, specifically genetic and constitutional factors (Eriksson & Lindström, 2005), and cultural factors (Gibson, 2003). Most recently, evaluations of the effectiveness of nursing interventions to mobilize GRR–RDs and enhance SOC have also been published. However, sampling has often failed to include highly vulnerable individuals lacking GRR–RDs, particularly across socioeconomic status and education levels. This is of concern, as it may be that the relationships of interest are most evident in these populations. Despite limitations, results to date continue to largely support empirical relationships between GRR–RDs and the SOC. There is further work to be accomplished in this area.

Numerous cross-sectional, correlational nursing studies have reported significant relationships between SOC and GRR–RDs, including social support (Wolff & Ratner, 1999), spirituality (Humphreys, 2000), education (Richardson, Adner, & Nordström, 2001), income (Leino-Loison, Gien, Katajisto, & Välimäki, 2004), and objective health (e.g., fatigue in Falk, Swedberg, Gaston-Johansson, & Ekman, 2007). Specifically, three recent studies have examined the relationship between SOC and GRR–RDs using descriptive correlational designs and bivariate analyses. First, Motzer, Hertig, Jarrett, and Heitkemper (2003) examined SOC and symptoms in adults with irritable bowel syndrome (IBS). Differences between women with ($n = 235$) and without IBS ($n = 89$) were examined. SOC scores were lower in women with IBS ($p < .001$), while women without IBS had higher levels of GRR–RDs, including satisfaction with physical health ($p < .001$), relationships with family or social support ($p = .002$), and learning or education ($p = .001$). The authors identified a need to examine these resources further, and reported that it was undetermined whether psychosocial interventions aimed at improving SOC and GRR–RDs would be effective for this population (Motzer et al., 2003).

Leino-Loison et al. (2004) studied SOC in unemployed nurses ($n = 183$). They reported income ($r = 0.21$, $P < .005$) and mental health resources ($r = -0.57$, $P < .0001$) had the greatest impact on nurses' SOC: A higher average family income and better state of mental health correlated with a higher SOC score during unemployment (Leino-Loison et al., 2004). The authors suggested that interventions, such as professional development workshops and opportunities to work abroad, may help unemployed nurses maintain a high SOC, mental confidence, and professionalism (Leino-Loison et al., 2004). Empirical evaluation of such interventions would be required.

The third descriptive, correlational study is from Fok, Chair, and Lopez (2005). They examined SOC in critically ill patients recently discharged from an intensive care unit ($n = 88$) in China. They reported GRR–RDs including higher household income (> $25,000) ($P = .04$) and social support from adult children ($P = .01$) significantly correlated to higher SOC scores. The authors recommend longitudinally examining SOC in a larger sample of critically ill patients. Fok et al. (2005) further recommend examining the effectiveness of nursing interventions targeted at improving SOC for critically ill individuals.

Most recently, Ekwall, Sivberg, and Hallberg (2007) examined older caregivers' coping strategies and SOC. Stronger SOC scores were correlated with better mental health ($p < .001$), those who were independent or "self-sustaining" ($P = .018$), and those who were better off economically ($P = .026$). This study found that a lack of social support was detrimental for individuals with caregiving responsibilities.

Stronger research methodologies have been recently used to examine GRR–RDs and SOC in adults with cancer. Koinberg, Languis-Eklöf, Holmberg, and Fridlund (2006) used a prospective, longitudinal study to examine the effectiveness of a multidisciplinary educational program (MEP) for women after breast cancer surgery. Fifty women participated in the MEP, while 46 (control group) participated in a traditional physician follow-up program. There were no statistically significant differences reported for the SOC scores at baseline or at 1 year follow-up for either the control or the study sample. Despite designing the program from a salutogenic perspective, this intervention aimed at improving knowledge resources did not improve overall SOC.

Another example is from nurse researchers Delbar and Benor (2001). They applied a quasi-experimental design to examine SOC and GRR–RDs in cancer patients ($n = 94$). The intervention group ($n = 48$) received additional support to enhance psychological, social, and cultural resources from nurses. Overall SOC was significantly increased in the intervention group ($p < .001$). Specifically, manageability ($p < .001$), meaningfulness ($p < .01$), and comprehensibility ($p < .01$) were all significantly increased after the intervention. Patients with an initially high SOC responded better to the intervention than those with initially lower scores. Familial resources including the dimensions of pain support ($p < .001$), psychological support ($p < .01$), social support ($p < .001$), and physical support ($p < .05$), all correlated with SOC. Further, knowledge resources for pain ($p < .01$), psychological understanding ($p < .01$), and social understanding ($p < .05$) had a beneficial relationship with SOC. The strength of this study was a stronger experimental, longitudinal design. The intervention was also modeled after the key concepts within the SOC construct.

This body of nursing literature has identified significant relationships between GRR–RDs and the SOC. However, it is difficult to aggregate findings across nursing studies because researchers have used varying sample populations and measures of GRR–RDs. Multivariate, prospective designs provide a richer understanding of the interplay of GRR–RDs—particularly as these may be related to specific disease states and disease trajectories. It would be important to establish the clinical relevance of a weak SOC. Is there a point below which children, youth, and adults are particularly vulnerable and prone to poor outcomes when faced with a chronic illness or disability? Are some GRR–RDs more salient to patient outcomes than others, and if so, how might nursing interventions be designed to reflect these differences? Much work remains to be done in these areas.

Antonovsky (1996) emphasized that effective interventions should be guided by the SOC construct, aiming to strengthen comprehensibility, manageability, and/or meaningfulness of life experiences. Further, he proposed that interventions should be guided by the model, for example, by holistically viewing the individual beyond their disease and by seeking to strengthen the individual's capacity to understand their total life situation as "making sense." For example, Langeland, Wahl, Kristoffersen, and Hanestad (2007) published a theoretical, salutogenic intervention to promote SOC, coping, and mental health in individuals with mental health disability. Therapy sessions, consisting of story sharing and strategizing, were implemented to enhance SOC and mobilize GRRs. The authors identified crucial GRRs to effective tension management as including material, relational, cultural, physical, biochemical, and attitudinal resources. The intervention they outlined prompted participants to describe their lives, reach a higher awareness of their situation, and come to reach recovery on their own terms (Langeland et al., 2007). At the time of publishing, this intervention had not been implemented and tested in clinical practice. However, it is an example of the rigorous use of Antonovsky's salutogenic theory, framework, and principles to guide development of a nursing intervention.

In summary, empirical examination of relationships between GRR–RDs and SOC are supported in nursing literature. Further empirical work is required to determine whether nursing interventions can enhance individuals' application of GRR–RDs and improve SOC and positive patient outcomes. To date there has not been a coherent program of research of sufficient substance to direct the allocation of nursing resources. A thorough examination of findings within the literature on "health equity" may provide relevant insights to those seeking to design helpful nursing interventions. Issues related to education, employment/poverty, and adequate housing are relevant to Antonovsky's (1979, 1987) notions of GRR–RDs, and these social determinants are increasingly being linked empirically to improved health outcomes for vulnerable populations across the life span and across cultures.

Relationships Between the Sense of Coherence and Symptoms and Distress

The salutogenic model (Antonovsky, 1979, 1987) proposes a positive relationship between SOC and an individual's perception of symptoms and distress. Antonovsky (1987) notes that "the person with a strong SOC is more likely to define stimuli as non-stressors" (p. 132). Furthermore, when a stimulus is appraised as a stressor, it is likely to be viewed as less burdensome by persons with a strong SOC.

The empirical findings in recent nursing literature are largely supportive of the hypothesized relationship between a low SOC and distress. In general, individuals with a stronger SOC have reported lower distress. Yet, results of investigations of the relationship between SOC and stress-related symptomology (distress) have been mixed. In general, a higher SOC has been related with lower stress-related symptoms (distress) in community-based samples. However with samples of clinical participants, SOC has been correlated with symptomology in participants with some clinical conditions, but not others. Further work is warranted, including systematic, prospective, longitudinal evaluations comparing the relationship between SOC and stress-related symptomology amongst participants with the same disease state, across the disease trajectory.

Harri (1998) examined SOC in a healthy sample of nurse educators ($n = 477$). Using multiple regression analysis, significant relationships between SOC and negative stress ($P < .001$), as well as between SOC and symptoms of diseases ($P < .001$) were reported. Nurse educators with a high SOC reported significantly lower symptoms of disease and lower levels of stress.

Similar findings were reported using a large Canadian sample. Wolff and Ratner (1999) carried out a secondary analysis of stress data from the 1994 Canadian National Population Health Survey ($n = 20,725$). A random sample of participants ($n = 17,626$) were selected to complete the SOC questionnaire. Negative correlations between SOC and both chronic stress ($p < .01$) and personal stress ($p < .01$) were reported. Individuals with higher personal and chronic stress had a lower SOC.

In a clinical, descriptive correlational study, A. Richardson et al. (2001) reported relationships between symptoms and SOC with a random sample of 107 insulin-dependent, diabetic participants. SOC was significantly stronger for participants with only one or no complications associated with their diabetes ($P < .05$). SOC was not significantly correlated with objective, metabolic control data.

Motzer et al. (2003) similarly examined SOC, symptoms, and distress in women with and without irritable bowel syndrome (IBS). SOC was significantly lower in women with (IBS) than the healthy controls ($P < .001$). A moderate negative relationship between SOC and psychological distress was reported. Weak relationships were reported between SOC and the stress-related symptoms of alternating constipation and diarrhea, while having a regular bowel cycle was strongly correlated with a higher SOC ($P < .001$) (Motzer et al., 2003).

Falk et al. (2007) used multiple regression analysis to examine the relationship between SOC and symptoms of fatigue in adults with chronic heart failure ($n = 96$). Together, SOC and the New York Heart Association functional classification criteria explained 31% of the variance in reported fatigue, with SOC accounting for 20%. Participants with chronic heart failure and a low SOC reported difficulty concentrating and were especially affected by mental fatigue causing distress (Falk et al., 2007).

Weissbecker et al. (2002) employed a prospective randomized trial to explore SOC and distress in 91 women with fibromyalgia. This study provided rigorous evidence linking SOC and reported stress/distress. Individuals with a strong SOC reported significantly less stress ($r = \sim.64$, $p < .01$) and depression ($r = \sim.65$, $p < .01$). However, no relationship was supported between SOC and fibromyalgia symptoms or bodily functioning.

Delbar and Benor (2001) used a quasi-experimental study to examine the relationships between SOC and symptoms in cancer patients ($n = 94$). Before the intervention, negative relationships were reported between SOC and the intensity of 16 symptoms measured by a symptom control assessment tool. The assessment tool included basic universal symptoms as well as additional items, including health-pain, anxiety, self-image, and sexuality (Delbar & Benor, 2001). Intensity of symptoms, including pain ($p < .03$), psychological symptoms ($p < .001$), and social symptoms ($p < .001$) were negatively correlated with SOC.

In summary, empirical nursing research generally supports the hypothesized benefit of a strong SOC on individuals' perceptions of distress. Empirical evidence for the relationship between SOC and disease symptoms and objective indicators of disease management are inconclusive.

Relationship Between the Sense of Coherence and Tension Management and Coping Behaviors

The salutogenic model proposes a positive relationship between SOC and individual coping behavior or tension management. When confronted with an acute or chronic stressor, a person with a stronger SOC "is more likely to respond behaviorally with adaptive health behavior" (Antonovsky, 1987, p. 153). The benefit of a stronger SOC on coping has been examined in nursing studies, and results are supportive. In general, individuals with a stronger SOC reported "better" coping behavior or tension management. Most of the research in this area has focused on adult clinical populations using descriptive, correlational, cross-sectional designs. Additional longitudinal and experimental studies are needed to further examine coping behavior in both healthy and clinical populations, as well as in children and youth. Furthermore, piloting the SOC scale as a clinical indicator may help to identity individuals with a clinically relevant SOC who are at risk for poor coping and tension management.

Richardson et al. (2001) described relationships between coping and SOC in a random sample of 107 individuals diagnosed with insulin-dependent diabetes mellitus. In this descriptive study, higher SOC scores significantly correlated with greater disease acceptance ($P < .001$). The authors indicated that individuals with a stronger degree of acceptance reported more ability to cope with this condition. Richardson et al. (2001) recommended that nurses use the SOC scale as a clinical indicator to identify patients' ability to accept and cope with chronic diseases.

Nurse researchers Fok et al. (2005) examined SOC in a Chinese sample of critically ill, adult patients coping after a chronic illness ($n = 88$). In their descriptive, correlational study, patients with a higher SOC reported a greater ability to cope with illness-related stress after discharge. The authors recommended that prior to discharge, nurses assess patients' SOC and abilities; they also urged the development of nurse interventions to enhance coping skills for individuals experiencing a high severity of illness (Fok et al., 2005).

In a cross-sectional study, Ekwall et al. (2007) examined older caregiver's ($n = 171$) coping strategies and SOC. Caregivers with a high SOC were better able to cope and "handle demanding situations" (p. 592). Further, caregivers with a lower SOC were discussed as most vulnerable to burnout and strain, therefore needing enhanced caregiving supports and education on coping strategies (Ekwall et al., 2007).

SOC and coping behaviors are empirically linked, particularly in relation to health-related behaviors of interest to nursing (e.g., self-care, care giving, and quality of life). Longitudinal, multivariate, cohort designs that consider these relationships across the life span and illness trajectories in clinical populations would be particularly useful. It would be desirable to measure relevant GRR–RDs within these studies, so that the relationships among GRR–RDs, the SOC, coping, and stress-related symptoms can be examined together; the inclusion of objective measures of disease management, and cost–benefit analyses, would further strengthen the relevance of findings—particularly in the current climate of fiscal restraint.

Relationships Among the Sense of Coherence, Subjective and Objective Health, and Well-Being

The salutogenic model (Antonovsky, 1979, 1987) states that by managing tension and coping well with stress, the person with a strong SOC will "reinforce or improve his or her health status" (1987, p. 152). Hence, a positive relationship between SOC and health and well-being is posited.

Numerous studies, nursing and non-nursing, have examined the hypothesized relationship between SOC and subjective/objective health. SOC is empirically linked to perceived health and mental health in particular. Eriksson and Lindström's (2006) systematic review of the SOC–health relationship found 458 relevant scientific articles and 13 relevant theses. Overall, a strong SOC correlated with positive perceived health, regardless of age, sex, ethnicity, and nationality (Eriksson & Lindström, 2006). SOC was found to predict and protect health, although it is unsure where the threshold lies and where SOC loses this capacity. Eriksson and Lindström (2006) agree with criticisms to the model that SOC does not completely explain overall health, and they agree that other factors play a role (e.g., mastery, inner strength, resiliency, and hardiness). Still, Eriksson and Lindström concluded that the SOC plays a unique, comprehensive, salutary role in explaining the development and maintenance of health and well-being. They also concluded that the SOC concept provides a unique contribution to understanding health promotion (Eriksson & Lindström, 2006). Selected nursing empirical examinations are now presented that illustrate this area of inquiry.

Nurse researchers Berglund, Mattiasson, and Nordström (2003) used a correlational study to assess functional health status and SOC in 77 individuals with a rare genetic connective tissue disorder, Ehlers-Danlos syndrome ($n = 77$). A strong SOC was correlated with better functional health status ($p < .05$) and better psychosocial health ($p < .01$). The authors encouraged nurses to engage in health promotion and assess the factors that impact overall health. Identifying individuals with a low SOC was encouraged, in order to provide enhanced supports for better functioning and overall health for this population (Berglund et al., 2003).

Cole (2007) described the SOC and functional health status of residents of nursing homes. Measurements were taken at baseline (T1) and 10 to 12 weeks follow-up (T2) to examine functional decline. Pearson product correlations supported a significant relationship between SOC and functional health status at T2 ($p = .039$). Functional status of individuals with a lower SOC at T1 was found to decline at T2. Although not significant, individuals with a stronger SOC at T1 had a slightly improved mean functional health score at T2. This study suggested that residents with lower SOC scores are at a higher risk for functional health decline.

Drageset et al. (2009) used a cross-sectional, descriptive, correlational design to examine SOC and subjective and objective health as measured by the SF-36 Health Survey. The SF-36 examines physical, mental, and general health, as well as bodily pain, role limitation due to physical and emotional problems, social functioning, and vitality. They sampled 20 nursing homes in western Norway and obtained questionnaires from 227 long-term nursing home residents aged 65 and older. The SOC-13 was correlated with all SF-36 subscales ($p < .0001$); stronger SOCs were related to fewer limitations and higher function.

As these studies suggest, empirical support for the relationship between SOC and self-perceived health and well-being is strong. However, psychometric work is warranted to examine the unique contribution of SOC on health, compared to other similar constructs such as mastery, hardiness, neuroticism, and other personality traits and states (see Forbes, 2001). Further work is also warranted to study the threshold where SOC no longer protects and predicts health; it is quite likely that at least some of these relationships are not linear—and

may be manifested primarily below or above some "threshold." As noted previously, longitudinal, health-promotion nursing interventions aimed at increasing SOC and facilitating disease acceptance, management, and positive health behavior are an identified direction for contemporary nursing research (Koinberg et al., 2006; Langeland et al., 2007; Wainwright et al., 2007).

USEFULNESS OF THE SALUTOGENIC MODEL IN NURSING

The current and future usefulness of the salutogenic model is somewhat limited by issues of stability and persistent, unexplained variance in the central construct, SOC (Lindström & Eriksson, 2006). There is a need to differentiate SOC from similar phenomena, such as neuroticism, hardiness, self-efficacy, self-transcendence, hope, inner strength, and life satisfaction (Lindström & Eriksson, 2006; Lundman et al., 2010; Sullivan, 1993). Comparative studies that examine the relative contribution of these constructs to outcomes of interest for nursing are imperative because it makes little sense to fund two or more research programs if the central constructs of these programs cannot be meaningfully distinguished from one another. Further, discrepancies in the literature for SOC stability across age, gender, culture, and during significant negative life events indicates a need for rigorous comparative research (Bruscia, Shultis, Dennery, & Dileo, 2008; K. W. Nilsson et al., 2010).

The most prominent issue affecting the current and future usefulness of the salutogenic model is its application and evaluation in clinical nursing practice (Lindström & Eriksson, 2006). Many authors have stressed the need for practical implementation and evaluation of the salutogenesis framework in real-life scenarios (Morrison, Stosz, & Clift, 2008). Becker et al. (2010) suggested that the "time has come for more salutogenic thinking, research and practices" (p. 4). The future usefulness of the model appears to rely on nurses using the SOC as a clinical indicator and applying the salutogenic model as a framework for clinical interventions.

Nurses can mediate the link between health and stressful circumstances by applying the salutogenic model in nursing practice, education, and research. Antonovsky did not overtly define or recognize nursing in his model—though nursing is recognized as a GRR in recent literature (Menzies, 2000; Sullivan, 1989). Nurses have the ability to protect against stressors, aid in managing tension, and promote positive health practices.

All nurses have encountered clients who have reached higher levels of health and well-being despite severe adversity (e.g., chronic illness, poverty, and war). The salutogenic model (Antonovsky, 1979, 1987), which is based on human strengths rather than weaknesses, frames a revolutionary perspective and possesses intuitive appeal. It is not surprising that it continues to receive attention within nursing.

The GRR–RDs support a multicausal perspective that recognizes the contributions of cultural, historical, psychosocial, spiritual, and biological factors to health. This broad perspective reminds nurses that issues of war, unemployment, education, housing, cultural instability, and poverty are integral to health promotion and disease prevention and supports a renewed impetus for social activism within the nursing profession.

The salutogenic model (Antonovsky, 1979, 1987) stresses the importance of fostering a strong sense of coherence during childhood and adolescence. It supports diverse health-promotion programs across the life span and for clinical populations—across the illness trajectory. Although the model suggests that nursing interventions to facilitate a strong SOC in older adults will have limited impact, it urges the identification of adults who are at risk for poor tension management, stress, and negative health outcomes. The SOC scale has been suggested as a highly useful clinical indicator to identify vulnerable subpopulations. Individuals with a weak SOC may be identified and offered more supportive nursing interventions (e.g., counseling, behavior management, emotional support, home follow-up) maintained over longer periods of time. Likewise, individuals with a strong SOC may be effectively managed through technology-mediated self-management programs and virtual, online supportive communities.

GENERALIZABILITY OF THE SALUTOGENIC MODEL IN NURSING

Overall, generalizability of the salutogenic model in nursing includes reasonably sentient children, youth, and adults across cultures—inclusive of both community-based and clinical populations. Research has shown the importance of childhood levels of GRR–RDs and how they impact a strong SOC in adolescence and adulthood. A strong SOC has been linked to tension and stress management processes as well as both subjective and objective health and placement on the ease/dis-ease continuum. The salutogenic model suggests that nursing and allied health interventions, targeted toward enhancing childhood exposure to positive GRR–RDs, may be particularly useful in promoting healthy lifestyles and healthy populations. More research is needed to examine the model with populations evidencing low levels of generalized resistance resources (e.g., material resources and knowledge and intelligence). This is an important gap because GRR–RDs may negatively influence SOC and placement on the ease/dis-ease continuum primarily when they are manifested at low levels.

The salutogenic model has been studied around the world. A remaining gap is to examine genetic and constitutional factors in relation to the other GRR–RDs and the development of the SOC—particularly as genomics and personalized medicine are predicted to play an ever-increasing role in health care over the coming decades. Indeed, cross-disciplinary work that brings together researchers across the basic, clinical and social/population–health sciences may be best positioned to carry out such work. New, longitudinal panel studies such as the Canadian Longitudinal Study of Aging and the Canadian Cancer Research Alliance present excellent opportunities to examine the salutogenic model in concert with other, rival theoretical perspectives, to begin to develop more parsimonious, measurable models comprised of a manageable number of relatively orthogonal constructs that will account for at least ~70% of the variance in subjective and objective outcomes of importance to nursing and of importance to the communities nurses care for.

PARSIMONY OF THE SALUTOGENIC MODEL

The salutogenic model (Antonovsky, 1979, 1987), as depicted in Figure 8.1, is not parsimonious. Because the model seeks to explain complex and abstract human phenomena, however, a high degree of complexity is not surprising.

Antonovsky's work has yielded many testable hypotheses with a high degree of relevance for nursing. As noted previously, the major barrier to the determination of the heuristic relevance of the model, and its further development, is the need for practical applications of the model. It can be anticipated that applied research efforts devoted to this issue will yield high dividends for nursing practice and health promotion as the nursing profession, and other health professions, seek to understand factors that facilitate human health and well-being in the face of life stress.

References

Antonovsky, A. (1972). Breakdown: A needed fourth step in the conceptual armamentarium of modern medicine. *Social Science and Medicine, 6*, 537–544.

Antonovsky, A. (1979). *Health, stress, and coping.* San Francisco, CA: Jossey-Bass.

Antonovsky, A. (1987). *Unraveling the mystery of health: How people manage stress and stay well,* San Francisco, CA: Jossey-Bass.

Antonovsky, A. (1993). The structure and properties of the sense of coherence scale. *Social Science Medicine, 36*, 725–733.

Antonovsky, A. (1996). The salutogenic model as a theory to guide health promotion. *Health Promotion International, 11*(1), 11–18.

Becker, C., Glascoff, M. A., & Felts, W. M. (2010). Salutogenesis 30 years later: Where do we go from here? *International Electronic Journal of Health Education, 13*, 25–32.

Bengtsson-Tops, A., & Hansson, L. (2001). The validity of Antonovsky's Sense of Coherence measure in a sample of schizophrenic patients living in the community. *Journal of Advanced Nursing, 33*(4), 432–438.

Berglund, B., Mattiasson, A.-C., & Nordström, G. (2003). Acceptance of disability and sense of coherence in individuals with Ehlers-Danlos syndrome. *Journal of Clinical Nursing, 12*, 770–777.

Boscaglia, N., & Clarke, D. M. (2007). Sense of coherence as a protective factor for demoralisation in women with a recent diagnosis of gynaecological cancer. *Psycho-Oncology, 16*, 189–195.

Bowman, B. J. (1996). Cross-cultural validation of Antonovsky's sense of coherence scale. *Journal of Clinical Psychology, 52*(5), 547–549.

Bowman, B. J. (1997). Cultural pathways toward Antonovsky's sense of coherence. *Journal of Clinical Psychology, 53*(2), 139–142.

Bronikowski, M., & Bronikowska, M. (2009). Salutogenesis as a framework for improving health resources of adolescent boys. *Scandinavian Journal of Public Health, 37*, 525–531.

Bruscia, K., Shultis, C., Dennery, K., & Dileo, C. (2008). The sense of coherence in hospitalized cardiac and cancer patients. *Journal of Holistic Nursing, 26*, 286–294.

Cole, C. S. (2007). Nursing home residents sense of coherence and functional status decline. *Journal of Holistic Nursing, 25*(2), 96–103.

Delbar, V., & Benor, D. E. (2001). Impact of a nursing intervention on cancer patients' ability to cope. *Journal of Psychosocial Oncology, 19*(2), 57–75.

Drageset, J., Eide, G. E., Nygaard, H. A., Bondevik, M., Nortvedt, M. W., & Natvig, G. K. (2009). The impact of social support and sense of coherence on health-related quality of life among nursing home residents—A questionnaire survey in Bergen, Norway. *International Journal of Nursing Studies, 46*, 66–76.

Dubos, R. J. (1960). *The mirage of health.* London, England: Allen & Unwin.

Dubos, R. J. (1968). *Man, medicine and environment.* New York, NY: Praeger.

Ekman, I., Fagerberg, B., & Lundman, B. (2002). Health-related quality of life and sense of coherence among elderly patients with severe chronic heart failure in comparison with healthy controls. *Heart & Lung, 31*(2), 94–101.

Ekwall, A. K., Sivberg, B., & Hallberg, I. R. (2007). Older caregivers' coping strategies and sense of coherence in relation to quality of life. *Journal of Advanced Nursing, 57*(6), 584–596.

Eriksson, M., & Lindström, B. (2005). Validity of Antonovsky's sense of coherence scale: A systematic review. *Journal of Epidemiology & Community Health, 59*, 460–466.

Eriksson, M., & Lindström, B. (2006). Antonovsky's sense of coherence scale and the relation with health: A systematic review. *Journal of Epidemiology & Community Health, 60*, 376–381.

Evans, W. P., Marsh, S. C., & Weigel, D. J. (2010). Promoting adolescent sense of coherence: Testing models of risk, protection, and resiliency. *Journal of Community & Applied Social Psychology, 20*, 30–43.

Falk, K., Swedberg, K., Gaston-Johansson, F., & Ekman, I. (2007). Fatigue is prevalent and severe symptom associated with uncertainty and sense of coherence in patients with chronic heart failure. *European Journal of Cardiovascular Nursing, 6*, 99–104.

Feldt, T., Lintula, H., Suominen, S., Koskenvuo, M., Vahtera, J., & Kivimäki, M. (2007). Structural validity and temporal stability of the 13-item sense of coherence scale: Prospective evidence from the population-based HeSSup Study. *Quality of Life Research, 16,* 483–493.

Fok, S. K., Chair, S. Y., & Lopez, V. (2005). Sense of coherence, coping and quality of life following critical illness. *Journal of Advanced Nursing, 49*(2), 173–181.

Forbes, D. A. (2001). Enhancing mastery and sense of coherence: important determinants of health in older adults. *Geriatric Nursing, 22*(1), 29–32.

Frankl, V. E. (1959). *Man's search for meaning.* New York, NY: Washington Square Press.

Gibson, L. M. (2003). Inter-relationships among sense of coherence, hope, and spiritual perspective (inner resources) of African-American and European-American breast cancer survivors. *Applied Nursing Research, 16*(4), 236–244.

Gustavsson-Lilius, M., Julkunen, J., Keskivaara, P., & Hietanen, P. (2007). Sense of coherence and distress in cancer patients and their partners. *Psycho-Oncology, 16,* 1100–1110.

Harri, M. (1998). The sense of coherence among nurse educators in Finland. *Nurse Education Today, 18,* 202–212.

Hawley, D. J., Wolfe, F., & Cathey, M. A. (1992). The Sense of Coherence Questionnaire in patients with rheumatic disorders. *Journal of Rheumatology, 19,* 1912–1918.

Hittner, J. B. (2007). Factorial invariance of the 13-item sense of coherence scale across gender. *Journal of Health Psychology, 12*(2), 273–280.

Honkinen, P., Aromaa, M., Suominen, S., Rautava, P., Sourander, A., Helenius, H., & Sillanpaa, M. (2009). Early childhood psychological problems predict a poor sense of coherence in adolescents: A 15-year follow-up study. *Journal of Health Psychology, 14*(4), 587–600.

Honkinen, P. K., Suominen, S. B., Välimaa, R. S., Helenius, H. Y., & Rautava, P. T. (2005). Factors associated with perceived health among 12-year-old school children. Relevance of physical exercise and sense of coherence. *Scandinavian Journal of Public Health, 33*(1), 35–41.

Horsburgh, M. E. (2000). Salutogenesis: Origins of Health and Sense of Coherence. In V. H. Rice (Ed.), *Handbook of stress, coping, and health: Implications for nursing research, theory, and practice* (pp. 175–194). Thousand Oaks, CA: Sage.

Humphreys, J. (2000). Spirituality and distress in sheltered battered women. *Journal of Nursing Scholarship, 32*(3), 273–278.

Ing, J. D., & Reutter, L. (2003). Socioeconomic status, sense of coherence and health in Canadian women. *Canadian Journal of Public Health, 94*(3), 224–228.

Koinberg, I., Languis-Eklöf, A., Holmberg, L., & Fridlund, B. (2006). The usefulness of a multidisciplinary educational programme after breast cancer surgery: A prospective and comparative study. *European Journal of Oncology Nursing, 10,* 273–282.

Langeland, E., Wahl, A. K., Kristoffersen, K., & Hanestad, B. R. (2007). Promoting coping: Salutogenesis among people with mental health problems. *Issues in Mental Health Nursing, 28,* 275–295.

Lazarus, R. S., & Folkman, S. (1984). *Stress, appraisal, and coping.* New York, NY: Springer.

Leino-Loison, K., Gien, L. T., Katajisto, J., & Välimäki, M. (2004). Sense of coherence among unemployed nurses. *Journal of Advanced Nursing, 48*(4), 413–422.

Lindström, B., & Eriksson, M. (2006). Contextualizing salutogenesis and Antonovsky in public health development. *Health Promotion International, 21*(3), 238–244.

Lundman, B., Aléx, L., Jonsén, E., Norberg, A., Nygren, B., Santamäki Fischer, R., & Strandberg, G. (2010). Inner strength—A theoretical analysis of salutogenic concepts. *International Journal of Nursing Studies, 47,* 251–260.

Menzies, V. (2000). Depression in schizophrenia: nursing care as a generalized resistance resource. *Issues in Mental Health Nursing, 21,* 605–617.

Moons, P., & Norekvål, T. M. (2006). Is sense of coherence a pathway for improving the quality of life of patients who grow up with chronic diseases? *European Journal of Cardiovascular Nursing, 5,* 16–20.

Morrison, I., Stosz, L. M., & Clift, S. M. (2008). An evidence base for mental health promotion through supported education: A practical application of Antonovsky's salutogenic model of health. *International Journal of Health Promotion & Education, 46*(1), 11–20.

Motzer, S. A., Hertig, V., Jarrett, M., & Heitkemper, M. M. (2003). Sense of coherence and quality of life in women with and without irritable bowel syndrome. *Nursing Research, 52*(5), 329–337.

Myrin, B., & Lagerström, M. (2008). Sense of coherence and psychosocial factors among adolescents. *Acta Paediatrica, 97,* 805–811.

Nilsson, B., Holmgren, L., Stegmayr, B., & Westman, G. (2003). Sense of coherence—stability over time and relation to health, disease, and psychological changes in a general population: A longitudinal study. *Scandinavian Journal of Public Health, 31,* 297–304.

Nilsson, K. W., Leppert, J., Simonsson, B., & Starrin, B. (2010). Sense of coherence and psychological well-being: Improvement with age. *Journal of Epidemiology & Community Health, 64,* 347–352.

Olsson, M., Gassne, J., & Hansson, K. (2009). Do different scales measure the same construct? Three sense of coherence scales. *Journal of Epidemiology & Community Health, 63,* 166–167.

Rabin, S., Matalon, A., Maoz, B., & Shiber, A. (2005). Keeping doctors healthy: A salutogenic perspective. *Families, Systems, & Health, 23*(1), 94–102.

Richardson, A., Adner, N., & Nordström, G. (2001). Persons with insulin-dependent diabetes mellitus: Acceptance and coping ability. *Journal of Advanced Nursing, 33*(6), 758–763.

Richardson, C. G., & Ratner, P. A. (2005). Sense of coherence as a moderator of the effects of stressful life events on health. *Journal of Epidemiology & Community Health, 59,* 979–984.

Richardson, C. G., Ratner, P. A., & Zumbo, B. D. (2007). A test of the age-based measurement invariance and temporal stability of Antonovsky's sense of coherence scale. *Educational and Psychological Measurement, 67*(4), 679–696.

Ristkari, T., Sourander, A., Rønning, Piha, J., Kumpulainen, K., Tamminen, T., Moilanen, I., & Almqvist, F. (2009). Childhood psychopathology and sense of coherence at age 18: Findings from the Finnish from a boy to a man study. *Social Psychiatry and Psychiatric Epidemiology, 44,* 1097–1105.

Sandell, R., Blomberg, J., & Lazar, A. (1998). The factor structure of Antonovsky's sense of coherence scale in Swedish clinical and non-clinical samples. *Personality and Individual Differences, 24,* 710–711.

Schmitt, F., Santalahti, P., Saarelainen, S., Savonlahti, E., Romer, G., & Piha, J. (2008). Cancer families with children: factors associated with family functioning—a comparative study in Finland. *Psycho-Oncology, 17,* 363–372.

Schnyder, U., Büchi, S., Sensky, T., & Klaghofer, R. (2000). Antonovsky's Sense of Coherence: trait or state? *Psychotherapy and Psychosomatics 69,* 296–302.

Selye, H. (1956). *The stress of life.* New York, NY: McGraw-Hill.

Sullivan, G. C. (1989). Evaluating Antonovsky's salutogenic model for its adaptability to nursing. *Journal of Advanced Nursing, 14,* 336–342.

Sullivan, G. C. (1993). Towards clarification of convergent concepts: sense of coherence, will to meaning, locus of control, learned helplessness and hardiness. *Journal of Advanced Nursing, 18,* 1772–1778.

Surtees, P., Wainwright, N., Luben, R., Khaw, K.-T., & Day, N. (2003). Sense of coherence and mortality in men and women in the EPIC-Norfolk United Kingdom prospective cohort study. *American Journal of Epidemiology, 158*(12), 1202–1209.

Vastamäki, J., Moser, K., & Ingmar Paul, K. (2009). How stable is sense of coherence? Changes following an intervention for unemployed individuals. *Scandinavian Journal of Psychology, 50,* 161–171.

Wainwright, N. W. J., Surtees, P. G., Welch, A. A., Luben, R. N., Khaw, K., & Bingham, S. A. (2007). Healthy lifestyle choices: Could sense of coherence aid health promotion? *Journal of Epidemiology & Community Health, 61,* 871–876.

Walker, L. O., & Avant, K. C. (1995). *Strategies for theory construction in nursing* (3rd ed.). Norwalk, CT: Appleton & Lange.

Weissbecker, I., Salmon, P., Studts, J. L., Floyd, A. R., Dedert, E. A., & Sephton, S. E. (2002). Mindfulness-based stress reduction and sense of coherence among women with fibromyalgia. *Journal of Clinical Psychology in Medical Settings, 9*(4), 297–307.

Wolff, A. C., & Ratner, P. A. (1999). Stress, social support, and sense of coherence. *Western Journal of Nursing Research, 21*(2), 182–197.

Evolution of a Model of Stress, Coping, and Discrete Emotions

Richard S. Lazarus

Because I am writing for two kinds of readers in nursing, those who are familiar with my work and ideas and those who are not, what I present in this chapter follows a historical perspective of the emergence over the years of my basic ideas about psychosocial stress and emotion. Both of these topics also include the coping process as an essential component. The content of this chapter is divided into my early work and ideas (beginning in the 1950s), transitional views in the 1960s and 1970s (some of which occurred again quite recently), and present themes in the 1980s and 1990s (that flow from my increasing recognition that stress and emotion are two interdependent themes that should be combined as one). [Lastly, nursing research conducted in the last decade (2000–2010) using Lazarus's theoretical perspective will be identified.]

A fundamental theme of my approach is that stress and emotion can no longer be divided into two separate research and theoretical literatures (Lazarus, 1993). Readers interested in my latest views about stress and emotion, including my espousal of a narrative approach to research and theory in contrast to a system theory approach, should review my latest books (Lazarus, 1999; Lazarus & Lazarus, 1994).

Although first proposed in ancient Greece, cognitive-mediational approaches to the mind,

and my own views too, were greatly influenced by the work of a substantial number of distinguished modern psychologists. Largely oriented to personality, social, and clinical issues, two generations of psychological scholars deviated sharply from the radical behaviorist stance that had dominated and severely limited psychological theory and research for more than 50 years.

One generation, which included Gordon Allport, Kurt Lewin, Henry Murray, and Edward Tolman, articulated their main theoretical and metatheoretical outlooks in the 1930s. The second generation, which included Solomon Asch, Jerome Bruner, Harry Harlow, Fritz Heider, George Kelly, David McClelland, Gardner Murphy, Julian Rotter, Mutzafer Sherif, and Robert White, published their main work in the late 1940s and 1950s.

Both generations were enormously influential in moving many scientific scholars toward an approach to mind and behavior that was epistemologically more open and congenial to theory and inference and a wide variety of methodological approaches to obtaining knowledge. This also led to a more modern definition of psychology as the science of mind, which broke away from the severely constricting radical behavioristic-positivist tradition of defining it as the science of behavior.

Even this distinguished list of psychological mavericks is substantially incomplete because

---

EDITOR'S NOTE: Richard S. Lazarus died November 2002.

there were also many frankly phenomenological psychologists who had considerable influence in personality and clinical psychology in those days. Along with members of many deviant movements of European origin, such as the *'gestaltists'* and the *'existentialists';* these mavericks set the stage for renewed interest in cognitive mediation and value-expectancy theory.

MY EARLY WORK AND IDEAS

In this section, I discuss the origins and terminology of the appraisal construct and my version of appraisal and coping theory as applied to psychological stress. I will later show that these concepts—and that of relational meaning—are also central concepts in my motivational-cognitive-relational approach to the emotions, within which stress is properly encompassed.

In my earliest monograph dealing with stress and coping theory and research (Lazarus, 1966), appraisal was the centerpiece of my approach. At that time, stress had little if any cachet in social science; this was to change greatly, however, during the 1970s. Selye's (1956/1976) approach to physiological stress helped greatly to influence this change. Janis's (1951, 1958) works on the stress experienced by surgical patients had not yet achieved much notice but were to be treated later as classics. Mechanic's (1962/1978) monograph about students under stress also gained major attention in the 1970s. Although there had been important theoretical contributions even before the 1960s, such as those of Leeper (1948) and McReynolds (1956), emotion as a topic of research and theory burgeoned mainly during the 1980s and 1990s.

Origins and Terminology of the Appraisal Construct

How did appraisal first emerge as the main mediational construct of psychological stress and emotion? Because I am one of the earliest contributors, I first portray my role in this topic. I first began to think programmatically about individual differences in psychological stress in the early 1950s when my research was sponsored by the military and focused on the effects of stress on skilled performance. Early on, and based on research data, it seemed obvious that the arousal and effects of stress depended on how different individuals evaluated and coped with the personal significance of what was occurring.

I was greatly impressed by a World War II monograph written by two research-oriented psychiatrists, Grinker and Spiegel (1945), about how flight crews managed the constant stress of air battles and flak from antiaircraft guns on the ground. These authors were among the first to refer to "appraisal," although the term was employed only casually. They wrote,

> The emotional reaction aroused by a threat of loss is at first an undifferentiated combination of fear and anger, subjectively felt as increased tension, alertness, or awareness of danger. The whole organism is keyed up for trouble, a process whose physiological components have been well studied. Fear and anger are still undifferentiated, or at least mixed, as long as it is not known what action can be taken in the face of the threatened loss. If the loss can be averted, or the threat dealt with in active ways by being driven off or destroyed, aggressive activity accompanied by anger is called forth. This appraisal [italics added] of the situation requires mental activity involving judgment, discrimination, and choice of activity, based largely on past experience. (p. 122)

Appraisal aside, Grinker and Spiegel's (1945) monograph contains most of the important basic themes of a theory of stress and emotion. Their work is centered mainly on anger and fear, the characteristics of which are not typical of all emotions. Their approach centered on how soldiers construe what is happening to them, thereby adopting a phenomenological or subjective outlook. The authors' reference to actions that can be taken in the face of threat, and defense mechanisms implies the important role of coping.

One can see in the Grinker and Spiegel's (1945) work that stress and emotion concern the personal meaning of what was happening, which in military combat was the imminent danger of being killed or maimed. In addition, what a soldier could do to cope with this danger was severely constrained by debilitating guilt or shame about letting one's buddies down, the potential accusation of cowardice for refusing voluntarily to commit to battle, and the threat of punishment or death. Because this was an intractable conflict, the only viable way to escape was to depend on intra-psychic forms of coping, such as denial, avoidance, detachment, and magical thinking, which in those days were considered both pathological and pathogenic.

In a published review that emphasized the individual differences observed in stress research, Lazarus, Deese, and Osler (1952, p. 294) wrote that *"the situation will be more or less stressful for the individual members of the group, and it is likely that differences in the meaning of the situation will appear in [their] performance."* My concern with individual differences in motives, beliefs, coping, and relational meaning in the stress process was articulated often in those days and thereafter.

Lazarus, Deese, and Osler (1952, p. 295), for example, wrote that "stress occurs when a particular situation threatens the *attainment of some goal* [italics added]." Lazarus and Baker (1956a, p. 23) stated that stress and emotion depend on "the degree of *relevance of the situation to the motive state* [italics added]," which is a statement about the person-environment relationship. In another article, Lazarus and Baker (1956b, p. 267) wrote that "relatively few studies have attempted to define stress in terms of internal psychological processes which may vary from *individual to individual* [italics added] and which determine the *subjects' definition of the situation* [italics added]."

In those days, I made the same mistake that William James (1890) made in his discussion of the relationship of emotion to action—that is, I used the term "perception" instead of appraisal. Thus, Lazarus and Baker (1956a, p. 22) wrote that "psychological stress occurs when a situation is perceived as thwarting or potentially thwarting to some motive state, thus resulting in affective arousal and in the elicitation of *regulative processes* aimed at the management of the affect" (italics added). The expression "regulative processes" refers to coping.

The word *perception* is ambiguous because it does not explicitly indicate an evaluation of the personal significance of what is happening for well-being. *Apperception* would have been more apt because it implies thinking through the implications of an event. John Dewey (1894) was quite clear on this score, but William James (1890) failed to indicate that perception meant more than the mere registration of what is occurring.

One reason for the terminological lapse was the influence of the New Look movement. In its usage, the term perception was given much broader connotations than it had in classical perception psychology. When New Look psychologists spoke of perception, it also encompassed the personal meaning of what was being perceived. In other words, how people construe events was said to depend on variations in motivation and beliefs. Much more clearly than perception, the term *appraisal* connotes an evaluation of the significance to the individual of what is happening for well-being.

Influenced by Magda Arnold's (1960) monograph on emotion and personality, I first began to use *appraisal* for this evaluation in Lazarus (1964) and Speisman, Lazarus, Mordkoff, and Davison (1964). Arnold had developed an impressive programmatic case for a cognitive-mediational approach to the emotions, with appraisal being her central construct. Tolman's (1932) book—courageous in those days because it spoke of purposive behavior—preceded all other work in turning attention from a past-directed mind (centered on what had been learned) to a future-directed focus on the possible outcomes of motivated action.

Those who favor a cognitive-mediational approach must also recognize that Aristotle's (1941) *Rhetoric* more than 2,000 years ago applied this approach to many emotions in terms that seem remarkably modern. More than a century ago, Robertson (1877) also put the same basic ingredients together—namely, evaluative thought, motivation (or a personal stake), beliefs (or knowledge), and degree of excitement—in a *Rashomon*-like[1] description of individual differences in emotion. Robertson wrote,

> Four persons of much the same age and temperament are traveling in the same vehicle. At a particular stopping place it is intimated to them that a certain person has just died suddenly and unexpectedly. One of the company looks perfectly stolid. A second comprehends what has taken place, but is in no way affected. The third looks and evidently feels sad. The fourth is overwhelmed with grief which finds expression in tears, sobs, and exclamations. Whence the difference of the four individuals before us? In one respect they are all alike: An announcement has been made to them. The first is a foreigner and has not understood the communication. The second has never met with the deceased, and could have no special regard for him. The third had often met with him in

social intercourse and business transactions, and been led to cherish a great esteem for him. The fourth was the brother of the departed, and was bound to him by native affection and a thousand ties earlier and later. From such a case we may notice that [to experience an emotion] there is need first of some understanding or apprehension; the foreigner had no feeling because he had no idea or belief. We may observe further that there must secondly be an affection of some kind; for the stranger was not interested in the occurrence. The emotion flows forth from a well, and is strong in proportion to the waters; it is stronger in the brother than in the friend. It is evident, thirdly, that the persons affected are in a moved or excited state. A fourth peculiarity has appeared in the sadness of the countenance and the agitations of the bodily frame. Four elements have thus come forth to view. (p. 413)

The premise of appraisal theory is that people (and infrahuman animals) are constantly evaluating relationships with the environment with respect to their implications for personal well-being (Lazarus, 1981; Lazarus & Folkman, 1984; Lazarus & Launier, 1978). Although my theory is subjective in outlook, it is not classical phenomenology but a modified subjectivism. In my view of appraisal, people negotiate between two complementary frames of reference: First, wanting to view what is happening as realistically as possible to cope with it and, second, wanting to put the best possible light on events so as not to lose hope or sanguinity. In effect, appraisal is a compromise between life as it is and what one wishes it to be, and efficacious coping depends on both.

Dissident voices still argue against the scientific adequacy of a cognitive-mediational approach to stress and the emotions, thereby demonstrating what might be regarded as residual behaviorism. For example, Hobfoll (1998) has regularly expressed scientific disdain about a subjective epistemology and metatheory, even when it is only partial as in my version noted previously. This is evident in his emphasis on loss as an objective antecedent condition of stress and his principle of conservation of resources as the basis of stress. What is a loss, however, or a threat of loss is not adequately defined before the fact of the emotional reaction without reference to a person's values, goal

hierarchy, beliefs, resources, and coping styles and processes. What individuals consider important or unimportant to their well-being influences how emotionally devastating any loss will be and what coping choices must be made to manage it—therefore affecting the details of the observed emotional reaction and subjective experience. This is true even when loss is normatively defined, which refers, of course, to a collective average. With regard to any given individual rather than some epidemiological (probabilistic) estimate, an average value is of little predictive utility. The concept of loss without detailed specification of its personal significance for various individuals or types of individuals offers less precision than when personality is taken into account. Therefore, Hobfoll's (and anyone else's) claim that an analysis of stress in terms of objective stimulus conditions is more scientific than a cognitive-mediational analysis is specious.

About my own work with Folkman, and that of Bandura, Meichenbaum, and Seligman, Hobfoll (1998) writes,

> I argue against a strictly cognitive view of stress. I suggest from the outset that the cognitive revolution has misled us in our understanding of the stress process. But this should not be construed to mean that elements of the stress phenomenon are not cognitive, or that cognitive psychology does not provide valuable insights into our understanding of stress. Rather, I will argue that cognitive notions have colonized too much of inquiry into stress, have misinterpreted elements of the stress process that are environmental as being a matter of appraisal (as opposed to objective reality that is perceived), and have served a Western view of the world that emphasizes control, freedom, and individual determinism. I suggest that resources, not cognitions, are the primum mobile on which stress is hinged. . . . Cognition is the player not the play. (pp. 21-22)

Unfortunately, what Hobfoll says about cognitive mediation is a red herring, suggesting that he has not read carefully what I and other cognitive-mediationists have written, so he ends up co-opting what has already been said and passing it off as his own. Nor does he seem to understand what it means to speak of relational meaning, or that the theory is cognitive, motivational, and relational. He presents a stereotypical and erroneous view of what such a theory is about, despite the vagueness and internal inconsistency of his own position. What he proposes is no substitute at all because, in the main, it remains just as circular as traditional stimulus-response psychology.

This circularity stems from the fact that what makes a so-called stressor stressful is not adequately spelled out before the fact but depends on the quality, intensity, and duration of the stressor stimulus, which varies greatly from person to person even in very similar environmental circumstances. (For more detail, see Lazarus and Folkman (1984), and Lazarus (1999); also see Parkinson and Manstead (1992), for another critique of appraisal theory.) In general, most epistemically focused criticisms of appraisal theory seem to be a case of the pot, which has historically been overzealous of the need to demonstrate its scientific credentials, calling the kettle black.

Appraising in Stress Theory

Early on (Lazarus, 1966), my theorizing about stress drew on concepts of appraisal and coping. Before proceeding with the role of appraisal in stress theory, however, it is useful to distinguish linguistically between the verb form, *appraising*, which refers to the act of making an evaluation, and the noun form, *appraisal*, which stands for the evaluative product. The former usage offers the advantage of emphasizing the appraisal process as a set of cognitive actions, and I use this convention here. I first suggested this in Lazarus and commentators (1995). McAdams (1996) also employed it with respect to the concept of self. He referred to the process by which a person constructs selfhood developmentally with the accurate but awkward verb form "selfing" and the product of this construction with the noun "self."

In my treatment of psychological stress, I emphasize two kinds of appraising, primary and secondary. Figure 9.1 presents a schematization

Figure 9.1   A Systems Theoretical Schematization of Stress, Coping, and Adaptation

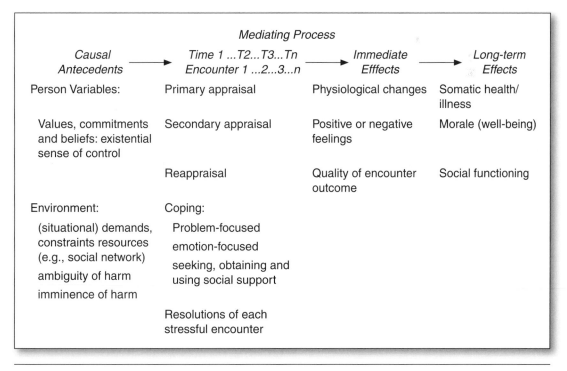

SOURCE: Reproduced with permission from Lazarus and Folkman (1984, p. 305).

of the main variables of the system that were originally presented by Lazarus and Folkman (1984).

Primary Appraising

This process has to do with whether or not what is happening is relevant to one's values, goal commitments, beliefs about self and world, and situational intentions and, if so, in what way. Because we do not always act on them, values and beliefs are apt to be weaker factors in mobilizing action and emotion than goal commitments. Thus, one may think it is good to have wealth but not worth making a major sacrifice to obtain it. The term *goal commitment* implies that a person will strive hard to attain the goal despite discouragement and adversity.

I have always stood by the widely acknowledged principle that if there is no goal commitment, there is nothing of adaptational importance at stake in an encounter to arouse emotions. The person goes about dealing with routine matters until there is an indication that something of greater adaptational importance is taking place, which will interrupt the routine because it has more potential for harm, threat, or challenge (Mandler, 1984).

What questions does one ask in primary appraising in any transaction? Fundamental is whether anything is at stake—in effect, one asks "Are any of my goals, important personal relationships, or core beliefs and values represented here?" and "If I do have a stake, what might the expected outcome be?" If the answer to the fundamental primary appraisal question is "no stake"—in other words, the transaction is not relevant to one's well-being—there is nothing further to consider.

Secondary Appraising

This process focuses on what can be done about a troubled person-environment relationship—that is, the coping options and the social and intrapsychic constraints against acting them out. Such an evaluation and the personal meanings a person constructs from the relationship are the essential cognitive underpinnings of coping actions.

In any stressful transaction, one must evaluate coping options, decide which ones to choose, and decide how to set them in motion (Lazarus & Launier, 1978). This is the function of secondary appraisal. The questions addressed vary with the circumstances, but they concern diverse issues, such as the following: Do I need to act? What can be done? Is it feasible? Which option is best? Am I capable of carrying it out? What are the costs and benefits of each option? Is it better not to act? What might be the consequences of acting or not acting? When should I act? Decisions about coping actions are not usually etched in stone. They must often be changed in accordance with the flow of events, although they may be unchangeable once matters go beyond a given point. I shall address coping after concluding the discussion of appraisal.

The qualifying adjective, secondary, does not connote a process of less importance than primary, but it suggests only that primary appraising is a judgment about whether what is happening is worthy of attention and, perhaps, mobilization. Primary appraising never operates independently of secondary appraising, which is needed to attain an understanding of one's total plight. In effect, there is always an active interplay of both. The distinctly different contents of each type of appraisal justify treating them separately, but each should be regarded as integral meaning components of a more complex process.

The main appraisal variants of psychological stress are harm and loss, threat, or challenge (Lazarus, 1966, 1981; Lazarus & Launier, 1978). Harm and loss consists of damage that has already occurred. Threat consists of the possibility of such damage in the future. Challenge is similar to Selye's (1974) eustress in that people who feel challenged pit themselves enthusiastically against obstacles and feel expansive—even joyous—about the struggle that will ensue. Performers of all sort, whether musicians, entertainers, actors, or public speakers, love the liberating effects of challenge and hate the constricting effects of threat.

These three types of stress reactions should be separated only for convenience of analysis. For example, harm appraisals, which concern the past, also have implications for the future. Therefore, they usually contain components of threat; challenge appraisals do too. Threat and challenge are mostly focused on the future, and we are usually in a state of uncertainty because we have no clear idea about what will actually happen.

Threat and challenge can occur in the same situation, although one or the other usually predominates. In some situations, we are more threatened than challenged, and in other situations the reverse may be true. Although threat appraisals may be subordinated to challenge in a particular situation, favorable personal resources capable of producing a desired outcome may reverse the balance between the two appraisals, which could quickly change in the face of shifting fortunes or the need to cope. Thus, threat and challenge are not immutable states of mind. As a result of appraising and reappraising, threat can be transformed into challenge and vice versa.

Antecedents of Appraisal

The two main sets of variables jointly influencing whether the appraisal is that of threat or challenge are environmental and personality centered. Some environmental circumstances impose too great a demand on a person's resources, whereas others provide considerable latitude for available skills and persistence, thereby influencing whether threat or challenge will occur. The substantive environmental content variables having an influence consist of diverse situational demands, constraints, and opportunities. Formal environmental variables consist of situational dimensions, such as novelty versus familiarity, predictability versus unpredictability, clarity of meaning versus ambiguity, and temporal factors such as imminence, timing, and duration.

Personality dispositions influencing whether a person is more prone to threat or to challenge include self-confidence or self-efficacy (Bandura, 1977, 1989, 1997). The more confident we are of our capacity to overcome dangers and obstacles, the more likely we are to be challenged rather than threatened; a sense of inadequacy, however, promotes threat. Nevertheless, and consistent with a relational analysis of stress, in any transaction both the environmental circumstances and the personality dispositions combine in determining whether there will be a threat or challenge appraisal.

Coping in Stress Theory

Lazarus and Folkman (1984, p. 141) offer the following process view of coping: "We define coping as constantly changing cognitive and behavioral efforts to manage specific external and/or internal demands that are appraised as taxing or exceeding the resources of the person."

Simply stated, coping is the effort to manage psychological stress. I present three main themes of a process approach to coping.

First, there is no universally effective or ineffective coping strategy. Coping must be measured separately from its outcomes so that the effectiveness of each coping strategy can be properly evaluated. Efficacy depends on the type of person, the type of threat, the stage of the stressful encounter, and the outcome modality—that is, subjective well-being, social functioning, or somatic health. Because the focus is on flux or change over time and diverse life conditions, a process formulation is also inherently contextual.

Thus, denial, which was once thought to be harmful and signify pathology, can be quite beneficial in certain circumstances but harmful in others. I illustrate this using diseases of several kinds which are especially stressful when life threatening or handicapping. (See Maes, Leventhal, and de Ridder [1996] for a recent review of research on coping with chronic diseases.)

In a heart attack, denial is dangerous if it occurs while the person is deciding whether or not to seek medical help. This is a period in the attack in which the person is most vulnerable, and delay in treatment as a result of denial can be deadly. Denial is useful during hospitalization, however, because it is an antidote to so-called cardiac neuroses, a syndrome in which the patient is inordinately fearful of dying suddenly. This fear prevents the patient from engaging in activity that would facilitate recovery. Denial again becomes dangerous when the patient returns home and must reestablish normal life activities. The danger at this clinical stage is that denial will lead the patient to take on too much, including stressful work and too much recreational pressure, which may have contributed to the cardiovascular disease in the first place.

There is also much research (Lazarus, 1983) suggesting that denial is useful in elective surgery (Cohen & Lazarus, 1973) but counterproductive in other diseases such as asthma, in which being vigilant has value (Staudenmeyer et al., 1979). Hospitals infantalize patients, so vigilance is not very useful, whereas denial is just what the doctor ordered: "Depend on me or my nurses and you will be fine." The danger in asthma is that a person who begins to experience an asthmatic attack must be vigilant enough to take medication or seek medical help. Denial defeats any effort to ward off the attack, so deniers often wind up in a hospitalized asthmatic crisis compared with more vigilant asthmatics.

All this suggests that we need to understand when denial and other forms of coping are beneficial or harmful. The explanatory principle I favor is that, when nothing can be done to alter the condition or prevent further harm, denial can be beneficial. When denial or any other defense or illusion prevents necessary adaptive action, however, it will be harmful (Lazarus, 1983, 1985).

Consider another illness, prostate cancer, which is very common in older men. The idea that one has a dangerous cancer provides an ever-present stressful background of life and death concerns, which potentiate many specific threats. For example, there is the threat posed by having to make a decision about how to treat the disease—especially in light of the conflicting judgments about what to do by physicians.

Another threat concerns the periodic need after surgery to determine whether cancer cells are still present or have spread to other organs. After surgery, there may be a period of low anxiety until the patient is again examined for medical evidence about the current status of the cancer. This period of low anxiety is the result of having survived surgery and, perhaps, good news from the pathology report. It could also be the result of coping by avoidance or distancing since all the patient can really do at this stage is wait, and vigilance and high anxiety would serve no useful purpose at such a time. As the time for the diagnostic examination nears, however, avoidance or distancing are no longer likely to be effective, and anxiety will increase. If there is evidence of a recurrence or spread of the cancer, the patient is forced to cope in new ways to deal with the changed set of life-threatening options. Life now may depend on radiation treatment.

Another threat is uncertainty about what to tell others, such as acquaintances, friends, and loved ones, about one's situation. Avoidance and silence are frequent coping strategies. A contrasting strategy is to tell everyone, or selected persons, such as acquaintances, friends, and loved ones, the truth about what is happening in an effort to gain social support and to be honest and open. Collective coping in the United States has for a long time involved the maintenance of silence about a disease that, like breast cancer, was considered a social embarrassment. The result was that few men and their loved ones knew much about the disease, and most were ill prepared to deal with it. This secrecy is rapidly diminishing, with the useful result that increasingly more men and their loved ones now have the necessary understanding, which enables them to deal more effectively with the serious threats that the disease imposes.

The threats previously mentioned, and the coping processes they generate, apply to any potentially fatal or disabling disease. Consider the following examples, which involve two other diseases. In the first, an unmarried, 35-year-old woman with multiple sclerosis must decide whether or not to announce to the men she is dating that she has a progressive, debilitating ailment. Not to do so would be unfair to them, but being open about it might chase them away. Also, in the case of breast cancer, men with whom a woman might be intimate might, without forewarning, discover with distress that the woman has lost one or both breasts. What is the woman's best coping strategy? Should she tell them in advance? How should this be evaluated? These are difficult questions for patients who must face these decisions and for coping researchers.

It is not valid to assume that the way an individual copes with one threat will be the same as that chosen for a different threat. The evidence, in fact, indicates otherwise. A key principle is that the choice of coping strategy will usually vary with the adaptational significance and requirements of each threat and its status as a disease, which will change over time.

Let me assure you that what I am saying about coping with a health crisis, such as cancer, is not solely a dispassionate intellectual analysis. I have an intimate personal knowledge about it, having recently been a patient with prostate cancer. The disease was discovered more than 4 years ago, and I had to decide what to do about it. I had major surgery and am now fine, free of this cancer I hope permanently.

The second theme is that to study the coping process requires that we describe in detail what the person is thinking and doing at each stage with each specific threat. In the late 1970s and 1980s, I, as well as many others in the United States and Europe, developed measurement scales and research designs for this purpose (Folkman & Lazarus, 1988a).

Research on the coping process requires an intra-individual research design, nested within inter-individual comparisons in which the same individuals are studied in different contexts and at different times. Many individuals must be compared to avoid dependence on a single case. This is the only way to observe change and stability in what is happening within any individual across conditions and over time. The best generic research design for this kind of research is longitudinal.

The following is the third theme of a process approach to coping: There are at least two major functions of coping, which I refer to as problem focused and emotion focused. With respect to the problem-focused function, a person obtains information on which to act and mobilizes actions for the purpose of changing the reality of the troubled person-environment relationship. The coping actions may be directed at either the self or the environment. To illustrate using my own health crisis, when I sought the opinions of different medical specialists about what treatment to select, and which surgeon was the best available, I was engaging in what seems to be problem-focused coping.

The emotion-focused function is aimed at regulating the emotions tied to the stress situation—for example, by avoiding thinking about the threat or reappraising it without changing the realities of the stressful situation. To again illustrate, I first approached my prostate problem vigilantly rather than with avoidance. After the decision had been made to have surgery, however, because there was nothing further I could do I made an effort to distance myself from the potential dangers that lay ahead. I also reassured myself that I had chosen the right course and secured the best surgeon available. These efforts constitute a pattern of emotion-focused coping.

When we reappraise a threat, we are altering our emotions by constructing a new relational meaning of the stressful encounter. Although at first I was very anxious at the discovery of the disease (my father died of it), I reassured myself that all the medical tests pointed to a cancer that was localized within the prostate gland and had not yet spread, so I was a good candidate for surgery. I was convinced—or more accurately, I tried to convince myself—that my surgeon was one of the best in the area, and that much more was now known about the surgical procedure than in the past so that my chances were very good. Also, as I mentioned previously, I distanced myself from threats I could not do anything about, so the initial anxiety was lessened.

Reappraisal is an extremely effective way to cope with a stressful situation. It is often difficult, however, to distinguish it from an ego defense, such as denial. When the personal meaning of what is happening fits the evidence, it is not an ego defense but rather one of the most durable and powerful ways of controlling destructive emotions.

An example of reappraisal that serves as a form of coping and involves important interpersonal relationships can be seen in efforts to manage the emotion of anger. If one's spouse or lover has managed to offend by what he or she has said and done, instead of retaliating to repair one's wounded self-esteem, one might be able to recognize that, being under great stress, the spouse or lover could not realistically be held responsible; in effect, he or she was not in control of himself or herself, and it would be advantageous to assume that the basic intention was not malevolent.

This reappraisal of another's intentions makes it possible to empathize with the loved one's plight and excuse the outburst. This should defuse or prevent the anger that would ordinarily have been felt in response to the assault. Also, it is hoped that the other person would do the same if one behaves badly under pressure. To construct a benign reappraisal is easier said than done. This example, however, illustrates the power of this form of cognitive coping to lessen or turn negative emotions into positive ones by changing the relational meaning of the encounter.

At the risk of adding further complications, I offer an important qualification to what I have just said about the two most important coping functions. The way I have spoken about them invites certain errors, or bad habits of thought, about the distinction between problem-focused and emotion-focused coping. This distinction, which has been widely endorsed in the field of coping measurement and research, leads to their treatment as distinctive coping action types, which is an over simple and too literal conception of how coping works.

One error is that when we allow ourselves to slip into the language of action types, we often end up speaking as if it is easy to decide which thought or action belongs in the problem-focused or emotion-focused category. On the surface, some coping factors, such as confrontive coping and planful problem solving, seem to represent the problem-focused function, whereas others, such as distancing, escape avoidance, and positive reappraisal, seem to represent emotion-focused coping.

This way of thinking is too simple, however. For example, if a person takes a Valium before an exam because of distressing and disabling test anxiety, we could be convinced that this act serves both functions, not just one. Although the emotion and its physiological sequelae, such as excessive arousal, dry mouth, trembling, and intrusive thoughts about failing, can be reduced by the drug, performance is also likely to improve because these symptoms will now interfere less with the performance. We should have learned by now that the same act may have more than one function and usually does.

A second error is that we contrast the two functions, and even try to determine which is more useful. In a culture centered on control over the environment, it is easy to come to the erroneous conclusion, which is common in the research literature, that problem-focused coping is always or usually a more useful strategy. There is evidence, however, that in certain circumstances problem-focused coping can be detrimental to health and well-being (Collins, Baum, & Singer, 1983). In the study by Collins et al., people who continued to struggle to change conditions that could not be changed, thus relying rigidly on problem-focused coping, were far more troubled over the long haul than those who accepted the reality and relied more on emotion-focused coping.

Although it is legitimate to ask which coping strategies produce the best adaptational outcomes under different sets of conditions, this way of thinking fails to recognize that in virtually all stressful encounters the person draws on both functions. In nature, the two functions of coping are never separated. Both are essential parts of the total coping effort, and ideally each facilitates the other.

It is the fit between thinking, wanting, emotion, action, and the environmental realities that determines whether coping is efficacious or not. However seductive it is to think of the two functions as separate and distinct, coping should never be thought of in either-or terms but as a complex of thoughts and actions aimed at improving the troubled relationship with the environment—in other words, a process of seeking the most serviceable meaning available in the situation, one that supports realistic actions while also viewing the situation in the most favorable way possible.

TRANSITIONAL VIEWS

What I refer to as transitional views grew gradually out of my analysis of stress and coping, and these do not represent positions that, strictly speaking, I have reached very recently. These positions deal with two awkward and unresolved conceptual and methodological issues about the difference between appraising and coping and how appraisal works. My thoughts about them, which I discuss in the following sections, span the period between the 1980s and the mid-1990s and reflect my efforts to think through problems of appraisal theory.

Confusions About Appraising and Coping

Conceptually, appraising and coping go hand in hand and overlap, which results in uncertainty about whether, in any given instance, a stress-related thought or action is an appraisal, a coping process, or both. The uncertainty stems from the fact that cognitive coping (like an ego defense) is basically a reappraisal, which is difficult to distinguish from the original appraisal except for its history. The answer about which process is taking place—secondary appraising or coping—must always be based on a full exploration of what is going on in the mind of a particular individual and the context in which the person-environment transaction occurs. My solution is to say an appraisal is the result of a coping process when it constitutes a motivated search for information and the constructed meanings on which to act under stress.

When thinking of appraisal decisions, it is important to recognize that the traditional appraisal questions I listed previously have been posed in very general terms, and additional details about the transaction are usually required to make a decision about what to do (Janis & Mann, 1977). Because conditions vary greatly with respect to a harm or loss, threat, challenge, and benefit, to make decisions and take action we need to ask more detailed questions. In effect, these broad types of stress reactions must be narrowed to much more specific ones.

For example, on the negative affective side, the harm or loss might be bereavement, a rejection, or a minor or serious slight; the threat may be a life-threatening or terminal illness; and challenge could arise from an uncertain job opportunity. On the positive affective side, the relevant decisions and actions might have to do with an achievement, reward, or honor that justifies, for example, joy or pride.

Even these more narrowly defined damaging, threatening, challenging, and beneficial subconditions might have to be broken down further to identify the requirements for making coping decisions. For example, it is likely that different versions of bereavement, such as how the person died or the quality of the relationship before the death, influence the emotional state to be experienced and what can or must be done to cope effectively. Also, if the source of pride could be seen by an important other as a competitive putdown, one might decide to soft-pedal it to preserve the interpersonal relationship. Just as individuals take these small but significant details into account in their own coping efforts, the scientific study of appraising and coping, and clinical efforts to help people cope more effectively, must consider them in the search for workable principles.

How Appraisals Are Constructed

The issue of how appraisal works is important if we are to make a thorough examination of the validity and utility of appraisal theory. Magda Arnold (1960) viewed appraising as instantaneous rather than deliberate. She wrote,

> The appraisal that arouses an emotion is not abstract; it is not the result of reflection. It is immediate and undeliberate. If we see somebody stab at our eye with his finger, we avoid the threat instantly, even though we may know that he does not intend to hurt or even to touch us. Before we can make such an instant response, we must have estimated somehow that the stabbing finger could hurt. Since the movement is immediate, unwitting, or even contrary to our better knowledge, this appraisal of possible harm must be similarly immediate, (p. 172)

Originally (Lazarus, 1966), I thought that Arnold had underemphasized the complexity of evaluative judgments that are often called for in garden-variety stress emotions, and I still do. I am now more impressed with the instantaneity

of much appraising, however, even in complex and abstract cases. Appraisals are usually dependent on many subtle cues in the environment, previous experience, and a host of personality variables, such as goals, situational intentions, personal resources, and liabilities.

All these sources of input, and probably additional ones, are involved in the decision about how to evaluate adaptational demands, constraints, and opportunities and how to cope, which makes the speed of many or most appraisals seem quite remarkable. Little is known about how the process works. I am inclined to believe the necessary information is often at the tips of our fingers, operating as tacit knowledge (Polanyi, 1966) about ourselves and our environment (see Merleau-Ponty, 1962, for the concept of embodied thought). Therefore, scanning inputs in an analogy to a digital computer is probably not the way appraisal actually works.

When Arnold (1960) wrote her monograph, psychology was just beginning to think in terms of stepwise information processing. This is one reason why my own treatment of appraising was considerably more abstract than Arnold's and also more conscious and deliberate. Despite the redundancy of the expression, I used the term "cognitive appraisal" to emphasize the complex, judgmental, and conscious process that must often be involved in appraising (Lazarus, 1966).

There is considerable agreement about the two main ways in which an appraisal might be made. First, the process of appraising can be deliberate and largely conscious. Second, it can be intuitive, automatic, and unconscious. Under some conditions, a slow, deliberate search for information is required on which to predicate a judgment about what is at stake and what should be done to cope with the situation. At other times, a very rapid appraisal is more adaptive.

Most of the scenarios resulting in an emotion are recurrences of basic human dilemmas of living, including triumph, attainment of a goal, loss, disappointment, uncertain threat, violating a moral stricture, and being insulted or subtly demeaned. Most of us, especially if we have lived long enough, have already experienced these more than once, an example of the wisdom of the ages (Lazarus, 1991). A recurrence can never be identical in detail, but its personal significance can remain the same.

I have referred to this latter principle as the short-circuiting of threat (Lazarus & Alfert, 1964;

Lazarus & Launier, 1978; Opton, Rankin, Nomikos, & Lazarus, 1965). The metaphor is the electrical short circuit in which the original route to the end of the wire is shortened by something that cuts the circuit at a much earlier point. At the psychological level, in contrast to having always to deliberate and learn anew about the import of threatening events, which would be a very inefficient way of monitoring our relationships with the environment, we are enabled to respond quickly and automatically to an adaptational crisis, even without awareness of the process, as a result of what we have already learned.

There is widespread acceptance of the idea that many of our appraisals are the result of unconscious processes. One of the most remarkable changes in outlook that has taken place since the 1950s is the attitude of psychologists toward unconscious processes. In earlier times, psychology was mostly nihilistic about the ability of the science to deal with the unconscious mind (Eriksen, 1960, 1962). The question at that time mainly concerned whether an appraisal can be unconscious rather than about the dynamics of unconscious psychological processes.

In addition to their influence on social actions, present-day thinking asks about how unconscious processes work—for example, whether they are smart or dumb. This is an allusion to the primitive and wishful thinking that Freud suggested characterizes unconscious (id) processes. This issue, among others, is still being debated (see a special section of *American Psychologist* edited by Loftus, 1992, that included brief articles by Bruner; Erdelyi; Greenwald; Jacoby, Lindsay, & Toth; Kihlstrom, Barnhardt, & Tataryn; Lewicki, Hill, & Czyzewska; Loftus & Klinger; and Merikle).

The 1980s and 1990s produced an explosion of interest in the unconscious (Lazarus & commentators, 1995). This interest and research centers mainly on what might be called the cognitive unconscious—that is, what we fail to attend to and how unconscious processes influence our thoughts, feelings, and actions. Articles and books by Bargh (1990), Bowers (1987), Brewin (1989), Brody (1987), Buck (1985), Epstein (1990), Kihlstrom (1987, 1990), LeDoux (1989), Leventhal (1984), Shepard (1984), Uleman and Bargh (1989), and others attest to this interest.

Another kind of unconsciousness, which is the result of ego-defense processes, is usually referred to as the dynamic unconscious (Erdelyi, 1985). It receives far less attention compared to the cognitive unconscious, especially in nonclinical circles. Unconscious appraising based on casual inattentiveness should be distinguished from defensive reappraisal, which involves motivated self-deception (Lazarus, 1991; Lazarus & commentators, 1995; Lazarus & Folkman, 1984).

Does an unconscious appraisal based on ego defense differ from appraisals that are based on inattention? The answer to this question is not known for sure, but the main theoretical difference is that, compared with the dynamic unconscious, the contents of the cognitive unconscious should be relatively easy to make conscious by drawing attention to the conditions under which they have occurred. Making the dynamic unconscious conscious, however, is another matter. Because, presumably, the person does not wish to confront threatening thoughts, especially those related to socially proscribed goals, their exclusion from consciousness must be intentional—that is, they are a means of coping with threat. In such a case, awareness would defeat the function of the defensive maneuver.

Mental contents that result from ego defense pose another serious problem. They distort what a person can tell us about the relational meaning of an encounter with the environment. This makes the task of assessing how the person is appraising the encounter very difficult because what is reported about the inner mental life cannot be accepted at face value. It is difficult to identify the truth, but the solution need not be completely refractory. Skilled clinicians, and even laypersons, are often able to make reasonable and, it is hoped, accurate inferences about defenses and what is being concealed by them. They draw on observed contradictions of three kinds to alert themselves to defensive distortions in self-reported appraisals (Lazarus & commentators, 1995).

One such contradiction is between what a person says at one moment and what he or she says at another moment. A second is the contrast between what is said and contrary behavioral and physiological evidence—for example, voice quality and gestures that give evidence of discomfort, physical flushing or paling, and willful acts that belie what is being said. A third contradiction is between what is said and the normative response to the same provocative situation. If most people would be angered or made fearful in the same situation, we can use this knowledge clinically to second-guess the person who denies one or another of these emotions. We need to be wary of this strategy, however, because in many cases individuals have different motives and perspectives on the events of interest, so we could be wrong in any particular instance. A comparable strategy in research is the use of multiple levels of observation, such as self-reports, actions, and bodily changes.

The problem with depending on contradictions among different response measures to second-guess the truth is that we do not know the natural correlation among these measures. Because each has somewhat different causal antecedents—physiological measures being captive of energy mobilization; verbal reports depending on knowledge, willingness, and ability to expose the truth; and actions being influenced by social opportunities and constraints—the correlations among the measures are usually low, even when intraindividual analysis is employed. Thus, response discrepancies are a somewhat unreliable source of evidence about defense.

This correlation problem should also indicate why no single response measure, such as facial expressions or physiological arousal, can be regarded as criterial about a person's inner emotional state. There is a need for evidence to confirm one or another interpretation when we observe a discrepancy as well as basic research on how response measures are correlated under diverse conditions, which has not been undertaken programmatically.

In my judgment, introspective or self-report data about subjective experience tend to be viewed too negatively by psychologically oriented scientists. Under certain conditions, this kind of data can certainly be seriously flawed as a source of information about personal meanings. The negative general opinion about the validity of such data, however, is not fully justified for two reasons. First, little or no effort is usually made to maximize accuracy and minimize the sources of error. Second, problems of validity and how to interpret what is observed are no less daunting for behavioral and psychophysiological data compared with introspection. Despite the claim that they are more objective response measures than self-report, both have their own validity problems, which must be taken just as seriously as those involved in self-report. There is no simple, guaranteed route to

the truth of what is in our minds—only fragmentary clues that we must investigate carefully through hard work.

Casually constructed questionnaires, such as those used in survey research, are particularly vulnerable to error when we want to examine accurately and in-depth what people want, think, and feel and the contexts in which they do so. This has led me to propose that in-depth studies of individuals over time and across circumstances, which is an adaptation of the clinical method, must be employed in the study of appraisal and coping in the emotions (Lazarus & commentators, 1990, 1995).

PRESENT THEMES

The analysis of appraising in the context of stress and coping can be readily applied to the emotions by making some modifications (Lazarus, 1966, 1968, 1981, 1999; Lazarus, Averill, & Opton, 1970). Also, as noted previously, the concepts of stress and emotion need to be conjoined, with emotion being the more inclusive concept. To understand positively toned emotional states, the analysis must be expanded from a focus solely on harm, threat, and challenge to a focus on a variety of benefits—each associated with its own emotion. Each of the negatively toned emotions also has its own special pattern of appraisal and relational meaning.

As in the case of stress, emotions are tied jointly or interactively to social and physical conditions of importance and person variables, such as goals, goal hierarchies, personal values, belief systems, and personal resources. What changes as we shift our attention from stress to the emotions are the primary and secondary appraisal judgments and relational meanings that must be added to accommodate each of the emotions we wish to understand.

In this section, which covers the 1990s, I discuss my cognitive-motivational-relational theory of the emotions (Lazarus, 1991), focusing especially on the distinctive features of the approach. Most of the ideas expressed here are more recent than those previously discussed, although they are not inconsistent with the earlier positions I took when my main focus was stress and coping. I refer to this theory as cognitive-motivational-relational because motivation and cognition and the meanings constructed about the person-environment relationship are conjoined in the emotion process and serve as crucial concepts.

Despite some important differences in detail, there is remarkable agreement among theorists about what a person is supposed to think to react with many of the diverse emotions. In the 1980s and 1990s, many emotion theorists with a cognitive-mediational perspective sought to analyze what a person must want and think to feel one or another of the various emotions. In addition to my own work, some of the most active and visible theorists and researchers include Conway and Bekerian (1987), Dalkvist and Rollenhagen (1989), de Rivera (1977), de Sousa (1987), Frijda (1986), Oatley and Johnson-Laird (1987), Ortony, Clore, and Collins (1988), Reisenzein (1995), Roseman (1984), Scherer (1984), Smith and Ellsworth (1985), Solomon (1976), and Weiner (1985, 1986).

The main appraisal variables common to cognitive-mediational theories include having a goal at stake, whether the goal is facilitated or thwarted, and locus of control or responsibility for what happened, typically referred to as accountability, legitimacy, and controllability. Pleasantness is also viewed by some as an appraisal variable, but I consider it to be a response to, rather than an antecedent of, appraisal. Figure 9.2 provides an updated schematization of the psychosocial system of the discrete emotions, with stress integrated within it, which is discussed in Lazarus (1999). The reader might want to compare it with the earlier schematization, emphasizing stress from Lazarus and Folkman (1984).

Distinctive Features of My Theoretical Approach

Despite substantial agreement, my current view of appraisal processes differs from other theoretical positions in at least six main ways: (a) I point to a motivational basis of the choice of a discrete emotion—that is, its quality in addition to its intensity; (b) I treat appraisals as hot rather than cold cognitions; (c) more than most others, I emphasize coping as an integral feature of the emotion process; (d) I assume that emotions have an implacable logic and reject the widespread penchant for thinking of emotions as irrational; (e) I believe that the division of emotions into positive and negative

can be misleading—positively toned and negatively toned emotional states are interdependent; and (f) perhaps most important, I treat relational meanings as core relational themes that are derived from the process of appraising. In effect, I view appraisal in holistic terms as a synthesis, in contrast with the dominant reductive science outlook seeking to separate causes of phenomena, each of which constitutes only a part of the whole.

The differences between my views and those of other appraisal theorists are reprised throughout the following sections. I also interweave my theoretical stance about the appraisals involved in each of the emotions, thereby outlining my theoretical approach along with discussions of the distinctions between my approach and other appraisal-based approaches.

The Motivational Basis of Emotion Quality

Few appraisal theorists advocate a major role for diverse personal goals in shaping the quality of an emotion, although they all recognize the importance of the fate of antecedent goals in emotional intensity and the new goals that each emotion generates. I take the position that many ego involvements—that is, goal commitments focused on one's ego identity or self—influence the quality of an emotional experience. These ego involvements include self- or social esteem, moral values, ego ideals, important meanings and ideas, the well-being of other persons, and life goals.

For example, shame, pride, and anger are the result of the fate of our desire to preserve or enhance self- or social esteem; guilt is about moral issues; and anxiety, which is par excellence an existential emotion having to do with one's being in the world and personal fate (e.g., life and death), and so forth. Table 9.1 presents a list of ego involvements and some of the discrete emotions they help shape. For a developmental analysis of emergent goals in the shaping of the self-conscious emotions, namely, shame, guilt, embarrassment, and pride, see Mascolo & Fischer, 1995.

One can see the role of goals in the emotions in the following analysis of the main appraisal components I propose for each emotion. For a fuller account, see Lazarus (1991). The following are the main appraisal components of the discrete emotions I tend to examine:

Figure 9.2 Revised Model of Stress and Coping

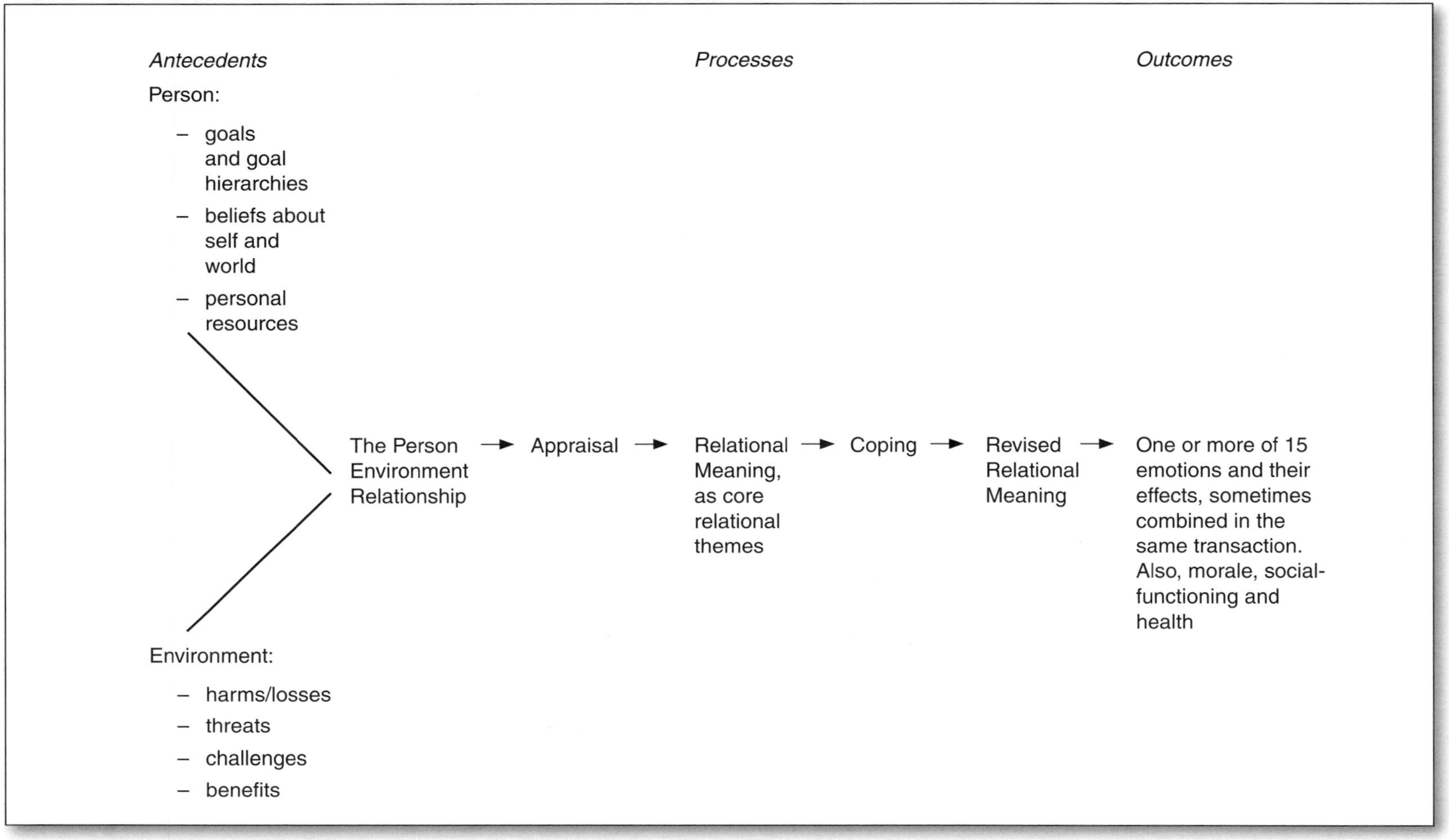

Antecedents

Person:

– goals and goal hierarchies

– beliefs about self and world

– personal resources

Environment:

– harms/losses

– threats

– challenges

– benefits

Processes

The Person Environment Relationship → Appraisal → Relational Meaning, as core relational themes → Coping → Revised Relational Meaning →

Outcomes

One or more of 15 emotions and their effects, sometimes combined in the same transaction. Also, morale, social-functioning and health

SOURCE: Reproduced with permission of Lazarus (1991).

Table 9.1   Types of Ego Involvement and the Emotions They Influence[a]

Ego involvement		Emotions
Self- and social esteem	———	Anger, pride
Moral values	———	Guilt
Ego ideals	———	Shame
Meanings and ideas	———	Anxiety
Other persons and their well-being	———	All emotions
Life goals	———	All emotions

SOURCE: From Lazarus (1991).

a. Ego involvements refer to commitments, which might be thought of as goals that fall within the rubric of what we usually mean by ego identity.

Primary appraising: The three primary appraisal components are goal relevance, goal congruence, and type of ego involvement.

Goal relevance is fundamental to whether an encounter is viewed by a person as relevant to well-being. In effect, there is no emotion without a goal at stake.

Goal congruence or incongruence refer to whether the conditions of an encounter facilitate or thwart what the person wants. If conditions are favorable, a positively toned emotion is likely to be aroused. If unfavorable, a negatively toned emotion follows.

Secondary appraising: As in the case of stress emotions, this has to do with options for coping with emotional encounters. Three basic judgments are involved: blame or credit for an outcome, coping potential, and future expectations. They complete the primary appraisal decisions leading to each of the positive and negative emotions.

Both blame and credit require a judgment about who or what is responsible for a harm, threat, challenge, or benefit. Two kinds of information influence this judgment. The first is that the outcome of the transaction is the result of an action that was under the control of the provocateur or perpetrator. If what occurred could not have been avoided, it is more difficult to attribute blame or credit. The second is the attribution of a malevolent or benign intention to the other person, which increases the odds of blame or credit being attributed.

Coping potential arises from the personal conviction that we can or cannot act successfully to ameliorate or eliminate a harm or threat or bring to fruition a challenge or benefit.

Future expectations may be positive or negative—that is, the troubled person-environment relationship will change for better or worse.

Hot Versus Cold Cognitions

I consider appraisals as hot or emotional cognitions (Lazarus & Smith, 1988) and attributions as cold and abstract (Smith, Haynes, Lazarus, & Pope, 1993). The attributional dimensions explored by Weiner (1985, 1986), such as locus of causality, stability, controllability, intentionality, and globality, represent what I consider cold information rather than hot or emotional appraisals.

The important point for cognitive psychology is that information is not meaning. Meaning or, more precisely, relational meaning refers to the personal significance of information that is constructed by the person. Meaning or personal significance is what gives an appraisal its emotional quality. Thus, whereas locus of causality (or responsibility) is a factor in blaming someone, which depends on the situational context, responsibility is neutral or coolly distanced. Attributing blame or credit to someone rather than responsibility carries the immediate relational heat, which of course is a metaphor for emotion.

Coping Is an Integral Feature of the Emotion Process

Coping is central to my approach to the emotions, just as it originally was for stress. Unfortunately, the importance of coping is often understated and sometimes ignored in appraisal theories of emotion. It is as if coping is conceived as having been brought about through an entirely separate process only after an emotion has occurred rather than, as I see it, being an integral part of the emotion-generating process. It also plays a role at the earliest possible moments of the emotion process. In other words, the cognitive and motivational underpinnings of coping—that is, secondary appraising of coping options—originate with the first recognition of one's trouble or good fortune. The resulting coping thoughts and actions serve as bridges between the relational meaning of the encounter and how the person acts and feels. In effect, appraisal unites coping with the emotion process.

We cannot properly understand an emotion without reference to coping thoughts and actions. If the transaction is appraised as posing a great danger—for example, the person believes he or she could not safely cope with retaliation for attack on another—anxiety or fright is a more likely emotional reaction than anger, or the aroused anger will be suffused with anxiety. In effect, coping prospects and coping consequences have a strong influence on which emotion will be experienced; they serve as mediators of subsequent emotions (Folkman & Lazarus, 1988a, 1988b).

The Implacable Logic of Emotion: Rationality and Irrationality

People in Western society, including many of its scholars, regard emotions as irrational. Typically, we think of emotions as a form of craziness and believe they do not follow logical rules. We constantly pit emotion against reason, as if they are inevitably in opposition. Our culture says that it was emotions that made us act foolishly and that emotions make us abandon reason.

In writing about the public attitude toward the death penalty, columnist Anthony Lewis

(1998), whom I respect and admire for his consistently thoughtful analyses of human fashions and foibles, nevertheless wrote the following sentence that epitomizes this tendency: "People want the death penalty, I am convinced, for emotional rather than rational reasons" (p. A15). I would change this sentence to say "for reasons that are not thoughtful or wise."

I acknowledge that sometimes emotions interfere with the thoughtful examination of an issue, but it is the quality of thought that should usually be blamed, not our emotions. Even when we suspect direct emotional interference, this does not allow us to predict the direction of the reasoning, as in the previous example about the death penalty. It is no more irrational to desire the death penalty than to rue the penalty, as many people do. Rather, it is the reasoning that Lewis should castigate, not the emotions involved in the issue. This is a very common type of reasoning error in today's media.

Another example appeared in a psychology best-seller, *Emotional Intelligence,* in which Daniel Goleman (1995), previously the science writer for the *New York Times,* speaks of two separate minds—one devoted to emotions and the other to reason. He states, "In a very real sense we have two minds, one that thinks and one that feels" (p. 8). He also says, "Our emotions have a mind of their own, one which can hold views quite independently of our rational mind" (p. 20). I am sure that this was written to appeal to the untutored layperson. It is bad science and misleading, however, especially as applied to what is known about the brain, which Goleman continuously refers to as the arbiter of our actions. It is the mind that is the arbiter; the brain is the organ that merely makes reason and emotion possible.

My argument is a hard sell in that it is difficult to shake off more than 2,000 years of Western habits of thought, with its roots in ancient Greece. Plato's views about cognition, motivation, and emotion were taken over in the Middle Ages by the Catholic Church, which emphasized the antithesis between reason and emotion and the need to regulate its parishioner's emotions and animal instincts by reason and an act of will. Despite the fact that such a struggle implies conflict between thought, motivation, and reason, this is no reason to perpetuate an outlook in which emotion is reified as always separate from reason. The position taken by Aristotle (1941) in the *Rhetoric*, which the Church and Western civilization largely ignored, is a wiser but less familiar view—namely, that although conflict can take place between these two agencies of mind, emotion depends on reason.

Integration Versus Disconnection in the Mind. A mentally healthy person may suffer from conflicts, but the mind is, in the main, integrated and its parts work in harmony if we are to function well. Otherwise, we could not engage in coordinated planning and make decisions about what we want and what is good for us. We have one mind, not three, and when this is not so we are dysfunctional or mentally ill. Only when we are at war with ourselves do thought, motivation, and emotion diverge importantly, but this dissociation is pathological rather than a healthy state of mind (Lazarus, 1989). Cognition, motivation, and emotion are parts of a larger, integrated subsystem (the mind), which in turn is embedded in even larger systems—for example, the family, social group, society, nation, or ecosystem.

To the extent that the emotion process is individualized—that is, dependent on a person's goals, beliefs, and personal resources—we would have no hope of understanding it without detailed knowledge of the person. Emotions would be unpredictable. Although it is correct to say that we employ reason to keep destructive emotions from getting out of control, the arousal of emotion depends on reason, as Aristotle maintained, although it might be bad reasoning. Our emotions follow clear, normative cognitive rules, as does their regulation, although the variables we need to consider depend on the individual being considered.

The key principle here is that emotions flow from the way we appraise what is happening in our lives. Despite the great appeal that blaming human folly on our emotions has had in much of Western thought, emotions follow an implacable logic, as long as we view them from the standpoint of an individual's premises about self and world, even when they are not realistic. It is this logic that we need to understand.

Economists think of rationality as making decisions that maximize self-interest in any transaction. One problem with this presumption is that to do so requires that we know what our self-interests are, and often we cannot say or are incorrect about these. Another problem is that economists venerate self-interest compared with other important human values, such as sharing our bounty with the community, sacrificing for our children, manifesting loyalty even when it could place us in jeopardy, and being concerned with fairness, justice, and compassion—in other words, the very values we call idealistic (often as a putdown), which should be hallmarks of a civilized society. Self-interest as a value can be greatly overdone, and it has consistently produced extensive worldwide misery along with great wealth for a limited segment of the population.

Of course, it is foolish to act constantly against one's best interests, although people often do so. In a fit of anger, for example, we attack powerful and threatening others or, worse, alienate those whom we love with angry and cutting assaults. It is also unwise and counterproductive not to appraise danger when it is present or to appraise it when it is not present, although people often do both. This is not so much because we think illogically but because we have appraised events in a particular way, based perhaps on unwise or inaccurate assumptions and goals. Inappropriate assumptions result in emotions that present a poor fit with the realities of the situation being faced. It is reason, which depends on the confluence of our ancestral and ontogenetic past and present realities, that has failed us and not our emotions. The main occasions in which emotions get in the way of reason are when they distract or misdirect our attention.

Emotions Reflect the Fate of Our Goal Striving. We have many goals, however, not just one, and actions seeking attainment of one goal often end up, perforce, defeating other goals. This is what it means to speak of conflict, which adds greatly to emotional distress because it complicates finding a maximally desirable solution. If we are convinced people are out to harm us, it is reasonable to feel frightened or angry. Diagnosing this as paranoia—that is, as delusions of persecution or grandeur—does not help us understand these feelings but rather the lack of realism in our thoughts and feelings. It is necessary to identify the operating assumptions that the paranoid person is making about self and world, and the reasons, to understand the fear and anger; in other words, the delusions must be examined from the individual's personal perspective.

We all live by making many foolish assumptions about the world, which program us to experience inappropriate emotions in our daily lives. We do this for many reasons, which I will discuss later. Once it is clear that we have made the wrong assumption, our feelings can readily be explained because they follow from what we have assumed, however erroneous that assumption might be. There is a sensible logic to the emotions that flows from the erroneous premise, and this logic provides an opportunity to understand and even predict emotions. Calling them irrational or an indication of mental illness merely denigrates someone else's reasoning without helping us understand the assumptive basis on which it rests and how it came into being.

Main Causes of Poor Reasoning. My wife Bernice and I (Lazarus & Lazarus, 1994) noted five common causes of erroneous judgments that influence our emotions. The first consists of physical ailments, such as damage to the brain, mental retardation, and psychosis. Such persons are unable to think normally, so their emotions are likely to have inadequate foundations. Pointing to these ailments is not enough to understand why they think and feel as they do. Despite their ailments, we need to identify the beliefs, motives, and thoughts about the life situation to which they are displaying inappropriate emotions. For example, why do they feel anger rather than anxiety or shame? Suggesting merely that there is brain damage does not provide the answer; one needs to understand the individual's psychosocial dynamics and perhaps developmental history.

The second cause of judgmental error is a lack of knowledge about the situation in which we have a stake. With an opaqueness similar to the distortion that results from ego defense, ignorance can distort our relationship with the environment, leading to actions and emotions that make sense only from the standpoint of what we think to be true.

For example, knowing nothing about microorganisms as causes of disease, physicians in the 19th century carried germs from cadavers they had recently dissected to the wombs of women delivering babies, thereby spreading a deadly disease called childbed fever. It was ignorance, not emotion or irrationality, that led them to engage in actions that today we would abhor from the standpoint of our improved

knowledge. Ironically, physicians today, who tend to blame germs that have become resistant to antibiotics instead of thinking preventively, still spread infection in modern hospitals by failing to wash their hands often enough. Also, antibiotics are still being overprescribed, thereby adding to the problem.

The third cause of inappropriate emotion and action is that we have not paid attention to the correct aspects in our social relationships. In most social relationships, there is too much to take into account, and we must decide what is useful and important and what is not. Often, we make a bad guess. Our attention can also be intentionally misdirected. For example, magicians create their magic by misdirecting the audience's attention. Also, we may judge that the other person is lying on the basis of faulty assumptions about how to tell (Ekman, 1985/1992), and we put our trust in people who are skillfully concealing their real motives and exhibiting false ones.

Fourth, when we are dealing with a personal crisis, such as a life-threatening disease, we may be unable to face the truth so we cope using ego defenses, such as denial. We should feel threatened and anxious and act accordingly, but because of our need to believe otherwise we sell ourselves on the idea that we are well or that the illness is temporary and minor and we will get better. This kind of self-deception is not always harmful because when we are not able to change the situation there may be nothing better to think and do about our plight than what is needed to preserve our morale. Defenses can be dangerous, however, when they prevent us from doing what is necessary to save our lives or well-being (Lazarus, 1983).

Fifth, when we make errors in judgment, it is often the result of ambiguity about what is going on. Our social relationships are filled with uncertainty about what other people are thinking, wanting, intending, and feeling, and it is easy to make the wrong guess. We see malevolence where it does not exist or good intentions where there is venality or evil, so we react with an inappropriate emotion. The cause lies in faulty reasoning and not emotion, which merely reflects that reasoning.

In summary, the theory of appraising and appraisal provides a set of propositions about what one must think to feel a given emotion. This is the implacable logic of which I previously spoke. If the theory is sound, we should to some degree be able to tell what a person has been thinking, assuming we know what that person is feeling. Also, we should be modestly able to predict the emotional reaction if we know beforehand what is thought by the person about the encounter or the life situation. This principle gives us considerable power over our emotions because it states the cognitive principles that lie behind each emotion. Knowledge, when it is sound, is power; when it is unsound, it results in foolishness, not only in actions but also in the emotions we experience.

The Interdependence of the Emotions

It is common in the psychology of emotion to distinguish sharply between negative and positively toned emotions and to treat them as if they were opposites. I consider this trend to be unfortunate. Dividing emotions into two types, negative and positive, distorts their individual substantive qualities and the complex meanings inherent in each discrete emotion.

Occasionally, even positively toned emotions involve harms and threats and sometimes originate in negative life conditions. For example, relief occurs when we are dealing with a threat that has abated or disappeared. Hope commonly occurs in a situation in which we are threatened but hope for the best. Consider, for example, what happens when we are awaiting a biopsy for a suspected cancer or when we fear we will do poorly on an exam or interview for an important job. In both instances, we hope our fear has been misguided.

The same reasoning also applies to happiness and pride. For example, although happy about something, we may fear that the favorable conditions provoking our happiness will soon end, so we engage in anticipatory coping to prevent this from happening. We may also fear that when conditions of life are favorable, others will resent our good fortune and try to undermine our well-being. In addition, when pride is viewed by another as the result of having taken too much credit for our success or that of our child or student protegé, or when our pride is viewed by others as a competitive putdown, we may be wise to keep it to ourselves. Biblical language expresses this in the aphorisms "pride goeth before a fall" and "overweening pride."

Love is commonly viewed as a positive emotional experience, but it can be very negative when unrequited or when we have reason to believe our lover is losing interest. When gratitude violates our beliefs and values, the social necessity of displaying it even when it is grudging can be quite negative. Finally, compassion is aversive when we fail to control our emotional reaction to the suffering of others. In effect, we should avoid the tendency to keep the emotions separate and inviolate when, in reality, they are interdependent.

This theme emphasizes the close relationships among emotions and not just their separateness. This is often not recognized in appraisal-centered theoretical approaches because these theorists are mainly concerned with distinguishing the cognitive-motivational-relational antecedents of each discrete emotion, which is a valid concern that should not blind us to their interdependence. It might be wiser not to study a single emotion by itself but rather to examine closely related clusters of emotion—that is, those emotions that are readily transformed into others by virtue of a change in the appraised relational meaning.

For example, pride and shame are closely related because they have cognate relational meanings; their meanings are opposite—that is, being credited with a socially valued outcome versus being slighted or demeaned. Furthermore, anger can also be a way of coping with shame, which is often an extremely distressing emotion because it requires accepting the blame for a serious failing that impugns one's character. In the context of shame, anger involves shifting the blame to another, which helps one feel more in command of oneself and one's relationships. The important point here is that a sudden change in what has been happening or self-generated reappraisal can transform one emotion into another. If we study the emotions separately, we will miss this interdependence.

The Core Relational Themes for Each Emotion

One of my major metatheoretical positions is that the standard examination of appraisal components is conducted at too elemental a level of analysis to be adequate for thorough understanding. In searching for psychological causes, we run the risk of losing the forest for the trees—that is, we ignore the phenomenon as it occurs in nature in favor of its component parts (Lazarus, 1998a, 1998b).

Most appraisal theories are good at distinguishing the separate components of meaning on which the emotion rests, but they do not address how they are organized into the basic relational meaning for each emotion, as in the six primary and secondary appraisals I noted earlier. The partial meanings must be combined to produce the final, integrated gestalt, which characterizes emotional phenomena in nature and defines their overall meanings. In other words, the process of appraising must be examined at a higher level of abstraction, to which I refer as the core relational theme for each emotion. This theme is a terse synthesis of the separate appraisal components into a complex meaning-centered whole. It is one of the features that make my appraisal theory distinctive.

There is no contradiction between the two levels of abstraction—namely, the separate appraisal components and the core relational themes. The same ideas are dealt with as partial meanings and as synthesized wholes. Table 9.2 presents what I think is a plausible list of core relational themes for each of the 15 emotions with which I deal, which is not an exhaustive list of all the emotions of interest.

I conclude the presentation of my appraisal theory by asking whether appraisal theory makes the emotions too cognitive and cold to be realistic. The best answer depends on what a person who had no emotions would be like. Dreikurs (1967) provided the following interesting and revealing answer, which addresses

Table 9.2   Core Relational Themes for Each Emotion

Emotion	Relational Theme
Anger	A demeaning offense against me and mine
Anxiety	Facing uncertain, existential threat
Fright	An immediate, concrete, and overwhelming physical danger
Guilt	Having transgressed a moral imperative
Shame	Failing to live up to an ego ideal
Sadness	Having experienced an irrevocable loss
Envy	Wanting what someone else has
Jealousy	Resenting a third party for loss or threat to another's affection or favor
Disgust	Taking in or being too close to an indigestible object or idea
Happiness	Making reasonable progress toward the realization of a goal
	Enhancement of one's ego identity by taking credit for a valued object or achievement—either one's own or that of someone or a group with
Pride	Enchantment of one's ego identity by taking credit for a valued object or achievement—either one's own or that of someone or a group with which we identify
Belief	A distressing goal-incongruent condition that has changed for the better or gone away
Hope	Fearing the worst but yearning for better and believing a favorable outcome is possible
Love	Desiring or participating in affection, usually but not necessarily reciprocated
Gratitude	Appreciation for an altruistic gift that provides personal benefit
Compassion	Being moved by another's suffering and wanting to help
Aesthetic	Emotions aroused by these experiences can be any of those

only one side of the matter. In dichotomizing reason and emotion, and by emphasizing Dionysian-like commitment, enthusiasm, and excitement in contrast with Appollonian reasonableness, Dreikurs seems to forget that both excitement and reason are conjoined in most emotions. He writes,

> We may easily discover the purpose of emotions when we try to visualize a person who has no emotions. His thinking ability could provide him with much information. He could figure out what he should do, but never would be certain as to what is right and wrong in a complicated situation. He would not be able to take a definite stand, to act with force, with conviction, because complete objectivity is not inducive to forceful actions. This requires a strong personal bias, an elimination of certain factors that logically may contradict opposing factors. Such a person would be cold, almost inhuman. He could not experience any association that would make him biased and one-sided in his perspectives. He could not want anything very much and could not go after it. In short, he would be completely ineffectual as a human being. (p. 207)

Such a person would not be a flesh-and-blood biological creature but a machine like Lieutenant Commander Data on *Star Trek, the Next Generation* or the nonhuman Vulcan, Mr. Spock, in the original television series. They are creatures that are incapable of responding emotionally. We should, however, reject the idea that an ideal human would be one who only thinks rather than feels, although I believe thought can occur without significant emotion but not vice versa. Emotions are complex, organized subsystems consisting of thoughts, beliefs, motives, meanings, subjective experiences, and physiological states. They depend on appraisals, which arise from and facilitate our struggles to survive and flourish in the world.

I am confident that appraisal as a psychological construct, especially as applied to our emotional life, will continue to be a productive idea. Nevertheless, much more must be learned about how appraisals work and affect social relationships. Although the concept makes some psychologists uneasy, I believe it is central to an understanding of how we survive and flourish during the course of our lives.

NOTE

1. *Rashomon* was a Japanese movie that became a classic. It viewed the same major emotional altercation from the disparate viewpoints of four different persons. The movie highlighted the distinctive experience and outlook of these individuals.

REFERENCES

Aristotle. (1941). Rhetoric. In R. McKeon (Ed.). *The basic works of Aristotle.* New York, NY: Random House.

Arnold, M. B. (1960). *Emotion and personality* (Vols. 1 & 2). New York, NY: Columbia University Press.

Bandura, A. (1977). Self-efficacy: Toward a unifying theory of behavioral change. *Psychological Review, 84,* 191–215.

Bandura, A. (1989). Human agency in social cognitive theory. *American Psychologist, 44,* 1175–1184.

Bandura, A. (1997). *Self-efficacy: The exercise of control.* New York, NY: Freeman.

Bargh, J. A. (1990). Auto-motives: Preconscious determinants of social interaction. In E. T. Higgins & R. M. Sorrentino (Eds.), *Handbook of motivation and cognition* (Vol. 2, pp. 93–130). New York, NY: Guilford.

Bowers, K. S. (1987). Revisioning the unconscious. *Canadian Psychology/Psychologie Canadienne, 28,* 93–132.

Brewin, C. R. (1989). Cognitive change processes in psychotherapy. *Psychological Review, 96,* 379–394.

Brody, N. (Ed.). (1987). The unconscious [Special issue]. *Personality and Social Psychology Bulletin,* 13.

Bruner, J. (1992). Another look at New Look 1. *American Psychologist, 47,* 780–783.

Buck, R. (1985). Prime theory: An integrated view of motivation and emotion. *Psychological Review, 92,* 389–413.

Cohen, F., & Lazarus, R. S. (1973). Active coping processes, coping dispositions, and recovery from surgery. *Psychosomatic Medicine, 35,* 375–398.

Collins, D. L., Baum, A., & Singer, J. E. (1983). Coping with chronic stress at Three Mile Island. *Health Psychology, 2,* 149–166.

Conway, M. A., & Bekerian, D. A. (1987). Situational knowledge and emotions. *Cognition and Emotion, 1,* 145–188.

Dalkvist, J., & Rollenhagen, C. (1989, September). *On the cognitive aspect of emotions: A review and model.* Reports from the Department of Psychology, University of Stockholm, No. 703.

de Rivera, J. (1977). A structural theory of the emotions. *Psychological Issues, 10,* 9–169.

de Sousa, R. (1987). *The rationality of emotion.* Cambridge, MA: MIT Press/Bradford.

Dewey, J. (1894). The theory of emotion. *Psychological Review, 1,* 553–569.

Dreikurs, R. (1967). *Psychodynamics and counseling.* Chicago, IL: Adler School of Professional Psychology.

Ekman, P. (1992). *Telling lies: Clues to deceit in the marketplace, politics, and marriage.* New York, NY: Norton. (Original work published 1985)

Epstein, S. (1990). Cognitive experiential self-theory. In L. A. Pervin (Ed.), *Handbook of personality theory and research* (pp. 165–192). New York, NY: Guilford.

Erdelyi, M. H. (1985). *Psychoanalysis: Freud's cognitive psychology.* New York, NY: Freeman.

Erdelyi, M. H. (1992). Psychodynamics and the unconscious. *American Psychologist, 47,* 784–787.

Eriksen, C. W. (1960). Discrimination and learning without awareness: A methodological survey and evaluation. *Psychological Review, 67,* 379–400.

Eriksen, C. W. (Ed.). (1962). *Behavior and awareness—A symposium of research and interpretation* (pp. 3–26). Durham, NC: Duke University Press.

Folkman, S., & Lazarus, R. S. (1988a). Manual for the Ways of Coping Questionnaire. Palo Alto, CA: Consulting Psychologists Press.

Folkman, S., & Lazarus, R. S. (1988b). Coping as a mediator of emotion. *Journal of Personality and Social Psychology, 54,* 466–475.

Frijda, N. H. (1986). *The emotions.* Cambridge, UK: Cambridge University Press.

Goleman, D. (1995). *Emotional intelligence: Why it can matter more than IQ.* New York, NY: Bantam.

Greenwald, A. G. (1992). New Look 3: Unconscious cognition reclaimed. *American Psychologist, 47,* 766–779.

Grinker, R. R., & Spiegel, J. P. (1945). *Men under stress.* New York, NY: McGraw-Hill.

Hobfoll, S. E. (1998). *Stress, culture, and community: The psychology and philosophy of stress.* New York, NY: Plenum.

Jacoby, L. L., Lindsay, D. S., & Toth, J. P. (1992). Unconscious influences revealed: Attention, awareness, and control. *American Psychologist, 47,* 802–809.

James, W. (1890). *Principles of psychology.* New York, NY: Holt.

Janis, I. L. (1951). *Air war and emotional stress.* New York, NY: McGraw-Hill.

Janis, I. L. (1958). *Psychological stress: Psychoanalytic and behavioral studies of surgical patients.* New York, NY: John Wiley.

Janis, I. L., & Mann, L. (1977). *Decision making.* New York, NY: Free Press.

Kihlstrom, J. F. (1987). The cognitive unconscious. *Science, 237,* 1445–1452.

Kihlstrom, J. F. (1990). The psychological unconscious. In L. A. Pervin (Ed.), *Handbook of personality: Theory and research* (pp. 445–464). New York, NY: Guilford.

Kihlstrom, J. F., Barnhardt, T. M., & Tataryn, D. J. (1992). The psychological unconscious: Found, lost, regained. *American Psychologist, 47,* 788–791.

Lazarus, R. S. (1964). A laboratory approach to the dynamics of psychological stress. *American Psychologist, 19,* 400–411.

Lazarus, R. S. (1966). *Psychological stress and the coping process.* New York, NY: McGraw-Hill.

Lazarus, R. S. (1968). Emotions and adaptation: Conceptual and empirical relations. In W. J. Arnold (Ed.), *Nebraska Symposium on Motivation* (pp. 175–266). Lincoln: University of Nebraska Press.

Lazarus, R. S. (1981). The stress and coping paradigm. In C. Eisdorfer, D. Cohen, A. Kleinman, & P. Maxim (Eds.), *Models for clinical psychopathology* (pp. 177–214). New York, NY: Spectrum.

Lazarus, R. S. (1983). The costs and benefits of denial. In S. Breznitz (Ed.), *The denial of stress* (pp. 1–30). New York, NY: International Universities Press.

Lazarus, R. S. (1985). The trivialization of distress. In J. C. Rosen & L. J. Solomon (Eds.), *Preventing health risk behaviors and promoting coping with illness* (Vol. 8, Vermont conference on the primary prevention of psychopathology, pp. 279–298). Hanover, NH: University Press of New England. (Reprinted from The master lecture series, Vol. 3, pp. 121–144, by B. L. Hammonds & C. J. Scheier, Eds., 1983, Washington, DC: American Psychological Association)

Lazarus, R. S. (1989). Constructs of the mind in mental health and psychotherapy. In A. Freeman, K. M. Simon, L. E. Beuktler, & H. Arkowitz (Eds.), *Comprehensive handbook of cognitive therapy* (pp. 99–121). New York, NY: Plenum.

Lazarus, R. S. (1991). *Emotion and adaptation.* New York, NY: Oxford University Press.

Lazarus, R. S. (1993). From psychological stress to the emotions: A history of changing outlooks. In *Annual review of psychology* (pp. 1–21). Palo Alto, CA: Annual Reviews, Inc.

Lazarus, R. S. (1998a). *Fifty years of the research and theory of R. S. Lazarus: An analysis of historical and perennial issues.* Mahway, NJ: Lawrence Erlbaum.

Lazarus, R. S. (1998b). The cognition-emotion debate: A bit of history. In T. Dalgleish & M. Power (Eds.), *The handbook of cognition and emotion* (pp. 3–19). Cambridge, UK: Wiley.

Lazarus, R. S. (1999). *Stress and emotion: A new synthesis.* New York, NY: Springer.

Lazarus, R. S. (in press). Relational meaning and discrete emotions. In K. R. Scherer, A. Schorr, & T. Johnstone (Eds.), *Appraisal processes in emotion: Theory, methods, research.* New York, NY: Oxford University Press.

Lazarus, R. S., & Alfert, E. (1964). The short-circuiting of threat by experimentally altering cognitive appraisal. *Journal of Abnormal and Social Psychology, 69,* 195–205.

Lazarus, R. S., Averill, J. R., & Opton, E. M., Jr. (1970). Towards a cognitive theory of emotion. In M. Arnold (Ed.), *Feelings and emotions* (pp. 207–232). New York, NY: Academic Press.

Lazarus, R. S., & Baker, R. W. (1956a). Personality and psychological stress—A theoretical and methodological framework. *Psychological Newsletter, 8,* 21–32.

Lazarus, R. S., & Baker, R. W. (1956b). Psychology. *Progress in Neurology and Psychiatry, 11,* 253–271.

Lazarus, R. S., & commentators. (1990). Theory based stress measurement. Psychological Inquiry, 1, 3–51.

Lazarus, R. S., & commentators. (1995). Vexing research problems inherent in cognitive-mediational theories of emotion, and some solutions. *Psychological Inquiry, 6,* 183–265.

Lazarus, R. S., Deese, J., & Osier, S. F. (1952). The effects of psychological stress upon performance. *Psychological Bulletin. 49,* 293–317.

Lazarus, R. S., & Folkman, S. (1984). *Stress, appraisal. and coping.* New York, NY: Springer.

Lazarus, R. S., & Launier, R. (1978). Stress-related transactions between person and environment. In L. A. Pervin & M. Lewis (Eds.), *Perspectives in interactional psychology* (pp. 287–327). New York, NY: Plenum.

Lazarus, R. S., & Lazarus, B. N. (1994). *Passion and reason: Making sense of our emotions.* New York, NY: Oxford University Press.

Lazarus, R. S., & Smith, C. A. (1988). Knowledge and appraisal in the cognition-emotion relationship. *Cognition and Emotion, 2,* 281–300.

LeDoux, J. W. (1989). Cognitive-emotional interactions in the brain. *Cognition and Emotion, 3,* 267–289.

Leeper, R. W. (1948). A motivational theory of emotion to replace "emotion as a disorganized response." *Psychological Review, 55,* 5–21.

Leventhal, H. (1984). *A perceptual motor theory of emotion* (pp. 271–291). Hillsdale, NJ: Lawrence Erlbaum.

Lewicki, P., Hill, T., & Czyzewska, M. (1992). Nonconscious acquisition of information. *American Psychologist, 47,* 796–801.

Lewis, A. (1998, January 2). *New York Times,* p. A15.

Loftus, E. F. (Guest Ed.). (1992). Science watch. *American Psychologist, 47,* 761–809.

Loftus, E. F., & Klinger, M. R. (1992). Is the unconscious smart or dumb? *American Psychologist, 47,* 761–765.

Maes, S., Leventhal, H., & de Ridder, D. T. D. (1996). Coping with chronic diseases. In M. Zeidner & N. S. Endler (Eds.), *Handbook of coping: Theory, research, applications* (pp. 221–252). New York, NY: John Wiley.

Mandler, G. (1984). *Mind and body: Psychology of emotion and stress.* New York, NY: Norton.

Mascolo, M. F., & Fischer, K. W. (1995). Developmental transformations in appraisals for pride, shame, and guilt. In J. P. Tangney & I. W. Fischer (Eds.), *Self-conscious emotions: The psychology of shame, guilt, embarrassment, and pride* (pp. 64–113). New York, NY: Guilford.

McAdams, D. P. (1996). Personality, modernity, and the storied self: A contemporary framework for studying persons. *Psychological Inquiry, 7,* 295–321.

McReynolds, P. (1956). A restricted conceptualization of human anxiety and motivation. *Psychological Reports, Monograph Supplements, 6,* 293–312.

Mechanic, D. (1978). *Students under stress: A study in the social psychology of adaptation.* New York, NY: Free Press. (Original work published 1962)

Merikle, P. M. (1992). Perception without awareness: Critical issues. *American Psychologist, 47,* 792–795.

Merleau-Ponty, M. (1962). *Phenomenology of perception* (C. Smith, Trans.). London, England: Routledge & Kegan Paul.

Oatley, K., & Johnson-Laird, P. N. (1987). Towards a cognitive theory of emotions. *Cognition and Emotion, 1,* 29–50.

Opton, E. M., Jr., Rankin, N., Nomikos, M., & Lazarus, R. S. (1965). The principle of short-circuiting of threat: Further evidence. *Journal of Personality, 33,* 622–635.

Ortony, A., Clore, G. L., & Collins, A. (1988). *The cognitive structure of emotions.* New York, NY: Cambridge University Press.

Parkinson, B., & Manstead, A. S. R. (1992). Appraisal as a cause of emotion. *Review of Personality and Social Psychology, 13,* 122–149.

Polanyi, M. (1966). *The tacit dimension.* Garden City, NY: Doubleday.

Reisenzein, R. (1995). On appraisal as causes of emotions. *Psychological Inquiry, 6,* 233–237.

Robertson, G. C. (1877). Notes. *Mind: A Quarterly Review, 2,* 413–415.

Roseman, I. J. (1984). Cognitive determinants of emotion: A structural theory. In P. Shaver (Ed.), *Review of personality and social psychology: Vol. 5. Emotions, relationships, and health* (pp. 11–36). Beverly Hills, CA: Sage.

Scherer, K. R. (1984). On the nature and function of emotion: A component process approach. In K. R. Scherer & P. Ekman (Eds.), *Approaches to emotion* (pp. 293–317). Hillsdale, NJ: Lawrence Erlbaum.

Selye, H. (1974). *Stress without distress.* Philadelphia, PA: J. B. Lippincott.

Selye, H. (1976). *The stress of life.* New York, NY: McGraw-Hill. (Original work published 1956)

Shepard, R. N. (1984). Ecological constraints on internal representation: Resonant kinematics of perceiving, imagining, thinking, and dreaming. *Psychological Review, 91,* 417–447.

Smith, C. A., & Ellsworth, P. C. (1985). Patterns of cognitive appraisal in emotion. *Journal of Personality and Social Psychology, 48,* 813–838.

Smith, C. A., Haynes, K. N., Lazarus, R. S., & Pope, L. K. (1993). In search of the "hot" cognitions: Attributions, appraisals, and their relation to emotion. *Journal of Personality and Social Psychology, 65,* 916–929.

Solomon, R. C. (1976). *The passions: The myth and nature of human emotion.* Garden City, NY: Doubleday.

Speisman, J. C., Lazarus, R. S., Mordkoff, A. M., & Davison, L. A. (1964). The experimental reduction of stress based on ego-defense theory. *Journal of Abnormal and Social Psychology, 68,* 367–380.

Staudenmeyer, H., Kinsman, R. S., Dirks, J. F., Spector, S. L., & Wangaard, C. (1979). Medical outcome in asthmatic patients. Effects of airways hyperactivity and symptom-focused anxiety. *Psychosomatic Medicine, 41,* 109–118.

Tolman, E. C. (1932). *Purposive behavior in animals and man.* New York, NY: Appleton.

Uleman, J. S., & Bargh, J. A. (Eds.). (1989). *Unintended thought.* New York, NY: Guilford.

Weiner, B. (1985). An attributional theory of motivation, achievement, and emotion. *Psychological Review, 92,* 548–573.

Weiner, B. (1986). *An attributional theory of motivation and emotion.* New York, NY: Springer-Verlag.

CHAPTER 9 Addendum

NURSING RESEARCH USING LAZARUS'S TRANSACTIONAL THEORY OF STRESS AND COPING AND THE WAYS OF COPING SCALE 2000–2010

VIRGINIA HILL RICE, EDITOR

Although Lazarus's Transactional Theory of Stress and Coping (TTSC) has been evolving and studied for more than 40 years and has been used in a number of different disciplines, nursing continues to find it most relevant and useful for addressing its concerns. The following provides information on the nursing research studies published in the last decade (2000–2010) using the TTSC model. Constructs and components studied include primary appraisal, secondary appraisal, reappraisal, and coping (including problem and emotion focused). Studies using the Ways of Coping Scale (Folkman & Lazarus, 1988) will also be cited.

Sixteen nursing research studies using the TTSC model were identified in a recent Cumulative Index to Nursing and Allied Health (CINAHL) search for the years 2000 to 2010. Gold, Treadmill, Weissman, and Vichinsky (2008) examined stress and coping in the siblings of children with sickle cell disease, and Gibbons, Dempster, and Moutray (2009) surveyed nursing students on their sources of stress. Stress was assessed in a sample of professional Australian nurses (Healy & McKay, 2000), and job uncertainty in nursing was evaluated in Alberta, Canada (Maurier & Northcott, 2000). Clinical studies

EDITOR'S NOTE: *It is my privilege to report on the extensive use of Lazarus's Transactional Theory of Stress and Coping (TTSC) and his Ways of Coping Scale by so many nurse researchers in the last decade (2000–2010). In 1999, at one of our very early meetings for the first edition of this text, Dr. Lazarus indicated how honored he was that his work was so useful for patients, professional nursing practice, and for nursing research. Richard S. Lazarus, a distinguished scholar, researcher, and professor emeritus of psychology at the University of California, Berkeley, died on November 24, 2002, leaving a remarkable legacy for all in the field of stress, coping, and health.*

documented coping with chronic heart failure (Yu, Lee, Kwong, Thompson, & Woo, 2008), asthma (Vinson, 2002), chronic illnesses among HIV-infected women (Bova, 2001), chronic pain (Dysvik, Natvig, Eikeland, & Lindstrøm, 2005; Knussen & McParland, 2009; Richardson & Poole, 2001), and the intensive care unit experience (Cronqvist, Theorell, Burns, & Lutzen, 2001). Gill and Loh (2010) examined health-promoting behaviors in new primiparous mothers, and Shaw (2001) documented depression and grief post-miscarriage. Ducharme and Trudeau (2002) studied an individual stress management intervention for caregivers of the elderly, and Sherwood and colleagues (2004) developed a conceptual framework for the care-giving of persons with a brain tumor. Lazarus's TTSC model was foundational to understanding stress in the recovery of persons with psychiatric disabilities (Provencher, 2007). In addition to the studies cited above, 16 nursing research dissertations were guided by the TTSC model in the same period of time.

The following nursing research studies used the Ways of Coping Scale in the last 10 years. It is a 66-item questionnaire with a wide range of thoughts and actions that people commonly use to deal with stressful encounters. It measures coping processes, not coping dispositions or coping style. The stressor or demand is first described in an interview or in a briefly written statement. The revised Ways of Coping (Folkman & Lazarus, 1985) differs from the original Ways of Coping Checklist (Folkman & Lazarus, 1980) in its scoring. The response format in the original version was a dichotomous "Yes or No." On the revised version the subject responds on a 4-point Likert scale (0 = does not apply and/or not used to 3 = used a great deal).

A number of studies in the last decade have assessed Ways of Coping by nurses (Golbasi, Kelleci, & Dogan, 2008; Hays, All, Mannahan, Cuaderes, & Wallace, 2006; LeSergent & Haney, 2005; Payne, 2001; Timmermann, Naziri, & Etienne, 2009; West, Ahern, Byrnes, & Kwanten, 2007) and nursing students (Gibbons, Dempster, & Moutray, 2009; Lo, 2002; Pryjmachuk & Richards, 2007; Tully, 2004). Clinical studies have assessed patients' ways of coping with alcohol use (Boyd, Baliko, Cox, & Tavakoli, 2007) urinary incontinence (Criner, 2006), chronic obstructive pulmonary disease (Andenaes, Kalfoss, & Wahl, 2004), chronic fatigue syndrome (Tuck, Wallace, Casalenuovo, & May, 2000), and prostate cancer (Eller et al., 2006). Assessment of coping by caregivers of family members with childhood diabetes mellitus (Azar & Solomon, 2001) and skull base tumors (Wyness, Durity, & Durity, 2002) were also determined. International studies using the Ways of Coping Scale have been numerous, including those completed in China (Xianyu & Lambert, 2006), Sweden (Ahlström & Wadensten, 2010), and Japan (Filazoglu & Griva, 2008).

References

Ahlström, G., & Wadensten, B. (2010). Encounters in close care relations from the perspective of personal assistants working with persons with severe disability. *Health & Social Care in the Community, 18*(2), 180–188.

Andenaes, R., Kalfoss, M. H., & Wahl, A. (2004). Psychological distress and quality of life in hospitalized patients with chronic obstructive pulmonary disease. *Journal of Advanced Nursing, 46*(5), 523–530.

Azar, R., & Solomon, C. R. (2001). Coping strategies of parents facing child diabetes mellitus. *Journal of Pediatric Nursing, 16*(6), 418–428.

Bova, C. (2001). Adjustment to chronic illness among HIV-infected women. *Journal of Nursing Scholarship, 33*(3), 217–223.

Boyd, M. R., Baliko, B., Cox, M. F., & Tavakoli, A. (2007). Stress, coping, and alcohol expectancies in rural African-American women. *Archives of Psychiatric Nursing, 21*(2), 70–79.

Criner, J. A. (2006). *An exploratory study of the psychosocial effects of stress urinary incontinence and coping strategies among military women* [Doctoral dissertation]. The University of Texas at Austin.

Cronqvist, A., Theorell, T., Burns, T., & Lutzen, K. (2001). Dissonant imperatives in nursing: A conceptualization of stress in intensive care in Sweden. *Intensive and Critical Care Nursing, 17*(4), 228–236.

Ducharme, F., & Trudeau, D. (2002). Qualitative evaluation of a stress management intervention for elderly caregivers at home: A constructivist approach. *Issues in Mental Health Nursing, 23*(7), 691–713.

Dysvik, E., Natvig, G. K., Eikeland, O. J., & Lindstrøm, T. C (2005). Coping with chronic pain. *International Journal of Nursing Studies 42,* 297–305.

Eller, L. S., Lev, E. L., Gejerman, G., Colella, J., Esposito, M., Lanteri, V., . . . Sawczuk, I. (2006). Prospective study of quality of life of patients receiving treatment for prostate cancer. *Nursing Research, 55*(2), S23–S36.

Filazoglu, G., & Griva, K. (2008). Coping and social support and health-related quality of life in women with breast cancer in Turkey. *Psychology, Health and Medicine, 13*(5), 559–573.

Folkman, S., & Lazarus, R. S. (1980). An analysis of coping in a middle-aged community sample. *Journal of Health and Social Behavior, 21,* 219–239.

Folkman, S., & Lazarus, R. S. (1985). If it changes it must be a process: Study of emotion and coping during three stages of a college examination. *Journal of Personality and Social Psychology, 48,* 150–170.

Folkman, S., & Lazarus, R. S. (1988). Coping as a mediator of emotion. *Journal of Personality and Social Psychology, 54,* 466–475.

Gibbons, C., Dempster, M., & Moutray, M. (2009). Stress, coping and satisfaction in nursing students. *Journal of Advanced Nursing, 67*(3), 621–632.

Gill, R. M., & Loh, J. (2010). The role of optimism in health-promoting behaviors in new primiparous mothers. *Nursing Research, 59*(5), 348–355.

Golbasi, Z., Kelleci, M., & Dogan, S. (2008). Relationships between coping strategies, individual characteristics and job satisfaction in a sample of hospital nurses: Cross-sectional questionnaire survey. *Anesthesiology Clinics, 45*(12), 1800–1806.

Gold, J. I., Treadmill, M., Weissman, L., & Vichinsky, E. (2008). An expanded Transactional Stress and Coping Model for siblings of children with sickle cell disease: Family functioning and sibling coping, self-efficacy and perceived social support. *Child: Care, Health and Development, 34*(4), 491–502.

Hays, M. A., All, A. C., Mannahan, C., Cuaderes, E., & Wallace, D. (2006). Reported stressors and ways of coping utilized by intensive care unit nurses. *Dimensions of Critical Care Nursing, 25*(4), 185–193.

Healy, C., & McKay, M. F. (2000). Nursing stress: The effect of coping strategies and job satisfaction in a sample of Australian nurses. *Journal of Advanced Nursing 31,* 681–688.

Knussen, C., & McParland, J. (2009). Catastrophizing, ways of coping and pain beliefs in relation to pain intensity and pain-related disability. *Journal of Pain Management, 2*(2), 203–215.

LeSergent, C., & Haney, C. (2005). Rural hospital nurse's stressors and coping strategies: A survey. *International Journal of Nursing Studies, 42,* 315–325.

Lo, R. (2002). A longitudinal study of perceived level of stress, coping and self-esteem of undergraduate nursing students: an Australian case study. *Journal of Advanced Nursing, 39*(2), 119–126.

Maurier, W. L., & Northcott, H. C. (2000). Self-reported risk factors and perceived chance of getting HIV/AIDS in the 1990s in Alberta. *Canadian Journal of Public Health, 91,* 340–344.

Payne, N. (2001). Occupational stressors and coping as determinants of burnout in female hospice nurses. *Journal of Advanced Nursing, 3*(3), 396–405.

Provencher, H. L. (2007). Role of psychological factors in studying recovery from a transactional stress-coping approach: Implications for mental health nursing practices. International *Journal of Mental Health Nursing, 16*(3), 188–197.

Pryjmachuk, S., & Richards, D. A. (2007). Predicting stress in pre-registration nursing students. *British Journal of Health Psychology, 12,* 125–144.

Richardson, C., & Poole, H. (2001). Chronic pain and coping: A proposed role for nurses and nursing models. *Journal of Advanced Nursing, 34*(5), 659–667.

Shaw, C. (2001). A framework for the study of coping, illness behavior and outcomes. *Journal of Advanced Nursing, 29*(5), 1246–1255.

Sherwood, P., Given, B., Given, C., Schiffman, R., Murman, D., & Lovely, M. (2004). Caregivers of persons with a brain tumor: A conceptual model. *Nursing Inquiry, 11*(1), 43–53.

Timmermann, M., Naziri, D., & Etienne, A.M. (2009). Defence mechanisms and coping strategies among caregivers in palliative care units. *Journal of Palliative Care, 25*(3), 181–190.

Tuck, I., Wallace, D., Casalenuovo, G., & May, B. (2000). Psychosocial responses of sufferers of chronic fatigue syndrome. *Journal of Chronic Fatigue Syndrome, 7*(3), 49–63.

Tully, A. (2004). Stress, sources of stress and ways of coping among psychiatric nursing students. *Journal of Psychiatric and Mental Health Nursing, 11,* 43–47.

Vinson, J. A. (2002). Children with asthma: Initial development of the Child Resilience Model. *Journal of Pediatric Nursing, 28*(2), 149–158.

West, S., Ahern, M., Byrnes, M., & Kwanten, L. (2007). New graduate nurse adaptation to shift work: Can we help? *Collegian, 14*(1), 23–30.

Wyness, M. A., Durity, M. B., & Durity, F. (2002). Narratives of patients with skullbase tumors and their family members: Lessons for nursing practice. *Axone, 24,* 18–35.

Xianyu, Y., & Lambert, V. A. (2006). Investigation of the relationships among workplace stressors, ways of coping, and the mental health of Chinese head nurses. *Nursing Health Science, 8*(3), 147–155.

Yu, D., Lee, D., Kwong, A., Thompson, D. R., & Woo, J. (2008). Living with chronic heart failure: A review of qualitative studies of older people. *Journal of Advanced Nursing, 61*(5), 474–483.

10

STRESS, COPING, AND HEALTH IN CHILDREN

NANCY A. RYAN-WENGER, VICKI L. (SHARRER) WILSON, AND
ALEXANDRA G. BROUSSARD

Stressful situations and attempts to cope with these experiences have a direct and observable impact on an individual's psychological, behavioral, and physiological systems. Therefore, these experiences are of interest to nursing and other health care professionals. Effective coping strategies may help prevent or minimize maladaptive stress responses. Because lifelong patterns for coping with stress are begun in childhood, it is important to understand children's stressors, coping patterns, outcomes, and the environmental and individual factors that influence the stress-coping process (Compas, Connor-Smith, Saltzman, Thomsen, & Wadsworth, 2001). For simplicity, in this chapter, a *child* is generally defined as a person between the ages of 6 and 21 years, unless otherwise noted. Extant knowledge about children's stress-coping processes is derived primarily from the disciplines of nursing, psychology, sociology, and medicine. This chapter, although not all-inclusive, is a synthesis of key findings from these disciplines.

THEORETICAL FRAMEWORK

There are no specific models or theories to explain the entire process of children's development and their stress and coping, therefore, this chapter is based on an integration of three theoretical perspectives: (1) growth and development

theories, (2) Lazarus's (2000) transactional model of stress and coping, and (3) Bronfenbrenner's (1979) ecological model. Within a developmental context, sources of stress are closely related to age, gender, and developmental level. In addition, growth, maturation, and expansion of environmental influences that occur with increasing age change the nature of stressful experiences (Berk, 2008). The literature reveals two major categories of stressors in children normative and non-normative. *Normative* refers to the common, developmental stressors of daily life (e.g., being overweight, feeling left out of the group, parents fighting, or getting bad grades). *Non-normative* stressors arise from unusual or traumatic experiences (e.g., serious illness of the child or parent, child abuse, or community disasters). Age and gender influence what is most stressful, for example, "being larger than others your age" is more stressful for adolescent girls than for adolescent boys. Troubled peer relationships with same-sex friends are very stressful for school-age children, whereas the most stressful relationships for adolescents are usually with the opposite sex. From an ecological perspective, human behavior demands an examination of multiple systems across different settings (Bronfenbrenner, 1979). The ecological environment is best presented by a nested, concentric model with the individual system at the core of relationship, community, and societal systems (see Figure 10.1).

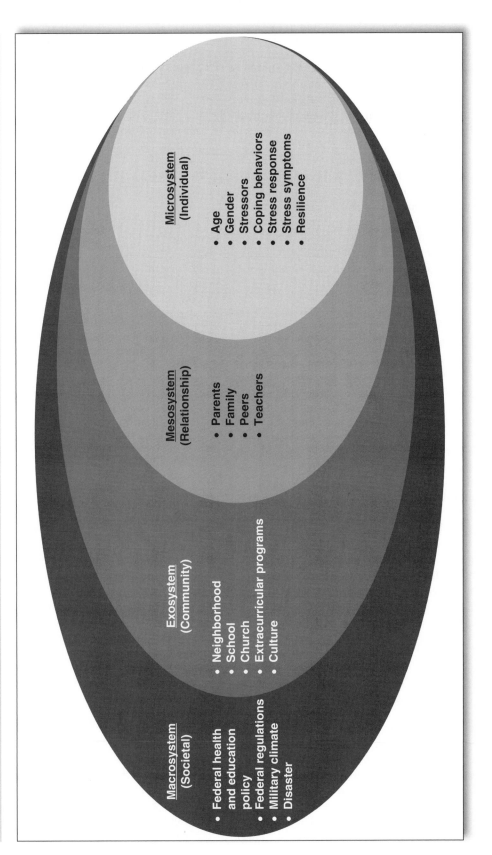

Figure 10.1 An Ecological Model (Bronfenbrenner, 1979) Adapted to Illustrate Potential Sources of Stress, Protective Factors, and Modifying Factors That Influence Children's Coping Behaviors and Stress-Related Responses

The microsystem of the child includes characteristics and internal traits such as age, gender, and personality; stressors related to the self; coping behaviors; and stress responses. The mesosystem encompasses the quality of the child's relationships with parents, other family members, close friends, and teachers. The exosystem is the community environment that may directly or indirectly affect the child. Examples include exposure to community stressors such as violence, drugs, or homelessness, or the effects of after-school programs and religious influences. The macrosystem includes the impact of societal influences on the child such as educational and health care policy, government, the country's military climate, and natural disasters.

Sources of Stress in Children and Adolescents

Sources of stress in preschool, elementary, junior high, and high school children were first quantified by Coddington (1972), who developed the widely used Life Event Scales for children (LES) consisting of 36 stressful life events, 78% of which are non-normative. The events were derived from the literature about adult coping behavior, the popular Holmes and Rahe (1967) Social Readjustment Rating Scale, and the authors' experience with children. The amount of "life change" likely to be incurred by each stressful event was estimated by other professionals who worked with children. "Death of a parent" was assigned the highest number of "life change units." A total stress score was the sum of life change units for each stressor experienced in the past year. Other instruments with items derived from adults' perspective were developed, including a revision of the Life Events Scale (LES) (Table 10.1).

Research designed to examine children's responses to "life stress" requires instruments that tap the range of stressors that are most relevant to children. New instruments were developed from events that children identified as stressful to them e.g., the Feel Bad Scale (Lewis, Siegel, & Lewis, 1984), and the Children's Sources of Stress Scale (Ryan-Wenger, Sharrer, & Campbell, 2005). To obtain stressors for a new instrument, children were asked to identify events that were stressful or made them "feel bad, nervous, or worried" (Lewis et al., 1984).

Children's responses were incorporated into the 20-item Feel Bad Scale (FBS) consisting of 17 (85%) normative stressors and 3 (15%) non-normative stressors. In fact, there are only 5 items in common between the adult-generated LES and the child-generated FBS (Ryan, 1988). To identify sources of stress that are most salient to school-age children for the new Children's Sources of Stress Scale (CSSS), Ryan-Wenger et al. (2005) conducted studies with 688 children, second grade through eighth grade, from Ohio and Washington in the year 2000. Children were asked to identify stressors, stress symptoms, and coping behaviors. The 494 children from Washington responded to the question, "What is the worst thing that has happened to you lately?" The 194 children from Ohio responded to the question, "What are some of the things that make you feel bad, nervous, or worried?" The children in Ohio reported 414 stressful situations which were inductively sorted into 54 mutually exclusive categories. The 494 responses from the children in Washington were deductively sorted into 45 of the 54 original categories.

The 54 CSSS stressor categories were compared to six similar instruments and the literature published between 1972 and 1997 (Ryan-Wenger et al., 2005). Twenty-three of the stressors were represented in instruments published in the '70s, including problems related to parents or family members, getting in trouble, bad grades, feeling left out, being lost, and their appearance. Nine more stressors emerged in the 1980s, all of which were normative developmental stressors, for example, feeling bad about oneself, and being pressured by friends and parents.

In the 1990s, 16 new stressors were identified, most of which are normative (e.g., fighting with friends, being made fun of, and doing things in front of others). Several stressors related to the socioeconomic climate of the '90s included being bullied, violence, disasters, and war or terrorism. In the 2000s, six normative stressors were added. School-aged children identified stressors such as too much homework, playing sports and games, and too many things to do. These findings are validated by David Elkind (2001) in the third edition of his book called *The Hurried Child: Growing Up Too Fast Too Soon*, in which he states that parents feel compelled to enroll their children in extracurricular activities as well as excel in school,

Table 10.1 Instruments for Measurement of Stressors in Children and Adolescents

Author	Instrument	Target group	Original source of items	Format	Completed by	Meaning of scores
Coddington (1972)	Life Event Record	Preschool, elementary, junior high, senior high	Author, literature (life change units determined by adults)	30–42 items; checked if experienced in past 12 months	Parent or adolescent	Total number of life change units = amount of social readjustment
Yamamoto (1979)	Stressful Experiences Scale	7- to 11-year-olds	Literature, classroom teachers	20 items; rated on scale of 1 to 7 for severity and frequency	Children	Sum of scores for each subscale = stress severity and frequency
Monaghan, Robinson, & Dodge (1979)	Children's Life Events Inventory	Children	Coddington Scales and authors (Life change units determined by adults)	40 items; checked if experienced in past 12 months	Parent or child	Total number of life change units = amount of social readjustment
Yeaworth, York, Hussey, Ingle, & Goodwin (1980)	Adolescent Life Change Event Scale	Junior high, senior high	Authors (life change units determined by adolescents)	31 items; checked if occurred in past 12 months	Adolescents	Sum of life change units = amount of life change
Johnson & McCutcheon (1980)	Life Events Checklist	12- to 17-year-olds	Coddington scales and authors	46 items; checked if occurred in past 12 months; circled if good or bad; impact of the event on life rated on 0 to 3 scale	Adolescents	Sum of impact ratings for positive & negative events = positive & negative change scores
Newcomb, Huba, & Bentler (1981)	Life Events Questionnaire	7th–12th grades	Literature	39 items; rated 1 to 5 on a "happiness" scale; yes/no in past 12 months and before the past 12 months	Adolescents	Sum of item scores = severity score; total number of items selected = frequency score
Coddington (1984)	Life Event Scale for Children Life Event Scale for Adolescents	School-age children	Adults, literature	31 to 47 items; yes/no in 3-month intervals (summer, fall, autumn, and spring)	Children	Total number of life change units = amount of social readjustment

(Continued)

Table 10.1 (Continued)

Author	Instrument	Target group	Original source of items	Format	Completed by	Meaning of scores
Beall & Schmidt (1984)	Youth Adaptation Rating Scale	Junior high, high school	Adolescents determined the items and severity ratings for each one	59 items; checked if stressor occurred; severity rated; time period not specified	Adolescents	Sum of severity ratings = degree of adaptation required
Lewis, Siegel, & Lewis (1984)	Feel Bad Scale	8- to 12-year-olds	Children	20 items; rated on scale of 1 to 5 for how bad it is, and how often it happens	Children	Product of total scores for severity subscale × frequency subscale = total level of stress
Bobo, Gilchrist, Elmer, Snow, & Schinke (1986)	Adolescent Hassles Inventory	11- to 13-year-olds (6th graders)	Borrowed from Kanner, Coyne, Schaefer, & Lazarus (1981); some were investigator developed	69 items; rated on scale of 1 to 3 for severity of hassle if experienced within the last week (1 = small/minor hassle, 3 = large /major hassle)	Adolescents	Sum of all nonzero item scores = frequency of daily hassles; sum of all items = severity of daily hassles
Elwood (1987)	Stressor Inventories	4th and 7th grades	Children	Items include 7 or 8 major events & 16 to 24 daily hassles; rated on scale of 0 to 4 for amount of upsettingness	Children, adolescents	Sum of scores for each event = level of stressfulness
Compas, Davis, Forsythe, & Wagner (1987)	Adolescent Perceived Events Scale—Jr. High version	Junior high	Junior high school students	142 items; checked if experienced during this school year; rated from −4 to +4 on bad to good scale (desirability)	Adolescents	Total weights of positive and negative events = cognitive appraisal of stressors
Compas et al. (1987)	Adolescent Perceived Events Scale—High School version; College version	High school–college	High school and college students	200 to 210 items; checked if experienced in past 3 months; rated from −4 to +4 on desirability, impact, and frequency	Adolescents	Sum of product of desirability ratings × impact ratings = cognitive appraisal of stressors
McCubbin & Patterson (1987)	A-FILE: Adolescent-Family Inventory of Life Events and Changes	12- to 18-year-olds	Other stress scales, group of 11th graders	50 items; checked if experienced in past 12 months and before the past 12 months	Adolescents	Sum of checked responses = amount of stressful change in family

Author	Instrument	Target group	Original source of items	Format	Completed by	Meaning of scores
Dise-Lewis (1988)	Life Events and Coping Inventory	12- to 15-year-olds	Adolescents	125 items; scored on scale of 1 to 9 for amount of stress it caused	Young adolescents	Sum of item scores = amount of stress
Broome, Hellier, Wilson, Dale, & Glanville (1988)	Child Medical Fear Scale	5- to 12-year-olds	Clinical experience of children	17 items; rated on scale of 0 to 2 for level of fear	Children; parent version also available	Sum of item scores = level of medical fear
Reed, Thompson, Brannick, & Sacco (1991)	Physical Appearance State and Trait Anxiety Scale (PASTAS)	Undergraduate females	Author derived	48 weight-related appearance items and 48 non-weight related appearance items; level of anxiety about each body part rated from 1 = never to 5 = almost always	Young adults	Sum of item scores = level of disturbance
Grych, Sied, & Fincham (1992)	Children's Perception of Interparental Conflict Scale	4th and 5th grades	Investigator-developed or borrowed from Emery & O'Leary's (1982) Personal Data Form	51 items scored as 1 = True, 2 = Sort of true, or 3 = False	Children	Sum of scores on 9 subscales: frequency, intensity, child-focused, threat, self-blame, triangulation, resolution, coping efficacy, marital stability
Gullone & King (1993), Burnham & Gullone (1997)	Fear Survey Schedule for Children	2nd through 12th grades	Theory, clinical experience, literature	80 items; scale of 0–2 for amount of fear perceived for each event	Children, adolescents	Sum of item scores = total level of fear
Thompson, Cattarin, Fowler & Fisher, (1995)	Perception of Teasing Scale	5- to 16-year-olds	Investigator-developed	11 items; frequency scored on scale of 1 to 5 (1 = never, 5 = very often); severity scored on scale of 1 to 5 (1 = not upset, 5 = very upset)	Children, adolescents	Sum of item scores = frequency of perceptions of teasing about weight and competency

(Continued)

Table 10.1 (Continued)

Author	Instrument	Target group	Original source of items	Format	Completed by	Meaning of scores
Hockenberry-Eaton, Manteuffel, & Bottomley (1997)	Childhood Cancer Stressors Inventory	7- to 13-year-olds	Literature, clinical experience	18 items; true/false for experience of each stressor; scale of 0 to 3 for bothersomeness of each stressor	Children, adolescents	Number of stressors = frequency of stress; sum of bothersome scores = intensity of stress; sum of frequency × intensity scores = total perceived stress
Dumont & Provost (1999)	Adolescent Hassles Inventory	8th and 11th graders	French version of 68 items (Bobo, Gilchrist, Elmer, Snow, & Stevens [1986])	59 items scored as yes/no; yes items scored on scale of 1 = not annoyed at all, to 4 = very annoyed	Adolescents	Mean of item scores = severity of daily hassles
Hyman & Snook (2002)	My Worst Experience Scale (MWES)	9- to 18-year-olds	Investigator-developed	Part I: 21 events; child checks the worst one that was experienced and writes a description. Part II: 105 items (thoughts, behaviors, emotions) rated on scale 0 to 5 for frequency (0 = did not happen; 5 = all the time)	Children, adolescents	Sum of total raw scores and T-scores for 7 symptom or general psychopathology subscales; total T-score = PTSD symptom score
Ryan-Wenger, Sharrer, & Campbell (2005)	Children's Source of Stress Scale (CSSS)	7- to 12-year-olds (2nd to 6th graders)	Children, put together by investigators	51 item self-report checklist that identifies sources of acute and chronic stress	Children	Sum of all nonzero item scores = frequency of stressors experienced by child
Goodman & Scott (1999)	Strengths & Difficulties Questionnaire (DSQ)	3- to 16-year-olds	Theory and diagnostic concepts	25 items	children, adolescents, parents, teachers	Five subscales: emotional symptoms, conflict problems, hyperactivity/ inattention, peer relationships, and pro-social behavior

resulting in over-booked, overwhelmed children. In the 2000s, children reported that girlfriend/boyfriend problems were stressful for them. This source of stress is developmentally beyond the maturity level of school-aged children who should be focusing more on same-sex peer relationships rather than opposite-sex relationships.

Table 10.1 describes many instruments developed during the past 38 years to measure stressors in children from preschool age to adolescence. Despite the many instruments available to measure sources of stress in children, most were developed for and tested on largely White, middle-class children, and published more than a decade ago. New research is needed to identify sources of stress that are most salient to children of different racial, ethnic, geographic, and socioeconomic backgrounds.

Contemporary Sources of Stress for Children and Adolescents

Between 2000 and 2010, sociopolitical changes in the United States negatively affected more and more children and adolescents, including homelessness, illicit drug use, and bullying (Sparrow, 2007a); community violence; and war (Carroll & Ryan-Wenger, 1999; Gullone & King, 1993; Neff & Dale, 1996; Wang, Iannotti, Luk, & Nansel, 2010). In addition, the Centers for Disease Control and Prevention (CDC, 2000) and Capuzzi and Gross (2008) report that 500,000 juveniles are homeless, 27 million juveniles live in poverty, and 1.5 million juveniles are reported to be abused every year. McWhirter, McWhirter, McWhirter, and McWhirter (2007) predict that approximately 77% of juveniles will have used alcohol by age 14, and 25% will acquire a sexually transmitted disease during high school. These and other contemporary sources of stress are discussed below, according to the originating ecological system.

Illicit Drug Use—An Endosystem Stressor

Alcohol is the most common drug of choice for adolescents, despite the minimum legal drinking age of 21 in most states. Teenage alcohol consumption is associated with motor vehicle crashes, injuries, death, fighting, and crime (Centers for Disease Control and Prevention [CDC], 2006). In 2005, 15% of eleventh and twelfth graders reported driving after drinking alcohol. In addition to the accessibility of alcohol, 55% of 12- to 17-year-olds report that marijuana is easy to obtain, according to the Substance Abuse and Mental Health Services Administration (2001). Marijuana use may have a profound negative effect on the development of very young teenagers. Other illicit drugs such as cocaine and amphetamines are linked with cardiovascular problems such as heart attack and stroke (National Institute on Drug Abuse, 2005; MacKay & Duran, 2008; CDC, 2006).

The relationship between childhood stressors and illicit drug use cannot be ignored. Drug use and abuse are associated with sexually transmitted diseases, unintentional injuries, interpersonal violence, and crime; adverse childhood experiences (ACEs) may lead to drug abuse as well. In a retrospective study of 8,613 adults, the number and type of ACEs were examined in association with early initiation of drug use (Dube et al., 2003). Results indicated that each ACE increased the likelihood of illicit drug initiation 2- to 4-fold by the age of 14, as well as increased the likelihood of lifetime drug use. While the 14 and under age group showed the strongest relationship, the other age categories (15 to 18 years, and 19 or older) were also related.

Bullying—A Mesosystem Stressor

While childhood bullying has tormented children for quite a long time, its effects on children's physical and psychological health continue to raise concern. The prevalence of how often a child bullies or is bullied and the methods used to do so were studied in a sample of 1,211 primary and secondary school students from the Netherlands (Dehue, Bolman, & Völlink, 2008). Results showed that 16% of the children had bullied someone and nearly a quarter (22%) had reported being bullied. In both instances, the percentages were higher among primary students than secondary students (17.1% vs. 13.5%; 23.4% vs. 18.6%, respectively). The most frequent methods used to bully others included chatting on the Internet (13.0%) and name-calling (11.7%). A study by Aricak and colleagues (2008) found that of a sample of 269 Turkish 12- to 19-year-olds, more than half (59.5%) reported saying things about peers online they would not say face to face. Over one-third of them (35.3%) had introduced themselves as someone else on the Internet.

The consequences of all types of bullying can be devastating. Victims of bullying suffer high levels of depression, social anxiety, and loneliness in comparison with their uninvolved counterparts, and teachers rated them as more disengaged in school (Juvonen, Graham, & Schuster, 2003). Furthermore, victims suffer from emotional distress and social marginalization more than their uninvolved classmates and the bullies themselves. According to Sparrow (2007b), the sustained stress of bullying can have long-term effects on metabolism, cardiovascular and immune system functioning, and brain development. The fear of future and recurrent stress incurred from bullying may also interfere with a child's healthy development of self-esteem. Anxiety often manifests itself in physical maladies. In a study of 2,588 Swedish children 10 to 18 years old conducted by Hjern, Alfven, & Östberg (2008), an average of 8.3% of this sample reported being subjected to one type of harassment weekly; the frequency of harassment was highest in grades 3 through 6 and decreased significantly in grades 7 to 9 and upper secondary schools. An average of 3.5% of children reported several forms of harassment weekly. Children who reported harassment were 1.7 to 3.8 times more likely to report headaches and/or stomachaches weekly.

Current research identifies four specific types of bullying (Smokowski & Kopasz, 2005). Physical bullies participate in direct bullying behaviors such as hitting and kicking, and are more likely to be boys. The second type, verbal bullies, hurt their victims emotionally by calling them names and humiliating them. Relational bullies often exclude and/or ignore certain children from activities, isolating them from their own peer group. Finally, reactive bullies taunt and provoke others into fighting them, then claim self-defense when they retaliate. A study conducted by Hampel, Manhal, and Hayer (2009) found, in a sample of 409 German children ages 10 to 16 years, that 68 (16.3%) of them reported that they were bullied by other children. Of the 68 victims, 27 (39.7%) received direct physical or verbal bullying, 23 (33.8%) received relational bullying, and 18 (26.5%) encountered physical, verbal, and relational bullying. Victims of direct physical or verbal bullying reported more antisocial behaviors, anger

control problems, emotional distress, and negative view of self than nonvictimized students, while children who were relationally victimized had higher scores on anger control problems, emotional distress, and negative self-esteem than their nonvictimized counterparts.

With the advent of computers and cellular telephone technology, the most recent method of bullying is known as cyberbullying. Now, bullies can tease and ridicule their victims from the comfort of home while children being bullied have difficulty escaping from their tormenters. Instruments to measure cyberbullying are emerging in the literature, but none have established reliability or validity psychometrics. The Cyberbullying Questionnaire (CBQ) was administered to 1,431 adolescents aged 12 to 17 years old in Spain (Calvete, Orue, Estévez, Villardón, & Padilla, 2010). The items represent 16 different forms of cyberbullying. They found that 44.1% of 12- to 17-year-olds "sometimes" or "often" participated in cyberbullying. Some of the most prevalent types of Internet harassment included deliberately excluding someone from an online group (20.2%); writing embarrassing jokes, rumors, gossip, or comments about a classmate on the Internet (20.1%); hacking to send messages by e-mail that could make trouble for the other person (18.1%); and sending threatening or insulting messages by e-mail (15.8%).

Juvonen and Gross (2008) used a 5-point scale ranging from "never" to "more than 12 times" to describe how frequently youth experienced name-calling or insults, threats, the spreading of embarrassing or private pictures, the sharing of private communications, and password theft. Respondents also mentioned whether they experienced such things through e-mail, instant messaging, text messages, chat rooms, blogs, personal profile websites, and message boards. Another study modified the Revised Peer Experiences Questionnaire (RPEQ) and added four self-report questions to the victimization subscales (Dempsey, Sulkowski, Nichols, & Storch, 2009) including text/instant messaging, comments on their web space, e-mail, and creation of disparaging web pages. Increases in the prevalence of cyberbullying among children and adolescents have led to the question of whether such victimization may lead to increased suicide rates of children. However, as of yet, no research has demonstrated a causal relationship between the two (David-Ferdon & Hertz, 2009).

Community Violence— An Exosystem Stressor

Yet another source of stress for children and adolescents is exposure to violence within their own communities. The National Center for Children Exposed to Violence (NCCEV, 2006) defines community violence as "exposure to acts of interpersonal violence committed by individuals who are not intimately related to the victim." An estimated 41% (10.4 million) of adolescents from the ages of 12 to 17 years have witnessed violence (Zinzow et al., 2009). The repercussions of witnessing community violence include mental health issues and an increased propensity to use violence. This study by Zinzow et al. (2009) found that community violence was significantly associated with post-traumatic stress disorder (PTSD) as well as major depressive episodes (MDE) in adolescents. Within a sixth-grade sample of 702 children living in or near public housing, there was a positive correlation between exposure to/victimization by violence in the community and intent to use violence ($r = 0.29$, $p \le .0001$), along with an increased frequency during the past 3 months of drug use such as alcohol, cigarettes, and crack cocaine ($r = 0.11$ to 0.29, $p < .05$) (Barkin, Kreiter, & DuRant, 2001).

Another study conducted by Skybo (2005) investigated children's appraisal of violence and the biopsychosocial symptoms they experience due to encounters with violence. The sample consisted of 62 children between the ages of 7 and 14 years from a metropolitan area where murders, rapes, robberies, and vehicle theft increased from 2000 to 2002. Among the 62 children, 60 (97%) had witnessed some form of violence. Out of 24 stress symptoms that may be experienced during a stressful event, children reported experiencing an average of 11 symptoms ($SD = 10$), with the most common symptoms being confused, afraid, mad, and cry. These symptoms also were ranked as having the most impact on children. It was also discovered that the number of witnessed violent encounters correlated with the impact of such encounters ($r = .850$, $p < .01$) as well as the impact of the stress symptoms ($r = .293$, $p < .05$). Children witnessing more violent episodes experienced a greater impact from the encounters and displayed more stress symptoms than their counterparts.

War—A Macrosystem Stressor

Since 2003, the United States' war on terror in Afghanistan and Iraq has resulted in deployment of over 2 million men and women, and thousands have experienced multiple-return deployments. The consequences of combat on servicemen's and servicewomen's health have been well documented. However, the effects on their families, more specifically, the close to 1 million children waiting for their return, are not so widely researched (Manos, 2010). The behavioral effects of parental deployment on school-age children were examined in 272 children of parents who were currently deployed ($n = 85$) or recently returned from combat ($n = 187$) (Lester et al., 2010). The prevalence of clinically significant depression and internalizing or externalizing symptoms was similar to community norms. Clinically significant anxiety levels, however, were above community norms for both deployment groups, primarily due to high scores in separation anxiety and physical symptoms of anxiety in 31.9% of children with recently returned parents and 24.7% with currently deployed parents. Mothers who remained at home with the children ($n = 163$) and 65 recently returned fathers also reported on their symptoms of emotional distress. On average, both parents demonstrated significantly higher global severity of symptoms, depression, and anxiety compared to community norms ($p < .01$) (Lester et al., 2010). Regression analysis indicated that the longer a parent was deployed, the higher the children scored on depression and externalizing symptoms ($t = 2.46$ and 3.48, respectively, $p < .01$). Mothers' depression, anxiety, and symptom severity were significant predictors of high internalizing and externalizing symptoms in the children ($t = 3.63$ to 5.73, $p < .001$). Higher depression scores in mothers was predictive of higher depression scores in the children ($t = 2.93$, $p < .01$). High levels of separation anxiety in children are consistent with lengthy absence of a parent from the home. Additionally, the threat that parents are experiencing during combat deployments is reflected in the high levels of physiological stress symptoms of their children.

In a different study, 1,507 children 11 to 17 years old were recruited from the National

Military Family Association Operation Purple applicant pool to evaluate the health and well-being of children from military families from their own perspective and the perspective of their caregivers (Chandra et al., 2010). The investigators sought to determine the relationship between parental deployment and the experience of deployment on children. *Experience* was defined as academics, peer and family relationships, emotional difficulties, and problem behaviors. Using the Strengths and Difficulties Questionnaire (SDQ), girls 11 to 14 years old had significantly higher scores than the national sample, with higher scores indicating more emotional difficulties. Regression analyses revealed age and gender differences regarding child well-being. Academic and behavioral problems became worse as age increased ($\beta = .36$, $p < .01$ and $\beta = .87$, $p < .01$, respectively) while peer functioning (according to the primary caregiver) improved with age ($\beta = -0.16$, $p < .01$). There was also a marked decrease in anxiety symptoms as age increased ($\beta = -0.15$, $p < .01$).

While a parent was deployed, girls reported having more difficulties with the deployment than their male counterparts ($\beta = 0.35$, $p < .01$) and caregivers reported their older children had more problems with deployment ($\beta = 0.12$, $p < .01$) (Chandra et al., 2010). Length of service played an important role in the number of child difficulties as well. According to caregivers, there was a positive association between months deployed in the past 3 years and increased childhood difficulties ($\beta = 0.04$, $p < 0.01$). Not only was deployment a point of contention for children and their at-home caretakers, but reintegration of the deployed parent into the home proved to be tumultuous for children, specifically older children and girls according to the children themselves ($\beta = 0.10$, $p < .01$ and $\beta = .54$, $p < .01$, respectively). Finally, the mental health status of the caregiver significantly determined child difficulties when reported by the child ($\beta = 0.04$, $p < .01$). There is little evidence that the number of military conflicts will diminish, and numerous redeployments are guaranteed. Therefore, preventive and therapeutic interventions for military children are imperative to their healthy development.

Appraisal of Stressors. Lazarus (2000) categorized an individual's cognitive appraisal of person-environment interactions (stressors) as irrelevant, benign-positive, or stressful. If the encounter is appraised as stressful or potentially stressful, the individual further appraises it as harm or loss, threat or challenge. These categories are not necessarily mutually exclusive, which further illustrates the importance of considering the individual perspective when studying the stress-coping process. It is this appraisal that helps to determine the actual effects of the stressor on the individual. It makes little sense to ask one individual to appraise or evaluate "stress" for another. Three studies illustrate this assertion. Yamamoto (1979) asked fourth, fifth, and sixth graders and their parents to rate academic and personal stressors for level of *upsettingness*. Children ranked 2 events as much more stressful for them, 4 events were much less stressful, and 1 event was approximately the same (death of a parent) as the adults' ranking. Rende and Plomin (1991) compared parents' perception of the upsettingness of 25 life events to their first-grade children's perceptions of the same events. Parents rated 4 events as significantly higher in upsettingness than did the children. Total scores were also significantly higher for parents, suggesting that overall parents overestimated their children's level of stress. A third study showed the opposite; that is, children reported higher stress levels than did their parents (Bagdi & Pfister, 2006).

MEASUREMENT OF COPING BEHAVIOR IN CHILDREN

Coping behaviors or coping strategies are "constantly changing cognitive and behavioral efforts" to manage stressors (Lazarus & Folkman, 1984, p. 141). Coping strategies are inherently neutral; they can be viewed as positive or negative only in the context of the situation and outcomes. In other words, "ignore it" may be the best strategy for a stressor a child cannot change but is relatively short lived, such as being ridiculed by a group of children at summer camp. A pattern of stressful peer relationships at school, however, is not a stressor that should be ignored. Coping strategies are learned in infancy and childhood, and many continue into adulthood.

Bruce Compas is the leading expert on stress and coping in children and adolescents. In his work, *coping* is conceptualized as one component of self-regulatory processes, and defined as "conscious, volitional efforts to regulate emotion, cognition, behavior, physiology, and the environment in response to stressful events or circumstances" (Compas et al., 2001, p. 87). Children's resources for coping are limited by their developmental level. A key characteristic of coping is that it is a voluntary response to stressors, as distinguished from an automatic or involuntary response to stressors.

A distinction was made in Lazarus's early work between problem-focused and emotion-focused coping strategies (Lazarus & Launier, 1978). Problem-focused strategies are used to manage or change the stressor, whereas emotion-focused strategies are used to manage the emotions generated by the stressor. Implementation of these definitions is difficult without knowing the *intent* behind the strategy—that is, coping strategies are not inherently problem focused or emotion focused. For example, "talk to someone" could be a strategy intended to obtain advice about how to handle the problem or to complain bitterly about the problem, and "think about it" could focus on ways to handle the problem or ways to "get even" with the perpetrators. In our view, categorizing coping strategies as either problem- or emotion-focused is not a particularly useful exercise. Nevertheless, "active coping" strategies that include problem solving, assertive communication, and social support are often valued more than other types of strategies by clinicians and researchers alike.

Clarke (2006) conducted a meta-analysis of 40 studies of children and adolescents to evaluate the strength of the relationship between active coping strategies and psychosocial health in the context of interpersonal stress. Mean effect sizes were small, ranging from 0.02 for internalizing behavior, 0.06 for externalizing behavior, 0.11 for social competence ($z = 2.17$, $p < .05$), and 0.12 for academic performance. Active coping strategies account for less than 2% of the variance in psychosocial health. The extent to which interpersonal stressors were perceived as controllable or not controllable proved to be an important distinction. Controllability was a significant predictor of mean effects of active coping on social competence (0.22, $p < .01$) and externalizing behavior (0.09, $p < .01$), such that the more controllable the stressors, the more useful active coping is for improving social competence and minimizing externalizing symptoms. Still, active coping explained only 3.7% of the variances.

A nonhierarchical taxonomy of children's coping behaviors was developed from a synthesis of 16 published research studies of primarily healthy children (N. M. Ryan-Wenger, 1992). All coping strategies mentioned in the research studies were inductively sorted into categories, resulting in 15 mutually exclusive categories. The categories, their definitions, and examples are shown in Table 10.2.

Table 10.2   Taxonomy of Children's Coping Strategies

Category	Definition	Examples of coping strategies
Aggressive activities	Verbal or motor activities that may be hurtful to persons, animals, or objects	Aggression, motor aggression, heavy-handed persuasion Moderate persuasion, indirect display of anger, attacks Physical attacks, destroy, verbal aggression, yell, argue
Behavioral avoidance	Behavior other than isolating that is a deliberate attempt to keep oneself away from a stressor	Escape, escape from family contact, temporary escape Escape from social contact, avoidance, go somewhere else Don't do anything about it, sleep, leave the situation Try to get out of it, change the topic, look away Limit setting, inhibition of action
Behavioral distraction	Behavior other than isolating or avoidance that delays the need to deal with a stressor	Distraction, do something else, watch TV Strenuous activities, quiet activities, animals Motor distraction, play, play alone Group activities, music, inanimate objects

(Continued)

Table 10.2 (Continued)

Category	Definition	Examples of coping strategies
Cognitive avoidance	Deliberate cognitive attempts to avoid acknowledging the existence of a stressor	Deny that situation exists, don't think about it Reject it, information limiting, ignore it Forget about it Thought stopping
Cognitive distraction	Deliberate cognitive attempts to keep thoughts away from a stressor	Diversionary thinking, visual distraction Cognitive distraction, think about something else Read, fantasy, humor
Cognitive problem solving	Thoughts focused on ways to modify, prevent, or eliminate the stressor	Focus on the situation, processing information Analyze, learn, problem solving Reality-oriented working through, think, reason Stress recognition, decision making
Cognitive restructuring	Thoughts that alter one's perception of the characteristics of the stressor	Positive restructuring, emphasize the positive Think about a reward, reward-oriented cognition Wishful thinking, tell self it's OK, convince self Defensive reappraisal, hope enhancement
Emotional expression	Behavior other than aggressive motor and verbal activities that expresses feelings or emotions	Ventilate feelings, act the way you want to feel Cry, empathize
Endurance	Behavior that causes one to face the stressor and accept its consequences	Expose self to fear, peaceful acquiescence Comply/cooperate, submit, endurance Relinquish control
Information seeking	Behavior that involves obtaining information about the stressor	Information seeking, programs, media, parents Explore, investigate, touch, clarify other's feelings Questioning, vigilant behavior, orienting
Isolating activities	Behavior that serves to separate the individual from the presence of others	Solitary, time-out, go to a special place Exclusion, isolate self
Self-controlling activities	Behavior or cognitions that serve to reduce tension or control one's behavior or emotions	Behavior-regulating cognitions Emotion-regulating cognitions, emotion management Self-soothing activities, think about relaxing Self-destruction, repetitive actions/habits Self-protection, tension reducing, eating, drinking Self-focusing, relax
Spiritual support	Behavior that suggests an appeal to a higher being	Spiritual support, pray
Stressor modification	Non-cognitive behavior that eliminates the stressor or modifies the characteristics of the stressor	Propose a compromise, alter the situation Conflict mitigation

A similar review of research studies on coping behavior of children with acute or chronic illness showed that the children used the same 15 categories of coping strategies (N. A. Ryan-Wenger, 1996). In a study to understand children's experiences of hospitalization in a pediatric intensive care unit (PICU), 21 children ages 7 to 12 years were interviewed after transfer from the PICU to a general care unit (Board, 2005). They reported on their experience and completed a coping strategies inventory. The three most frequently used coping strategies were also evaluated as the most effective: sleep or take a nap, talk to someone, and try to relax and stay calm.

The development of instruments to measure children's coping has followed a similar pattern as that of measurement of children's stressors, beginning with items derived from adults' perspective, literature on adult coping behavior, or observation of children. Later, instruments began to include coping strategies that children say they use. Table 10.3 lists instruments used in research or clinical practice to measure coping behavior in children.

Longitudinal, prospective studies are needed to examine the mechanisms by which coping strategies are acquired, retained, and abandoned. The cognitive processes involved in deciding which coping behaviors will be used to manage stressors are also largely unknown. Additional research is needed to differentiate coping behavior from psychological and physical stress responses, for example, "throwing things" is a coping behavior, while the psychological stress response is "anger." Compas (2009) asserts that research on coping and stress, and the primarily self-report methodology, is stagnating the growth of science in these areas. He proposed four challenges for interdisciplinary researchers that must be addressed in order to make progress on our understanding of coping behavior: (1) Integration of research on coping and regulation is required to remove the artificial boundaries between these two related constructs; (2) integration of context and neurobiology, to understand relationships between brain development, executive function, and coping, and emotion regulation; (3) integration of automatic stress responses (i.e., stress reactivity) and controlled stress responses (i.e., coping behavior); and (4) development of more in-depth study of how coping behaviors differ depending upon the goal of coping, that is, self-protection versus action against the stressor, affiliation versus protection of others, and controllability of stressors.

PERSONAL FACTORS THAT INFLUENCE COPING BEHAVIOR

A variety of individual and environmental factors play a moderating or mediating role in determining the stress-coping process and outcomes, and it is outside the scope of this chapter to describe them all. These factors include age, gender, developmental level, coping styles, resilience, socioeconomic status, parental support, health status, and personality characteristics. Two factors that will be briefly reviewed here are coping style and resilience.

Coping Styles

An individual's repertoire of coping strategies is probably partially determined by the individual's coping *style,* which is not to be confused with coping *behavior.* Coping style is a relatively stable personality characteristic that typifies one's style of managing person–environment interactions (Compas et al., 2001; Thomas & Chess, 1984). Coping styles are usually described in unidimensional, dichotomous terms, such as monitors versus blunters (Miller, 1989), avoidant versus vigilant (Cohen & Lazarus, 1973), internalizers versus externalizers (Boyd & Johnson, 1981), primary versus secondary control, and engagement versus disengagement (Compas et al., 2001). Temperament is a coping style that is usually defined in terms of nine characteristic ways of responding to one's environment: activity, rhythmicity, approach or withdrawal, adaptability, threshold of responsiveness, intensity of reaction, mood, distractibility, and persistence. Difficult infants tend to have biological irregularity, withdrawal, slow adaptability, and negative reactions of high intensity (Chess, 1990). Difficult school-aged children are those with low adaptability and negative mood (Hegvik, McDevitt, & Carey, 1982).

Many instruments exist to measure coping styles of children of all ages, as shown in Table 10.4. Little is known, however, about how coping strategies, styles, and outcomes interact. In a critical review of the literature, Compas, Connor-Smith, and Jaser (2004) examined the

Table 10.3 Instruments for Measurement of Coping Styles in Children and Adolescents

Author	Instrument	Target group	Original source of items	Format	Completed by	Meaning of scores
Rose (1972)	Level of Involvement in the Coping Process	1½- to 7-year-olds, at a home and hospital	Theory, literature	Observation of child's coping behaviors	Observer	Observations sorted into three categories: pre-coping, active coping, inactive coping
Murphy & Moriarty (1976)	Comprehensive Coping Inventory	3- to 5-year-olds	Theory, literature, clinical practice	999 items; scoring methods not reported	Children, parents, and professional team	Scores represent typical coping style
Carey & McDevitt (1978)	Infant Temperament Questionnaire	4- to 8-month-olds	Theory	95 items; scale of 1 to 6 for frequency of behavior	Mother	Sum of item scores for nine subscales = child's typical temperament or coping style
McDevitt & Carey (1978)	Behavioral Style Questionnaire	3- to 7-year-olds	Theory	100 items; scale of 1 to 6 for frequency of behavior	Mother	Sum of item scores for nine subscales = child's typical temperament or coping style
Zeitlan (1980, 1985a)	Coping Inventory-Observation	3- to 5-year-olds	Theory	48 items; scale of 1 to 5 for frequency of behavior	Observation by parent, teacher	Sum of item scores = subscale scores on three dimensions: productive/nonproductive, flexible/rigid, active/passive
Boyd & Johnson (1981)	Analysis of Coping Style	Form C: 8–12 years Form Y: 13–18 years	Theory	Projective test; children's reactions to 20 drawings	Interviewer, child	Responses sorted into six categories: internalized attack, denial, and avoidance and externalized attack, denial, and avoidance
Hegvik, McDevitt, & Carey (1982)	Middle Childhood Temperament Questionnaire	8- to 12-year-olds	Theory	99 items; scale of 1–6 for frequency of behavioral occurrence	Mother	Sum of item scores for nine subscales = child's typical temperament or coping style
Fullard, McDevitt, & Carey (1984)	Toddler Temperament Scale	12- to 36-month-olds	Theory	97 items; scale of 1 to 6 for frequency of behavior	Mother	Sum of item scores for nine subscales = child's typical temperament or coping style

Author	Instrument	Target group	Original source of items	Format	Completed by	Meaning of scores
LaMontagne (1984, 1987)	Preoperative Mode of Coping Interview	8- to 18-year-olds hospitalized, prior to surgery	Theory	Structured interview; character of responses reduced to a score from 1 to 10	Interviewer, child	Low score = avoidant; high score = active coping style
Zeitlan (1985b)	Coping Inventory: Self-Related Form	Adolescents, adults	Theory	48 items; scale of 1 to 5 for frequency of behavior	Observation by parent, teacher	Sum of item scores = three subscales: productive/nonproductive, flexible/rigid, active/passive
Peterson & Toler (1986)	Coping Strategies Interview	5- to 11-year-olds hospitalized, prior to surgery	Literature, theory, children	Structured interview	Interviewer, child	Compare number of information-seeking versus avoiding responses
Meisgeier & Murphy (1987)	Murphy-Meisgeier Type Indicator for Children	2nd to 8th grade	Theory	70 items; forced choice between two responses	Children	Responses profiled into 16 type dimensions
Zeitlan, Williamson, & Szczepanski (1988)	Early Coping Inventory	4- to 36- month-olds	Theory	48 items; scale of 1 to 5 for frequency of behavior	Observation by parent, teacher	Sum of item scores = subscale scores on three dichotomous dimensions: productive/ nonproductive, flexible/rigid, active/passive
Martin (1988)	Temperament Assessment Battery for Children	3- to 7-year-olds	Theory	48 items; scale of 1–7 for frequency of behaviors	Parent, teacher, and clinician	Sum of item scores = subscale scores; standardized into T scores; profile plots for temperament style
Miller (1989)	Kiddie Choice Survey (Monitoring-Blunting Scale for Children)	Not stated	Theory	Structured interview	Interviewer, child	Compare number of responses in categories of blunting versus monitoring

literature on relationships among temperament, stress reactivity, coping, and depression in childhood and adolescence. The evidence suggests that "temperamental characteristics may moderate and be moderated by stress responses and coping in their effects on depression" (p. 21). Clinicians who desire to help children acquire more effective coping strategies would probably benefit by examining the compatibility of new coping strategies with the child's inherent coping style. To advance theory about the origin and maintenance of coping strategies, and inform practice, it is essential to study the contribution of coping style to this process.

Stress Resistance (Resilience) and Stress Vulnerability

Research in the area of stress and coping in children has focused on positive outcomes of stress as well as negative outcomes. Some research concerns a special subset of *resilient* children who have experienced many unusually severe stressors and yet function exceptionally well despite the great odds against them (Masten, Best, & Garmezy, 1990). Other children appear to be more vulnerable to stressful situations and environments. *Stress vulnerability* is defined as a "condition of unusual or exaggerated susceptibility to the environmental agents of disease or disorder, including psychosocial stressors" (Boyce, 1992, p. 4).

Resilience

Many definitions of resilience exist (Ahern, Kiehl, Sole, & Byers, 2006; Collishaw et al., 2007; Masten, 2001; Preits & Dimova, 2008; Richardson, 2002; Rutter, 1993; Thompkins & Swartz, 2009). We have synthesized the definition of resilience as "the ability to overcome an adversity that involves an internal process of adaptive coping in combination with protective individual, family or community factors." (Table 10.2.) Examples of protective factors within the child include strong cognitive abilities and problem-solving skills, viewing change or stress as an opportunity, proactive approach to dealing with stressors and recognizing one's own limitations to control the stressor, closer and more secure attachment to others, easy temperament in infancy and adaptability in childhood and adolescence, positive self perceptions, self-efficacy, having a sense of faith and meaning, optimism and hope, strong self-regulation skills, sense of humor, and sense of empowerment (Connor & Davidson, 2003; Masten & Reed, 2002; Rutter, 1985; Scudder, Sullivan, & Copeland-Linder, 2008; Thompkins & Swartz, 2009). One or more of these child characteristics in combination with one or more family and/or community factors contributes to development of resilience over time. Family protective factors include close relationships among family members, low discord between parents, warm parenting style that is structured and sets clear expectations, socioeconomic advantage, parental involvement in child's education, parents with cognitive strengths such as optimism and self-regulation, and parents who see the child as appealing and value the child's talents (Masten & Reed, 2002; Preits & Dimova, 2008; Scudder et al., 2008). Community factors that promote resilience include: the child's closest peers and adults model responsible behavior, neighbors who are caring and take responsibility for monitoring children's behavior, school provides a caring and encouraging environment and teachers encourage the children to do well, and a community that values youth.

Stress Vulnerability

We argue that "ineffective coping strategies" contribute to internalization of stress. In his work with adults, Lazarus stated that the ways that people cope with stress are probably more directly related to health and illness than are the frequency and severity of stressors (Lazarus & Launier, 1978). The effectiveness (and social acceptability) of children's coping strategies may determine the extent to which children are vulnerable or resilient to current and future stressful situations. Even successful coping takes a psychological toll on children; therefore, it is important to examine the amount of coping children have to do over time (Emery & Coiro, 1997). It may be that although emotional regulation buffers against certain stressors, it also increases vulnerability to others, and successful coping in one realm may not be indicative of positive coping and overall psychological well-being (Thompson & Calkins, 1996). It is important to identify factors that cause children to be resistant to stress. It is tempting to assume that protective factors are simply the opposite of risk

Table 10.4 Instruments for Measurement of Coping Strategies in Children and Adolescents

Author	Instrument	Target group	Original source of items	Format	Completed by	Meaning of scores
Mooney, Graziano, & Katz (1984)	Nighttime Fears Coping Checklist	8- to 13-year-olds	Literature, children, parents	36 items; scored yes/no	Children	Sum of items scores for five subscales = frequency and variety of coping strategies used
Wertlieb, Weigel, & Feldstein (1987)	Stress and Coping Interview	7- to 10-year-olds	Scoring method derived from theory	Semi-structured interview; 10 categories of coping behavior	Interviewer and child	Child's responses sorted into 1 of 10 categories reflecting focus, function, and mode of child's coping behavior
Patterson & McCubbin (1987)	A-COPE: Adolescent Coping Orientation for Problem Experiences	12- to 18-year-olds	10th- to 12th-grade students	95 items; scale of 1–5 for frequency of use	Adolescents	Sum of item scores for 12 subscales = frequency and variety of coping strategies used
Ritchie, Caty, & Ellerton (1988)	Children's Coping Strategies Checklist	Hospitalized 2- to 6-year-olds	Scoring method derived from literature, theory	Observation of hospitalized preschoolers; 40 behaviors scored as yes/no	Observer	Total number of coping behaviors observed for each of six subscales = variety and type of coping behavior
Spirito, Stark, & Williams (1988)	KIDCOPE (Brief Coping Checklist) School-age version Adolescent version	7- to 12-year-olds 13- to 18-year-olds	Adult coping scales	School-age: 15 items; yes/ no for frequency; 0 to 2 for efficacy Adolescent: 10 items; scale of 0 to 3 for frequency and efficacy	Children, adolescents	Sum of item scores = total frequency and efficacy of coping strategies
Hammer (1988)	Coping Resources Inventory	High schoolers	Clinical practice, literature	60 items; scale of 0 to 3 for extent to which strategies used during the past 6 months	Adolescents	Sum of item scores = amount of resources; standard scores profile plots of five dimensions

Table 10.4 (Continued)

Author	Instrument	Target group	Original source of items	Format	Completed by	Meaning of scores
Dise-Lewis (1988)	Life Events and Coping Inventory	12- to 14-year-olds	Junior high students	52 items; scale of 1 to 9 for likelihood that one would use each strategy	Children	Sum of item scores = amount of coping strategies that are likely to be used
N. M. Ryan-Wenger (1990)	Schoolagers' Coping Strategies Inventory	8- to 12-year-olds	Elementary school children	26 items; scale of 0 to 3 for frequency of use and effectiveness	Children	Sum of item scores = frequency of use and effectiveness of coping strategies used
Austin, Patterson, & Huberty (1991)	Coping Health Inventory for Children	8- to 12-year-olds with chronic illness	Theory, literature, parents, children	45 items; scale of 1 to 5 for frequency of use	Parents of children with chronic illness	Sum of item scores for five subscales = frequency and variety of coping strategies
Gil, Abrams, Phillips, & Keefe (1989)	Coping Strategies Questionnaire for Sickle Cell Disease (SCD)	Children and adolescents with chronic pain due to SCD	Adult instrument, clinical practice	42 items; scale of 0 to 6 for frequency of use, amount of pain control, and effectiveness	Children, adolescents	Item scores converted to composite scores on two factors: coping attempts and pain control/rational thinking Overall level of control over pain and overall effectiveness of each strategy

factors, and that stress resistance and vulnerability are opposite poles of a single dimension. In the absence of a body of research to support either assumption, Rutter (1996) suggests that in the search for causality, stress resistance and stress vulnerability should be treated as separate constructs, and that exploration of causal factors include physical, psychological, social, and environmental variables. Little is known about many aspects of children's appraisal of coping effectiveness, including when and how often this appraisal occurs, the criteria that they use to define "effectiveness," how these criteria differ from adults' definitions of effectiveness, or how children alter their coping behaviors based on periodic appraisal of their effectiveness.

STRESS RESPONSES—SHORT-TERM AND LONG-TERM OUTCOMES

Stress is known to cause physiologic changes in the hypothalamic-pituitary-adrenocortical (HPA) system. Some children develop frequent or exaggerated psychological symptoms, illnesses, social isolation, or other long-term manifestations of the internalization of stress. Instruments to measure these short- and long-term outcomes are listed in Table 10.5.

Physiologic Changes

In infants and children, as well as adults, experiences of stressful situations and attempts to cope with stressors have a direct and observable impact on physiological systems. Stressful experiences activate the HPA system (Kharmandari, Tsigos, & Khrousos, 2005; King & Hegadoren, 2002). The HPA system enhances stress resistance by increasing energy needed to cope and by modulating other body systems that are sensitive to stress, including emotions. Studies of laboratory-induced stress provide useful data for examination of the physiologic impact of real-life stressors on children. Salivary cortisol is often used as a noninvasive physiologic measure of stress in children. Normal patterns of salivary cortisol in adults and children have a circadian rhythm (diurnal pattern of a morning high, followed by a peak about 30 minutes after wake-up, a rapid decrease the next 1 to 2 hours, and a more gradual decrease throughout the rest of the day

to a nadir at bedtime (Gunnar & Cheatham, 2003; King & Hegadorian, 2002; Kudielka, Buske-Kirschbaum, Hellhammer, & Kirschbaum, 2004). Research demonstrates that production of cortisol increases when adults and children are presented with stressful stimuli (Bruce, Davis, & Gunnar, 2002; Gunnar, Bruce, & Hickman, 2001; Kudielka et al., 2004).

Norms for cortisol levels in children are not well established, but a recent study has begun to fill that gap (McCarthy et al., 2009). McCarthy et al. conducted a descriptive study to establish normative time-specific salivary cortisol levels in children ($n = 384$) ages 4 to 10 years (mean age 7.2 years) and to assess cortisol level changes after a stressful procedure of IV insertion compared to baseline levels. Children were recruited from pediatric specialty clinics of three Midwestern children's hospitals. The sample was nearly equally divided between boys (49%) and girls (51%); the racial and ethnic distribution was 81% Caucasian, 7% African Americans, 1% Asians, 2% Hispanics or Latinos, and 9% unknown race. A total of four salivary cortisol samples were obtained. Time 1 was upon arrival to the clinic; Time 2 was 20 minutes after IV insertion (allowing the HPA axis time to respond). To compare the stress response to cortisol levels on a nonstressful day at least 24 hours after the IV placement, Time 1 and Time 2 baseline cortisol samples were collected at home at the same time of day that they were collected in the clinic. As hypothesized, elevated salivary cortisol levels were found on the day of the IV insertion. Compared to baseline levels at home, cortisol levels prior to IV insertion increased 33.6% (+ 10.1, $p = .004$), and 69.3% (+ 14.1, $p < .0001$). These results support the use of salivary cortisol levels as an objective biological measure of childhood distress.

During chronic stress, the HPA axis does not have a chance to reset, such that cortisol may remain high across the day and into the evenings when it should be decreasing to its lowest level (Cicchetti & Rogosch, 2001; McCabe & Schneider, 2009). This pattern was demonstrated in a study of children in foster care. Foster care is considered a chronic stressor because early child care was often inadequate and inconsistent, compounded by separation from their primary caregiver and oftentimes multiple placements (Dozier et al., 2006). Daytime patterns of cortisol levels were examined in 55 children placed in

Table 10.5 Instruments for Measurement of Stress Responses in Children and Adolescents

Author	Instrument	Target group	Original source of items	Format	Completed by	Meaning of scores
Horowitz, Wilner, & Alvarez (1979)	Impact of Event Scale (for post-traumatic stress disorder [PTSD])	Children, adults who have experienced a traumatic event	Theory, clinical practice	30 items; scale of 0 to 3 for extent to which symptoms are experienced	Children, adults	Sum of item scores = subscale scores on intrusiveness and avoidance (PTSD)
Chandler, Shermis, & Marsh (1985)	Stress Response Scale	5- to 14-year-olds	Derived from theory and DSM-III categories	40 behavioral items; scale of 0 to 5 for frequency of occurrence	Children	Sum of frequency scores = total and subscale scores = amount of stress response; profiles indicate four common response patterns
Hockenberry-Eaton, Manteuffel, & Bottomley (1997)	Children's Adjustment to Cancer Index	7- to 13-year-olds	Derived from literature and experience of primary author	30 items; scale of 1 to 5 for frequency of ability to do things	Children	Sum of item scores = level of adjustment to cancer
Achenbach & Edelbrock (1983)	Child Behavior Checklist: Behavior Problem Scale	2- or 3-year-olds; 4- to 16-year-olds	Theory, clinical practice, literature	113 items; scale of 0 to 2 for extent to which item is true for the child	Parent, teacher, adolescent	Sum of item scores = subscale scores on nine dimensions; standardized scores profiled for specific behavior problem areas
Achenbach & Edelbrock (1983)	Child Behavior Checklist: Social Competence Scale	2- or 3-year-olds; 4- to 16-year-olds	Theory, clinical practice, literature	Eight sections; multiple-response choices for characteristics descriptive of the child	Parent, teacher, adolescent	Sum of item scores = subscale scores on six dimensions; standardized scores profiled for specific social competence areas
Elliott, Jay, & Woody (1987)	Observation Scale for Behavioral Distress	3- to 13-year-olds undergoing medical procedures	Literature, other observation instruments	Eight behavior categories	Observation by health care provider	Modal categories of observed behaviors most descriptive of child's response to medical procedures
Merrell & Walters (1998)	Internalizing Symptoms Scale for Children	8- to 13-year-olds	Theory, literature, clinical practice	48 items; scale of 0–3 for extent to which statement is true of the child	Child, adolescent	Sum of item scores = subscale scores; standardized and plotted on profile for Negative Affect/General Distress and Positive Affect

foster care and 104 children who lived continuously with their parents. The sample included 28 boys and 27 girls ages 20 to 60 months (mean = 32.7 months). Time in foster care ranged from 2 to 45 months, and the number of placements ranged from 1 to 4 times (mean 1.5). The primary cause of placement was neglect (86%). Results showed that young children who first entered foster care in infancy displayed atypical patterns of cortisol across the day compared to controls. Authors speculated that instability of foster children's caregiving situation played a role in this effect. Wake-up values that are normally high were significantly lower for foster children versus controls ($F = 8.43$, $p < .01$). Differences were not significant between afternoon and bedtime levels. Several years after placement in foster care, many young children fail to show a typical pattern of cortisol production.

Compas (2006) calls for expansion of research on the effects of chronic stress on children and adolescents, with particular attention to longitudinal psychobiological processes involving the brain's cortex, hippocampus and amygdale, the HPA axis, and the sympathetic-adrenal-medullary axis. An example of recent research is a study to test the hypothesis that hyper-secretion of glucocorticoids associated with post-traumatic stress disorder results in diminished size of the hippocampus, which is a portion of the brain that regulates long-term memory and spatial navigation. A pilot study of 15 children who experienced maltreatment showed that PTSD symptoms and cortisol levels predicted levels of hippocampal reductions over 12 to 18 months (Carrion, Weems, & Reiss, 2007).

Sharrer and Ryan-Wenger (2002) asked 194 children, ages 7 to 12 years, to describe what they think and feel when something stressful happens to them. They named 507 symptoms that were inductively categorized into 11 cognitive/emotional symptoms (56.4%) and 13 physiological symptoms (43.6%). The top five cognitive/emotional symptoms were mad, worried, sad, nervous, and afraid; the top five physiological symptoms were headache, stomachache, sweaty, heart beating fast, and feeling sick. All of the instruments currently used to measure children's responses to stress contain items derived from theory, literature, and professional clinical practice (Table 10.5). These instruments capture only 36% to 55% of the cognitive/emotional symptoms and 0 to 33% of the physiological

symptoms that were reported by the children in our study. Future instrument development should include items that were developed from the children's perspective.

Somatic Health and Illness

Numerous studies summarized by Boyce (1992) and others indicate that consistently, and across settings, a small portion (15% to 20%) of the child population accounts for most of the school absentee rate, more than half of the morbidity, and half of the health services utilization of that population (Kornguth, 1990; Weitzman, Walker, & Gortmaker, 1986). Children with chronic illnesses or disabilities account for only approximately 5%; the remainder comprises children with frequent and various physical and psychological morbidity conditions. One longitudinal study showed that the same childhood patterns of illness and health services utilization persist into adulthood (Lewis & Lewis, 1989). Some hypothesized determinants of frequent illnesses are parental anxiety regarding the child's health, constitutional vulnerability to stress (illness-prone), or internalization of stress (Boyce, 1992). Research on children with frequent illnesses, frequent absence from school due to illness, and frequent use of health services is needed to examine their relationships to coping behavior.

IMPLICATIONS FOR THEORY DEVELOPMENT, RESEARCH, AND PRACTICE

New stress-coping-response theories developed specifically for children are overdue. Although researchers have typically applied theories that explain adult stress and coping behavior to research and practice with children, children's cognitive, physical, and social realities are dramatically different from those of adults. If one accepts that appraisal plays a significant role in the stress-coping process, then theories are needed to explain differences in appraisal as children move through stages of cognitive development. Children's stressors are not the same as adults' stressors, nor is their level of control over stressors the same. Theories should account for endosystem sources of stress such as height, weight, appearance, and agility, which are of extreme importance to children and adolescents when peer acceptance begins to take priority over family relationships or relationships with significant others. It may be helpful to begin by comprehensively analyzing and perhaps revising each proposition of an adult-level theory with respect to obvious differences between children and adults.

Stress, coping, and outcome models are based on the assumption that the relative effectiveness of coping strategies influences psychological behavior, social functioning, and somatic health of individuals. To date, little empirical research has adequately tested this proposition. More research is needed to understand children's appraisal of stressors and coping resources; children's motivations for selecting coping strategies; linkages between stressors, coping behavior, and outcomes; and interventions to decrease vulnerability or increase children's stress resistance. Future research must be multidisciplinary, in which multiple perspectives are synthesized into one approach (problem, design, method) and results are interpreted by the research team.

Nurses and other health care providers should always consider potential interactions among stress, coping, health, and illness. Include in history-taking the sources of stress and typical coping strategies from the child's and the parents' perspectives. Children can be taught new coping strategies in individual or group settings. Helping children relate specific coping strategies to desirable and undesirable outcomes may be the first step in assisting children to manage their own stress-related responses. In addition, health care professionals can support parents in building their child's resiliency by assisting parents to set realistic goals for their children, as well as help them provide numerous opportunities for their child to succeed at reaching those goals (Scudder et al., 2008). It is imperative to create an environment that encourages hope and optimism, while also fostering a persistent sense of belief in the child's potential.

Reivich and Gilham (2010) discuss a number of their own strategies intended to increase resiliency in children, including (1) teaching to think accurately about causes and implications of problems, (2) teaching to think more "flexibly," (3) helping to put stressors into perspective, (4) educating on setting goals and developing plans for reaching them, (5) providing assertiveness and negotiation training (speaking up and asking others for help are useful and beneficial coping skills when dealing with stress), and (6) finding ways to instruct on decision making and creative problem solving to increase the child's self-efficacy, optimism, impulse control, and empathy. As health care providers, it is important to recognize the role that resiliency plays in children's responses to stressful events.

REFERENCES

Achenbach, T. M., & Edelbrock, C. (1983). *Manual for the Child Behavior Checklist and Revised Child Behavior Profile.* Burlington: University of Vermont, Department of Psychiatry.

Ahern, N. R., Kiehl, E. M., Sole, M. L., & Byers, J. (2006). A review of instruments measuring resilience. *Issues in Comprehensive Pediatric Nursing, 29*(2), 103–125.

Aricak, T., Siyahhan, S., Uzunhasanoglu, A., Saribeyoglu, S., Ciplak, S., Yilmaz, N., et al. (2008). Cyberbullying among Turkish adolescents. *CyberPsychology and Behavior, 11*(3), 253–261.

Austin, J. K., Patterson, J. M., & Huberty, T. J. (1991). Development of the coping health inventory for children. *Journal of Pediatric Nursing, 6*(3), 166–174.

Bagdi, A., & Pfister, I. (2006). Childhood stressors and coping actions: A comparison of children and parents' perspectives. *Child & Youth Care Forum, 35*(1), 21–40.

Barkin, S., Kreiter, S., & DuRant, R. H. (2001). Exposure to violence and intentions to engage in moralistic violence during early adolescence. *Journal of Adolescence, 24*(6), 777–789.

Beall, S., & Schmidt, G. (1984). Development of a youth adaptation rating scale. *Journal of School Health, 54*(5), 197–200.

Berk, L. E. (2008). *Child development* (8th ed.). Boston, MA: Allyn & Beacon.

Board, R. (2005). School-age children's perceptions of their PICU hospitalization. *Pediatric Nursing, 31*(3), 166–175.

Bobo, J. K., Gilchrist, L. D., Elmer, J. F., Snow, W. H., & Schinke, S. P. (1986). Hassles, role strain, and peer relations in young adolescents. *The Journal of Early Adolescence, 6*(4), 339–352.

Boyce, W. T. (1992). The vulnerable child: New evidence, new approaches. *Advances in Pediatrics, 39*, 1–33.

Boyd, H. F., & Johnson, G. O. (1981). *Analysis of coping style: A cognitive-behavioral approach to behavior management.* Columbus, OH: Merrill.

Bronfenbrenner, U. (1979). *The ecology of human development.* Cambridge, MA: Harvard University Press.

Broome, M. E., Hellier, A., Wilson, T., Dale, S., & Glanville, C. (1988). Measuring children's fears of medical experiences. In C. F. Waltz & O. L. Strickland (Eds.), *Measurement of nursing outcomes: Vol. 1. Measuring client outcomes* (pp. 201–214). New York, NY: Springer.

Bruce, J., Davis, E. P., & Gunnar, M. R. (2002). Individual differences in children's cortisol response to the beginning of a new school year. *Psychoneuroendocrinology, 27*(6), 635–650.

Burnham, J. J., & Gullone, E. (1997). The Fear Survey Schedule for Children—II: A psychometric investigation with American data. *Behaviour, Research, and Therapy, 35*(2), 165–173.

Calvete, E., Orue, I., Estévez, Villardón, L., & Padilla, P. (2010). Cyberbullying in adolescents: Modalities and aggressors' profile. *Computers in Human Behavior, 26,* 1128–1135.

Capuzzi, D., & Gross, D. R. (2008). *Youth at risk: A prevention resource for counselors, teachers, and parents* (5th ed.). Alexandria, VA: American Counseling Association.

Carey, W. B., & McDevitt, S. C. (1978). Revision of the Infant Temperament Questionnaire. *Pediatrics, 61*(5), 735–739.

Carrion, V. G., Weems, C. F., & Reiss, A. L. (2007). Stress predicts brain changes in children: A pilot longitudinal study on youth stress, posttraumatic stress disorder, and the hippocampus. *Pediatrics, 119*(3), 509–516.

Carroll, M. K., & Ryan-Wenger, N. A. (1999). School-age children's fears, anxiety, and human figure drawings. *Journal of Pediatric Health Care, 13*(1), 24–31.

Centers for Disease Control and Prevention (CDC) & National Center for Chronic Disease Prevention and Health Promotion. (2006). *Youth Risk Behavior Survey. Unpublished analysis.*

Chandler, L. A., Shermis, M. D., & Marsh, J. (1985). The use of the Stress Response Scale in diagnostic assessment with children. *Journal of Psychoeducational Assessment, 3*(1), 15–29.

Chandra, A., Lara-Cinisomo, S., Jaycox, L. H., Tanielian, T., Burns, R. M., Ruder, T., et al. (2010). Children on the homefront: The experience of children from military families. *Pediatrics, 125*(1), 16–25.

Chess, S. (1990). Studies in temperament: A paradigm in psychosocial research. *Yale Journal of Biology and Medicine, 63*(4), 313–324.

Cicchetti, D., & Rogosch, F. A. (2001). The impact of child maltreatment and psychopathology on neuroendocrine functioning. *Development and Psychopathology, 13*(4), 783–804.

Clarke, A. T. (2006). Coping with interpersonal stress and psychosocial health among children and adolescents: A meta-analysis. *Journal of Youth and Adolescence, 35*(1), 11–24.

Coddington, R. D. (1972). The significance of life events as etiologic factors in the diseases of children. II. A study of a normal population. *Journal of Psychosomatic Research, 16*(3), 205–213.

Coddington, R. D. (1984). Measuring the stressfulness of a child's environment. In J. H. Humphrey (Ed.), *Stress in childhood* (pp. 97–126). New York, NY: AMS Press.

Cohen, F., & Lazarus, R. S. (1973). Active coping processes, coping dispositions, and recovery from surgery. *Psychosomatic Medicine, 35*(5), 375–389.

Collishaw, S., Pickles, A., Messer, J., Rutter, M., Shearer, C., & Maughan, B. (2007). Resilience to adult psychopathology following childhood maltreatment: Evidence from a community sample. *Child Abuse & Neglect, 31*(3), 211–229.

Compas, B. E. (2006). Psychobiological processes of stress and coping: Implications for resilience in children and adolescents—comments on the papers of Romeo & McEwen and Fisher et al. *Annals of the New York Academy of Sciences, 1094,* 226–234.

Compas, B. E. (2009). Coping, regulation, and development during childhood and adolescence. *New Directions for Child and Adolescent Development, 2009*(124), 87–99.

Compas, B. E., Connor-Smith, J., & Jaser, S. S. (2004). Temperament, stress reactivity, and coping: Implications for depression in childhood and adolescence. *Journal of Clinical Child and Adolescent Psychology, 33*(1), 21–31.

Compas, B. E., Connor-Smith, J. K., Saltzman, H., Thomsen, A. H., & Wadsworth, M. E. (2001). Coping with stress during childhood and adolescence: Problems, progress, and potential in theory and research. *Psychological Bulletin, 127*(1), 87–127.

Compas, B. E., Davis, G. E., Forsythe, C. J., & Wagner, B. M. (1987). Assessment of major and daily stressful events during adolescence: The Adolescent Perceived Events Scale. *Journal of Consulting and Clinical Psychology, 55*(4), 534–541.

Connor, K. M., & Davidson, J. R. (2003). Development of a new resilience scale: The Connor-Davidson Resilience Scale (CD-RISC). *Depression and Anxiety, 18*(2), 76–82.

David-Ferdon, C., & Hertz, M. (2009). *Electronic media and youth violence: A CDC issue brief for researchers.* Atlanta, GA: Centers for Disease Control and Prevention.

Dehue, F., Bolman, C., & Völlink, T. (2008). Cyberbullying: Youngsters' experiences and parental perception. *CyberPsychology and Behavior, 11*(2), 217–223.

Dempsey, A. G., Sulkowski, M. L., Nichols, R., & Storch, E. A. (2009). Differences between peer victimization in cyber and physical settings and associated psychosocial adjustment in early adolescence. *Psychology in the Schools, 46*(10), 962–972.

Dise-Lewis, J. E. (1988). The life events and coping inventory: An assessment of stress in children. *Psychosomatic Medicine, 50*(5), 484–499.

Dozier, M., Manni, M., Gordon, M. K., Peloso, E., Gunnar, M. R., Stovall-McClough, K. C., et al. (2006). Foster children's diurnal production of cortisol: An exploratory study. *Child Maltreatment, 11*(2), 189–197.

Dube, S. R., Felitti, V. J., Dong, M., Chapman, D. P., Giles, W. H., & Anda, R. F. (2003). Childhood abuse, neglect, and household dysfunction and the risk of illicit drug use: The adverse childhood experiences study. *Pediatrics, 111*(3), 564–572.

Dumont, M., & Provost, M. A. (1999). Resilience in adolescents: Protective role of social support, coping strategies, self-esteem, and social activities on experience of stress and depression. *Journal of Youth and Adolescence, 28*(3), 343–363.

Elkind, D. (2001). *The hurried child: Growing up too fast too soon* (3rd ed.). Reading, MA: Perseus Publishing.

Elliott, C. H., Jay, S. M., & Woody, P. (1987). An observation scale for measuring children's distress during medical procedures. *Journal of Pediatric Psychology, 12*(4), 543–551.

Elwood, S. W. (1987). Stressor and coping response inventories for children. *Psychological Reports, 60*(3, Pt 1), 931–947.

Emery, R. E., & Coiro, M. J. (1997). Some costs of coping: Stress and distress among children from divorced families. In D. Ciccetti & S. L. Toth (Eds.), *Developmental perspectives on trauma: Theory, research and intervention* (pp. 435–462). Rochester, NY: University of Rochester Press.

Fullard, W., McDevitt, S. C., & Carey, W. B. (1984). Assessing temperament in one- to three-year-old children. *Journal of Pediatric Psychology, 9*(2), 205–217.

Gil, K. M., Abrams, M. R., Phillips, G., & Keefe, F. J. (1989). Sickle cell disease pain: Relation of coping strategies to adjustment. *Journal of Consulting and Clinical Psychology, 57*(6), 725–731.

Goodman, R., & Scott, S. (1999). Comparing the Strengths and Difficulties Questionnaire and the Child Behavior Checklist: Is small beautiful? *Journal of Abnormal Child Psychology, 27*(1), 17–24.

Grych, J. H., Seid, M., & Fincham, F. D. (1992). Assessing marital conflict from the child's perspective: The children's perception of interparental conflict scale. *Child Development, 63*(3), 558–572.

Gullone, E., & King, N. J. (1993). The fears of youth in the 1990s: Contemporary normative data. *Journal of Genetic Psychology, 154*(2), 137–153.

Gunnar, M. R., Bruce, J., & Hickman, S. E. (2001). Salivary cortisol response to stress in children. *Advances in Psychosomatic Medicine, 22*, 52–60.

Gunnar, M. R., & Cheatham, C. L. (2003). Brain and behavior interface: Stress and the developing brain. *Infant Mental Health Journal, 24*, 195–211.

Hammer, A. L. (1988). *Manual for the Coping Resources Inventory.* Palo Alto, CA: Consulting Psychologists Press.

Hampel, P., Manhal, S., & Hayer, T. (2009). Direct and relational bullying among children and adolescents: Coping and psychological adjustment. *School Psychology International, 30*(5), 474–490.

Hegvik, R. L., McDevitt, S. C., & Carey, W. B. (1982). The middle childhood temperament questionnaire. *Journal of Developmental & Behavioral Pediatrics, 3*(4), 197–200.

Hjern, A., Alfven, G., & Ostberg, V. (2008). School stressors, psychological complaints and psychosomatic pain. *Acta Paediatrica, 97*(1), 112–117.

Hockenberry-Eaton, M., Manteuffel, B., & Bottomley, S. (1997). Development of two instruments examining stress and adjustment in children with cancer. *Journal of Pediatric Oncology Nursing, 14*(3), 178–185.

Holmes, T. H., & Rahe, R. H. (1967). The Social Readjustment Rating Scale. *Journal of Psychosomatic Research, 11*(2), 213–218.

Horowitz, M., Wilner, N., & Alvarez, W. (1979). Impact of Event Scale: A measure of subjective stress. *Psychosomatic Medicine, 41*(3), 209–218.

Hyman, I. A., & Snook, P. (2002). *My Worst School Experience Scale (MWSE).* Los Angeles, CA: Western Psychological Services.

Johnson, J. H., & McCutcheon, S. (1980). Assessing life stress in older children and adolescents: Preliminary findings with the Life Events Checklist. In I. G. Sarason & C. D. Spielberger (Eds.), *Stress and anxiety, Vol. 7* (pp. 111–125). Washington, DC: Hemisphere.

Juvonen, J., Graham, S., & Schuster, M. A. (2003). Bullying among young adolescents: The strong, the weak, and the troubled. *Pediatrics, 112*(6, Pt 1), 1231–1237.

Juvonen, J., & Gross, E. F. (2008). Extending the school grounds?—Bullying experiences in cyberspace. *Journal of School Health, 78*(9), 496–505.

Kharmandari, E., Tsigos, C., & Khrousos, G. (2005). Endocrinology of the stress response. *Annual Review of Physiology, 67,* 259–284.

King, S. L., & Hegadoren, K. M. (2002). Stress hormones: How do they measure up? *Biological Research for Nursing, 4*(2), 92–103.

Kornguth, M. L. (1990). School illnesses: Who's absent and why? *Pediatric Nursing, 16*(1), 95–99.

Kudielka, B. M., Buske-Kirschbaum, A., Hellhammer, D. H., & Kirschbaum, C. (2004). Differential heart rate reactivity and recovery after psychosocial stress (TSST) in healthy children, younger adults, and elderly adults: The impact of age and gender. *International Journal of Behavioral Medicine, 11*(2), 116–121.

LaMontagne, L. L. (1984). Children's locus of control beliefs as predictors of preoperative coping behavior. *Nursing Research, 33*(2), 76–79, 85.

LaMontagne, L. L. (1987). Children's preoperative coping: Replication and extension. *Nursing Research, 36*(3), 163–167.

Lazarus, R. S. (2000). Toward better research on stress and coping. *American Psychologist, 55*(6), 665–673.

Lazarus, R. S., & Folkman, S. (1984). *Stress, appraisal and coping.* New York, NY: Springer.

Lazarus, R. S., & Launier, M. R. (1978). Stress related transaction between person and environment. In L. A. Pervin & M. Lewis (Eds.), *Perspectives in interactional psychology.* New York, NY: Plenum.

Lester, P., Peterson, K., Reeves, J., Knauss, L., Glover, D., Mogil, C., et al. (2010). The long war and parental combat deployment: Effects on military children and at-home spouses. *Journal of the American Academy of Child and Adolescent Psychiatry, 49*(4), 310–320.

Lewis, C. E., & Lewis, M. A. (1989). Educational outcomes and illness behaviors of participants in a child-initiated care system: A 12-year follow-up study. *Pediatrics, 84*(5), 845–850.

Lewis, C. E., Siegel, J. M., & Lewis, M. A. (1984). Feeling bad: Exploring sources of distress among pre-adolescent children. *American Journal of Public Health, 74*(2), 117–122.

MacKay, A. P., & Duran, C. (2008). *Adolescent health in the United States, 2007.* Washington, DC: U.S. Department of Health & Human Services.

Manos, G. H. (2010). War and the military family. *Journal of the American Academy of Child and Adolescent Psychiatry, 49*(4), 297–299.

Martin, R. P. (1988). *The Temperament Assessment Battery for Children.* Brandon, VT: Clinical Psychology Press.

Masten, A. S. (2001). Ordinary magic. Resilience processes in development. *American Psychologist, 56*(3), 227–238.

Masten, A. S., Best, K. M., & Garmezy, N. (1990). Resilience and development: Contributions from the study of children who overcome adversity. *Development and Psychopathology, 2,* 425–444.

Masten, A. S., & Reed, M. G. (2002). Resilience in development. In C. R. Snyder & S. J. Lopez (Eds.), *Handbook of positive psychology* (pp. 74–88). New York, NY: Oxford University Press.

McCabe, P., & Schneider, M. (2009). What does their saliva say? Salivary cortisol levels in children exposed to severe stressors. *Communique, 37*(8), 26–28.

McCarthy, A. M., Hanrahan, K., Kleiber, C., Zimmerman, M. B., Lutgendorf, S., & Tsalikian, E. (2009). Normative salivary cortisol values and responsivity in children. *Applied Nursing Research, 22*(1), 54–62.

McCubbin, H. I., & Patterson, J. M. (1987). A-FILE: Adolescent Family Inventory of Life Events and Changes. In H. I. McCubbin & A. I. Thompson (Eds.), *Family assessment inventories for research and practice* (pp. 100–109). Madison: University of Wisconsin Press.

McDevitt, S. C., & Carey, W. B. (1978). The measurement of temperament in 3–7 year old children. *Journal of Child Psychology and Psychiatry, 19*(3), 245–253.

McWhirter, J. J., McWhirter, B. T., McWhirter, E. H., & McWhirter, R. J. (2007). *At-risk youth: A comprehensive response for counselors, teachers, psychologists, and human service professionals* (3rd ed.). Belmont, CA: Brooks/Cole.

Meisgeier, C., & Murphy, E. (1987). *Murphy-Meisgeier Type Indicator for Children.* Palo Alto, CA: Consulting Psychologists Press.

Merrell, K. W., & Walters, A. S. (1998). *Internalizing Symptoms Scale for Children.* Austin, TX: Pro-Ed.

Miller, S. M. (1989). Cognitive informational styles in the process of coping with threat and frustration. *Advances in Behavioural Research and Therapy, 11,* 223–234.

Monaghan, J. H., Robinson, J. O., & Dodge, J. A. (1979). The children's Life Events Inventory. *Journal of Psychosomatic Research, 23*(1), 63–68.

Mooney, K. C., Graziano, A. M., & Katz, J. N. (1984). A factor-analytic investigation of children's nighttime fear and coping responses. *Journal of Genetic Psychology, 111,* 205–215.

Murphy, L. B., & Moriarty, A. E. (1976). *Vulnerability, coping and growth.* New Haven, CT: Yale University Press.

National Center for Children Exposed to Violence. (2006). *Community violence.* Retrieved June 29, 2010, from http://www.nccev.org/violence/community.html

National Institute on Drug Abuse. (2005). *Marijuana abuse.* Bethesda, MD: National Institutes of Health.

Neff, E. J., & Dale, J. C. (1996). Worries of school-age children. *Journal of the Society of Pediatric Nurses, 1*(1), 27–32; quiz 33–24.

Newcomb, M. D., Huba, G. J., & Bentler, P. M. (1981). A multidimensional assessment of stressful life events among adolescents: Derivation and correlates. *Journal of Health and Social Behavior, 22,* 400–415.

Patterson, J. M., & McCubbin, H. I. (1987). A-COPE: Adolescent Coping Orientation for Problem Experiences. In H. I. McCubbin & A. I. Thompson (Eds.), *Family assessment inventories for research and practice* (pp. 226–241). Madison: University of Wisconsin Press.

Peterson, L., & Toler, S. M. (1986). An information seeking disposition in child surgery patients. *Health Psychology, 5*(4), 343–358.

Preits, M., & Dimova, A. (2008). Vulnerable children of mentally ill parents: Towards evidence-based support for improving resilience. *Support for Learning, 23*(3), 152–159.

Reed, D. L., Thompson, J. K., Brannick, M. T., & Sacco, W. P. (1991). Development and validation of the Physical Appearance State and Trait Anxiety Scale (PASTAS). *Journal of Anxiety Disorders, 5*(5), 323–332.

Reivich, K., & Gillham, J. (2010). Building resilience in youth: The Penn Resiliency Program. *Communique, 18*(6), 17–19.

Rende, R. D., & Plomin, R. (1991). Child and parent perceptions of the upsettingness of major life events. *Journal of Child Psychology and Psychiatry, 32*(4), 627–633.

Richardson, G. E. (2002). The metatheory of resilience and resiliency. *Journal of Clinical Psychology, 58*(3), 307–321.

Ritchie, J. A., Caty, S., & Ellerton, M. L. (1988). Coping behaviors of hospitalized preschool children. *Maternal-Child Nursing Journal, 17*(3), 153–171.

Rose, M. H. (1972). *The effects of hospitalization on coping behaviors of children.* Chicago, IL: University of Chicago.

Rutter, M. (1985). Resilience in the face of adversity. Protective factors and resistance to psychiatric disorder. *British Journal of Psychiatry, 147,* 598–611.

Rutter, M. (1993). Resilience: Some conceptual considerations. *Journal of Adolescent Health, 14*(8), 626–631, 690–696.

Rutter, M. (1996). Stress research: Accomplishments and tasks ahead. In R. J. Haggerty, L. R. Sherrod, N. Garmezy, & M. Rutter (Eds.), *Stress, risk and resilience in children and adolescents: Processes, mechanisms, and interventions* (pp. 354–385). New York, NY: Cambridge University Press.

Ryan-Wenger, N. A. (1996). Children, coping, and the stress of illness: A synthesis of the research.

Journal of the Society of Pediatric Nurses, 1(3), 126–138.

Ryan-Wenger, N. A., Sharrer, V. W., & Campbell, K. K. (2005). Changes in children's stressors over the past 30 years. *Pediatric Nursing, 31*(4), 282–288, 291.

Ryan, N. M. (1988). The stress-coping process in school-age children: Gaps in the knowledge needed for health promotion. *ANS: Advances in Nursing Science, 11*(1), 1–12.

Ryan-Wenger, N. M. (1990). Development and psychometric properties of the Schoolagers' Coping Strategies Inventory. *Nursing Research, 39*(6), 344–349.

Ryan-Wenger, N. M. (1992). A taxonomy of children's coping strategies: A step toward theory development. *American Journal of Orthopsychiatry, 62*(2), 256–263.

Scudder, L., Sullivan, K., & Copeland-Linder, N. (2008). Adolescent resilience: Lessons for primary care. *The Journal for Nurse Practitioners, 4*(7), 535–543.

Sharrer, V. W., & Ryan-Wenger, N. A. (2002). School-age children's self-reported stress symptoms. *Pediatric Nursing, 28*(1), 21–27.

Skybo, T. (2005). Witnessing violence: Biopsychosocial impact on children. *Pediatric Nursing, 31*(4), 263–270.

Smokowski, P. R., & Kopasz, K. H. (2005). Bullying in school: An overview of types, effects, family characteristics, and intervention strategies. *Children & Schools, 27*(2), 101–110.

Sparrow, J. D. (2007a). From developmental to catastrophic: Contexts and meanings of childhood stress. *Psychiatric Annals, 37*(6), 397–401.

Sparrow, J. D. (2007b). Understanding stress in children. *Pediatric Annals, 36*(4), 187–194.

Spirito, A., Stark, L. J., & Williams, C. (1988). Development of a brief coping checklist for use with pediatric populations. *Journal of Pediatric Psychology, 13*(4), 555–574.

Substance Abuse and Mental Health Services Administration. (2001). *Summary of findings from the 2000 national household survey on drug abuse.* Rockville, MD: Office of Applied Studies.

Thomas, A., & Chess, S. (1984). *Temperament and development.* New York, NY: Brunner/Mazel.

Thompkins, S. M., & Swartz, R. C. (2009). Enhancing resilience in youth at risk: Implications for psychotherapists. *Annals of the American Psychotherapy Association, 12*(4), 32–39.

Thompson, J. K., Cattarin, J., Fowler, B., & Fisher, E. (1995). The Perception of Teasing Scale (POTS): A revision and extension of the Physical Appearance Related Teasing Scale (PARTS). *Journal of Personality Assessment, 65*(1), 146–157.

Thompson, R. A., & Calkins, S. D. (1996). The double-edged sword: Emotional regulation for children at risk. *Development and Psychopathology, 8,* 163–182.

Wang, J., Iannotti, R. J., Luk, J. W., & Nansel, T. R. (2010). Co-occurrence of victimization from five subtypes of bullying: Physical, verbal, social exclusion, spreading rumors, and cyber. *Journal of Pediatric Psychology, 35(10),* 1103–1112.

Weitzman, M., Walker, D. K., & Gortmaker, S. (1986). Chronic illness, psychosocial problems, and school absences. Results of a survey of one county. *Clinical Pediatrics (Phila), 25*(3), 137–141.

Wertlieb, D., Weigel, C., & Feldstein, M. (1987). Measuring children's coping. *American Journal of Orthopsychiatry, 57*(4), 548–560.

Yamamoto, K. (1979). Children's ratings of the stressfulness of experiences. *Developmental Psychology, 15,* 581–582.

Yeaworth, R. C., York, J., Hussey, M. A., Ingle, M. E., & Goodwin, T. (1980). The development of an adolescent life change event scale. *Adolescence, 15*(57), 91–97.

Zeitlin, S. (1980). Assessing coping behavior. *American Journal of Orthopsychiatry, 50*(1), 139–144.

Zeitlin, S. (1985a). *Coping inventory: A measure of adaptive behavior (observation form).* Bensenville, IL: Scholastic Testing Service.

Zeitlin, S. (1985b). *Coping inventory: A measure of adaptive behavior (self-rated form).* Bensenville, IL: Scholastic Testing Service.

Zeitlin, S., Williamson, G. G., & Szczepanski, M. (1988). *Early Coping Inventory: A measure of adaptive behavior.* Bensenville, IL: Scholastic Testing Service.

Zinzow, H. M., Ruggiero, K. J., Resnick, H., Hanson, R., Smith, D., Saunders, B., et al. (2009). Prevalence and mental health correlates of witnessed parental and community violence in a national sample of adolescents. *Journal of Child Psychology and Psychiatry, 50*(4), 441–450.

11

STRESS, COPING, AND ADOLESCENT HEALTH

CAROLYN MARIE GARCÍA AND JESSIE KEMMICK PINTOR

U pon entering their second decade of life, adolescents say good-bye to childhood and welcome increasing physical, emotional, and social maturity. Through processes that occur over several years, adolescents are growing substantially; for example, leading research has demonstrated the dramatic changes that occur in an adolescent's brain between the "tween" years (10–13) and young adulthood (18–24). There is no doubt these changes are concurrent with challenges, and the extent to which an adolescent can successfully maneuver through these changes will determine whether she or he will thrive, struggle, or do a bit of both thriving and struggling.

Attention toward adolescent coping is in part the result of enhanced understanding about risk and protective factors that can be intervened on to enhance well-being. It is thought that if an adolescent's coping skills can be improved, she or he may perceive and react to stressors in ways that yield positive health outcomes. *Coping*, broadly, is behavior that uses available resources in response to something stressful; resources can be healthy (e.g., caring adult) or unhealthy (e.g., substances) and subsequently, coping can also be healthy or unhealthy. Certainly, it is an important behavior, because coping has a direct influence on how an adolescent comes through stressful experiences. Adolescents experience many stressful situations, ranging from pubertal changes or chronic diseases to family and peer relationship conflicts. In this chapter we explore adolescent stress and coping in the context of this developmental stage, and present a synthesis of literature, specifically the conceptualization and measurement of adolescent coping. Recommendations are offered with respect to advancing science on adolescent coping.

OVERVIEW OF ADOLESCENT DEVELOPMENT

An overview of adolescent development is necessary to provide context for the unique experience of stress and coping in this developmental

AUTHORS' NOTE: Thank you to the following individuals who assisted in compiling the articles reviewed: Elizabeth Kinder, Christie Martin, and Eve Shapiro. Effort on this book chapter was supported by a Building Interdisciplinary Research Careers in Women's Health Grant administered by the Deborah E. Powell Center for Women's Health at the University of Minnesota, Grant K12HD055887 from the National Institute of Child Health and Human Development. The content is solely the responsibility of the author and does not necessarily represent the official views of the National Institute of Child Health and Human Development, or the National Institutes of Health.

phase. Adolescence is marked by growth on many levels; holistically one can appreciate the intertwined development of an adolescent in physical, psychological, social, and spiritual domains (Rew, 2005). The rate by which an adolescent develops in these domains varies, and development in one domain does not imply parallel development in other domains. In this way, adolescents reflect unique developmental patterns that can be broadly categorized into predictable patterns of change. For example, the pubertal development of boys and girls occurs in a relatively sequential manner within a range of time such that there are "early" or "late" developers but very few who have not developed most physical changes by a certain age.

Psychologically, adolescence is a decade of cognitive and moral development. Piaget's theoretical work identified four cognitive developmental phases and three processes an adolescent undertakes to reach a new phase (Piaget & Inhelder, 1969). According to Piaget, a pre-adolescent, at 12 years of age, is capable of the fourth stage and therefore, most adolescents will reach adult-like thinking in their adolescent years. Critical thinking and information processing develop a great deal during adolescence, with older adolescents demonstrating greater abilities to remember (short- and long-term memory) and to reason (deductively and inductively). Adolescent moral development has been conceptualized in three phases by Kohlberg (1978). Gilligan (1993) advanced understanding of morality by exploring observed differences in how boys and girls approach moral dilemmas, demonstrating that, generally, boys seek direct resolution and girls will avoid conflict to maintain a relationship (Rew, 2005). These differences are likely reflected in how boys and girls cope with stressors.

Socially, adolescence has been characterized by Erikson (1968) as the developmental period in which "identity" is the primary psychosocial crisis. Indeed, as adolescents migrate toward peer relationships and begin to separate from their parents, their perspectives are broadened and they are faced with the task to form their own identity. Identity development is critical to how the adolescent perceives "self," and perceives how social interaction and the future are "conferred or constructed" (Rew, 2005, p. 112; Marcia, 1980). A healthy identity is one that is constructed by the adolescent (rather than conferred by others onto the adolescent), as she or he formulates opinions as simple as whom to spend time with and as complex as what to believe (Rew, 2005).

Adolescent spiritual development has been explored theoretically despite lacking a consistent definition of what "spiritual" comprises. It is acknowledged that spiritual development should not be overlooked and is integral to holistic adolescent development, as evidenced in the growing research addressing spirituality and newly developed models to explain adolescent spiritual development (e.g., Cole's Model of Spiritual Development and Fowler's Stages of Faith Consciousness Theory) (Rew, 2005). For example, Fowler (1991) proposed seven stages of faith consciousness, two of which can occur during adolescence as formal thinking and identity formation are occurring. In these stages, the adolescent establishes a set of beliefs, in the context of identity formation, and then is able to re-evaluate beliefs in order to more clearly explicate his or her beliefs.

The complexity of adolescent development, and the variability in which this development occurs, makes obvious the challenges inherent in specifying what coping is for adolescents, and how it should be measured in research. Similar to the spectrums of development, the concept of adolescent coping reflects a range of behaviors, experiences, triggers, and actions. And as with theories of development, theories of stress and coping have been developed, refined, and challenged as the field, and understanding, advances.

STRESS AND COPING THEORETICAL DEVELOPMENT

Lazarus and Folkman (1984) used the term *coping* to describe the "cognitive and behavioral efforts" a person employs to manage stress, generally categorized as emotion-focused or problem-focused coping. Not an individual trait, coping is instead conceptualized by Lazarus and Folkman as a process (Rew, 2005). Stress and coping models such as Lazarus's transactional stress-coping process (1990) and Moos's model of context, coping, and adaptation (transactional model) (2002), and the theoretical work of Carver (1997), Carver, Scheier, and Weintraub (1989), and Frydenberg and Lewis (1990) have advanced the science regarding stress, coping, and the measurement of these constructs. Frydenberg's work (2008), in particular, has had a great impact upon how coping is conceptualized and measured in adolescents. As opposed to characterizing distinct coping patterns in terms of the actual strategies employed, Frydenberg conceptualizes coping strategies based upon their effectiveness in helping adolescents successfully manage stressors, labeling patterns as either productive or nonproductive.

Theorists have built upon the original work of Selye (1978), who proposed the term *stress* to explain responses being observed in the general adaptation syndrome (GAS), a syndrome identified as an "initial alarm reaction followed by a state of adaptation . . . called the stage of resistance" (Rew, 2005, p. 136). Selye was also the first to identify a *stressor*, or cause of subsequent stress. A healthy response to stress resulted in adaptation, according to Selye, whereas an unhealthy or resistant response would lead to exhaustion.

In adolescent stress and coping research, specifically, there are stressors that coincide with this developmental stage, for example, stressors associated with identity development, a process involving growing independence from parent figures whilst establishing stronger associations with peer groups. Numerous factors influence the extent to which this and the other developmental milestones introduce stress for an adolescent, including intrapersonal and environmental factors. Bronfenbrenner's ecological model (1979) demonstrates the complex and numerous sources of potential stress or security in the life of an adolescent, influences that may be protective or harmful (see Figure 11.1). Family, school, and peers are examples of microsystem-level factors

that present direct influences, whilst macrosystem-level factors (e.g., societal values, economic circumstances) are distal influences. These external forces are particularly recognized in Moos's (2002) model of context, coping, and adaptation in adolescence, in that Moos emphasizes the necessity of understanding them (e.g., family, social context) in order to realize how an adolescent adapts and subsequently copes. One can see how an adolescent's appraisal of a stressor involves both subtle and obvious factors contributing to how an adolescent acts, or copes, with the stressor. It becomes clear, as well, that assessment of coping, resources, and responses is complex. However, with insights about adolescent coping, interventions such as school- or clinic-based programs can be structured to strategically reinforce environmental factors that promote healthy coping. This is an ideal but challenged scenario, given the complexity of the existing science regarding coping conceptualization and measurement.

State of the Science: Relevant Reviews of Coping Measurement

Over 15 years ago, Parker and Endler (1992) conducted a critical review of coping assessment and concluded that the empirical weaknesses in coping assessment significantly challenged and limited the applicability and relevance of coping data. In 2001, Compas, Connor-Smith, Saltzman, Thomsen, and Wadsworth completed a critical review of coping with specific attention to the coping of children and adolescents. Similar to Parker and Endler, Compas et al. concluded that a gap continues to exist between the acknowledged need

---

Figure 11.1   Example Stressors at Ecological Levels

Individual level	Microsystem level (family, school, work, peers)	Macrosystem level
• Pubertal changes • Chronic disease • Acute injury or illness • Lack of sleep or poor diet • Abuse	• Relationship conflicts • Schedule demands • Family disruptions (e.g., parent job loss, divorce, home foreclosure) • Neighborhood safety • Occupational exposures • Access to health care	• Immigration policy • Economic climate • Cultural conflicts • Racism or discrimination

for identifying ways individuals cope or sub-types of coping behaviors and the development of measures that can distinguish these sub-types for children and adolescents. More recently, Skinner, Edge, Altman, and Sherwood (2003) completed an evaluation of 100 coping assessment tools used with young people and adults. They identified over 400 ways of coping that were measured in these tools, demonstrating the breadth and depth of coping measurement and the resultant challenges in interpreting, generalizing, and acting on coping data. Decker (2006) conducted a review of coping among adolescents with cancer. Her review of 12 articles yielded a consistent theme; namely, that although the studies used validated instruments to measure coping, few used the same measure, which made comparisons difficult. As a result, "comparison of the coping strategies of younger children and adolescents yielded conflicting results as did the gender comparisons" (Decker, p. 135). Nicholls and Polman (2007a) conducted a systematic review of the coping literature on sports and athletes. The review confirmed a variety of coping strategies were used, as well as age and sex differences in coping. Finally, Sveinbjornsdottir and Thorsteinsson (2008) conducted an analysis examining six adolescent coping scales and their psychometric properties, specifically considering their design and construction against "best classical test-theoretical practice" criteria. Each of the six were found to perform poorly against the criteria, yet are among the more popular scales used to assess adolescent coping.

The main goals of this review were to summarize how coping is being conceptualized and measured in adolescent research and to provide a synthesis of adolescent coping measures used since 2000. Our search was conducted between June and October 2010, using four scientific databases: Medline, CINAHL, HAPI, and PyschInfo. The key words used, purposefully broad, included adolescent(s), cope/coping, stress(ors), and adaptation/psychological (as alternative wording for stress in some of the databases). Reference lists of identified articles were also examined in order to identify relevant work that may not have surfaced in the database search. Finally, published reviews addressing adolescent coping and coping measurement were examined to identify additional relevant publications.

Identifying and Selecting Articles

A total of 1,548 articles were initially identified using the search strategy outlined above. Review of published abstracts yielded 446 empirical articles to retrieve and examine more closely for inclusion. Criteria for inclusion in the review were that the study (a) measured adolescent's self-report of coping, (b) presented original coping outcome data, (c) primarily targeted adolescents between the ages of 12 and 18, (d) was reported in English, and (e) was published between 2000 and September 2010. Articles with the primary purpose of validating an adolescent coping measure were not included. Articles in which coping was reported as a mediator, moderator, or predictor but was not a primary outcome were also excluded after careful review. These criteria yielded 145 articles. Articles were organized using a matrix approach (Garrard, 2007) that facilitated examination of study purpose, sample, outcomes, and instruments (see Table 11.1).

How Coping Was Conceptualized

Defined or Described. All but 38 studies included a specific statement defining coping. Twenty-three studies relied on Lazarus & Folkman's (1984) definition of coping as the "cognitive and behavioral efforts to manage internal and/or external demands appraised to be taxing or beyond the resources of the individual" (p. 141). Several articles explored unique ways of coping specific to certain populations, and as such, defined these ways of coping to reflect this uniqueness. For example, in their study on "Africultural" coping, Constantine, Donnelly, & Myers (2002) define this as "the degree to which African Americans utilize coping behaviors thought to be rooted in African American culture" (p. 699). Berg, Skinner, Ko, Butler, Palmer, et al. (2009) explored parent–adolescent dyadic coping in their study, which they conceptualized generally as collaborative coping wherein parents and adolescents pool resources and problem solve jointly.

Rather than providing a definition of coping, many authors *described* coping in the context of stress response by identifying particular types or ways of coping or naming specific coping strategies used. Ways of coping have been defined by Skinner et al. (2003) as, "the basic

Table 11.1 Articles Reviewed: Purpose, Sample, Coping Results, Coping Measures, and Definition of Coping (2000–2010)

Authors (alphabetical by year)	Purpose/aim	Sample size (Females and/ or males)	Age range (data provided in article)	Example coping results	Coping assessment* (number of items; Cronbach's alpha, if provided)	Coping definition
2010						
Bradshaw, Sudhinaraset, Mmari, & Blum	To describe efforts to help mobile military students cope with stress and identify strategies that schools can use to ease their transition	98 (F/M)	12–18	Students employed a variety of coping mechanisms including developing better communication skills, developing empathy for other "outsiders," taking on adult roles and responsibilities, participating in extracurricular activities, connecting with other students and military families, and confiding in peers.	Focus groups	No definition provided.
Braun-Lewensohn, Sagy, & Roth	To examine coping strategy use among Israeli Jewish and Arab adolescents who experienced missile attacks	303 (F/M)	12–19	Problem-solving coping was most common among both groups of teens. Differences were observed in how the Jewish and Arab youth used nonproductive and reference-to-others strategies.	Adolescent Coping Scale (ACS)-shortened (18 items; .49–.63)	Effort that is made to render a perceived stressor more tolerable and to minimize the distress induced by the situation.
De Boo & Spiering	To investigate relationships between temperament, coping, and depressive and aggressive mood in early adolescents, as well as gender differences in these relationships	404 (F/M)	8–12	Girls scored higher than boys on avoidant coping. For girls, effortful control and active problem solving accounted for variability in depressive mood, while for boys only effortful control accounted for this variance.	Children's Coping Strategies Checklist-Revised 1 (CCSC-R1 [54 items; .72–.88])	Effortful thoughts and behavior directed toward management of internal and external demands of situations that are appraised as stressful.

*Coping assessment refers to the mechanism by which coping data were collected in the study.

Author	Purpose	N	Age	Results	Measure	Definition/Description
Firth, Greaves, & Frydenberg	To compare reported coping among adolescents with learning disabilities to coping results obtained from the general Australian student population	98 (F/M)	12–15	"Ignoring the problem" and "not coping" were common among 12–13 year olds with learning disabilities. Higher rates of "not coping" or "ignoring the problem" existed among 14–15 year olds with learning disabilities but there were no differences in overall coping styles to the general population.	ACS (89 items; .44–.81)	Productive coping strategies focus on problem solving, optimism, and maintaining physical health. Nonproductive coping includes ignoring the problem, self-blame, not coping, or relieving tension. Reference to other includes strategies in which people seek the assistance of others.
Haraldsson, Lindgren, Hildingh, & Marklund	To describe adolescent girls' experiences and reflections about contributors to everyday life stress	15 (F)	17	Girls used three categories of strategies to reduce stress: "enjoyment and recovery" (such as leisure and cultural activities), "trust" (i.e., emotional support), and "insight and influence" (includes strategies such as problem solving).	In-depth interviews	Cognitive and behavioral efforts to manage stress.
Hoar, Crocker, Holt, & Tamminen	To examine gender differences in coping strategies adolescent athletes use to manage sport-related interpersonal stress	524 (F/M)	11–15; M = 13	Gender differences were revealed in select coping strategies. For example, females more often reported use of seeking social support and cognitive reappraisal, while males used more aggression.	Youth Coping Questionnaire (YCQ)	The cognitive and behavioral efforts to manage internal and external demands appraised to be taxing or beyond the resources of the individual.
Jones et al.	To evaluate impact of an interactive CD-ROM to educate adolescents about their cancer	130 (F/M)	12–18	No significant differences in coping scores were observed.	KIDCOPE	No definition provided.

(Continued)

Table 11.1 (Continued)

Authors (alphabetical by year)	Purpose/aim	Sample size (Females and/or males)	Age range (data provided in article)	Example coping results	Coping assessment* (number of items; Cronbach's alpha, if provided)	Coping definition
Kristiansen & Roberts	To examine how the Norwegian Olympic youth team experienced and coped with competitive and organizational stress	29 (F/M)	14–17	The athletes used cognitive coping strategies and relied on social support.	Interviews; open-ended questionnaires	A dynamic process following appraisal because of a challenging situation where an individual perceives an imbalance between the situation and resources.
Lepistö, Åstedt-Kurki, Joronen, Luukkaala, & Paavilainen	To describe the experiences of domestic violence and coping among ninth-grade adolescents	1393 (F/M)	14–17	The experience of violence was associated with the use of seeking to belong and self-blame as coping mechanisms.	ACS (79 items)	Coping divided into three domains: problem-focused coping, reference to others, and non-productive coping.
Orban et al.	To examine stressors and coping responses used by youth with HIV	166 (F/M)	13–21	Passive coping was reported as the most used and most helpful coping strategy. Youth with moderately advanced disease used a passive coping style more often than healthier youth, which was associated with greater emotional and behavioral problems.	KIDCOPE (11 items)	Passive strategies are emotion-focused and manage distress associated with uncontrollable events. Active strategies which take direct action to solve a problem are used when the stressor is more manageable.
Pendragon	To investigate how female youth perceive and respond to challenges related to late adolescence and a minority sexual orientation	15 (F)	18–23	Participants reported applying perseverance, tenacity, and appraisal and reappraisal, as well as engaging in avoidance to manage stress.	Interviews; focus groups	Universal elements of coping include perseverance, sustaining effort over time, and appraisal and reappraisal.

Ratcliff, Blount, & Mee	To examine adolescent renal transplant recipients' perceived adversity and its association with coping and medical nonadherence	33 (F/M)	11–20	Coping strategies used most often included using humor, investing in friends, and optimism. Those used least often included engaging in avoidance activities and seeking professional support. The perceived adversity of "feeling different from peers" was associated with greater total coping scores.	Adolescent-Coping Orientation for Problem Experience [A-COPE (54 items; .50–.75)]	Avoidance coping is denial or behavioral disengagement. Maladaptive coping is avoidance or denial.
Roesch, Duangado, Vaughn, Aldridge, & Villodas	To examine the predictive ability of components of dispositional hope in the consistent use of daily coping strategies among minority adolescents	126 (F/M)	14–18	Dimensions of dispositional hope were positively related to direct problem solving, planning, positive thinking, religious coping, distracting action, instrumental support for action, and overall coping use.	Daily diary method (8 items from CCSC and How I Cope Under Pressure Scale [HICUPS])	A strategy to alleviate stress or eliminate a stressful situation utilizing cognitive, behavioral, and material resources.
Sagar, Busch, & Jowett	To examine fear of failure and coping responses among youth soccer players	4 (M)	16–18	The athletes used problem-focused coping strategies to cope with failure. Other strategies were inconsistently used among the athletes.	In-depth interviews	A dynamic process that involves a person constantly changing cognitive and behavioral efforts to manage internal and external demands that are appraised as stressful.
Tamminen & Holt	To examine recurrent stressors and coping strategies over the course of the season, and to examine coping as a process in female adolescent athletes	13 (F)	$M = 16$	Coping strategies changed throughout the season. Proactive coping was distinguished from reactive coping by planning and evaluation.	Diary-audio	Proactive coping consists of efforts undertaken in advance of the occurrence of a potential stressor to avoid it or minimize its severity.

(Continued)

261

Table 11.1 (Continued)

Authors (alphabetical by year)	Purpose/aim	Sample size (Females and/ or males)	Age range (data provided in article)	Example coping results	Coping assessment* (number of items; Cronbach's alpha, if provided)	Coping definition
Zhang et al.	To investigate the stress-coping relationships among children and adolescents who survived the 2008 Chinese earthquake	423 (F/M)	M = 13	Certain coping styles were found to be significant determinants of mental health, with girls from the highly exposed areas appearing more vulnerable than males.	Coping Scale (CS [62 items; .884])	No definition provided.
2009						
Ben-Ari & Hirshberg	To examine the relationship between adolescents' attachment styles, conflict perceptions, and coping with peers	146 (F/M)	14–16; M = 15	Positive attitudes toward conflict and secure attachment were associated with cooperative strategies to cope with conflict.	Rahim Organizational Conflict Inventory (ROC II)	The dynamic process of responding to external events that are highly stressful or negative, with cognitive and behavioral components.
Berg et al.	To examine whether perceived coping effectiveness was higher when adolescents' dyadic coping was matched to shared stress appraisals	252 (F/M)	M = 12	Perceived coping effectiveness was enhanced when dyadic coping with mothers was consistent with stress appraisals.	Recalling stressful events, coping strategies, and parental involvement in coping.	Collaborative coping is defined as mothers and adolescents pooling resources and jointly problem solving together.
Berger & Dalton	To explore psychosocial adjustment in young people with a cleft	100 (F/M)	11–16; M = 13	Adolescents most often reported resignation, social support, and distraction. Youth perceived social support, cognitive restructuring, problem solving, and emotional regulation as most helpful coping strategies.	KIDCOPE	Initiation of a cognitive or behavior response in order to manage the situation.

Braun-Lewensohn et al.	To explore the use of coping strategies among adolescents in the context of ongoing terrorism	913 (F/M)	12–18	Adolescents use a wide variety of coping strategies. The most common are leisure activities, spend time with boyfriend/girlfriend, and think of what is good.	ACS [.56–.91], Youth Self Report (YSR [112 items])	The actual effort that is made in the attempt to render a perceived stressor more tolerable and minimize the distress induced by the situation.
Çengel-Kültür, Ulay, & Erda	To investigate ways of coping among adolescents with epilepsy	75 (F/M)	3–16	Problem behavior correlated with lower problem-focused coping. Use of problem-focused coping increases with self-esteem.	Turkish Ways of Coping Inventory (TWCI [30 items; .63–.72])	Problem-focused coping strategies include self-confidence, optimism, seeking social support. Emotion-focused coping strategies include submissiveness and helplessness.
Cotton et al.	To examine religious/spiritual coping, spirituality, and health-related quality of life in adolescents with sickle cell disease	48 (F/M)	11–19	Adolescents reported greater use of positive religious/spiritual coping strategies than negative strategies.	Religious/spiritual coping short form (Brief RCOPE [14 items])	How individuals may use religion/spirituality to deal with a stressor.
Eacott & Frydenberg	To explore the effects of a coping skill program	159 (F/M)	School level 10	Students at risk for depression significantly reduced non-productive coping	ACS (80 items)	Three coping styles: productive, non-productive, and reference to others.
Frydenberg & Lewis (a)	To examine the relationship between frequency and perceived efficacy of two coping styles, and their relationship to adolescent well-being and distress	870 (F/M)	12–16	Greater use of negative avoidant coping correlated with less well-being and greater distress. Active coping correlated positively with greater well-being and positively with distress for girls only.	ACS (23 items; > .7)	Cognitive and affective responses used by an individual to deal with problems encountered in everyday life.

(Continued)

Table 11.1 (Continued)

Authors (alphabetical by year)	Purpose/aim	Sample size (Females and/or males)	Age range (data provided in article)	Example coping results	Coping assessment* (number of items; Cronbach's alpha, if provided)	Coping definition
Frydenberg & Lewis (b)	To examine whether people who see themselves as less efficient problem-solvers use more maladaptive coping strategies	1917 (F/M)	12–18	Low efficacy was independent of the use of nonproductive strategies for boys and had only a moderate relationship for girls.	ACS (22 items; >.7)	Reduction of stress severity or number of stressors.
Grootenhuis, Maurice-Stam, Derks, & Last	To evaluate whether a psycho-educational group intervention for adolescents with inflammatory bowel disease can strengthen their coping efforts and positively impact their health-related quality of life	40 (F/M)	Intervention: $M = 15$; control: $M = 16$	The intervention group reported using more predictive control and optimism (predictive coping). Parents reported less behavioral–emotional problems 6–8 months post-intervention.	Cognitive Control Strategies Scale for pediatric patients (15 items; .74–.98)	Seeking information, using relaxation techniques, proactive behavior with peers, and positive thinking to increase self-worth and social–emotional functioning.
Hampel, Manhal, & Hayer	To investigate effects of different forms of bullying and victimization on coping with interpersonal stressors and psychological adjustment among children and adolescents	409 (F/M)	10–16; $M = 13$	Victimization was characterized by increased maladaptive coping.	German Coping Questionnaire for Children and Adolescents Stressverarbeitungsfragebogen für Kinder und Jugendliche (SVF-KJ [36 items; .56–.88])	Efforts to manage environmental and internal demands, and conflicts among them, which tax or exceed a person's resources.

Hema et al.	52 (F/M)	8–18	To qualitatively describe the daily stressors and coping responses of children and adolescents with type 1 diabetes using daily diaries	Coping responses included three general themes: submission, personal responsibility, and ambiguous. Younger children used more coping that involved choosing an alternate activity, helping others, and an emotional response, whereas adolescents used more coping that involved persistence, alternate thinking, and talking things over.	Diary prompts adapted from *Children's Stress and Coping: A Family Perspective* (Sorensen, 1993)	A conscious effort to regulate behavior, cognition, emotion, and the environment in response to stressful circumstances.
Jemtå, Fugl-Meyer, Öberg, & Dahl	138 (F/M)	7–18	To identify the impact of five self-esteem dimensions on well-being and coping strategies in children and adolescents with mobility impairment	Children and adolescents who estimated their "physical characteristics" lower used the coping strategy "distraction" more often.	CCSC (52 items)	No definition provided.
Kennedy & Lloyd-Williams	11 (F/M)	8–18	To explore how children cope, and to identify areas where there may be barriers to children accessing support to enable them to cope	Distraction and maintaining normality were the dominant coping strategies for children.	Semi-structured interviews	Effortful process of adaptation to a challenging, threatening, or harmful circumstances. Problem-focused coping is based on individual efforts to change aspects of the stressor. Emotion-focused coping is aimed at managing emotions caused by the stressor.

(Continued)

Table 11.1 (Continued)

Authors (alphabetical by year)	Purpose/aim	Sample size (Females and/ or males)	Age range (data provided in article)	Example coping results	Coping assessment* (number of items; Cronbach's alpha, if provided)	Coping definition
Martyn-Nemeth, Penckofer, Gulanick, Velsor-Friedrich, & Bryant	To examine the relationship of self-esteem, stress, social support, and coping related to unhealthy eating behavior and depressive mood in adolescents	102 (F/M)	14–18	Approach coping was endorsed by most participants (70%) followed by avoidant coping (30%). About 25% of the youth using food as a coping mechanism had positive correlation with higher body mass index.	Coping Across Situations Questionnaire (CASQ [6 items; .94])	Approach: active problem solving; avoidant: passive responses to withdraw.
Massey, Garnefski, Gebhardt, & van der Leeden	To investigate both concurrent and prospective relationships between daily frustration, cognitive coping, and coping efficacy with daily headache occurrence	89 (F/M)	13–21	Coping efficacy beliefs correlated with lower next day headache occurrence. No cognitive coping strategy used in response to daily frustration was related to same or next day headache occurrence.	Cognitive Emotion Regulation Questionnaire (CERQ [9 items])	Cognitive coping strategies are the thoughts (rather than the behaviors) employed to deal with the daily frustration or associated negative emotions.
Miranda & Claes	To find out whether three styles of coping by music listening are related to depression in adolescents and to examine whether peers' depression levels and coping by music listening are moderators of the relation between metal music preference and depression levels in adolescent girls	418 (F/M)	15–19; M = 16	Music preference and depression levels of participants are correlated with those of their closely affiliated peers (i.e., friends).	Not named (10 items; .69–.88)	Conscious volitional response to stressful events.

Murberg	259 (F/M)	14–16	Adolescents' coping styles were only moderately correlated with the personality traits of neuroticism and extraversion.	A-COPE (34 items; .67–.78)	Stable traits that influence perception of stressful events and consistently determine the individual's responses to stress that is experienced.
A. Nicholls, Polman, Morley, & Taylor	527 (F/M)	11–19; $M = 14$	The relationship between pubertal status and coping/effectiveness is different from the relationship between chronological age and coping/effectiveness.	Coping Inventory for Competitive Sport (CISC [39 items; .66–.87])	Conscious attempts individuals make to manage situations that they perceive as stressful and endangering their well-being.
A. R. Nicholls, Jones, Polman, & Borkoles	5 (M)	$M = 27$	Blocking was coping strategy most used on match days, while increased concentration was used most on training days. Coping effectiveness was higher during training.	Diary: open-ended coping response section, a Likert-type evaluation of coping effectiveness	No definition provided.
Pereda, Forns, Kirchner, & Muñoz	168 (F/M)	7–12; $M = 10$	Social support, emotional regulation, and wishful thinking were considered to be the most effective. Children from disadvantaged backgrounds used avoidant strategies to face uncontrollable stressors.	KIDCOPE (Spanish)	The use of cognitive, emotional, and behavioral strategies that intervene in responding to stressful situations.

(Continued)

Table 11.1 (Continued)

Authors (alphabetical by year)	Purpose/aim	Sample size (Females and/ or males)	Age range (data provided in article)	Example coping results	Coping assessment* (number of items; Cronbach's alpha, if provided)	Coping definition
Puskar, Grabiak, Bernardo, & Ren	To compare rural adolescents' coping responses before and after the behavioral intervention Teach Kids to Cope with Anger	179 (F/M)	14–18	The intervention group experienced a clinically significant, although not statistically significant, decrease in avoidant coping and increase in approach coping.	Coping Response Inventory-Youth (CRI-Y [.69–.79])	No definition provided.
Reeves, Nicholls, & McKenna	To describe stressors and coping among adolescent soccer players	40 (M)	12–18	Problem-focused coping strategies were most commonly observed among these adolescent athletes.	Semi-structured interviews	Problem-focused coping: a person's actions directed at either the self or the environment to change the situation; emotion-focused coping: regulating the emotional responses caused by stress; avoidance: includes behavioral and cognitive efforts to disengage from a stressful situation.
Seiffge-Krenke, Aunola, & Nurmi	To investigate the interplay between developmental changes in stress and coping during early and late adolescence	200 (F/M)	12–19	Throughout adolescent development, active and internal coping increased. High levels of perceived stress were associated with high active coping and low internal coping in particular situations.	CASQ (.76–.88)	An active, purposeful process in which an individual responds to stimuli appraised as taxing or exceeding his or her resources, including behavioral, emotional, and cognitive attempts to manage a stressor.

Author	Purpose	Sample	Age	Findings	Measure	Definition
Skovdal, Ogutu, Aoro, & Campbell	To explore how young caregivers in Western Kenya cope with challenging circumstances	48 (F/M)	11–17	Social support mobilization, generation of income, and positive social construction of caregiving were strategies used by young carers to cope.	Photography, drawing, interviews, group discussions	Engaging with protective factors such as social support, household cohesion, and personal attributes within their communities.
Steinhausen, Bearth-Carrari, & Winkler Metzke	To compare psychosocial adaptation in adolescent migrants, double-citizens, and native Swiss	1239 (F/M)	M = 14	Compared to natives, migrants showed more avoidant coping, having been exposed to a high number of negative life events.	CASQ German-Modified	No definition provided.
Stewart, Reutter, Letourneau, & Makwarimba	To create an intervention that optimized peer influence as social support for homeless youth	56 (F/M)	16–24	Participants reported increased support seeking, ability to cope with their lives.	Proactive Coping Inventory (28 items; .64–.85)	Coping strategies include problem-focused, support-seeking, and emotion-focused strategies.
Vliet & Andrews	To determine the feasibility and efficacy of a web-based stress management program for schools	464 (F/M)	Age not specified	Throughout the study, coping knowledge and support seeking coping increased and avoidant coping decreased.	CCSC; Strengths and Difficulties Questionnaire	No definition provided.
Wu, Chin, Haase, & Chen	To describe the essence of the coping experiences of Taiwanese adolescents with cancer	10 (F/M)	12–18	Coping experiences were marked by losing confidence (by physical and psychological suffering) and rebuilding hope (by thought restructuring, revaluing resources, and envisioning a hopeful future).	Open-ended interviews	Psychological coping strategies are antecedent to adjustments in adolescents as they appraise and reappraise stressful situations.
Yang, Lunt, & Sylva	To explore the peer stress-related coping strategies young adolescents adopt in asthma management	34 (F/M)	9–14	Adolescents used cognitive justifying, explaining, outsourcing, and un-disclosing.	Semi-structured storytelling protocols	Actions to relieve psychological stress.

(Continued)

Table 11.1 (Continued)

Authors (alphabetical by year)	Purpose/aim	Sample size (Females and/or males)	Age range (data provided in article)	Example coping results	Coping assessment* (number of items; Cronbach's alpha, if provided)	Coping definition
2008						
Alumran & Punamäki	To examine gender and age differences in emotional intelligence and coping styles amongst a sample of Bahraini adolescents and to investigate how gender, age, academic achievement, and emotional intelligence would explain the variations in the adolescents' coping styles	312 (F/M)	13–21	Gender was significantly associated with coping style. Girls showed higher levels of nonproductive coping styles than boys.	ACS-General Short Form (18 items, .62–.64)	To maintain, augment, and/or control external or internal stressors appraised as taxing the individual's resources, and to regulate one's behavior, emotions, and cognitive orientations under stress. Coping is also viewed as a dynamic multilevel and goal-directed activity aimed at either removing the source of stress and/or managing the emotional reactions evoked by stress.
Aymer	To explore the coping strategies of 10 adolescent males exposed to domestic violence perpetrated by a male parent	10 (M)	14–17	Healthy coping strategies included reading and getting professional help. Unhealthy coping strategies included fighting with peers, and using and selling drugs.	In-depth qualitative interviews	No definition provided.

Baigrie & Giráldez	To explore the relationship between binge eating and coping strategies in a sample of Spanish adolescents and to examine the adolescents' concept of binge eating	259 (F/M)	12–21	Adolescents reporting binge eating used more avoidance coping than those who did not binge eat.	ACS (80 items)	No definition provided.
Bolgar, Janelle, & Giacobbi	To describe the appraisal and coping strategies of high-trait-anger vs. low-trait-anger adolescent athletes	103 (F/M)	11–18	Athletes with higher anger control scores reported greater use of problem- and emotion-focused coping responses compared to those who scored lower.	Coping Flexibility Questionnaire (CFQ)	Constantly changing cognitive and behavioral efforts to manage specific external and/or internal demands that are appraised as taxing or exceeding the resources of the person.
Carlson & Grant	To examine relations among gender, psychological symptoms, stress, and coping in low-income African American urban early adolescents	1200 (F/M)	10–15; $M = 13$	Girls used more expressing feeling coping (co-rumination). Both boys and girl used rumination as a primary strategy, which was linked to higher symptom levels.	The Coping Checklist (52 items, .71–.87), Responses to Depression Questionnaire (Rumination scale [22 items, .85])	No definition provided.
Kaye	To describe strategies employed in coping with stress of pregnancy and motherhood	52 (F)	14–19	Participants showed four major themes of coping strategies: thriving, bargaining, surviving, and despairing.	In-depth interviews; focus groups	No definition provided.

(Continued)

Table 11.1 (Continued)

Authors (alphabetical by year)	Purpose/aim	Sample size (Females and/ or males)	Age range (data provided in article)	Example coping results	Coping assessment* (number of items; Cronbach's alpha, if provided)	Coping definition
A. R. Nicholls & Polman	To develop a way (think aloud) to measure high stress and coping during performance	5 (M)	M = 17	Coping strategies varied throughout the course. Golfers may experience up to five stressors before reporting a coping strategy.	Diary: open-ended coping response section, a Likert-type evaluation of coping effectiveness	Constantly changing cognitive and behavioral efforts to manage specific external and/or internal demands that are appraised as taxing or exceeding the resources of the person.
K. R. Puskar & Grabiak	To identify rural youth coping responses	193 (F/M)	14–17	Coping responses differed significantly by gender. Female participants reported the coping response of cognitive avoidance most often, where males most often reported use of logical analysis as a coping response.	CRI-Y (.69–.79)	Approach coping: cognitive and behavioral efforts to master or resolve problems; avoidance coping: cognitive and behavioral efforts to avoid thinking about a stressor.
Sanjari, Heidari, Shirazi, & Salemi	To examine the relationship between parental and adolescent coping in Iranian adolescents with cancer	120 (F/M)	11–18	There was a positive correlation between adolescents' engagement and disengagement coping and that of their parents.	Coping Strategies Inventory (CSI [32 items, .79])	Cognitive and behavioral strategies that individuals use to deal with different dimensions of stress.
Shelton & Harold	To examine adolescents' cognitive appraisals and coping strategies following exposure to interparental conflict	252 (F/M)	11–12	Marital conflict exerted direct effects on boys' coping behavior, while for girls effects were indirect through their self-blame and threat appraisals.	Four subscales of the Security in the Interparental Subsystem Scale (SIS)	Constantly changing cognitive and behavioral efforts to manage specific external and/or internal demands that are appraised as taxing or exceeding the resources of the person.

Yahav & Cohen	To describe the effect of a cognitive–behavioral intervention for coping with stress in nonclinical adolescents	225 (F/M)	14–16	The intervention was effective in reducing state anxiety, test anxiety, and behavior symptoms in the intervention groups as compared with the control groups.	Lapouse and Monk's (1964) list of 18 common behavior symptoms in children and adolescents (.9–.92)	Behavioral and cognitive efforts to deal with stressful encounters.
2007						
Callaghan	Case study to examine the coping of an adolescent with cancer	1 family (F/M)	14	The adolescent showed positive coping and adaptation through symptom control, hope, denial, and peer identity.	Case study	The constantly changing cognitive and behavioral efforts to manage specific external and internal demands that are determined to be taxing or exceeding the resources of the person.
Chagnon	To examine the relationship between coping mechanisms and suicide attempts among adolescents in Juvenile Justice and Child Welfare Services	84 (F/M)	14–17	Suicidal youths' coping strategies were inadequate compared to nonsuicidal youths. Negative cognitive reframing, anger, and blaming others were more frequently reported by suicidal youths.	In-depth interviews	Negative coping behavior includes avoidance and withdrawal.

(Continued)

Table 11.1 (Continued)

Authors (alphabetical by year)	Purpose/aim	Sample size (Females and/ or males)	Age range (data provided in article)	Example coping results	Coping assessment* (number of items; Cronbach's alpha, if provided)	Coping definition
Eschenbeck, Kohlmann, & Lohaus	To explore interactions between gender, type of stressful situation, and age group in coping strategies in childhood and adolescence	1990 (F/M)	7–16; M = 11	Girls reported using more social support and problem-solving strategies, while boys reported using more avoidant strategies. These gender differences were more salient in social situations.	German Stress and Coping Questionnaire for Children and Adolescents-Fragebogen zur Erhebung von Stress und Stressbewältigung im Kindesund Jugendalter (SSKJ [30 items, 68–.88])	No definition provided.
Gelhaar et al.	To compare problem-specific coping strategies and coping styles of European adolescents from seven nations	3030 (F/M)	11–20; M = 16	Patterns of strategy use were similar for all cultures, especially for self- and future-related problems. Cultural differences in coping style were revealed for specific stressors, especially for job-related problems.	CASQ (20 items, .79–.82)	Constantly changing cognitive and behavioral efforts to manage specific external and/or internal demands that are appraised as taxing or exceeding the resources of the person.
A. R. Nicholls & Polman	To examine stressors, coping strategies, and perceived coping effectiveness among international adolescent rugby players	111 (M)	M = 18	Blocking, increased effort, and taking advice were the most commonly reported coping strategies.	Daily diary, including Likert-type scale evaluation of coping effectiveness	Constantly changing cognitive and behavioral efforts to manage specific external and/or internal demands that are appraised as taxing or exceeding the resources of the person.

Author	Purpose	Sample	Age	Findings	Method	Coping description
A. R. Nicholls (a)	To examine the experiences of an internationally ranked golfer during a training program for coping	1 (M)	16	The participant adhered to effective coping strategies while also reducing his use of ineffective coping behaviors.	Audio diary	Cognitive: rationalizing, reappraising, blocking, and positive self-talk; behavioral: going through a pre-shot routine; emotional: breathing exercise, physical relaxation, and seeking social support.
A. R. Nicholls (b)	To explore coping effectiveness among international golfers	5 (M)	$M = 17$	Even when used to manage the same stressor, the same coping strategies were frequently reported as being both effective and ineffective.	Daily coping effectiveness diaries	Constantly changing cognitive and behavioral efforts to manage specific external and/or internal demands that are appraised as taxing or exceeding the resources of the person.
A. R. Nicholls, Polman, Levy, Taylor, & Cobley	To examine stressors, coping, and its effectiveness as a function of gender, sport played, and skill level	749 (F/M)	18–38	Males used blocking. Females used planning, technique-oriented coping. Individual sport athletes used emotion-focused coping. Team athletes used communication.	Concept and coping maps	Constantly changing cognitive and behavioral efforts to manage specific external and/or internal demands that are appraised as taxing or exceeding the resources of the person.
Sabiston, Sedgwick, Crocker, Kowalski, & Mack	To explore adolescent females' experiences of social physique anxiety and related coping strategies	31 (F)	13–18; $M = 15$	Most common coping categories included behavioral and cognitive avoidance, appearance management, diet, social support, physical activity, reappraisal, cognitive deflection and comparison to others, seeking sexual attention, and substance use.	Semi-structured interviews	A progression of behavioral and cognitive adaptations to the emotional process contingent on personal characteristics and resources.

(Continued)

275

Table 11.1 (Continued)

Authors (alphabetical by year)	Purpose/aim	Sample size (Females and/ or males)	Age range (data provided in article)	Example coping results	Coping assessment* (number of items; Cronbach's alpha, if provided)	Coping definition
Seaton	To examine the relationships between risk, stress, and coping for a sample of urban Black adolescent males and explore the role of fear in promotion of hypermasculine coping	125 (M)	Age not specified	Hypermasculine attitudes as a form of coping are a function of hypervulnerability.	Scale measuring hypermasculine attitudes as a form of coping—from Hypermasculinity Scale (HMS [30 items, .70])	Cognitive and behavioral efforts to manage specific external and/or internal demands that are appraised as taxing or exceeding the resources of the person.
Tatar & Amram	To examine coping strategies in Israeli adolescents in relation to terrorist attacks	330 (F/M)	12–18; M = 16	Adolescents used more productive than nonproductive coping strategies, but rarely sought professional help. Males use more non-productive strategies and females seek more social support.	14 of 18 categories from original ACS (Hebrew)	No definition provided.
Vashchenko Lambidoni, & Brody	To enhance understanding of adaptation to psychosocial stressors of adolescence	30 (F)	18–21; M = 19	External coping strategies were used more in conflicts with parents, while conciliatory coping strategies were used in peer conflicts. Coping strategies became more adaptive by end of third writing session.	Pennebaker's narrative disclosure task	A set of cognitive, affective, behavioral, and physiological processes that are consciously and/ or unconsciously used to deal with stress.
Zimmer-Gembeck & Locke	To examine associations between adolescents' relationships with families and teachers, and coping behaviors	487 (F/M)	M = 14	Adolescents with more positive family and teacher relationships used more active coping at home and school.	CCSC (12 items, .68–.87)	The repertoire of responses people employ when faced with problems that threaten to impinge upon their physical or emotional equilibrium.

2006

	Purpose	N	Age	Findings	Measure	Definition
Brown & Ireland	To describe the relationship between coping style and well-being in incarcerated adolescents	133 (M)	16–20	Adolescents adapt to the initial period of incarceration by changing coping style. For example, prisoners' shift from emotion-based coping toward detachment coping was associated with less distress.	Coping Strategies Questionnaire (CSQ [60 items])	Cognitive and behavioral efforts to mitigate the effects of stressors.
Hampel & Petermann	To investigate age and gender effects on perceived interpersonal stress, coping with interpersonal stressors, and psychological adjustment among early and middle adolescents	286 (F/M)	10–14; $M = 12$	Maladaptive coping was correlated with adjustment problems, and was more commonly reported among girls than boys. Younger students were less likely to use maladaptive coping strategies and more likely to use adaptive coping strategies than older students. Behavioral problems were negatively correlated with problem- and emotion-focused coping.	SVF-KJ (36 items, .70–.82)	Adaptive coping styles were defined as "emotion-focused coping" and "problem-focused coping." Emotion-focused coping was represented by minimization and distraction/recreation. Problem-focused coping was composed by situation control, positive self-instructions, and social support. "Maladaptive coping" consisted of passive avoidance, rumination, resignation, and aggression.
Israelashvili, Gilad-Osovitzki, & Asherov	To examine the relationship between female adolescents' suicidal behavior and their mothers' ways of coping	64 (F)	12–18	Mothers use more problem-focused coping while adolescents use more disengagement coping.	Coping Orientation for Problem Experiences (COPE [48 items; .65–.90]), Active Coping Test (30 items)	No definition provided.

(Continued)

Table 11.1 (Continued)

Authors (alphabetical by year)	Purpose/aim	Sample size (Females and/or males)	Age range (data provided in article)	Example coping results	Coping assessment* (number of items; Cronbach's alpha, if provided)	Coping definition
Kowalski, Mack, Crocker, Niefer, & Fleming	To explore how adolescents cope with social physique anxiety	621 (F/M)	13–19	Females had significantly higher emotion-focused coping than males. Behavioral avoidance, appearance management, social support, cognitive avoidance, and acceptance were the most common strategies.	Coping Function Questionnaire (CFQ [18 items, .80–.84])	Coping at the micro level is defined as specific coping strategies that an individual employs in a particular situation, whereas coping at the macro level is viewed as the primary functions that coping strategies serve (problem-focused, emotion-focused, and avoidance).
Lafferty & Dorrell	To examine how national junior-age-group swimmers cope with poor performance and explore whether coping strategy use changes with perceptions of parental support	104 (F/M)	M = 14	Swimmers used individually/internally focused behavioral and cognitive strategies. Low perception of parental support was correlated with less active mechanisms and more self-blame and venting of emotion.	Modified COPE Scale (48 items, .61–.94)	Constantly changing cognitive and behavioral efforts to manage specific external and/or internal demands or conflicts appraised as taxing or exceeding one's resources.

Li, DiGiuseppe, & Froh	To examine the roles of coping and masculinity in rates of depressive symptoms among girls compared to boys	246 (F/M)	14–18	Being female, high ruminative coping, and low distractive and problem-focused coping increase risk of depression.	ACS (79 items; .70–.84)	Problem-focused coping: thoughts/action initiated to deal directly with the stressor; emotion-focused coping: thoughts/actions initiated to deal with one's emotions associated with the stressor.
Sung, Puskar, & Sereika	To evaluate the coping levels of rural adolescents and gender differences of coping and psychosocial factors	72 (F/M)	14–18	Significant relationships were observed between coping strategies and psychosocial factors. Higher levels of avoidance coping were endorsed than in normative samples.	CRI-Y	No definition provided.
Turner, Kaplan, & Badger	To identify factors of adaptive functioning, well-being, roles of maternal mutuality, and after-school programming among outpatient and community Hispanic girls	31; 62 (F)	12–20	Outpatient Hispanic sample demonstrated fewer coping skills than community sample of adolescent Hispanic females.	KIDCOPE (10 items)	No definition provided.
2005						
Carbonell, Reinherz, & Beardslee	To explore the adaptation and coping strategies used over time by emerging adults	25 (F/M)	Cohort of 26-year-olds	Difficulty was dealt with using active evasion, seeking support, and "letting go."	In-depth interviews	A pattern of responses to adverse situations.

(Continued)

Table 11.1 (Continued)

Authors (alphabetical by year)	Purpose/aim	Sample size (Females and/ or males)	Age range (data provided in article)	Example coping results	Coping assessment* (number of items; Cronbach's alpha, if provided)	Coping definition
D'Anastasi & Frydenberg	To address cultural differences in coping in one school community and consider how students benefit from a coping skills program	105 (F/M)	12–15; M = 13	Use of spiritual support and taking social action was observed more often in students labeled "Australian minority group" (comprising of Asian, African, Pacific Islander, and Middle Eastern students) than in Anglo-Australian students. After participation in a school-based coping skills program, students in the Australian minority group significantly decreased their use of self-blame, whereas Anglo-Australian students increased their use of physical recreation as a coping strategy.	ACS-Long Form (80 items, .62–.87)	Intentional efforts to manage affective arousal in threatening situations or to change the situation.
Hampel & Petermann	To investigate age and gender effects of children and adolescents' coping with common stressors	1123 (F/M)	8–14; M = 11	Maladaptive coping scores were higher and adaptive coping lower among all adolescents and girls of all ages. No situational coping patterns were established with regard to age and gender.	SVF-KJ (36 items, .70–.82)	Problem-focused, approach, and primary control coping represent strategies directed towards modifying the stressful encounter or individual goals. Emotion-focused, avoidant, and secondary control coping reflect strategies directed towards regulating stress-related negative emotions.

Author	Purpose	N	Age	Findings	Instrument	Definition
Kowalski, Crocker, Hoar, & Niefer	To examine the relationship between perceived control and emotion-focused coping	344 (F/M)	12–18	In both males and females, problem-focused coping was related to control over changing the situation, but not control over emotions. Emotion-focused coping was related to control over emotions, but not control over changing the situation.	CFQ (18 items, .80–.84)	Coping strategies are used by the individual to mediate the amount of stress experienced and perceived situational demands.
Magaya, Asner-Self, & Schreiber	To report on the coping strategies of Zimbabwean adolescents and highlight some major stressors they face	101 (F/M)	16–19; $M = 18$	Emotion-focused strategies were more frequently reported than problem-solving strategies by Zimbabwean youth.	Ways of Coping Questionnaire (WCQ [66 items, .83–.91])	The manner in which one copes may mitigate or resolve the identified stressor.
A. R. Nicholls, Holt, Polman, & James	To establish stressors experienced and examine coping strategies used by elite adolescent golfers	11 (M)	$M = 16$	The most frequently reported strategy was blocking, along with increased concentration and technical adjustment. Problem-focused coping was reported more frequently than emotion-focused or avoidance coping.	Daily diary	Constantly changing cognitive and behavioral efforts to manage specific external and/or internal demands that are appraised as taxing or exceeding the resources of the person.
Puente-Diaz & Anshel	To identify sources of acute stress, cognitive appraisal, and the use of coping strategies as a function of culture among highly skilled tennis players from Mexico and the U.S.	112 (F/M)	13–18; $M = 16$	Perceived controllability and strategy use were predicted by culture.	COPE-modified, translated to Spanish (40 items)	Constantly changing cognitive and behavioral efforts to manage specific internal and/or external demands that are appraised as taxing or exceeding the resources of a person.

(Continued)

Table 11.1 (Continued)

Authors (alphabetical by year)	Purpose/aim	Sample size (Females and/ or males)	Age range (data provided in article)	Example coping results	Coping assessment* (number of items; Cronbach's alpha, if provided)	Coping definition
Remillard & Lamb	To examine coping strategies for relational aggression	98 (F)	6–12th graders	Passive and avoidant strategies were more likely to be used when girls felt more hurt by the aggression. Seeking social support was the strategy most often used when girls felt closer to their friends after the aggressive act.	Revised Ways of Coping Questionnaire (R-WCQ [66 items, .59–.88])	No definition provided.
Schneider & Phares	To address the process by which children and adolescents cope with severe acute stress of parental loss because of termination of parental rights	60 (F/M)	9–18; M = 12	Children used avoidant coping strategies more than emotion-focused coping strategies, which in turn, were used more than problem-focused coping strategies.	HICUPS (45 items, .57–.74)	The process of responding to stressors.
Scott & House	To examine the use of approach and avoidance strategies for coping with perceived racial discrimination and their relationship to feelings of distress evoked by perceived discrimination in Black youth	71 (F/M)	14–18; M = 16	Internalizing and externalizing coping strategies are correlated with greater feelings of distress, while perceived control is related to greater use of seeking social support and problem-solving coping strategies.	Self-Report Coping Scale (SRCS [34 items, .64–.87])	Coping strategies that are approach oriented include cognitive attempts to change the manner in which a stressor is understood or perceived and behavioral efforts to directly resolve a stressor or its consequences. In contrast, coping strategies that are avoidance oriented include cognitive attempts to minimize or deny a stressor and behavioral efforts to avoid or withdraw from a stressor.

Seiffge-Krenke & Beyers	To examine the links between coping and attachment	112 (F/M)	Followed from 14 to 21	Secure individuals used their social network to cope. Secure and dismissing individuals used more internal coping than preoccupied individuals.	CASQ (20 items, .73–.80)	An active, purposeful process of responding to stimuli appraised as taxing or exceeding the resources of the person.
Tam & Lam	To compare stress and coping among migrant and local-born Chinese adolescents in Hong Kong	1116 (F/M)	7th and 9th graders	Migrants were more likely to use withdrawal coping than local-born adolescents.	CASQ (20 items, .69–.77)	Three coping styles are identified: active coping refers to the mobilization of social resources to solve the problem; internal coping involves the acknowledgement, appraisal, and acceptance of the problem and the search for its solution; and withdrawal coping reflects a fatalistic approach to the problem and the inability to solve it, using displacement or avoidance strategies.
Tourigny, Hébert, Daigneault, & Simoneau	To measure the effects of a group therapy program for teenage girls reporting child sexual abuse	42 (F)	$M = 15$	Intervention subjects had significant improvements in coping strategies, empowerment, post-traumatic stress, behavior problems, and relationship with mother.	WOCQ (21 items)	No definition provided.
Yi, Smith, & Vitaliano	To evaluate how coping correlates with resilience in athletes.	404 (F)	$M = 16$	Resilient athletes endorsed problem-focused coping and seeking social support; non-resilient used avoidance.	WOCC (45 items)	Cognitive and behavioral measures designed to master, tolerate, or reduce external and internal demands and conflicts.

(Continued)

Table 11.1 (Continued)

Authors (alphabetical by year)	Purpose/aim	Sample size (Females and/or males)	Age range (data provided in article)	Example coping results	Coping assessment* (number of items; Cronbach's alpha, if provided)	Coping definition
Young, Chadwick, Heptinstall, Taylor, & Sonuga-Barke	To clarify the developmental risk for interpersonal relationship problems and ineffective coping strategies associated with hyperactive behavior in girls	70 (F)	Follow-up ages 14–16	Hyperactivity was related to ineffective coping strategies. Conduct problem girls rated their coping strategies to be ineffective.	KIDCOPE (10 items)	No definition provided.
Zanini, Forns, & Kirchner	To examine coping behavior in Spanish adolescents	1362 (F/M)	12–16	Girls endorsed approach, avoidance, and behavioral responses more than boys. Changes in coping preferences with increased age were observed for both sexes.	Coping Reactions Inventory (CRI [48 items; .71–.77])	The constantly changing cognitive and behavioral efforts made by the subject to manage the specific external or internal demands which arise between the person and the environment.
2004						
Cunningham, Werner, & Firth	To examine the interplay between school-, teacher-, and peer-connectedness, and mastery; coping self-efficacy, and coping behaviors in adolescents	300 (F/M)	14–17; $M = 15$	The effects of school connectedness factors on the utilization of nonproductive coping strategies were mediated by coping self-efficacy and mastery. Coping self-efficacy also partially mediated the relationships between school connectedness factors and productive coping behaviors, whereas mastery did not.	Children's Coping Scale (CCS [45 items, .52–.78])	Coping resources are those aspects of the self or the environment that are valued by the individual or that serve as a means to gain valued resources.

Frydenberg & Lewis	To identify coping strategies which characterize adolescents who profess the least ability to cope	976 (F/M)	11–18	Poor coping youth used nonproductive coping strategies. However, a range of productive strategies was sometimes used.	ACS (79 items, .70)	Coping can be categorized into three areas: problem-focused (dealing with the problem, e.g., working hard, solving the problem), emotion-focused (reference to others, e.g., seeking social support, fitting in with friends), and non-productive strategies, (e.g., self-blame, worry).
Goodman	To explore how unaccompanied refugee youths from Sudan, who grew up amid violence and loss, coped with trauma and hardship in their lives	14 (M)	16–18	Four themes were identified: collectivity and the communal self, suppression and distraction, making meaning, and emerging from hopelessness to hope.	Case-centered, comparative, narrative approach	No definition provided.
Howard & Medway	To examine how high school students cope with stress as a function of their attachment style	75 (F/M)	14–19; $M = 17$	Attachment security was negatively related to negative avoidance behaviors. Attachment insecurity was positively related to negative avoidance.	ACOPE-Revised (20 items, .67–.77)	Coping is a way to respond to stress and may be positive (appropriate and addressing the problem) or negative (unhelpful, unhealthy, or not directed toward problem resolution).

(Continued)

Table 11.1 (Continued)

Authors (alphabetical by year)	Purpose/aim	Sample size (Females and/or males)	Age range (data provided in article)	Example coping results	Coping assessment* (number of items; Cronbach's alpha, if provided)	Coping definition
Kausar & Munir	To examine the effect of parental loss and gender of adolescents on their coping with stress	80 (F/M)	14–17; M = 15	Girls tended to use more strategies than boys. Adolescents used avoidance-focused coping most frequently and active distractive coping least frequently. Active distractive coping, and religious-focused coping, were used by adolescents with both parents more than by those with one living parent.	CSQ (62 items, .70–.76)	Coping is a regulator of emotion and distress and management of the problem that causes distress.
Kendall, Safford, Flannery-Schroeder, & Webb	To evaluate the maintenance of outcomes of children who received a 16-week cognitive–behavioral treatment for anxiety	86 (F/M)	15–22	Significant improvements in coping were observed over time.	Coping Questionnaire for Children (CQ-C)	No definition provided.
Meesters & Muris	To examine relationships between parental rearing practices and coping styles	122 (F/M)	13–16; M = 15	Passive coping strategies were more likely to be used if parents were perceived to be rejecting. Active coping was related to perceived control by parents.	Utrecht Coping List for Adolescents (UCL-A [44 items])	The cognitive and behavioral strategies people use to deal with both the emotional and instrumental dimensions of stress.

Puotiniemi & Kyngäs	To describe the coping of an adolescent girl who had been in psychiatric inpatient care and her mother in everyday life	2 (F)	16	The most important coping resource for both mother and daughter was emotional support.	Interviews	The constantly changing totality of cognitive and behavioral efforts to manage specific external and/or internal demands that are appraised as taxing or exceeding a person's resources.
Rasmussen, Aber, & Bhana	To examine how African American and Latino adolescents coped with neighborhood danger in low, medium, and high crime neighborhoods throughout Chicago	140 (F/M)	16–19; $M = 17$	In low and medium crime rate areas, using confrontive strategies was significantly correlated with increased exposure to violence. Coping strategies were associated with perceived safety to a substantial degree only in high crime neighborhoods, and none were associated with exposure to violence.	Ways of Coping Scale–modified (WCS)	Constantly changing cognitive and behavioral efforts to manage specific external and/or internal demands that are appraised as taxing or exceeding the resources of the person.
Ruffolo, Sarri, & Goodkind	To identify risk and protective factors for high-risk adolescent girls	159 (F)	$M = 16$	Girls in the community-based closed residential settings used more negative coping behaviors.	Adolescence Interpersonal Competence Questionnaire (AICQ)	No definition provided.

(Continued)

287

Table 11.1 (Continued)

Authors (alphabetical by year)	Purpose/aim	Sample size (Females and/or males)	Age range (data provided in article)	Example coping results	Coping assessment* (number of items; Cronbach's alpha, if provided)	Coping definition
Scott	To examine the relation of background and race-related factors to the use of approach and avoidance strategies for coping with perceived discriminatory experiences among affluent African American adolescents	71 (F/M)	14–18; M = 16	Gender, family structure, socioeconomic status, perceived discriminatory distress, and racism-related socialization were correlates of coping with perceived discriminatory experiences.	SRCS (34 items, .64–.87)	Approach coping includes strategies such as seeking support or taking direct action, whereas avoidance coping includes strategies such as denying, accepting, or minimizing stressful situations or expressing one's feelings of anger verbally or behaviorally.
Seepersad	To examine the similarities between the way adolescents cope with loneliness both online and offline	429 (F/M)	14–23; M = 20	Online and offline coping behaviors are strongly related, especially if they are avoidant.	Compiled from three separate coping instruments (60 items)	No definition provided.
Snethen, Broome, Kelber, & Warady	To identify coping strategies that adolescents with end stage renal disease use to manage their chronic illness	35 (F/M)	13–18	Personal characteristics of gender, transplant status, age, and religious views were significantly related to coping strategies used.	A-COPE (54 items, .44–.81)	The actions one takes to alleviate the demands of a chronic illness.
Thabet, Tischler, & Vostanis	To establish the nature and extent of maltreatment experiences, coping strategies, and behavioral/emotional problems, and their relationships, in a sample of Palestinian adolescents	97 (M)	15–18; M = 17	Exposure to maltreatment was related to reliance on emotion-focused or avoidant strategies. Maladaptive coping predicted emotional difficulties in the respondents.	WCS (39 items)	Constantly changing cognitive and behavioral efforts to manage specific external and/or internal demands that are appraised as taxing or exceeding the resources of the person.

van der Zaag-Loonen, Grootenhuis, Last, & Derkx	To compare generic coping styles adopted by adolescents suffering from inflammatory bowel disease (IBD) to styles used by healthy peers	65 (F/M)	12–18	Adolescents with IBD are more likely to use avoidant coping strategies. Health-related quality of life is related to disease-related coping styles.	UCL-A (44 items, .45–.79— expression of emotions scale not used due to low alpha); CCSS-c (22 items)	Constantly changing cognitive and behavioral efforts to manage specific external and/or internal demands that are appraised as taxing or exceeding the resources of a person.
Wadsworth et al.	To examine age and gender differences in stress responses to similarities in stress responses to September 11	720 (F/M)	M = 12	Females used more emotion-based and fewer disengagement strategies than males. With age, emotion-based coping increased and disengagement coping and rumination decreased.	Responses to Stress Questionnaire (RSQ [57 items, .69–.90]), Coping Activities Checklist (CAC [12 items])	Coping is a subset of responses that an individual experiences when faced with stress; it is essential to simultaneously consider both effortful and involuntary stress responses.
Washburn-Ormachea, Hillman, & Sawilowsky	To explore gender and gender-role orientation differences on adolescents' coping with peer stressors	285 (F/M)	M = 14	Significant differences for gender-role orientation were found for active, acceptance, and emotion-focused coping.	COPE (60 items, .51–.87)	Flexible cognitive or behavioral actions that are changing constantly to meet an individual's demands.

(Continued)

Table 11.1 (Continued)

Authors (alphabetical by year)	Purpose/aim	Sample size (Females and/ or males)	Age range (data provided in article)	Example coping results	Coping assessment* (number of items; Cronbach's alpha, if provided)	Coping definition
2003						
Bal, Crombez, Van Oost, & Debourdeauduij	To investigate the role that social support plays in well-being and in coping after a stressful event in a group of nonclinical adolescents	820 (F/M)	11–18; M = 14	Avoidance was more common and support-seeking was less common among sexually abused adolescents. Nonsexually abused adolescents used less avoidance and more support-seeking when family support was high.	HICUPS (54 items, .57–.87)	Avoidance coping strategies include behavioral efforts to avoid stressful situations and efforts to avoid thinking about problems by using fantasy or wishful thinking, whereas active coping strategies include strategies such as positive thinking and problem solving.
Elgar, Arlett, & Groves	To compare rural and urban adolescents with regard to self-reported stress, coping, and behavioral problems	246 (F/M)	M = 12	Although stressors, conflicts, and behaviors differed between rural and urban adolescents, levels of stress and coping strategies were similar.	WOC-R (66 items, .72–.80)	Coping is a process by which an individual either deals directly with a conflict, daily hassle, or life event, or adapts to it by regulating emotional responses.
Frydenberg et al.	To examine how young people from a variety of cultures cope with their concerns, emphasizing positive psychology, rather than deficit	572 (F/M)	4 samples: mean ages 14–16	Australian and German students ranked culturally determined activities in their coping repertoires more than Colombians and Palestinians. Coping cannot be assumed across different student populations.	ACS (80 items)	Intentional efforts to manage the affective arousal in threatening situations, or changing of the situation.

Author	Purpose	N	Age	Findings	Measure	Definition of coping
Goldblatt	To understand the meaning of interparental violence for adolescents	21 (F/M)	13–18	Thematic analysis revealed coping strategies serving as survival mechanisms in a violent environment, and positive life outcomes in spite of adversity.	In-depth interviews	Constantly changing cognitive and behavioral efforts to manage specific external and/or internal demands (and conflicts between them) that are appraised as taxing or exceeding the resources of the person.
Harris & Franklin	To evaluate a cognitive–behavioral school-based group intervention for Mexican American pregnant and parenting adolescent girls	85 (F)	14–19; $M = 17$	Experimental and control groups differed significantly on the post-test measure of problem-focused coping, with a significant increase in problem-focused strategies observed in the experimental group.	A-COPE (18 items, .69–.75)	No definition provided.
Hess & Bundy	To investigate the relationship between playfulness and coping skills in adolescent males both typically developing and with severe emotional disturbance	30 (M)	13–17	Adolescents' level of playfulness positively correlated with their coping skills. Typically developing adolescents were more playful than those with severe emotional disturbance and scored higher in effective coping skills.	The Coping Inventory (48 items, 84–98)	An individual's resources that facilitate successful adaptation to life stress.
Piquet & Wagner	To compare the coping responses of hospitalized adolescent suicide attempters to those of hospitalized non-attempters matched on diagnosis and demographics	42 (F/M)	13–18; $M = 16$	Suicide attempters made fewer effortful-approach and more automatic-approach coping responses, and coped less effectively. In follow-up, increased coping effectiveness was related to decreased suicidal symptoms.	Modified version of Child and Adolescent Coping Scale	No definition provided.

(Continued)

Table 11.1 (Continued)

Authors (alphabetical by year)	Purpose/aim	Sample size (Females and/ or males)	Age range (data provided in article)	Example coping results	Coping assessment* (number of items; Cronbach's alpha, if provided)	Coping definition
Puskar, Sereika, & Tusaie-Mumford	To test the effectiveness of a group, CBT intervention for rural youth	89 (F/M)	14–18	Some improved coping skills and reduced depressive symptoms in intervention group.	CRI-Y (.69–.79)	Responses to stress.
Renk & Creasey	To examine the relationships among gender, gender identity, and coping in late adolescents	169 (F/M)	17–22; M = 20	Females used more emotion-focused coping strategies than males. High masculinity adolescents endorsed more problem-focused coping. High femininity adolescents endorsed more emotion-focused coping strategies. Neither gender nor masculinity/femininity predicted avoidant coping.	COPE (60 items, .83–.85)	The constantly changing cognitive and behavioral efforts to manage specific external and/or internal demands that are appraised as taxing or exceeding the resources of the person.
Scott (a)	To explore whether the resonance of certain orientations and dimensions asserted to be distinctive of Black culture were related to the strategies used by African American youth to cope with perceived discrimination	120 (F/M)	14–18; M = 16	Spirituality and effort optimism were related to greater use of self-reliance/problem-solving coping strategies, whereas communalism was related to lower use of externalizing coping strategies.	SRCS (34 items, .70–.88)	Approach coping involves cognitive and behavioral strategies that attempt to act on or modify stressors, whereas avoidance coping involves cognitive and behavioral strategies that attempt to escape, avoid, or deny stressors.

Scott (b)	To explore whether the strategies used by African American adolescents to cope with perceived discriminatory experiences were related to racial identity and socialization	88 (F/M)	$M = 16$	Importance of racial identity was unrelated to both approach and avoidance coping. Socialization messages about racism from parents/guardians were related to use of approach coping strategies.	SRCS (34 items, .68–.86)	With approach coping strategies, stressors are actively engaged in an effort to resolve them, whereas the use of strategies that avoid stressors or manage emotional reaction to stressors are considered avoidance coping strategies.
Seiffge-Krenke & Stemmler	To study coping with everyday stressors in a longitudinal sample of adolescents with insulin-dependent mellitus diabetes	98 (F/M)	Recruited at 14 years old	Maintenance of stable metabolism was negatively related to avoidant coping.	CASQ (20 items, .73–.88)	Process of managing stressors.
Trask et al.	To investigate the relationship between parental and adolescent adjustment and coping and their relationship to social support and family function in adolescents with cancer and one of their parents	56 (F/M)	11–18; $M = 14$	More adaptive than maladaptive coping strategies were used by both adolescents and parents. Adaptive coping was associated with distress.	CSI (72 items, .71–.94)	No definition provided.

(Continued)

Table 11.1 (Continued)

Authors (alphabetical by year)	Purpose/aim	Sample size (Females and/ or males)	Age range (data provided in article)	Example coping results	Coping assessment* (number of items; Cronbach's alpha, if provided)	Coping definition
Wolfradt, Hempel, & Miles	To investigate the relationship between perceived parenting styles, depersonalization, anxiety, and coping behavior in a normal high school student sample	276 (F/M)	14–17; M = 15	Perceived parental warmth was positively associated with active coping. Children of authoritative and permissive parents showed highest score on active problem coping.	Coping Questionnaire by Seiffge-Krenke (20 items, .48–.68)	Coping efforts can be divided into two groups: those intended to act on the stressor and those intended to regulate emotional states resulting from the stressful event.
2002						
Broderick & Korteland	To investigate the interrelationships among coping styles, gender roles, and level of depression for early adolescents	864 (F/M)	M = 11	Coping patterns of more depressed girls resembled those of depressed adolescent and adult women. Distraction, but not rumination, was determined to be an appropriate coping strategy for men.	Children's Coping Styles Questionnaire (15 items, .45–.76)	Coping is a subset of broader self-regulatory processes that involve "conscious, volitional efforts to regulate emotion, cognition, behavior, physiology, and the environment in response to stressful events or circumstances."
Browne	To highlight the coping strategies used by young people in foster care with histories of child abuse	21 (F/M)	12–19; M = 15	Individuals having experienced abuse and crisis foster placements were more likely to display less adaptive coping strategies than those who had not been abused, and more likely to cope alone rather than seek the help of others.	ACS (79 items)	No definition provided.

Clark, Novak, & Dupree	To examine the relationship of perceived parenting practices to anger and coping in African American adolescents	70 (F/M)	14–18; $M = 16$	Perceptions of parental strictness were negatively correlated with avoiding problems and positively correlated with engaging in demanding activities. Perceptions of parental involvement were positively correlated with seeking diversions.	A-COPE (23 items from 6 subscales, .62–.70)	No definition provided.
Constantine, Donnelly, & Myers	To examine the relationships between dimensions of collective self-esteem and Africultural coping styles in African American adolescents	106 (F/M)	14–17; $M = 15$	Adolescents with higher public collective self-esteem reported greater use of spiritual-centered Africultural coping styles. Higher importance of identity collective self-esteem correlated with greater use of collective coping strategies.	Africultural Coping Systems Inventory (30 items, .60–.81)	Africultural coping is defined as the degree to which African Americans utilize coping behaviors thought to be rooted in African American culture.
Führ	To examine the appearance of humor as a coping tool in early adolescence	1755 (F/M)	10–16	Boys tend to use more aggressive and sexual related coping humor. Girls prefer to be cheered up by humor. This trend increased with age for girls but not for boys.	Coping Humor Scale (CHS [7 items; .60–.70])	Contending with unpleasant aspects of reality based on cognitive processes that do not reject or ignore the demands of reality.
C. L. Lewis & Brown	To describe the coping strategies of female adolescents infected with HIV or AIDS	112 (F)	15–21	Coping strategies included listening to music, thinking about good things, making your own decisions, sleeping, trying to deal with problems on your own, eating, daydreaming, and praying.	A-COPE (.50–.75)	The things people do to master, tolerate, and minimize life strains or demands; a constantly changing process involving cognitive and behavioral efforts deployed to manage specific external and or internal demands that are appraised as stressful.

(Continued)

Table 11.1 (Continued)

Authors (alphabetical by year)	Purpose/aim	Sample size (Females and/ or males)	Age range (data provided in article)	Example coping results	Coping assessment* (number of items; Cronbach's alpha, if provided)	Coping definition
R. Lewis & Frydenberg	To examine the relationship between youths' failure to cope and coping styles	30 (F/M)	11–18	Young people who coped less successfully used more emotion-focused strategies.	ACS (.56–.86)	Coping and emotion are in a reciprocal dynamic relationship.
Rask, Kaunonen, & Paunonen-Illmonen	To describe adolescent coping after the death of a loved one	89 (F/M)	14–16; M = 15	Self-help and social support were the most helpful strategies for adolescents coping with grief. Official support systems, such as school health services, were not experienced as helpful, and loneliness and fears of death were reported to hinder coping.	Two questions about what helps and hinders coping	A process of managing specific external and/or internal demands that are appraised as taxing or exceeding the resources of the person.
2001						
Aysan, Thompson, & Hamarat	To examine the effects that major academic exam periods have on students, as shown by measures of test anxiety, coping, and perceived health status	113 (F/M)	11th & 12th graders	Students with high test anxiety used less effective coping mechanisms. Prior to tests juniors used less effective coping mechanisms than seniors.	Coping Strategies Scale (CSS [32 items, .71–.85])	Plans and actions for dealing with stressful situations to lower distress and serve as buffers to the potential harmful effects of stress.
Myors, Johnson, & Langdon	To examine the coping styles and strategies used by a group of pregnant adolescents attending an adolescent family support services	71 (F)	15–19; M = 17	Optimistic and confrontive coping styles were most frequently used and perceived as being the most effective.	Jalowiec Coping Scale-Revised (JCS-R [60 items, .86])	The cognitive and behavioral efforts made to master, tolerate, or reduce external and internal demands and conflicts among them.

2000					
Bowker, Bukowski, Hymel, & Sippola	To examine individual differences in adolescents' response to peer stress, integrating information from the social problem-solving literature with research on stress and coping in adolescence	249 (F/M)	7th graders	More unpopular, aggressive adolescents employed more negative coping strategies, whereas more problem-focused coping strategies were used by more popular, aggressive female adolescents. More withdrawn adolescents demonstrated fewer negative strategies and problem-focused strategies, but used more emotion-focused strategies.	Written accounts of coping strategies	No definition provided.
Chapman & Mullis	To examine coping strategies and self-esteem among two racial groups of adolescents	361 (F/M)	12–19; $M = 15$	Diversions, self-reliance, spiritual support, close friends, demanding activities, family problems, and relaxation were strategies used more often by African Americans than Caucasians.	A-COPE (54 items, .87)	No definition provided.
de Anda et al.	To examine stress and coping among urban 10th and 11th grade high school students	333 (F/M)	10th and 11th graders	Low levels of coping were reported. Coping strategies differed by gender and ethnicity.	Adolescent Stress, Stressor, and Coping Measure (143 items; .76–.94)	No definition provided.
Dellve Cernerud, & Halberg	To describe how siblings of children with deficits in attention, motor control and perception (DAMP), and Asperger syndrome cope with their life situations in their families	15 (F)	12–18	Four categories of coping were identified: gaining understanding, gaining independence, following a bonding responsibility, and balancing.	Interviews	Cognitive and behavioral efforts to master psychological stress.

(Continued)

Table 11.1 (Continued)

Authors (alphabetical by year)	Purpose/aim	Sample size (Females and/ or males)	Age range (data provided in article)	Example coping results	Coping assessment* (number of items; Cronbach's alpha, if provided)	Coping definition
Dundas	To explore how children experience and cope with interpersonal distance in families with an alcoholic parent	17 (F/M)	10–21	Physical and cognitive/affective distancing was utilized by children in situations where interaction may have been overwhelming.	Semi-structured interviews	No definition provided.
Frydenberg & Lewis	To document the changes in coping in adolescents over time	168 (F/M)	11–19	Between the ages of 12 and 14, both boys and girls remained relatively stable in their own "declared inability to cope." However, when looking at changes in coping between the ages of 14 and 16, girls reported significantly higher levels of "inability to cope," whereas boys reported almost the same low level.	ACS (80 items, .54–.80)	The behavioral and cognitive efforts used by individuals to deal with the person–environment relationship.
Hains, Davies, Parton, Totka, & Amoroso-Camarata	To examine the effectiveness of a stress management training program in helping adolescents with diabetes cope with stress	15 (F/M)	12–15; M = 13	No differences in coping were observed between the training (intervention) group and control group at posttest and follow-up. However, there were significant differences (improvements in coping) within the intervention group between pretest and posttest and pretest to follow-up, while there were no over-time differences for those in the control group.	KIDCOPE (10 items)	No definition provided.

	Purpose	Sample	Age	Findings	Measure	Definition
Kobus & Reyes	To assess the perceived stress, coping, and coping effectiveness of low-income, urban, Mexican American adolescents	158 (F/M)	M = 16	Active coping strategies, family social support, self-reliance, and behavioral avoidance were the strategies most frequently reported by participants. Venting emotions and seeking family support was more common among females. Participants found coping most helpful when dealing with stressful school events.	Open-ended and structured interviews	No definition provided.
Mullis & Chapman	To study the relationship between coping, gender, age, and self-esteem in adolescents	361 (F/M)	12–19	Adolescents with higher self-esteem used more problem-focused coping strategies, while those with lower self-esteem used more emotion-focused coping.	ACOPE	Cognitive and behavioral means used to deal with stress, both emotionally and instrumentally, during early and later adolescence.
Siqueira, Diab, Bodian, & Rolnitzky	To examine stress and coping methods by smoking status among an inner-city, clinic-based, adolescent population	437 (F/M)	12–21	Current smokers and experimenters were more likely to use negative coping methods and less likely to use positive coping strategies than never-smokers.	Coping Measures Scale (47 items)	No definition provided.

categories used to classify how people cope" (p. 216) such as problem-solving or help-seeking. These mechanisms vary across individuals and influence not only the coping response to an acute stressor but also the longitudinal health and well-being of the individual. Kowalski et al. (2006) conceptualize coping at both a micro and macro level and explain that coping at the micro level is the specific coping strategies that an individual employs in a particular situation, whereas coping at the macro level is viewed as the primary functions that coping strategies serve (e.g., problem focused, emotion focused, and avoidance).

Among the studies describing rather than defining coping, eight defined coping by highlighting ways of coping such as avoidant or active coping strategies per the conceptualizations of Ebata and Moos (1991). In addition to using Lazarus and Folkman's (1984) definition of coping, 12 studies also utilized their popular dichotomy for ways of coping: problem-focused (i.e., efforts to modify the stressor) or emotion-focused coping (i.e., regulation of emotion in response to stressor) strategies. Another 5 studies relied on the 3 dimensions of coping conceptualized by Frydenberg (2008): productive (i.e., strategies leading to positive outcomes), non-productive (i.e., strategies leading to adverse outcomes), and productive in reference to others (i.e., support-seeking strategies that lead to positive outcomes).

The existing literature is extremely sparse with respect to how coping conceptualization or definition might change with varying adolescent developmental stages (see Seiffge-Krenke et al., 2009). This could, in part, be due to general recognition that adolescent coping, as conceptualized and defined, remains broad enough to encompass the various stages of development that an adolescent experiences.

How Coping Was Measured

In this section, we briefly summarize findings specific to the study designs and populations (see Table 11.2).

Study purposes. A wide range of stress-related risks or conditions were examined in these studies, representing many of the ecological systems presented in Bronfenbrenner's model (1979). These included individual-level psychological stressors such as eating disorders, suicidal ideation, and depression, and physical stressors such as HIV infection, sports participation, violence, or sexual abuse. Several authors explored coping among sexual minority youth, migrant youth, and pregnant or parenting adolescents. Studies examined influences of micro-level stressors—for example, familial stressors such as domestic violence or interparental conflict and social stressors such as romantic relationships or difficulties in school, the juvenile justice system, or a homeless shelter. Micro-level stressors were also examined among youth residing in rural settings and in military families. Finally, some examined macro-level stressors such as racial discrimination. Although some studies examined stressors across populations in order to compare across different groups, as seen in Table 11.2, the majority examined stressors within particular adolescent groups, diversely defined.

Assessing coping. Most studies relied on self-report data collection using a coping measure; however, a range of additional mechanisms for assessing coping were identified, including audio and daily diaries, focus groups, interviews, narrative tasks, photography, and storytelling. The five most common measures of coping were the Adolescent Coping Scale (ACS), the Adolescent Coping Orientation for Problem Experiences (A-COPE), the Children's Coping Strategy Checklist (CCSC), the Coping Across Situations Questionnaire (CASQ), and the KIDCOPE. Reliability coefficients of internal consistency for the samples studied were reported for all but 41 of the 110 studies that used coping measures (see Table 11.1).

Study results. Generally, there are numerous challenges to synthesizing adolescent coping results across studies. One of these challenges is the use of different measures of coping. For example, coping outcomes were reported in many of the descriptive studies by using terms from the selected study measures, which limits meaningful interpretations across studies unless one has the time needed to manually synthesize different terms/similar concepts (e.g., terminology such as avoidance, problem-focused, ruminative, self-blame, approach, seeking social support, engagement, disengagement, emotion-based, negative, thriving, and despairing).

Table 11.2 Summary of Literature Review Results

Study characteristics	n (%)	Specific details
Design		
Descriptive	128 (88.3%)	
Intervention	12 (8.3%)	Cognitive–behavioral therapy interventions, coping skills programs, education/coping programs for adolescents' chronic conditions, school-based stress management programs
Longitudinal	5 (3.4%)	
Population		
Male and female	113 (77.9%)	
Female only	18 (12.4%)	
Athletes	16 (11%)	Basketball players, college athletes, golfers, Olympic athletes, professional rugby players, soccer players, swimmers, tennis players, varsity athletes
Non-U.S. sample	41 (28.3%)	Australia, Bahrain, Canada, China, Colombia, Croatia, Czech Republic, England, Germany, Iran, Israel, Italy, Kenya, Mexico, Netherlands, Norway, Palestine, Portugal, Scotland, Spain, Sudan, Sweden, Switzerland, Taiwan, Wales, Zimbabwe
Ethnic minority	14 (9.7%)	African American, Asian American, biracial, Hispanic/Latino, Mexican American, multiracial, Native American
Acute or chronic health conditions	20 (13.8%)	Asthma, cancer, cleft, end-stage renal disease, epilepsy, HIV/AIDS, inflammatory bowel disease, mobility impairment, renal transplant patients, severe emotional disturbance, sickle cell disease, type 1 diabetes

Independently, and in small clusters, the studies provide data that are informative and contribute to our understanding of the adolescents represented in the particular investigations.

IMPLICATIONS FOR FUTURE RESEARCH

Although research over the past two decades has solidified the importance of healthy coping strategies in stress response, substantial progress is yet to be made in consistently using coping measures that yield data that can be readily interpretable across studies. This review demonstrated the wealth of coping data that exists, addressing a variety of contextualized stressors for adolescents in many parts of the world. It is encouraging that there is clearly a global appreciation for the importance of coping in adolescents' health and well-being.

Advances in the science regarding adolescent coping may be strengthened by more consistent use of coping measures that have been developed specifically for adolescents and demonstrate reliable and valid measurement properties. Researchers might benefit from modifying and adapting those tools that already exist. For example, if a particular sub-scale does not demonstrate adequate reliability with a specific group of adolescents, the researcher might explore adapting the instrument (e.g., cultural expectations may preclude certain coping behaviors that are measured in a tool created using a different cultural group/adolescent population). Researchers using standardized adolescent coping measures might consider additional mechanisms of assessing coping strategies used by the adolescents. Open-ended and nontraditional data can offer insights about how adolescents in a specific location, context, and time frame are coping with common stressors and may clarify the extent to which their preferred coping strategies are represented in the quantitative coping measures.

Recommendations for Advancing Measurement of Adolescent Coping

1. **Validation of coping measures for diverse adolescent populations.** Growing awareness of the health and social disparities experienced by ethnic minority youth necessitates examination of and intervention toward protective factors, including healthy coping. Efforts are needed to ensure that the ways in which coping is measured are meaningful and valid for adolescents at various developmental stages as well as for those from a broad range of cultural backgrounds. Advancement in culturally and linguistically relevant coping measures will encourage researchers not only to describe coping among these youth but also to measure and report coping outcomes.

2. **Longitudinal studies examining coping trajectories over time.** Existing studies, the majority of which are cross-sectional or include information from two points in time, do not adequately capture the variability in coping behaviors with time, experience, and social context. Longitudinal studies which examine patterns of change and continuity in coping processes over time will help advance our understanding and measurement of adolescent coping, as trends can be observed within and across participants over several points in time. Importantly, longitudinal adolescent coping inquiries will also contribute to understanding how coping behaviors or preferences are impacted or altered over time.

3. **Intervention studies examining coping as a primary outcome.** Some researchers may be hesitant to measure coping because of measurement incongruity aforementioned in this review. In addition, even when the teaching of coping skills is the primary purpose of an intervention, researchers may attend to other measures of emotional health and fail to measure coping as an outcome itself (e.g., Conrod, Castellanos-Ryan, & Strang, 2010; Judge Santacroce, Asmus, Kadan-Lottick, & Grey, 2010). Because coping is linked to many health outcomes and behaviors, such as depression or substance use, it is a commonly measured mediator or moderator (e.g., Brady, Gorman-Smith, Henry, & Tolan, 2008;

Franko, Thompson, Affenito, Barton, & Striegel-Moore, 2008; Gaylord-Harden, Taylor, Campbell, Kesselring, & Grant, 2009; Rodrigues & Kitzmann, 2007; Sun, Tao, Hao, & Wan, 2010). Although these studies make contributions with respect to adolescent coping, additional studies are needed that demonstrate consistency among theory, intervention model, and outcome measures, so that when appropriate, coping is the primary outcome measure.

Conclusions

Coping is an important construct in understanding how adolescents react to the diverse stressors and adjustments they experience. It is a complex construct yet worthy of examination because it is a critical point of intervention in the health trajectory of adolescents. Advances in coping conceptualization and measurement will ideally inform development of successful interventions that build adolescents' protective coping behaviors.

References

Alumran, J. I. A., & Punamäki, R. (2008). Relationship between gender, age, academic achievement, emotional intelligence, and coping styles among Bahraini adolescents. *Individual Differences Research, 6*(2), 104–119.

Aymer, S. R. (2008). Adolescent males' coping responses to domestic violence: A qualitative study. *Children and Youth Services Review, 30*(6), 654–664.

Aysan, F., Thompson, D., & Hamarat, E. (2001). Test anxiety, coping strategies, and perceived health in a group of high school students: A Turkish sample. *Journal of Genetic Psychology, 162*(4), 402–411.

Baigrie, S. S., & Giráldez, S. L. (2008). Examining the relationship between binge eating and coping strategies and the definition of binge eating in a sample of Spanish adolescents. *The Spanish Journal of Psychology, 11*(1), 172–180.

Bal, S., Crombez, G., Van Oost, P., & Debourdeaudhuij, I. (2003). The role of social support in well-being and coping with self-reported stressful events in adolescents. *Child Abuse & Neglect, 27*(12), 1377–1395.

Ben-Ari, R., & Hirshberg, I. (2009). Attachment styles, conflict perception, and adolescents' strategies of coping with interpersonal conflict. *Negotiation Journal, 25*(1), 59–82.

Berg, C. A., Skinner, M., Ko, K., Butler, J. M., Palmer, D. L., Butner, J., et al. (2009). The fit between stress appraisal and dyadic coping in understanding perceived coping effectiveness for adolescents with type 1 diabetes. *Journal of Family Psychology, 23*(4), 521–530.

Berger, Z. E., & Dalton, L. J. (2009). Coping with a cleft: Psychosocial adjustment of adolescents with a cleft lip and palate and their parents. *Cleft Palate-Craniofacial Journal, 46*(4), 435–443.

Bolgar, M. R., Janelle, C., & Giacobbi, P. J. (2008). Trait anger, appraisal, and coping differences among adolescent tennis players. *Journal of Applied Sport Psychology, 20*(1), 73–87.

Bowker, A., Bukowski, W. M., Hymel, S., & Sippola, L. K. (2000). Coping with daily hassles in the peer group during early adolescence: Variations as a function of peer experience. *Journal of Research on Adolescence, 10*(2), 211–243.

Bradshaw, C. P., Sudhinaraset, M., Mmari, K., & Blum, R. W. (2010). School transitions among military adolescents: A qualitative study of stress and coping. *School Psychology Review, 39*(1), 84–105.

Brady, S. S., Gorman-Smith, D., Henry, D. B., & Tolan, P. H. (2008). Adaptive coping reduces the impact of community violence exposure on violent behavior among African American and Latino male adolescents. *Journal of Abnormal Child Psychology: An Official Publication of the International Society for Research in Child and Adolescent Psychopathology, 36*(1), 105–115.

Braun-Lewensohn, O., Celestin-Westreich, S., Celestin, L., Verleye, G., Verté, D., & Ponjaert-Kristoffersen, I. (2009). Coping styles as moderating the relationships between terrorist attacks and well-being outcomes. *Journal of Adolescence, 32*(3), 585–599.

Braun-Lewensohn, O., Sagy, S., & Roth, G. (2010). Coping strategies among adolescents: Israeli Jews and Arabs facing missile attacks. *Anxiety, Stress, & Coping, 23*(1), 35–51.

Broderick, P. C., & Korteland, C. (2002). Coping style and depression in early adolescence: Relationships to gender, gender role, and implicit beliefs. *Sex Roles, 46*(7–8), 201–213.

Bronfenbrenner, U. (1979). *The ecology of human development: Experiments by nature and design.* Cambridge, MA: Harvard University Press.

Brown, S. L., & Ireland, C. A. (2006). Coping style and distress in newly incarcerated male adolescents. *Journal of Adolescent Health, 38*(6), 656–661.

Browne, D. (2002). Coping alone: Examining the prospects of adolescent victims of child abuse placed in foster care. *Journal of Youth and Adolescence, 31*(1), 57–66.

Callaghan, E. E. (2007). Achieving balance: A case study examination of an adolescent coping with life-limiting cancer. *Journal of Pediatric Oncology Nursing, 24*(6), 334–339.

Carbonell, D. M., Reinherz, H. Z., & Beardslee, W. R. (2005). Adaptation and coping in childhood and adolescence for those at risk for depression in emerging adulthood. *Child & Adolescent Social Work Journal, 22*(5–6), 395–416.

Carlson, G. A., & Grant, K. E. (2008). The roles of stress and coping in explaining gender differences in risk for psychopathology among African American urban adolescents. *The Journal of Early Adolescence, 28*(3), 375–404.

Carver, C. S. (1997). You want to measure coping but your protocol's too long: Consider the brief COPE. *International Journal of Behavioral Medicine, 4*(1), 92.

Carver, C. S., Scheier, M. F., & Weintraub, J. K. (1989). Assessing coping strategies: A theoretically based approach. *Journal of Personality & Social Psychology, 56*(2), 267–283.

Cengel-Kültür, S. E., Ulay, H. T., & Erdağ, G. (2009). Ways of coping with epilepsy and related factors in adolescence. *Turkish Journal of Pediatrics, 51*(3), 238–247.

Chagnon, F. (2007). Coping mechanisms, stressful events and suicidal behavior among youth admitted to juvenile justice and child welfare services. *Suicide and Life-Threatening Behavior, 37*(4), 439–452.

Chapman, P. L., & Mullis, R. L. (2000). Racial differences in adolescent coping and self-esteem. *The Journal of Genetic Psychology: Research and Theory on Human Development, 161*(2), 152–160.

Clark, R., Novak, J. D., & Dupree, D. (2002). Relationship of perceived parenting practices to anger regulation and coping strategies in African-American adolescents. *Journal of Adolescence, 25*(4), 373–384.

Compas, B. E., Connor-Smith, J. K., Saltzman, H., Thomsen, A. H., & Wadsworth, M. E. (2001). Coping with stress during childhood and adolescence: Problems, progress, and potential in theory and research. *Psychological Bulletin, 127*(1), 87–127.

Conrod, P. J., Castellanos-Ryan, N., & Strang, J. (2010). Brief, personality-targeted coping skills interventions and survival as a non-drug user over a 2-year period during adolescence. *Archives of General Psychiatry, 67*(1), 85–93.

Constantine, M. G., Donnelly, P. C., & Myers, L. J. (2002). Collective self-esteem and agricultural coping styles in African American adolescents. *Journal of Black Studies, 32*(6), 698–710.

Cotton, S., Grossoehme, D., Rosenthal, S. L., McGrady, M. E., Roberts, Y. H., Hines, J., et al.

(2009). Religious/Spiritual coping in adolescents with sickle cell disease: A pilot study. *Journal of Pediatric Hematology/Oncology, 31*(5), 313–318.

Cunningham, E. G., Werner, S. C., & Firth, N. V. (2004). Control beliefs as mediators of school connectedness and coping outcomes in middle adolescence. *Australian Journal of Guidance & Counselling, 14*(2), 139–150.

D'Anastasi, T., & Frydenberg, E. (2005). Ethnicity and coping: What young people do and what young people learn. *Australian Journal of Guidance & Counselling, 15*(1), 43–59.

De Boo, G., & Spiering, M. (2010). Pre-adolescent gender differences in associations between temperament, coping, and mood. *Clinical Psychology & Psychotherapy, 17*(4), 313–320.

de Anda, D., Baroni, S., Boskin, L., Buchwald, L., Morgan, J., Ow, J., et al. (2000). Stress, stressors, and coping among high school students. *Children and Youth Services Review, 22*(6), 441–463.

Decker, C. L. (2006). Coping in adolescents with cancer. *Journal of Psychosocial Oncology, 24*(4), 123–140.

Dellve, L., Cernerud, L., & Hallberg, L. R. (2000). Harmonizing dilemmas: Siblings of children with DAMP and Asperger syndrome's experiences of coping with their life situations. *Scandinavian Journal of Caring Sciences, 14*(3), 172–178.

Dundas, I. (2000). Cognitive/affective distancing as a coping strategy of children of parents with a drinking problem. *Alcoholism Treatment Quarterly, 18*(4), 85–98.

Eacott, C., & Frydenberg, E. (2009). Promoting positive coping skills for rural youth: Benefits for at-risk young people. *Australian Journal of Rural Health, 17*(6), 338–345.

Ebata, A. T., & Moos, R. H. (1991). Coping and adjustment in distressed and healthy adolescents. *Journal of Applied Developmental Psychology, 12*(1), 33–54.

Elgar, F. J., Arlett, C., & Groves, R. (2003). Stress, coping, and behavioural problems among rural and urban adolescents. *Journal of Adolescence, 26*(5), 574–585.

Erikson, E. H. (1968). *Identity: Youth and crisis.* New York, NY: Norton.

Eschenbeck, H., Kohlmann, C., & Lohaus, A. (2007). Gender differences in coping strategies in children and adolescents. *Journal of Individual Differences, 28*(1), 18–26.

Firth, N., Greaves, D., & Frydenberg, E. (2010). Coping styles and strategies: A comparison of adolescent students with and without learning disabilities. *Journal of Learning Disabilities, 43*(1), 77–85.

Fowler, J. W. (1991). Stages in faith consciousness. In F. K. Oser, & W. G. Scarlett (Eds.), *New directions for child development: Religious development in childhood and adolescence* (pp. 27–45). New York, NY: Jossey-Bass.

Franko, D. L., Thompson, D., Affenito, S. G., Barton, B. A., & Striegel-Moore, R. (2008). What mediates the relationship between family meals and adolescent health issues? *Health Psychology, 27*(2), S109–17.

Frydenberg, E. (2008). *Adolescent coping: Advances in theory, research, and practice.* London, England: Routledge.

Frydenberg, E., & Lewis, R. (1990). How adolescents cope with different concerns: The development of the adolescent coping checklist (ACC). *Psychological Test Bulletin, 3*(2), 63–73.

Frydenberg, E., & Lewis, R. (2000). Teaching coping to adolescents: When and to whom? *American Educational Research Journal, 37*(3), 727–745.

Frydenberg, E., & Lewis, R. (2004). Adolescents least able to cope: How do they respond to their stresses? *British Journal of Guidance & Counselling, 32*(1), 25–37.

Frydenberg, E., & Lewis, R. (2009a). Relations among well-being, avoidant coping, and active coping in a large sample of Australian adolescents. *Psychological Reports, 104*(3), 745–758.

Frydenburg, E., & Lewis, R. (2009b). The relationship between problem-solving efficacy and coping amongst Australian adolescents. *British Journal of Guidance & Counselling, 37*(1), 51–64.

Frydenberg, E., Lewis, R., Kennedy, G., Ardila, R., Frindte, W., & Hannoun, R. (2003). Coping with concerns: An exploratory comparison of Australian, Colombian, German, and Palestinian adolescents. *Journal of Youth and Adolescence, 32*(1), 59–66.

Führ, M. (2002). Coping humor in early adolescence. *Humor: International Journal of Humor Research, 15*(3), 283.

Garrard, J. (2007). *Health sciences literature review made easy: The matrix method.* Sudbury, MA: Jones & Bartlett Publishers.

Gaylord-Harden, N. K., Taylor, J. J., Campbell, C. L., Kesselring, C. M., & Grant, K. E. (2009). Maternal attachment and depressive symptoms in urban adolescents: The influence of coping strategies and gender. *Journal of Clinical Child & Adolescent Psychology, 38*(5), 684–695.

Gelhaar, T., Seiffge-Krenke, I., Borge, A., Cicognani, E., Cunha, M., Loncaric, D., et al. (2007). Adolescent coping with everyday stressors: A seven-nation study of youth from central, eastern, southern, and northern Europe. *European Journal of Developmental Psychology, 4*(2), 129–156.

Gilligan, C. (1993). *In a different voice.* Cambridge, MA: Harvard University Press.

Goldblatt, H. (2003). Strategies of coping among adolescents experiencing interparental violence. *Journal of Interpersonal Violence, 18*(5), 532–552.

Goodman, J. H. (2004). Coping with trauma and hardship among unaccompanied refugee youths from Sudan. *Qualitative Health Research, 14*(9), 1177–1196.

Grootenhuis, M. A., Maurice-Stam, H., Derkx, B. H., & Last, B. F. (2009). Evaluation of a psychoeducational intervention for adolescents with inflammatory bowel disease. *European Journal of Gastroenterology & Hepatology, 21*(4), 430–435.

Hains, A. A., Davies, W. H., Parton, E., Totka, J., & Amoroso-Camarata, J. (2000). A stress management intervention for adolescents with type 1 diabetes. *Diabetes Educator, 26*(3), 417–424.

Hampel, P., Manhal, S., & Hayer, T. (2009). Direct and relational bullying among children and adolescents: Coping and psychological adjustment. *School Psychology International, 30*(5), 474–490.

Hampel, P., & Petermann, F. (2005). Age and gender effects on coping in children and adolescents. *Journal of Youth and Adolescence, 34*(2), 73–83.

Hampel, P., & Petermann, F. (2006). Perceived stress, coping, and adjustment in adolescents. *Journal of Adolescent Health, 38*(4), 409–415.

Haraldsson, K., Lindgren, E., Hildingh, C., & Marklund, B. (2010). What makes the everyday life of Swedish adolescent girls less stressful: A qualitative analysis. *Health Promotion International, 25*(2), 192–199.

Harris, M. B., & Franklin, C. G. (2003). Effects of a cognitive-behavioral, school-based, group intervention with Mexican American pregnant and parenting adolescents. *Social Work Research, 27*(2), 71–83.

Hema, D. A., Roper, S. O., Nehring, J. W., Call, A., Mandleco, B. L., & Dyches, T. T. (2009). Daily stressors and coping responses of children and adolescents with type 1 diabetes. *Child: Care, Health & Development, 35*(3), 330–339.

Hess, L. M., & Bundy, A. C. (2003). The association between playfulness and coping in adolescents. *Physical & Occupational Therapy in Pediatrics, 23*(2), 5–17.

Hoar, S. D., Crocker, P., Holt, N. L., & Tamminen, K. A. (2010). Gender differences in adolescent athletes' coping with interpersonal stressors in sport: More similarities than differences? *Journal of Applied Sport Psychology, 22*(2), 134–149.

Howard, M. S., & Medway, F. J. (2004). Adolescents' attachment and coping with stress. *Psychology in the Schools, 41*(3), 391–402.

Israelashvili, M., Gilad-Osovitzki, S., & Asherov, J. (2006). Female adolescents' suicidal behavior and mothers' ways of coping. *Journal of Mental Health, 15*(5), 533–542.

Jemtå, L., Fugl-Meyer, K. S., Öberg, K., & Dahl, M. (2009). Self-esteem in children and adolescents with mobility impairment: Impact on well-being and coping strategies. *Acta Paediatrica, 98*(3), 567–572.

Jones, J. K., Kamani, S. A., Bush, P. J., Hennessy, K. A., Marfatia, A., & Shad, A. T. (2010). Development and evaluation of an educational interactive CD-ROM for teens with cancer. *Pediatric Blood & Cancer, 55*(3), 512–519.

Judge Santacroce, S., Asmus, K., Kadan-Lottick, N., & Grey, M. (2010). Feasibility and preliminary outcomes from a pilot study of coping skills training for adolescent—young adult survivors of childhood cancer and their parents. *Journal of Pediatric Oncology Nursing, 27*(1), 10–20.

Kausar, R., & Munir, R. (2004). Pakistani adolescents' coping with stress: Effect of loss of a parent and gender of adolescents. *Journal of Adolescence, 27*(6), 599–610.

Kaye, D. K. (2008). Negotiating the transition from adolescence to motherhood: Coping with prenatal and parenting stress in teenage mothers in Mulago hospital, Uganda. *BMC Public Health, 8,* 83–83.

Kendall, P. C., Safford, S., Flannery-Schroeder, E., & Webb, A. (2004). Child anxiety treatment: Outcomes in adolescence and impact on substance use and depression at 7.4-year follow-up. *Journal of Consulting and Clinical Psychology, 72*(2), 276–287.

Kennedy, V. L., & Lloyd-Williams, M. (2009). How children cope when a parent has advanced cancer. *Psycho-Oncology, 18*(8), 886–892.

Kobus, K., & Reyes, O. (2000). A descriptive study of urban Mexican American adolescents' perceived stress and coping. *Hispanic Journal of Behavioral Sciences, 22*(2), 163–178.

Kohlberg, L. (1978). Revisions in the theory and practice of moral development. *New Directions for Child and Adolescent Development, 1978*(2), 83–87.

Kowalski, K. C., Crocker, P. R. E., Hoar, S. D., & Niefer, C. B. (2005). Adolescents' control beliefs and coping with stress in sport. *International Journal of Sport Psychology, 36*(4), 257–272.

Kowalski, K. C., Mack, D. E., Crocker, P. R. E., Niefer, C. B., & Fleming, T. (2006). Coping with social physique anxiety in adolescence. *Journal of Adolescent Health, 39*(2), e9–e16.

Kristiansen, E., & Roberts, G. C. (2010). Young elite athletes and social support: Coping with competitive and organizational stress in "Olympic" competition. *Scandinavian Journal of Medicine & Science in Sports, 20*(4), 686–695.

Lafferty, M. E., & Dorrell, K. (2006). Coping strategies and the influence of perceived parental support in junior national age swimmers. *Journal of Sports Sciences, 24*(3), 253–259.

Lapouse, R., & Monk, M. A. (1964). Behavior deviations in a representative sample of children: Variation by sex, age, race, social class, and family size. *American Journal of Orthopsychiatry, 34,* 436–446.

Lazarus, R. S. (1990). Theory-based stress measurement. *Psychological Inquiry, 1*(1), 3–13.

Lazarus, R. S., & Folkman, S. (1984). *Stress, appraisal, and coping.* New York, NY: Springer.

Lepistö, S., Åstedt-Kurki, P., Joronen, K., Luukkaala, T., & Paavilainen, E. (2010). Adolescents' experiences of coping with domestic violence. *Journal of Advanced Nursing, 66*(6), 1232–1245.

Lewis, C. L., & Brown, S. C. (2002). Coping strategies of female adolescents with HIV/AIDS. *ABNF Journal, 13*(4), 72–77.

Lewis, R., & Frydenberg, E. (2002). Concomitants of failure to cope: What we should teach adolescents about coping. *British Journal of Educational Psychology, 72*(Pt 3), 419–431.

Li, C. E., DiGiuseppe, R., & Froh, J. (2006). The roles of sex, gender, and coping in adolescent depression. *Adolescence, 41*(163), 409–415.

Magaya, L., Asner-Self, K. K., & Schreiber, J. B. (2005). Stress and coping strategies among Zimbabwean adolescents. *British Journal of Educational Psychology, 75*(4), 661–671.

Marcia, J. E. (1980). Identity in adolescence. In J. Adelson (Ed.), *Handbook of adolescent psychology* (pp. 159–187). New York, NY: John Wiley.

Martyn-Nemeth, P., Penckofer, S., Gulanick, M., Velsor-Friedrich, B., & Bryant, F. B. (2009). The relationships among self-esteem, stress, coping, eating behavior, and depressive mood in adolescents. *Research in Nursing & Health, 32*(1), 96–109.

Massey, E. K., Garnefski, N., Gebhardt, W. A., & van der Leeden, R. (2009). Daily frustration, cognitive coping and coping efficacy in adolescent headache: A daily diary study. *Headache, 49*(8), 1198–1205.

Meesters, C., & Muris, P. (2004). Perceived parental rearing behaviours and coping in young adolescents. *Personality and Individual Differences, 37*(3), 513–522.

Miranda, D., & Claes, M. (2009). Music listening, coping, peer affiliation and depression in adolescence. *Psychology of Music, 37*(2), 215–233.

Moos, R. H. (2002). Life stressors, social resources, and coping skills in youth: Applications to adolescents with chronic disorders. *Journal of Adolescent Health, 30*(4 Suppl), 22–29.

Mullis, R. L., & Chapman, P. (2000). Age, gender, and self-esteem differences in adolescent coping styles. *The Journal of Social Psychology, 140*(4), 539–541.

Murberg, T. A. (2009). Associations between personality and coping styles among Norwegian adolescents: A prospective study. *Journal of Individual Differences, 30*(2), 59–64.

Myors, K., Johnson, M., & Langdon, R. (2001). Coping styles of pregnant adolescents. *Public Health Nursing, 18*(1), 24–32.

Nicholls, A., Polman, R., Morley, D., & Taylor, N. J. (2009). Coping and coping effectiveness in relation to a competitive sport event: Pubertal status, chronological age, and gender among adolescent athletes. *Journal of Sport & Exercise Psychology, 31*(3), 299–317.

Nicholls, A. R. (2007a). Can an athlete be taught to cope more effectively? The experiences of an international-level adolescent golfer during a training program for coping. *Perceptual & Motor Skills, 104*(2), 494–500.

Nicholls, A. R. (2007b). A longitudinal phenomenological analysis of coping effectiveness among Scottish international adolescent golfers. *European Journal of Sport Science, 7*(3), 169–178.

Nicholls, A. R., Holt, N. L., Polman, R. C. J., & James, D. W. G. (2005). Stress and coping among international adolescent golfers. *Journal of Applied Sport Psychology, 17*(4), 333–340.

Nicholls, A. R., Jones, C. R., Polman, R. C. J., & Borkoles, E. (2009). Acute sport-related stressors, coping, and emotion among professional rugby union players during training and matches. *Scandinavian Journal of Medicine & Science in Sports, 19*(1), 113–120.

Nicholls, A. R., Polman, R., Levy, A. R., Taylor, J., & Cobley, S. (2007). Stressors, coping, and coping effectiveness: Gender, type of sport, and skill differences. *Journal of Sports Sciences, 25*(13), 1521–1530.

Nicholls, A. R., & Polman, R. C. (2007a). Coping in sport: A systematic review. *Journal of Sports Sciences, 25*(1), 11–31.

Nicholls, A. R., & Polman, R. C. J. (2007b). Stressors, coping, and coping effectiveness among players from the England under-18 rugby union team. *Journal of Sport Behavior, 30*(2), 199–218.

Nicholls, A. R., & Polman, R. C. (2008). Think aloud: Acute stress and coping strategies during golf performances. *Anxiety, Stress, & Coping, 21*(3), 283–294.

Orban, L. A., Stein, R., Koenig, L. J., Conner, L. C., Rexhouse, E. L., Lewis, J. V., et al. (2010). Coping strategies of adolescents living with HIV: Disease-specific stressors and responses. *AIDS Care, 22*(4), 420–430.

Parker, J. D., & Endler, N. S. (1992). Coping with coping assessment: A critical review. *European Journal of Personality, 6*(5), 321–344.

Pendragon, D. K. (2010). Coping behaviors among sexual minority female youth. *Journal of Lesbian Studies, 14*(1), 5–15.

Pereda, N., Forns, M., Kirchner, T., & Muñoz, D. (2009). Use of the KIDCOPE to identify socio-economically diverse Spanish school-age children's stressors and coping strategies. *Child: Care, Health & Development, 35*(6), 841–850.

Piaget, J., & Inhelder, B. (1969). *The psychology of the child.* New York, NY: Basic Books.

Piquet, M. L., & Wagner, B. M. (2003). Coping responses of adolescent suicide attempters and their relation to suicidal ideation across a 2-year follow-up: A preliminary study. *Suicide and Life-Threatening Behavior, 33*(3), 288–301.

Puente-Diaz, R., & Anshel, M. H. (2005). Sources of acute stress, cognitive appraisal, and coping strategies among highly skilled Mexican and U.S. competitive tennis players. *Journal of Social Psychology, 145*(4), 429–446.

Puotiniemi, T. A., & Kyngäs, H. A. (2004). The coping of an adolescent who has been in psychiatric inpatient care and her mother in everyday life. *Journal of Psychiatric and Mental Health Nursing, 11*(6), 675–682.

Puskar, K., Grabiak, B. R., Bernardo, L. M., & Ren, D. (2009). Adolescent coping across time: Implications for psychiatric mental health nurses. *Issues in Mental Health Nursing, 30*(9), 581–586.

Puskar, K., Sereika, S., & Tusaie-Mumford, K. (2003). Effect of the teaching kids to cope (TKC) program on outcomes of depression and coping among rural adolescents. *Journal of Child & Adolescent Psychiatric Nursing, 16*(2), 71–80.

Puskar, K. R., & Grabiak, B. R. (2008). Rural adolescents' coping responses: Implications for behavioral health nurses. *Issues in Mental Health Nursing, 29*(5), 523–535.

Rask, K., Kaunonen, M., & Paunonen-Ilmonen, M. (2002). Adolescent coping with grief after the death of a loved one. *International Journal of Nursing Practice, 8*(3), 137–142.

Rasmussen, A., Aber, M. S., & Bhana, A. (2004). Adolescent coping and neighborhood violence: Perceptions, exposure, and urban youths' efforts to deal with danger. *American Journal of Community Psychology, 33*(1–2), 61–75.

Ratcliff, M. B., Blount, R. L., & Mee, L. L. (2010). The relationship between adolescent renal transplant recipients' perceived adversity, coping, and medical adherence. *Journal of Clinical Psychology in Medical Settings, 17*(2), 116–124.

Reeves, C. W., Nicholls, A. R., & McKenna, J. (2009). Stressors and coping strategies among early and middle adolescent premier league academy soccer players: Differences according to age. *Journal of Applied Sport Psychology, 21*(1), 31–48.

Remillard, A. M., & Lamb, S. (2005). Adolescent girls' coping with relational aggression. *Sex Roles, 53*(3–4), 221–229.

Renk, K., & Creasey, G. (2003). The relationship of gender, gender identity and coping strategies in late adolescents. *Journal of Adolescence, 26*(2), 159–168.

Rew, L. (2005). *Adolescent health: A multidisciplinary approach to theory, research, and intervention.* Thousand Oaks, CA: Sage.

Rodrigues, L. N., & Kitzmann, K. M. (2007). Coping as a mediator between interparental conflict and adolescents' romantic attachment. *Journal of Social and Personal Relationships, 24*(3), 423–439.

Roesch, S. C., Duangado, K. M., Vaughn, A. A., Aldridge, A. A., & Villodas, F. (2010). Dispositional hope and the propensity to cope: A daily diary assessment of minority adolescents. *Cultural Diversity and Ethnic Minority Psychology, 16*(2), 191–198.

Ruffolo, M. C., Sarri, R., & Goodkind, S. (2004). Study of delinquent, diverted, and high-risk adolescent girls: Implications for mental health intervention. *Social Work Research, 28*(4), 237–245.

Sabiston, C. M., Sedgwick, W. A., Crocker, P. R. E., Kowalski, K. C., & Mack, D. E. (2007). Social physique anxiety in adolescence: An exploration of influences, coping strategies, and health behaviors. *Journal of Adolescent Research, 22*(1), 78–101.

Sagar, S. S., Busch, B. K., & Jowett, S. (2010). Success and failure, fear of failure, and coping responses of adolescent academy football players. *Journal of Applied Sport Psychology, 22*(2), 213–230.

Sanjari, M., Heidari, S., Shirazi, F., & Salemi, S. (2008). Comparison of coping strategies in Iranian adolescents with cancer and their parents. *Issues in Comprehensive Pediatric Nursing, 31*(4), 185–197.

Schneider, K. M., & Phares, V. (2005). Coping with parental loss because of termination of parental rights. *Child Welfare, 84*(6), 819–842.

Scott, L. D., Jr. (2003a). Cultural orientation and coping with perceived discrimination among

African American youth. *Journal of Black Psychology, 29*(3), 235–256.

Scott, L. D., Jr. (2003b). The relation of racial identity and racial socialization to coping with discrimination among African American adolescents. *Journal of Black Studies, 33*(4), 520–538.

Scott, L. D., Jr. (2004). Correlates of coping with perceived discriminatory experiences among African American adolescents. *Journal of Adolescence, 27*(2), 123–137.

Scott, L. D., Jr., & House, L. E. (2005). Relationship of distress and perceived control to coping with perceived racial discrimination among black youth. *Journal of Black Psychology, 31*(3), 254–272.

Seaton, G. (2007). Toward a theoretical understanding of hypermasculine coping among urban black adolescent males. *Journal of Human Behavior in the Social Environment, 15*(2–3), 367–390.

Seepersad, S. (2004). Coping with loneliness: Adolescent online and offline behavior. *CyberPsychology & Behavior, 7*(1), 35–39.

Seiffge-Krenke, I., Aunola, K., & Nurmi, J. E. (2009). Changes in stress perception and coping during adolescence: The role of situational and personal factors. *Child Development, 80*(1), 259–279.

Seiffge-Krenke, I., & Beyers, W. (2005). Coping trajectories from adolescence to young adulthood: Links to attachment state of mind. *Journal of Research on Adolescence, 15*(4), 561–582.

Seiffge-Krenke, I., & Stemmler, M. (2003). Coping with everyday stress and links to medical and psychosocial adaptation in diabetic adolescents. *Journal of Adolescent Health, 33*(3), 180–188.

Selye, H. (1978). *The stress of life* (revised edition). New York, NY: McGraw-Hill.

Shelton, K. H., & Harold, G. T. (2008). Pathways between interparental conflict and adolescent psychological adjustment: Bridging links through children's cognitive appraisals and coping strategies. *The Journal of Early Adolescence, 28*(4), 555–582.

Siqueira, L., Diab, M., Bodian, C., & Rolnitzky, L. (2000). Adolescents becoming smokers: The roles of stress and coping methods. *Journal of Adolescent Health, 27*(6), 399–408.

Skinner, E. A., Edge, K., Altman, J., & Sherwood, H. (2003). Searching for the structure of coping: A review and critique of category systems for classifying ways of coping. *Psychological Bulletin, 129*(2), 216–269.

Skovdal, M., Ogutu, V. O., Aoro, C., & Campbell, C. (2009). Young carers as social actors: Coping strategies of children caring for ailing or ageing guardians in western Kenya. *Social Science & Medicine, 69*(4), 587–595.

Snethen, J. A., Broome, M. E., Kelber, S., & Warady, B. A. (2004). Coping strategies utilized by adolescents with end stage renal disease. *Nephrology Nursing Journal, 31*(1), 41–49.

Sorensen, E. S. (1993). *Children's stress and coping: A family perspective.* New York, NY: Guilford.

Steinhausen, H. C., Bearth-Carrari, C., & Winkler Metzke, C. (2009). Psychosocial adaptation of adolescent migrants in a Swiss community survey. *Social Psychiatry & Psychiatric Epidemiology, 44*(4), 308–316.

Stewart, M., Reutter, L., Letourneau, N., & Makwarimba, E. (2009). A support intervention to promote health and coping among homeless youths. *Canadian Journal of Nursing Research, 41*(2), 55–77.

Sun, Y., Tao, F., Hao, J., & Wan, Y. (2010). The mediating effects of stress and coping on depression among adolescents in china. *Journal of Child and Adolescent Psychiatric Nursing, 23*(3), 173–180.

Sung, K. M., Puskar, K. R., & Sereika, S. (2006). Psychosocial factors and coping strategies of adolescents in a rural Pennsylvania high school. *Public Health Nursing, 23*(6), 523–530.

Sveinbjornsdottir, S., & Thorsteinsson, E. B. (2008). Adolescent coping scales: A critical psychometric review. *Scandinavian Journal of Psychology, 49*(6), 533–548.

Tam, V. C., & Lam, R. S. (2005). Stress and coping among migrant and local-born adolescents in Hong Kong. *Youth & Society, 36*(3), 312–332.

Tamminen, K. A., & Holt, N. L. (2010). Female adolescent athletes' coping: A season-long investigation. *Journal of Sports Sciences, 28*(1), 101–114.

Tatar, M., & Amram, S. (2007). Israeli adolescents' coping strategies in relation to terrorist attacks. *British Journal of Guidance & Counselling, 35*(2), 163–173.

Thabet, A. A. M., Tischler, V., & Vostanis, P. (2004). Maltreatment and coping strategies among male adolescents living in the Gaza strip. *Child Abuse & Neglect, 28*(1), 77–91.

Tourigny, M., Hébert, M., Daigneault, I., & Simoneau, A. C. (2005). Efficacy of a group therapy for sexually abused adolescent girls. *Journal of Child Sexual Abuse, 14*(4), 71–93.

Trask, P. C., Paterson, A. G., Trask, C. L., Bares, C. B., Birt, J., & Maan, C. (2003). Parent and adolescent adjustment to pediatric cancer: Associations with coping, social support, and family function. *Journal of Pediatric Oncology Nursing, 20*(1), 36–47.

Turner, S. G., Kaplan, C. P., & Badger, L. W. (2006). Adolescent Latinas' adaptive functioning and sense of well-being. *Affilia, 21*(3), 272–281.

van der Zaag-Loonen, H. J., Grootenhuis, M. A., Last, B. F., & Derkx, H. H. F. (2004). Coping strategies and quality of life of adolescents with inflammatory bowel disease. *Quality of Life Research: An International Journal of Quality of Life Aspects of Treatment, Care & Rehabilitation, 13*(5), 1011–1019.

Vashchenko, M., Lambidoni, E., & Brody, L. R. (2007). Late adolescents' coping styles in interpersonal and intrapersonal conflicts using the narrative disclosure task. *Clinical Social Work Journal, 35*(4), 245–255.

Vliet, H. V., & Andrews, G. (2009). Internet-based course for the management of stress for junior high schools. *Australian & New Zealand Journal of Psychiatry, 43*(4), 305–309.

Wadsworth, M. E., Gudmundsen, G. R., Raviv, T., Ahlkvist, J. A., McIntosh, D. N., Kline, G. H., et al. (2004). Coping with terrorism: Age and gender differences in effortful and involuntary responses to September 11th. *Applied Developmental Science, 8*(3), 143–157.

Washburn-Ormachea, J. M., Hillman, S. B., & Sawilowsky, S. S. (2004). Gender and gender-role orientation differences on adolescents' coping with peer stressors. *Journal of Youth and Adolescence, 33*(1), 31–40.

Wolfradt, U., Hempel, S., & Miles, J. N. V. (2003). Perceived parenting styles, depersonalisation, anxiety and coping behavior in adolescents. *Personality and Individual Differences, 34*(3), 521–532.

Wu, L. M., Chin, C. C., Haase, J. E., & Chen, C. H. (2009). Coping experiences of adolescents with cancer: A qualitative study. *Journal of Advanced Nursing, 65*(11), 2358–2366.

Yahav, R., & Cohen, M. (2008). Evaluation of a cognitive-behavioral intervention for adolescents. *International Journal of Stress Management, 15*(2), 173–188.

Yang, T. O., Lunt, I., & Sylva, K. (2009). Peer stress-related coping activities in young adolescents' asthma management. *Journal of Asthma, 46*(6), 613–617.

Yi, J. P., Smith, R. E., & Vitaliano, P. P. (2005). Stress-resilience, illness, and coping: A person-focused investigation of young women athletes. *Journal of Behavioral Medicine, 28*(3), 257–265.

Young, S., Chadwick, O., Heptinstall, E., Taylor, E., & Sonuga-Barke, E. J. S. (2005). The adolescent outcome of hyperactive girls: Self-reported interpersonal relationships and coping mechanism. *European Child & Adolescent Psychiatry, 14*(5), 245–253.

Zanini, D. S., Forns, M., & Kirchner, T. (2005). Coping responses and problem appraisal in Spanish adolescents. *Perceptual & Motor Skills, 100*(1), 153–166.

Zhang, Y., Kong, F., Wang, L., Chen, H., Gao, X., Tan, X., et al. (2010). Mental health and coping styles of children and adolescent survivors one year after the 2008 Chinese earthquake. *Children and Youth Services Review, 32*(10), 1403–1409.

Zimmer-Gembeck, M. J., & Locke, E. M. (2007). The socialization of adolescent coping behaviours: Relationships with families and teachers. *Journal of Adolescence, 30*(1), 1–16.

12

Stress and the Workplace

Theories and Models of Organizational Stress

Judith A. Cohen, Jill Mattuck Tarule, Betty A. Rambur, and Carol Vallett

During the last 50 years, society—and in particular the work environment—has been characterized by unprecedented change (Cooper, 1998). The 1960s were forever transformed by growing technology followed by work conflicts in the 1970s between employers and workers. The 1980s reflected a decade of mergers and acquisitions, reengineering work processes, privatization, and competitive, entrepreneurial free-market environments. The 1990s were dominated by recession and its subsequent downsizing efforts and flattening of organizational structures. Fewer employees were doing more work with fewer resources and often less job security. The exponential growth of technology further complicated the work environment and meant that workers had to cope with information overload and increased expectations of productivity (Cooper, Dewe, & O'Driscoll, 2001). The first decade of the new century has been characterized by continued growth in computer science and technology, virtual organizations, a dispersed workforce working from home, increased job insecurity, and economic globalization. Recession again has lead to a repeat of the downsizing efforts of the 1990s while still trying to compete in a global market. In addition to fewer employees working in a conventional work environment, new arrangements mean fewer core full-time employees and more outsourcing of work to contingent employees whose relationship with the organization depends upon particular tasks and expertise. Work today has been criticized for being driven predominantly by "the technological imperative rather than by holistic perspectives that also take into account personal, social, and cultural issues within societies" (Cooper et al., 2001, p. 235). As the pace of this organizational change has accelerated, stress within the work environment has become an increasing focus for governments, organizations, and employees. Organizational stress and its concomitant problems of "burnout," absenteeism, high turnover, decreased productivity, employee conflicts, and increased workers' compensation claims have been estimated to cost over $200 billion dollars a year (DeFrank & Ivancevich, 1998; Simmons & Nelson, 2001). Other estimates identify 20% of a typical company payroll goes to dealing with organizational stress factors such as heavy workloads, uncertain job expectations, and working long hours (Avey, Luthens, & Jensen, 2009).

This chapter focuses on stress in the workplace, generally, and in health care organizations, specifically. It begins with a review of the concept of stress and introduces the prevalent theories and models of organizational stress, highlighting both the positive (eustress) and negative (distress) responses to stress. The presentation of the theories and models reflects both a historical and cumulative understanding of stress, with a new theory/model building upon the earlier ones. The final model presented, the Moral Cascade Model, is newly developed by the authors (Rambur, Vallett, Cohen, & Tarule, 2010) of this chapter and focuses specifically on stress that is moral or ethical. Implications for ongoing stress research are explored. The chapter concludes with brief discussions about the implication of organizational stress in three domains: (a) interventions to reduce organizational stress, (b) understanding stress in health care organizations, specifically, and (c) the role of leadership in addressing stress.

THE CONCEPT OF STRESS

The research and knowledge development around the concept of stress reflects the diversity in how it has been defined and operationalized by the various disciplines such as medicine, psychology, sociology, and management (LeFevre, Matheny, & Kolt, 2003) and nursing (Rice, 2000). Stress has been defined as a dependent variable or response-based stimulus focused on the consequences of stress (Selye, 1976, 1987). Selye's work introduced the construct of stress-related illness and defined the general adaptation syndrome (GAS) for stress. The GAS has three stages: (a) an alarm stage of lowered resistance followed by defense mechanisms being activated *(fight or flight)*, (b) the resistance stage in which adaptation replaces alarm, and (c) exhaustion or death, which occurs when resistance or adaptation can no longer be maintained over extended periods of time (Selye, 1956; Szabo, 1998). Selye mainly focused on the physiological response to stress and did not necessarily consider environmental factors in the stress process. He did, however, emphasize that stress reactions were not inherently good or bad and, in fact, a certain level of stress is essential for growth and development. He defined the type of stress that is vital to life as "positive" stress or *eustress*. Stress from unmanageable situations, which were detrimental and damaging, was identified as *distress* (Selye, 1976). Selye (1987) later suggested that positive emotions such as hope, gratitude, and goodwill maximized eustress and minimized distress when encountering stressors.

The knowledge development of the stress concept shifted to a focus that explored the external conditions that led to it. With this evolution, stress was defined as an independent variable or as a stimulus-based model whereby potential sources of stress were identified. Industrialization provided the impetus for this approach, and many of the stimuli variables studied were environmental ones such heat, cold, noise, and social density. Other variables included work scheduling factors, workload, effects of technological changes, exposure to risks and hazards, work hours, organizational roles and their related demands, role ambiguity, conflict, overload, work relationships, personalities and leadership style, job insecurity, and opportunity for career advancement. Organizational factors included the organizational culture and management style that was prevalent, decision-making processes, and communication styles, as well as organizational politics (Cooper et al., 2001). This stimulus-based definition of stress did not recognize that individuals exposed to the same stimulus could or would react in different ways or that there were individual differences such as perception and cognition that underpinned the different responses (Sutherland & Cooper, 1990).

The stimulus-response definitions of stress focused on a single aspect of the relationship between stress and the workplace, such as the individual's stress response or the environmental stimuli. The interactional definition of stress recognized that both the stimulus and response needed to be explored. In this evolution of knowledge development about stress, moderating variables were introduced that achieved greater complexity in understanding the stress process and in identifying the causal pathways specific to the relationship between the stimuli and response. These moderating variables include personality/dispositional variables, and situational and social characteristics. For example, personality may play an important role by influencing one's response to exposure to stressful events (i.e., risk-taking), by affecting one's reactions to the events, or both and can influence which coping mechanisms people choose to manage their stress (Bolger & Zuckerman, 1995; Cooper et al., 2001). Examples of personality-moderating variables include the Type A personality behavior pattern (Rosenman et al., 1964), hardiness (Kobasa, 1979), and self-efficacy (Bandura, 1997).

Situational moderators include factors such as perceived control over the environment and social support. The job demands–control model (Karasek, 1979) highlights the importance of perceived control over the work environment in perceptions of stress, even with high job demands. Highly challenging work coupled with high control is considered an active job while low job demands and low levels of control, such as with repetitive tasks, are passive jobs. Thus, stress around highly challenging work is mitigated by the power to make decisions and have control over one's work as well as the skills to meet the demands. Social support can come from different sources (e.g., family, coworkers, supervisors, friends) as well as the quantity and type of support provided, such as work-related and nonwork-related support. A type of nonwork-related social support might be the backing that comes from discussing what is happening in the workers' personal lives. There can be both positive and negative work-related support. Positive support can focus on why the organization is a good place to work, while the negative support can focus on group discussions of the organization's parts which are difficult for the employee (Cooper et al., 2001).

Finally, a fourth definition of stress reflects stress as a transactional model that moves beyond investigating moderating variables and the statistical interaction among them. This model of stress *"endeavors to explore the essential nature of stressor-response-outcome relationships and to encapsulate an understanding of the dynamic stress process itself"* (Cooper et al., 2001, p. 11). Stress as a transaction recognizes that stress does not reside solely within the individual or within the environment, but in the relationship between the two and must be understood within the context of that process (Lazarus, 1991). The defining characteristic of stress as a transaction is its emphasis on the process—one which involves individuals interacting with their environments, making cognitive appraisals of these encounters, and using coping strategies to deal with the issues that arise. In essence, it involves a process of giving meaning, adjustment, and coping (Cooper et al., 2001).

THEORIES AND MODELS OF ORGANIZATIONAL STRESS

It is important to explicate central tenets that underlie the theories and models of organizational stress. These include:

- Demands or stressors are inherently neutral.

- Stressors are identified by the source and timing of the stressor and the perceived control over and desirability of the stressor.

- Individual differences can moderate how the stressor is perceived.

- Stress is the response to stressors (i.e., demands) in the environment and can be either eustress, distress, or a combination of both, depending upon individuals' interpretation and appraisal.

- Eustress and distress can differentially affect outcomes that are valued in the workplace.

- The relationship and interaction between responses and outcomes is moderated by both the stated and unstated organizational values of the organization (LeFevre et al., 2003; Rambur et al., 2010; Simmons & Nelson, 2007).

These central tenets are explored in the following discussion of the theories and models of organizational stress.

Person–Environment Fit Theory (P-E Fit)

The person–environment (P-E) fit model, developed in the early 1970s, states that strain develops when there is a discrepancy between the motives of the person and the supplies of the environment, or between the demands of the job and the abilities of the person to meet those demands. Motives include factors such as participation, income, and self-utilization. Demands include work load and job complexity (Caplan, Cobb, French, Harrison, & Pinneau, 1975; Harrison, 1978). (See Figure 12.1.)

A lack of fit can result from an imbalance between the characteristics of the person, such as their abilities, skill, energy, and values, and the environmental demands, such as job expectations, role, and organizational norms. As demands exceed the supply of individual abilities, stress likely occurs. Conversely, if demand decreases so that it does not match with the person's abilities and skills, stress may also increase or decrease, depending upon whether the level is such that it causes boredom or inhibits achievement needs (Edwards, 1991; Edwards, Caplan, & Harrison, 1998). There may also be a lack of fit between the

Figure 12.1 A Model of Stress as Person-Environment Fit

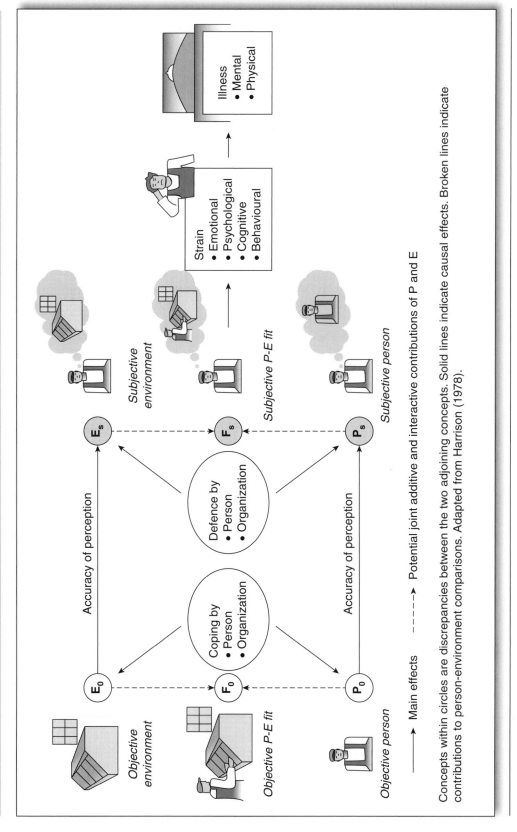

Concepts within circles are discrepancies between the two adjoining concepts. Solid lines indicate causal effects. Broken lines indicate contributions to person-environment comparisons. Adapted from Harrison (1978).

⟶ Main effects   ⟶ Potential joint additive and interactive contributions of P and E

SOURCE: Adapted from Harrison (1978).

313

individuals' perceptions of themselves and their environment and an objective representation of how the person and environment actually are in reality (Edwards et al., 1998; LeFevre et al., 2003). Theoretically, the P-E fit and resulting stress depend upon an individual's accurate self-assessment and good contact with reality which is subject to individual abilities and differences. The subjective assessment of fit (individuals' perceptions of themselves and their environment) was seen as a powerful determinant of stressors and perceptions of stress (LeFevre et al., 2003; Harrison, 1985).

The stress that results from a P-E misfit can be physiological, psychological, and/or behavioral. Physiological manifestations could include hypertension, increased cholesterolemia, and decreased immunity. Psychological signs and symptoms could include anxiety, restlessness, panic, and insomnia. Behavioral factors of absenteeism, use of health care services, or increased workers' compensation claims could be evident. Conversely, a good P-E fit can confer healthy outcomes physically, psychologically, and behaviorally (Edwards et al., 1998; Harrison, 1985). Another set of outcomes for this theory involves the individual's reactions to the misfit that includes coping or defense reactions. Coping could involve changing either the person or the environment through professional or skills development or negotiating a change in the environment. Defensive reactions involve reframing or cognitive restructuring of the stressors and changing one's own subjective perception/interpretation (Edwards et al., 1998; LeFevre et al., 2003).

Generally, the P-E fit theory distinguishes little between eustress and distress, and any misfit is characterized as distress. It does not test if an excess of individual ability or supply provided by the work environment leads to eustress. Additionally, the supply–demand model only focuses on the amount of stress or degree of misfit caused and does not provide any further understanding of the stressors themselves. Although the applications of this model imply the role and primacy of individual interpretation, there are limited links in the model between the concept of individual's abilities and needs to the concept of work supply and demands. In addition, the theory does not explicitly take into account the individual's personal appraisal or interpretation of the experience of stress (LeFevre et al., 2003).

In the last decade (2000–2010) 10 nursing research studies cited in the Cumulative Index to Nursing and Allied Health Literature (CINAHL) indicated use of the P-E fit model. These included the fit of job satisfaction and turnover intention and burnout (Takase, Maude, & Manias, 2005), nursing staff empowerment and work engagement/burnout (Greco, Lashinger & Wong, 2006), organizational commitment and generational differences in nursing faculty (Carver, 2008), career choices and available options (Price, 2009), and dietary choices and challenges (Evans, Crogan, & Shultz, 2004). An international study examined role discrepancies, depression, and turnover in the country of Jordan (Abualrub, 2007).

Cybernetic Model of Organizational Stress

Cummings and Cooper (1979) used the cybernetic approach as a framework to study organizational stress. This model focuses on the stress cycle as a process that involves the continuous interactions between person and environment. Its basic premise is that individuals seek to maintain equilibrium and will direct their behavior to reestablish equilibrium if some external force (stressor) disrupts it, consistent with the concepts of homeostasis and adaptation (Selye, 1956). The behavior involves the detection of stress because of a disparity or mismatch between the individual's actual and preferred state, the selection of an adjustment process, the implementation of coping behaviors, and an evaluation of those coping behaviors on the stressful encounter. The advantage of this model is its transactional framework, which emphasizes the temporal dimensions of stressful encounters and the need to consider the impact of time on person–environment interactions (Cooper et al., 2001). It extends the P-E fit model by incorporating the concept of perceived threat as a source of stress (Edwards, 1998). Not only is there an imbalance between the demands of the situation and the resources of the individual, but the mismatch must by perceived by the individual as a significant threat which requires some actions over and above the normal steady state. This focus on the appraisal process that Lazarus (1991) stressed in determining the significance of the threat (primary appraisal), and its potential impact along with actions necessary to cope with it (secondary appraisal), creates the transactional dimension of this model and could allow for the inclusion of the eustress because it accounts for the differences in individual reactions to situations that are objectively similar.

Similar to the P-E fit model, the cybernetic model addresses stress but does not distinguish between distress or eustress. While it infers the existence of the concept of eustress through the inclusion of an individual's capacity for interpretation of stressors and perceived threat and therefore extends the P-E fit model, the theory does not consider or provide any explicit links between this capacity and eustress. In the last decade (2000–2010), a cybernetic model was used to construct a multidisciplinary team approach to evidence-based practice (Porter-O'Grady, Alexander, Blaylock, Minkara, & Surel, 2006) and to develop a 14-item Cybernetic Coping Scale (CCS) that acknowledges the function of coping as both an independent variable and an outcome to predict psychological strain, and job and family satisfaction (Brough, O'Driscoll, & Kalliath, 2005). For a dissertation, it served as an organization model for determining characteristics of academic nursing centers (Williamson, 2000).

Theory of Organizational Burnout

It is well documented that many professionals (including nurses) experience high levels of stress that can lead to physical, psychological, and emotional problems, sometimes termed as burnout. The term *burnout* was first used by Freudenberger and Richelson (1980) to describe a psychological state of tiredness, disappointment, and hopelessness. Maslach and Goldberg (1998) further defined *it as a syndrome that includes depersonalization (D), emotional exhaustion (EE), and low personal accomplishment (PA) leading to decreased effectiveness in the work world.* They indicated that *EE* results from a decrease or loss of self-confidence and interest in one's profession as well as feelings of fatigue and weakness; *D* represents the interpersonal context or dimension of burnout; and *PA* describes low feelings of productivity, adequacy, and coping successfully. This definition of burnout, which is now being used widely in ongoing research, was not based on a theoretical model but was derived empirically. Several years of exploratory research provided the groundwork for the development of both the conceptual definition and a standardized measure, The Maslach Burnout Inventory (Maslach & Jackson, 1981a, 1981b). Burnout is often associated with decreased job performance and commitment and predicts stress-related health problems and low career satisfaction. It can be a response to job-related stressors such as chronic fatigue, high employee workload, compassion fatigue, and trying to maintain a balance between family and career demands. A number of studies have identified burnout in health care professionals (especially nurses) as both chronic and pervasive (Gabassi, Cervai, Rozbowsky, Semeraro, & Gregori, 2002; Weber & Jaekel-Reinhard, 2000; Weberg, 2010).

For the last 10 years (2000–2010), CINAHL documents more than 400 nursing research studies of burnout; in addition there are 40 reviews. The reviews have focused on burnout and mental health nursing (Dickinson & Wright, 2008; Gilbody et al., 2006; Edwards, Burnard, Coyle, Fothergill & Hannigan, 2000; Nakakris & Ouziuni, 2008); caregiving (Rundqvist, Sivonen, & Delmar, 2010; Sherman, Edwards, Simonton, & Mehta, 2006); cancer care (Cohen, Ferrell, Vrabel, Visovsky, & Babock, 2010; Zander, Hutton, & King, 2010); job satisfaction (Alarcon & Edwards, 2011; Gui, Barriball, & While, 2009; Lu, While, & Barriball, 2005; Takase et al., 2005); and medication errors (Garrett, 2008).

Control Theory of Organizational Stress

Control theory is based on the notion that the perception of stress may be moderated by the extent to which an individual experiences control over environmental stressors and the ability to make choices (Karasek, 1979; Spector, 1998). Control may range on a continuum from where there is complete autonomy in the workplace with personal control over workload and schedules to some degree of autonomy and personal control over schedule and workload to little if any autonomy and personal control. The model (Spector, 1998) proposes the concepts of *locus of control* and *self efficacy* (Bandura, 1997) as moderating factors on perception of control, which, with the individual's affective disposition, influences the perception of and emotional response to the stressor. The physical, psychological, and behavioral stress response therefore incorporates individual perception and affect.

The control model does not characterize the nature of the stressors nor the amount of stress, but acknowledges just the existence of environmental stressors. Similar to the other models discussed, there is no explicit discussion of eustress and distress when focusing on the stress response. The primacy of the individual's affective disposition and interpretation within the model and conception of stress, however, could allow for the individual to experience the stress as either distress or eustress (LeFevre et al., 2003), even though it is not explicitly addressed as an outcome.

LeFevre and colleagues suggested a parsimonious revision of Spector's (1998) control model to build upon Spector's emphasis on perception and the individual's key role as the interpreter of stressors. They present four concepts that capture the control model/theory: (1) the individual, characterized by perceptions of one's locus of control, efficacy, and affective disposition; (2) the stressor, an environmental stimulus characterized by the perceived source, timing, and desirability, impacting; (3) the perception of stressors, representing the interface of environmental stimuli and the individual's way of understanding, leading to; (4) the experience of stress, or what could be described as the eustress or distress experienced by the individual leading to behavioral, physical, and/or psychological outcomes.

Holistic Stress Model

The holistic stress model (Simmons & Nelson, 2007) is grounded in the positive psychology (Seligman & Csikszentmihalyi, 2000) and positive organizational behavior movement (Cameron, Dutton, & Quinn, 2003; Luthans, 2002; Nelson & Cooper, 2007). It acknowledges the positive qualities and traits of individuals and organizations and a commitment to building and applying these positive qualities for performance improvement in organizational settings. It highlights the primacy of the subjective experience in appraising and evaluating stressors, integrating Lazarus and Folkman's (1984) notion that people can have different responses to stressors depending upon whether they evaluate the stressor as positive or negative and its significance for their well-being. The model (see Figure 12.2) integrates the view that *challenge* (the potential for growth) and threat/harm responses can occur simultaneously from the same stressor and are separate but related constructs (Edwards & Cooper, 1988; Lazarus & Folkman, 1984; Simmons & Nelson, 2007). For

any given demand, an individual can have both a positive and negative response consisting of a variety of emotions, attitudes, and behaviors.

The model proposes that in addition to these responses being separate and distinct, they are complex, multivariate, and potentially interactive in nature (Simmons & Nelson, 2007). It, therefore, does not identify a stressor as challenging (positive) or threatening (negative) but seeks to understand how individual differences/traits (interdependence, self-esteem, optimism-pessimism, locus of control, hardiness) can affect the relationship between the stressors and response.

Empirical testing of this model has been done with hospital nurses, home health care nurses, university professors, and pastors and those who work in assisted living centers (Little, Simmons, & Nelson, 2007; Nelson & Simmons, 2003, 2004; Simmons, Gooty, Nelson, & Little, 2009; Simmons & Nelson, 2001; Simmons, Nelson, & Neal, 2001; Simmons, Nelson, & Quick, 2003). Demands/stressors studied were role ambiguity, death of a patient, workload, and work–family conflicts, and these showed no relationship between stressors and outcomes such as perception of health and performance (rated by supervisors). Researchers examined indicators of eustress such as the positive psychological states of hope, positive affect (PA), meaningfulness, and manageability, and indicators of distress, such as negative psychological states, including job alienation, negative affect (NA), anxiety, and anger. To date, hope (having the capacity and will to accomplish goals at work) has been the best indicator of eustress, with work satisfaction and supervisor satisfaction the best predictors of hope at work. The research has also validated a significant positive relationship between hope as an indicator of eustress and perception of health.

The individual trait that holds the most promise within the model is *interdependence,* or healthy attachment, which allows one to work both autonomously and to know when to ask for help from others (Quick, Nelson, & Quick, 1990; Simmons & Nelson, 2007). Hope mediated the relationship between interdependence and perception of health in home health care nurses in that those who were more interdependent were more likely to be hopeful and healthy (Simmons et al., 2003).

Indicators of eustress, such as positive affect, engagement, and forgiveness, have been examined with indicators of distress, such as negative

Figure 12.2 Holistic Stress Model

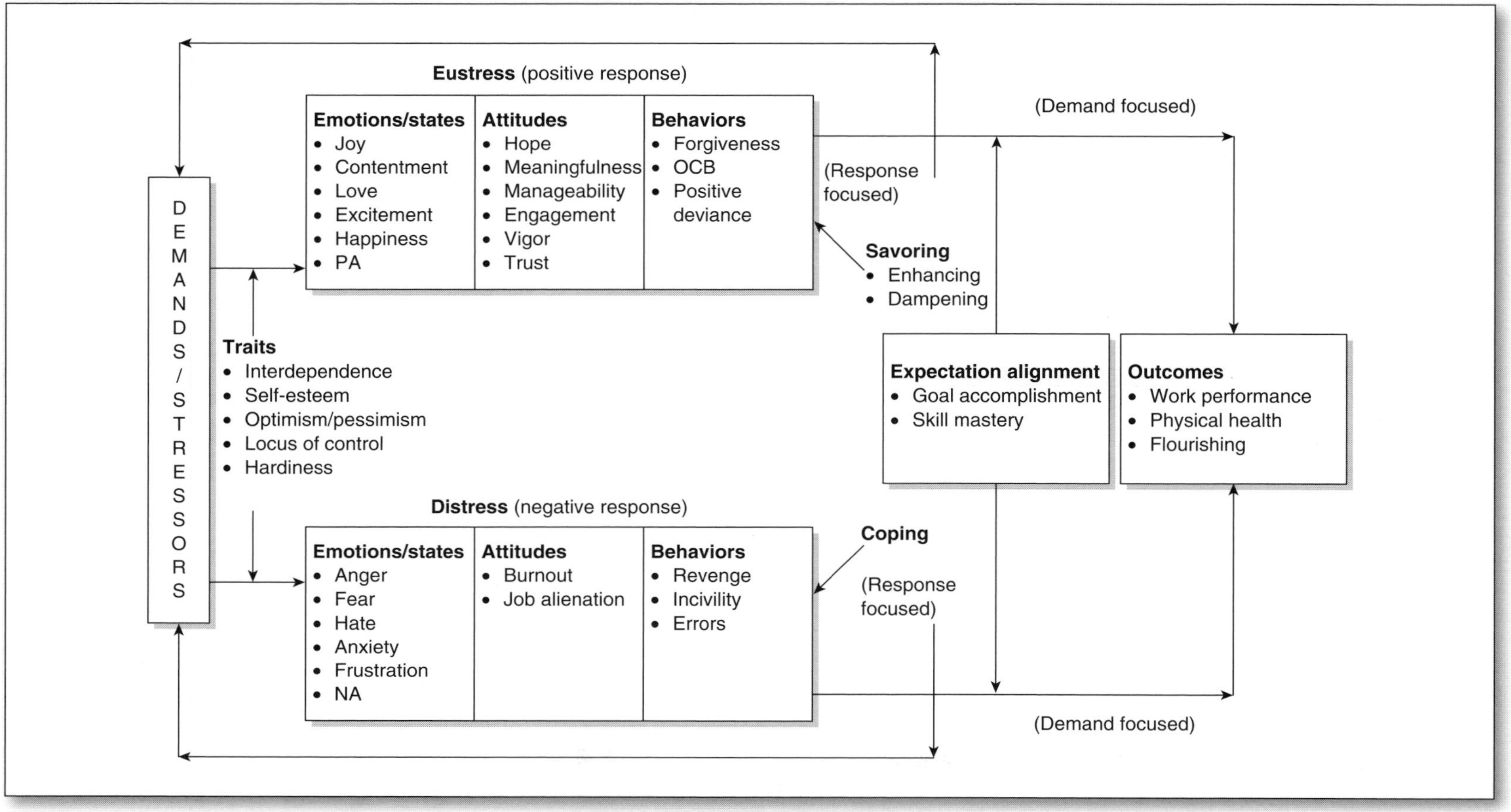

Eustress (positive response)

Emotions/states	**Attitudes**	**Behaviors**
• Joy	• Hope	• Forgiveness
• Contentment	• Meaningfulness	• OCB
• Love	• Manageability	• Positive deviance
• Excitement	• Engagement	
• Happiness	• Vigor	
• PA	• Trust	

Distress (negative response)

Emotions/states	**Attitudes**	**Behaviors**
• Anger	• Burnout	• Revenge
• Fear	• Job alienation	• Incivility
• Hate		• Errors
• Anxiety		
• Frustration		
• NA		

Traits
• Interdependence
• Self-esteem
• Optimism/pessimism
• Locus of control
• Hardiness

DEMANDS/STRESSORS

Savoring
• Enhancing
• Dampening
(Response focused)

Coping
(Response focused)

Expectation alignment
• Goal accomplishment
• Skill mastery

Outcomes
• Work performance
• Physical health
• Flourishing

(Demand focused)

SOURCE: Simmons & Nelson, 2007. Reprinted with permission.

317

affect, burnout, and revengeful behavior, in a study with pastors (Little et al., 2007). Only positive affect and revengeful behavior were identified as significant predictors of perceptions (positive or negative) of health. Engagement, or a strongly held commitment and responsibility to one's job, seemed to mitigate against revengeful behavior when faced with stressors. The model is undergoing further testing and development with the inclusion of emotions such as joy, love, contentment, fear, hate, frustration, identification of further behavioral indicators, and evaluating other variables which moderate eustress, distress, and positive outcomes.

Savoring eustress is another concept introduced by the model, which means enjoying and dwelling with the positive (Nelson & Simmons, 2004). It is seen in the model in contrast with problem-focused coping strategies designed to address the source of stress and emotion-focused strategies designed to deal with the perceived experience of distress (Lazarus & Folkman, 1984). These coping strategies are intended to deal with distress rather than enhancing positive emotions, attitudes, and behaviors. Savoring eustress could potentially link to outcomes through better work performance and health, which result from connection, resiliency, and receptivity. Simmons and Nelson's (2007) incorporation of the concept of expectation alignment into their model recognizes that the relationship between eustress and positive outcomes will be strongest when both supervisors and employees in an organization can come to a mutual understanding of what are important goals to each and common understandings of the expectations of work.

The concept of flourishing was newly added to the model as a positive outcome variable to include a more holistic view of individuals in organizational settings. It seeks to recognize that positive outcomes in organizations include more than the absence of disease and work performance but the building of organizations that are virtuous (Cameron, 2003) and encourage both individuals and organizations to thrive. This concept has not been tested in the model, but Simmons and Nelson (2007) caution about the empirical challenges in both conceptualizing and measuring the concept. Positive emotions, attitudes, and behaviors that make up eustress will have to be kept conceptually separate from the concept of flourishing—in other words,

since eustress can lead to flourishing, it is methodologically unsound to use these as indicators of flourishing.

Moral Cascade Model

The Moral Cascade Model (Figure 12.3) (Rambur et al., 2010) is a newly developed transactional model presently undergoing testing. It is grounded in positive organizational scholarship (POS) (Cameron, 2003; Cameron et al., 2003), and like positive psychology, it also focuses on the positive attributes (e.g., unselfishness, selflessness, altruism) of individuals and organizations, processes, and outcomes (e.g., vitality, meaningfulness, exhilaration, high-quality relationships). POS specifically explores "the dynamics that are typically described by words such as excellence, thriving, flourishing, abundance, resilience, or virtuousness" (Cameron et al., 2003, p. 3). Its values reflect the position that there is a universal desire to improve the human condition and while organizations have this capacity, it is usually latent (Cameron et al., 2003). By building capacity to understand and develop generative dynamics such as the cultivation of positive emotion, the creation of meaning, relationship transformation, and high-quality connections, organizations can produce sustained sources of collective capability that help organizations thrive (Cameron et al., 2003). It is this collective capacity, the overall organizational virtuousness, that sets a virtuous organization apart from others. Rather than merely a collection of virtuous individuals, it is the synergy produced by the collective that develops a moral trait unique to the organization (Park & Peterson, 2003).

In the Moral Cascade Model, the virtuous organization is defined as having a particular moral purpose that is known to members and nonmembers of the organization. The nonmembers might include community members, clients, or vendors. Furthermore, this virtuous organization would have alignment of the organization's moral purpose and its practices, regulations, and decision making. Rambur et al. (2010) conjecture that a virtuous organization also interacts and is shaped by the culture and events of its surroundings and environment. This interaction results in an organization that gradually develops a moral stance that is more encompassing and relevant to its environment. This evolving moral stance then allows for the enhancement of the ethical life for the organization and its members. In the ideal case "there is full alignment among: (1) the moral identity of individuals, which informs and shapes their behavior as they work in an organization, (2) the implicit values of the organization as embodied in the organizational culture and stated and unstated practices, and (3) the organization's explicit social purpose and stated mission" (Rambur et al., p. 41). The Moral Cascade Model (see Figure 12.3) proposes a schema for the interaction of moral identity, moral distress, moral eustress, and institutional moral practices, which is a framework for future inquiry as well as definitional within the model.

One goal of further inquiry is to expand the current understanding of moral distress—an idea commonly studied in health care organizational research—and moral eustress for broader extension to other types of contemporary organizations. A second goal is to examine how moral practices of individuals are shaped by organizational effectiveness and, in turn, how organizational effectiveness shapes individual moral practices. A third goal is to integrate the idea of the virtuous organization—a relatively new construct—with the concept of moral stress in order to highlight the interactive relationship between the moral workings of individuals and the organizational environment in which they are members. As discussed in Rambur et al. (2010), "The model, therefore, seeks to provide an understanding of the interactions among individual moral identity, the stated and unstated organizational values, and moral development of both the individual and the organization" (p. 42).

Moral stress and the cascade to moral eustress and moral distress. The moral identity of the individual is shaped by conceptions, construction, beliefs, and style (Weaver, 2006). Individuals may have several other moral sub-identities that combine to result in a distinctive moral identity (Malouf, 2003). Organizational awareness also varies from person to person and this, in turn, interacts with moral identity and helps to form individual moral agency.

A sense of personal harmony can result for individuals when there is alignment of individual moral identity and organizational awareness along with the values and actions of the stated or unstated organization. However, if organizational actions are in conflict with the explicit social purpose or stated mission of the institution, increasing discord between the moral identity of the individual and the unstated organization values can occur in those that are organizationally aware. *Moral prehension,* defined as "a vague, initial sense that an issue or situation has moral dimensions" (Rambur et al., 2010, p. 45) amplifies the stress state of vigilance and this in turn produces further consideration, appraisals, and judgments. Moral prehension is akin to Rest, Narvacz, Bebeau, and Thoma's (1999) "moral sensitivity" (p. 101) and to Cavanaugh and Moberg's (1999) idea about the start of ethical courage, which first requires "recognizing what potential behavior has ethical content" (p. 12). At the moral prehension stage, an organizational member may take several steps to clarify or solidify their thinking. They may take time to reflect on the issue, talk with colleagues, and report their concerns through organizational channels or to higher authorities. In any case, a crucial component of the model is that moral stress has resulted in capturing an individual's attention and energy that is then concentrated on action to achieve a solution. This action can then cascade in one of two directions, leading to either moral eustress or moral distress.

Thus, when an individual is being stressed, the person will move through a process to deal with the stress. This process usually involves considering a number of strategies and the potential outcomes of each strategy. In addition, the options and potential outcomes of the action or inaction are weighed and considered. Information, data, facts as well as personal experience can become the basis for movement to moral certainty. This moral certainty may confirm for an individual that although they might not know exactly how to proceed, the option of inaction is no longer a morally justifiable option. They are mobilized to "do something" to address the situation. As Rambur et al. (2010) state, if the individual's action is not impeded, it "instead becomes a moral transaction and discord decreases, the initial strain, dissonance and resulting stress, and action event have served to strengthen the moral identity of the individual" (p. 46). In turn, the individual and the stated as well as unstated organizational values are now more aligned. The individual, who had previously experienced moral stress, now feels the stress resolving and a fortifying of his or her moral identity. For the individual, this positive change in moral identity is termed *moral eustress* in the model.

Figure 12.3   The Moral Cascade Model

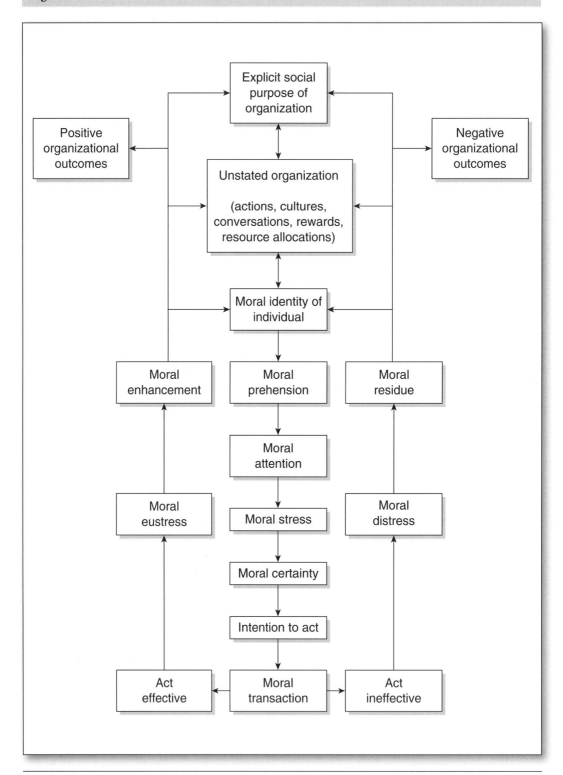

In the situation with an outcome involving moral eustress, conflict among the three arenas—the individual, the unstated organization, and the stated organizational purpose—provides the movement toward greater individual and organizational growth and, in turn, enhances the organization's public service outcomes. Experiencing moral eustress carries with it an increase in the capacity of both the individual and the organization to assess and resolve ever more complicated organizational challenges. This results in reinforcement of the positive feedback loop (see Figure 12.2) and an increasingly virtuous organization. Similar to Karasek's (1979) job demands–control model or Csikszentmihalyi's (1990) model of flow, when there are high degrees of moral challenge, moral skill, and individual control, a resulting positive state evolves. In order for this positive state to be induced, however, the individual must have the skill to respond and the organization needs the resources to respond. If this delicate balance is not in place, the moral stress results in a cascade to moral distress.

Moral distress results when one believes one knows how to act, but is thwarted by constraints (Austin, 2007). "There is a sense of being morally responsible, but unable to change what is happening" (p. 84). This moral distress in turn can lead to a scar in the individual's psyche, termed *moral residue* (Schluter, Winch, Holzhauser, & Henderson, 2008). Moral residue then affects a feedback loop that negatively influences the moral identity of the individual as well as dimensions of the organization. For the individual, a chronic state of moral distress and moral residue may lead to disengagement as an organizational member, with increasing sense of hopelessness, anger, and frustration. The impacts of moral distress are multifaceted and can involve additional emotional outcomes such as shame, sadness, powerlessness, guilt, and loss of integrity (Corley, 2002; Rushton, 1992; Sundin-Huard & Fahy, 1999). The individual may disengage from family, friends, and the organization while also manifesting physical symptoms such as neck pain, muscle and stomach aches, and headaches (Gutierrez, 2005).

Organizational disengagement may result in job dissatisfaction, decreased productivity, and withdrawal from patients (Gutierrez, 2005), with an end result of leaving the profession (Corley, 2002; Gutierrez, 2005; Hart, 2005; Joseph & Deshpande, 1997; Redman & Hill, 1997; Wilkinson, 1987). In health care settings, the terms *nurse suffering* and *wounded healers* have been used to characterize organizational members who experience chronic moral distress and resulting moral residue (Sundin-Huard & Fahy, 1999). The organization is also harmed, not only because it has a despondent worker and the organizational echoes this creates, but also because the issues that created the dissonance in the first place have not been addressed and reconciled. Organizational members who are distressed and disengaged may perform poorly in terms of quality, productivity, and their interactions with colleagues, clients, or patients may suffer. This in turn may lead to dissatisfied stakeholders as well as loss of positive public perceptions of the organization. These outcomes may also ultimately result in an erosion of both public support and the organization's financial health.

Health care literature often cite both resource issues (Corley, 2002; Sporrong, Hoglund, & Arnetz, 2006), cultural elements such as philosophy and goal differences between health care providers, perceived power differentials between disciplines, and conflicting moral and legal objectives (Corley, 2002; Schluter et al., 2008; Sporrong et al., 2006) as sources of stress, all of which could precipitate the moral cascade. It should not be surprising that the conception of moral distress originated in health care organizations given the nature and challenges in those environments. Outcomes in health care settings are often immediate and can have severe and long-lasting impacts on patients' lives and, perhaps, their deaths. Doctors and nurses see and touch their patients; the "clients" are personal and not abstract. Moral tensions are possibly more immediate and meaningful than in other types of organizations. Moral distress is so well recognized in health care that instruments have been developed (Corley, Elswickr, Gorman, & Clor, 2001) to assess and screen for the presence of moral distress. To date, there are no instruments measuring moral eustress in organizations, which will be one of the foci of ongoing research within the Moral Cascade Model.

IMPLICATIONS FOR ORGANIZATIONAL STRESS RESEARCH

Organizational stress theories and models have used a variety of definitions, research designs, and methods, which have led to confusing and oftentimes disjointed understanding of what is meant by organizational stress. The complex and dynamic processes of a transactional model of coping with stress require significant changes in how stress is conceptualized and measured. As described before, the P-E fit model provided a structural framework for understanding the stress–coping process but did not explicitly describe the processes through which the person and environment are linked and does not take into account the role of social context. A transactional model needs to recognize that the stress–coping process must go beyond the separate and interacting variables of person and environment and the static nature of their measurement. It needs to explore the characteristics that define the process, the interplay between the stressors, stress, and coping over time and recognize the role of subjective interpretation and context within that dynamic process (Cooper et al., 2001). This approach suggests use of qualitative and quantitative research methodologies or a combination of both, which allows for more vivid and enriched description of the interplay of these dynamic processes and a movement beyond the mere identification of different components of the stress process. Using a variety of research methods (or developing new ones) will help to address the validity question of whose reality are we measuring when we measure stress as well as the need to understand individual meanings and appraisals (Cooper et al., 2001). Other items in measurement tools, which examine work stressors such as the constructs of work, overload, and role ambiguity may need to be reexamined because they no longer represent the impact or reality of the current work environment. In other words, are we placing too much emphasis on reliability of measures to the detriment of their relevance to people's work lives? Are there other stressors such as the amount of change and insecurity within their jobs which reflect larger societal and other concerns?

While the health care literature has suggested relationships and linkages between moral distress and its negative impacts on the professional and the organization, there are many of these same methodological issues within this research that inspire further exploration of moral distress and eustress in both health care and other organizational contexts. These methodological issues include poorly defined terms, a lack of uniformity in design and data collection, and scant methodological descriptions, including sampling and analysis (Schluter et al., 2008). In addition, most of the research on virtuous organizations is relatively young and has targeted business and for-profit organizations, except for an important inquiry within the nonprofit sector of higher education (Vallett, 2010). Expanding the inquiry to include nonprofit organizations with an explicit mission to serve the public good, such as health, social service agencies, the military, and higher education institutions, holds promise for enhancing the theoretical power of Cameron et al.'s (2003) conception and for promoting further understanding of how virtuousness appears in the nonprofit sector.

It will be important to explore and understand the interplay of moral stress, the individual, and the organization, and how the cascade dynamic contributes to the vibrancy and growth of both employee and the organization or how it can instead lead to stagnation and/or dysfunction. Further research will need to illuminate the interactive individual and organizational dynamics as well as the effect of moral distress and eustress on organizational practices, development, change and transformation, or devolution and decline (Rambur et al., 2010). Some preliminary research questions are: How does the degree of organizational virtuousness impact the potential for moral eustress or distress? Do specific virtuousness factors predict the degree of moral response (eustress or distress)? How do individuals narrate their experiences of moral eustress and/or distress? Do those narratives differ within organizations with different levels of virtuousness? Do those narratives reveal different characteristics in individuals' moral conceptions (Gilligan, 1982; Kohlberg, 1984; N. Lyons, 1983) that illuminate the nature and quality of moral eustress and distress? Similarly, are there characteristics that define differences among an organization's moral stance and resulting organizational policies and practices? How do the narratives of organizational leaders illuminate which environments support organizational and individual moral development in terms of virtuousness and moral responses? Finally, how do these dynamics ultimately impact organizational performance and success?

Implications for Practice

This section will first examine the research on types of interventions to alleviate stress in organizations. The next discusses the specific issue of implications for and types of stress in health care settings. Lastly, the section examines the implications for leaders who seek to address stress in their organizations.

Interventions: A Preventative Stress Management Model to Alleviate Stress

An important and fairly recent approach, emerging at least in part from positive organizational theory, poses a new way to define and research different kinds of stress interventions. This orientation is based on a preventative medicine model (Quick & Macik-Frey, 2007; Quick, Quick, & Nelson, 1998). Quick et al. (1998), claim that "as a basic philosophy, preventive stress management consists of basic ideas, beliefs and principles to achieve good health and high performance in organizations" (p. 247). They further articulate five guiding principles:

1. Individual and organization health are interdependent.

2. Leaders have a responsibility for individual and organizational health.

3. Individual and organizational distress are not inevitable.

4. Each individual and organization reacts uniquely to stress.

5. Organizations are ever-changing, dynamic entities. (Quick et al., 1998, p. 247)

Grounded in this definition and these basic principles, they define a model of interventions to alleviate stress that they refer to as the Preventative Stress Management Model. It identifies primary, secondary, and tertiary prevention interventions, drawing on a tripartite model in preventative medicine. Using this framework, Cooper et al. (2001) observe that this model builds on the transactional model of stress for understanding the different interventions and their effect.

Primary interventions emphasize removing stressors from the environment so the individual is relieved of the stress. Using a person–environment fit model, they observe that the "focus of primary interventions is on modifying or adapting the physical or social-political environment to meet the needs of workers" (p. 189). Such interventions occur at the organizational level, ranging from redesigning jobs or tasks to creating more support for workers through changing organizational practices, better working environments, and the like.

Secondary interventions have as their focus the individual and employ techniques and strategies to diminish individuals' stress. These interventions usually fall into two general categories: 1) cognitive interventions, or 2) somatic ones, or a combination of both termed *multimodal* (LeFevre, Kolt, & Matheny, 2006). Cognitive interventions include teaching such things as conflict resolution, while somatic includes teaching relaxation techniques or meditation. Tertiary interventions are "concerned with the rehabilitation of individuals who have suffered ill health or reduced well-being as a result of strain in the workplace" (Cooper et al., 2001, p. 192). The moral residue in the Moral Cascade Model is an example of when a tertiary intervention might be appropriate.

Despite the efforts to identify and characterize different intervention approaches, the one that seems to be more prevalent in the current literature is the prevention model. Reviews of research that examine the effectiveness of primary or secondary interventions reveal what many observe: that empirical or other inquiries into the effectiveness of these approaches is relatively new and inconclusive (Cooper, 1998; Cooper et al., 2001; Lamontagne, Keegel, Louie, Ostry, & Landsbergis, 2007; LeFevre et al., 2006; Quick & Macik-Frey, 2007).

LeFevre et al. (2006) define stress management interventions, or SMIs, as "any purposeful action taken to reduce or alleviate the stress experience by organization citizens in the execution of their work functions" (p. 548). These authors examine empirical data on the effect of primary and secondary interventions. They note that individually focused interventions, or secondary interventions, appear to be most frequently used, but the literature focuses on primary interventions as being more desirable because they hold promise to remove stress from the environment, a more lasting solution than "treating" individual responses to stress.

Regardless of claims for what might be most effective, the empirical evidence, however, only weakly supports the claim. Examinations of both primary and secondary stress interventions are flawed by having poor follow-up, infrequent use of control groups, measurement issues, as well as inadequate and nonstandard definitions of what stress and stressors are (LeFevre et al., 2006). Further, it is noted that none of the empirical work includes any definition or study of eustress as an outcome from stress. LeFevre et al. argue that this absence may pose a serious limit in the research, may be what produces at least some of the variation in research results, and certainly impoverishes intervention designs because there is no effort toward helping individuals construct and sustain a positive approach to workplace stressors.

Examination of the effects of secondary interventions, despite the claims in favor of primary ones, reveals that overall they had positive effects. Again, the research is varied and demonstrates similar methodological limitations as the research on primary interventions. Further, it is suggested (LeFevre et al., 2006) that secondary interventions are frequently of shorter duration than primary ones, hence the outcomes may be more immediate and thus easier for the researcher to access. "This lack of clarity in the relationship between length of intervention and potential gain must raise questions in the minds of those who purchase and recommend stress management interventions in terms of cost relative to benefit" (LeFevre et al., p. 553). Additionally, to the extent that the intervention itself creates institutional change, it becomes a potential source of stress because organizational change has long been perceived as a stressor for all who work in the organization (LeFevre et al.).

The lack of clarity about what strategies are most effective leads LeFevre et al. (2006) to recommend that individually focused intervention ought to be viewed as the "first line of defence [*sic*]" (p. 562), with primary interventions following—at least until there is stronger empirical evidence that one intervention is more effective.

Implications for Stress in Health Care

The discussion about stress has looked at its role for individuals and organizations generally. This section focuses on stress in health care specifically, as a way to illuminate how stress and organizational interventions to address it can not only appear in the various and general

forms noted above, but can also occur in ways that are specific to health care professions and the organizations in which these professions are practiced.

Verhaeghe, Vlerick, Gemmel, Van Maele, and De Backer's study (2006) of 2,094 registered nurses (RNs) in 10 general hospitals found that recurrent minor changes in the work environment had a negative impact on RNs' psychological well-being, with resulting distress and an increase in absence frequency and duration. Notably, this outcome was found only when the changes were viewed as threatening. Conversely, changes viewed as challenging were positively related to eustress and well-being. Yet change is inevitable in any workplace setting and will likely accelerate in intensity in health care. Thus, creation of an environment in which changes, both large and small, can be viewed less as a threat and more as an opportunity is a worthy, evidence-based practice for those seeking to create sustainable health care environments that effectively address stress. Such efforts require great attention to nuance, as perceptions and their attendant threats vary markedly among individuals and age cohorts, as do out-of-workplace life stressors, as noted in many of the models defining stress. The heretofore mentioned study (Verhaeghe et al., 2006), for example, found that age cohort mattered dramatically, with the age category 31 to 45 being the most resilient. This differs from other studies that have found the oldest age cohorts in the nursing workforce to self-report highest levels of emotional well-being (Palumbo, Rambur, McIntosh, & Naud, 2010).

In addition to stress-related absenteeism, presenteeism is an increasingly reported stress-related outcome. In contrast to absenteeism, presenteeism is defined as "loss of productivity that occurs when employees come to work but perform below par due to any kind of illness" (Levin-Epstein, 2005). A relatively new construct, presenteeism may be more costly than absenteeism when considering direct and indirect costs (Stewart, Matousek, & Verdon, 2003). Estimates of organizations' lost productivity due to presenteeism range from 18% to as high as 61% (Goetzel et al., 2004). More recently, van den Heuvel, Geuskens, Hooftman, Koopes, and van den Bossche (2009), in a nationally representative study of 22,759 employees, found that the psychological factors and the very elements inherent to much of nursing—for example, physically demanding work including shift work and emotionally demanding work—were strongly associated with productivity loss. Similarly, in a study of 4,032 employees representative of the work population between the ages of 25 and 64, Wang, Schmitz, Smailes, Sareen, and Patten (2010) found that over 40% of employees at all job gradients demonstrated presenteeism. Stress, in particular distress, is a clear contributing factor. As one example, Lerner et al.'s (2010) exploration of workplace outcomes including presenteeism found that work stressors contribute to the impact of depression on related work absences and impaired work performance.

Health care is inherently team based. As such, stress-related presenteeism may exact a substantial toll. The impacts of presenteeism on health care quality, including medical errors and patient safety, however, are not fully known and to date largely unstudied as a specific, potentially correlated phenomenon. Nevertheless, additional work highlights the importance of attention to the creation of eustress rather than distress in the workplace. Gartner, Nieuwenhuijsen, van Dijk, and Sluiter (2010), in a comprehensive review on work function of nurses and allied health professionals, found firm evidence of a strong association between common mental disorders and general errors, medication errors, near misses, patient safety, and patient satisfaction.

Together, these overarching theories and findings suggest that managing the inevitable workplace stress in a manner that is life enhancing will have impacts far beyond the individual and the organization as a whole and touch every part of the institutional mission including patient safety. Opportunities for transformational organizational leaders to recontextualize change and its attendant stressors into a positive stimulus for growth have never been greater.

Implications for Leadership

As noted at the start of this chapter, the 21st century's first decade has demonstrated that there is reason for concern that the stressors in the workplace generally are increasing, becoming more complex, and, for some, becoming more morally and ethically challenging as evidenced by some of the leaders during the economic challenges of 2008 and beyond. Even

earlier in 1997, Cartwright and Cooper (1997) start their text on *Managing Workplace Stress* with an opening chapter titled "The Growing Epidemic of Stress" (p. 1).

Arguably, a significant and critical component in addressing workplace stress in health care and in other organizations lies with the leadership of the organization. In preventative interventions "leaders have a responsibility for individual and organizational health" (Quick et al., 1998, p. 247). Nevertheless, it is worth noting that as the workplace has become increasingly challenging, so has the job of being a leader in that setting. There is a vast and complex literature on leadership encompassing approaches from the philosophical to the empirical. Further, when an issue related to workplace stress (as well as other organizational issues) is identified, it is common to conclude at the end of a study or a narrative that leaders need to learn how to address the issue, whatever it is. Despite the vast array of literature on leadership, however, specific inquiry regarding how leadership influences the stress levels and types of stress in an organization is relatively slim. Still, it is reasonable to assert, based on existing studies of leadership and stress, that the kind of leadership and the values held by the leader can significantly impact how stress is experienced and managed in the workplace.

A commonly used definition of leadership style identifies three types of leaders, the laissez-faire leader, the transactional leader, and the transformational leader (Carli & Eagly, 2007; Johnson, 2001). The *laissez-faire leader*, as defined by the Multifactor Leadership Questionnaire, shows an "absence and lack of involvement during critical junctures" (Carli & Eagly, 2007, p. 137). The *transactional leader* focuses on rewards and tends to focus on when something goes wrong, otherwise not intervening until a problem is intense. *Transformational leaders*:

Engage in *charismatic leadership (idealized influence)* and *inspirational motivation*. They become role models for followers, set high standards and goals, create shared visions, provide meaning, and make emotional appeals. In addition, transforming leaders provide *intellectual stimulation* and *individual consideration*. They stimulate creativity by helping followers question their assumptions and develop new approaches to problems. They provide learning opportunities tailored to the needs of each individual. (Johnson, 2001, p. 124; also see Clarke & Cooper, 2004)

It is possible that the transactional leader will engage in addressing stress issues in the workplace, but given the intention and focus of this leadership style, those interventions are likely to be directed at individuals and may well be reactive rather than proactive. As such, they would be strategies for secondary or perhaps tertiary preventative interventions.

It is the transformational leader who has the style and capacity to create and sustain primary interventions to address both individual and organizational forms of stress. Transformational leaders are identified as having the capacity to create environments in which workers and teams have hope that they have both the will and the capacity to accomplish valued goals (Simmons & Nelson, 2007), feel well regarded, rewarded for their effort, appropriately engaged in organizational decisions, and supported to master their jobs both in terms of performance and in terms of emotional and personal strength (Cooper et al., 2001; Macik-Frey et al., 2009; Quick et al., 1998). The transformational leader may employ strategies at all three levels of intervention but is more likely to focus on those at the primary level since they hold the greatest promise for creating organizational change and practices to address stress that will be sustained.

In spite of both claims that it is the transformative leadership style that will be most effective on stress outcomes and the common sense conclusion that this should be true, there is slim empirical evidence to support this assertion. One empirical study found that leadership style correlated positively with influencing "task performance, social support perceptions, efficacy beliefs, change in negative affect and stressor appraisals" (J. Lyons & Schneider, 2008, p. 743). Both transactional and transformational leadership styles correlated with positive outcomes regarding stress. Significantly, subordinates report of experiencing social support from a transformative leader correlated with positive stress outcomes, that is, with the experience of less stress (J. Lyons & Schneider).

This effort for the leader is neither easy nor without its own impact on the leader as a person. That is, leaders and managers experience their

own form of stress, particularly when addressing and attempting to ameliorate stress experienced by their followers or subordinates. Looking specifically at leaders in the United Kingdom in human service organizations, Skagert, Delive, Edlof, Pousetts, and Albourg (2008) explored qualitatively how leaders reported their response to stress, which influenced their ability to address stress experienced by their followers. The leaders reported that they focused effort on handling workplace stress by acting as a "shock absorber" while simultaneously working to "sustain their own integrity" (p. 805). As a shock absorber, these leaders were aware of the need to "lead amidst continuous change" and to lead "whilst maintaining trust" (p. 806). Sustaining one's own integrity called upon leaders to identify with their role as leader and employ "distancing strategies" (pp. 806–807) to maintain distance between their leader identity and the rest of their life and identities (parent, partner, social life, etc.). The researchers concluded their analysis with a call for increased communication and structures designed to support leaders as they deal with the dilemmas of the workplace that produce stress for both them and the workers in the organization.

It is important to note that the work reviewed about leadership influence on stress does not address eustress. In short, and following LeFevre et al.'s (2006) lead, are there leadership styles or leadership strategies that create conditions that promote eustress for both the leader and the follower? Speculatively, it would seem that those leadership styles and capacities that are explicitly articulated in terms of moral and ethical principles and practices are more likely to create such conditions. It is beyond the scope of this chapter to explore this idea in any depth, but a brief examination will serve to inscribe the general ideas about leadership that might enhance the possibility for eustress outcomes.

It is likely that such a leader will practice what has been called authentic or ethical leadership (Johnson, 2001; May, Chan, Hodges, & Avolio, 2003; Trevino & Brown, 2007). These leaders may "take a stand that changes the course of history for others, be they organizations, departments or just other individuals" (May et al., 2003, p. 248). They are also enacting, on a daily or even moment-by-moment basis, a values-based approach to leadership that ultimately influences the work environment through maintaining and encouraging moral behaviors throughout the organization, and in modeling those in all decisions. Such leadership is characterized by the leader's capacity to recognize when a dilemma has moral or ethical components, being open and transparent about both the process and outcome of a decision, being self-aware and acting based on these considerations and values (May et al., 2003; Trevino & Brown, 2007). Such leaders are seen, at least theoretically, as being capable of creating workplaces that are characterized by vigor, vitality, and ongoing learning. These workplaces would, additionally, be capable of creativity and growth (Nelson & Cooper, 2007; Senge, Scharmer, Jaworski, & Flowers, 2004), would be demonstrably virtuous (Cameron, 2003), and would engage and demonstrate positive organizational behaviors (Nelson & Cooper, 2007).

It is reasonable to extrapolate from this form of leadership that the outcomes of the various strategies employed by the leader to shape the organization would result in eustress outcomes for the followers and leader alike. There is not yet qualitative or quantitative research, however, that further illuminates how the cascade to eustress, as defined in the Moral Cascade Model above, might be enhanced and encouraged by leader behavior, beliefs, and strategies.

Conclusion

It seems likely that stress is here to stay in health care professions, as well as other professions and the workplace generally. As a result, it is imperative that leaders and workers alike come to understand the nature and forms of stress that they may experience, and together work toward fashioning practices that promote transformed workplaces. Moreover, until very recently, stress has been cast as a negative force, and there is plenty of evidence that stress can indeed be deleterious to the individual, the organization, and by implication the professions and society. On the other hand, increasingly stress is also cast as an indicator of tensions that, if handled well, can lead to individuals experiencing eustress, feeling empowered and in control, and to organizations characterized by positive practices and outcomes. It is this transactional and dynamic view of stress within individuals and organizations, incorporating both the positive and negative aspects of

stress, which must serve as the foundation for future research and a more holistic understanding of the stress process within organizations.

References

Abualrub, R. F. (2007). Nursing shortage in Jordan: What is the solution? *Journal of Professional Nursing, 23*(2), 117–120.

Alarcon, G. M., & Edwards, J. M. (2011). The relationship of engagement, job satisfaction and turnover intentions. *Stress & Health, 27*(3), e294–e298.

Austin, W. (2007). The ethics of everyday practice: Healthcare environments as moral communities. *Advances in Nursing Science, 30*(1), 81–88.

Avey, J., Luthens, F., & Jensen, S. (2009). Psychological capital: A positive resource for combating employee stress and turnover. *Human Resource Management, 48*(5), 677–693.

Bandura, A. (1997). *Self-efficacy in changing societies*. Cambridge, UK: Cambridge University Press.

Bolger, N., & Zuckerman, A. (1995). A framework for studying personality in the stress process. *Journal of Personality and Social Psychology, 69*, 890–902.

Brough, P., O'Driscoll, M. P., & Kalliath, T. J. (2005). The ability of "family friendly" organisational resources to predict work–family conflict and job and family satisfaction. *Stress and Health, 21*, 223–234.

Cameron, K. (2003). Organizational virtuousness and performance. In K. Cameron, J. Dutton, & R. Quinn (Eds.), *Positive organizational scholarship* (pp. 48–65). San Francisco, CA: Berrett-Koehler.

Cameron, K., Dutton, J., & Quinn, R. (2003). Foundations of positive organizational scholarship. In K. Cameron, J. Dutton, & R. Quinn (Eds.), *Positive organizational scholarship* (pp. 3–13). San Francisco, CA: Berrett-Koehler.

Caplan, R. D, Cobb, S., French, J. R. P., Harrison, R. V., & Pinneau, S. R. (1975). *Job demands and worker health*. Cincinnati, OH: National Institute for Occupational Safety and Health. (Publication No. 75–168).

Carli, L., & Eagly, A. (2007). Overcoming resistance to women leaders: The importance of leadership style. In B. Kellerman & D. Rhode (Eds.), *Women and leadership: The state of play and strategies for change* (pp. 127–148). San Francisco, CA: Jossey-Bass.

Cartwright, S., & Cooper, C. (1997). *Managing workplace stress.* Thousand Oaks, CA: Sage.

Carver, L. L. (2008). *Organizational commitment and generational differences in nursing faculty* (Dissertation). University of Nevada, Las Vegas. Accessed August 31, 2011, from http://gateway .proquest.com/openurl%3furl_ver=Z39.88- 2004%26res_dat=xri:pqdiss%26rft_val_ fmt=info:ofi/fmt:kev:mtx:dissertation% 26rft_dat=xri:pqdiss:3319124

Cavanaugh, G., & Moberg, D. (1999). The virtue of courage within the organization. *Research in Ethical Issues in Organizations, 1,* 1–27.

Clarke, S., & Cooper, C. L. (2004). *Managing the risk of workplace stress: Health and safety hazards.* New York, NY: Routledge.

Cohen, M. Z., Ferrell, B. R., Vrabel, M., Visovsky, C., & Babcock, B. (2010). What does it mean to be an oncology nurse? Reexamining the life cycle concepts. *Oncology Nursing Forum, 37*(5), 561–570.

Cooper, C. (1998). The psychological implications of the changing nature of work. *Royal Society of Arts Journal, 1,* 71–84.

Cooper, C. L., Dewe, P., & O'Driscoll, M. P. (2001). *Organizational stress: A review and critique of theory, research, and applications.* Thousand Oaks, CA: Sage.

Corley, M. (2002). Nurse moral distress: A proposed theory and research agenda. *Nursing Ethics, 9*(6), 636–650.

Corley, M., Elswickr, K., Gorman, M., & Clor, T. (2001). Development and evaluation of a moral distress scale. *Journal of Advanced Nursing, 33*(2), 250–256.

Csikszentmihalyi, M. (1990). *Flow: The psychology of optimal experience.* New York, NY: Harper Row.

Cummings, T.G., & Cooper, C.L. (1979). A cybernetic framework for studying occupational stress. *Human Relations, 32*(5), 395-418.

DeFrank, R., & Ivancevich, J. (1998). Stress on the job: An executive update. *Academy of Management Executive, 12,* 55–66.

Dickinson T., & Wright, K. M. (2008). Stress and burnout in forensic mental health nursing: A literature review. *British Journal of Nursing, 17*(2), 82–87.

Edwards, D., Burnard, P., Coyle, D., Fothergill, A., & Hannigan, B. (2000). Stress and burnout in community mental health nursing: A review of the literature. *Journal of Psychiatric and Mental Health Nursing, 7*(1), 7–14.

Edwards, J. (1991). Person-job fit: A conceptual integration, literature review, and methodological critique. *International Review of Industrial and Organizational Psychology, 6,* 283–357.

Edwards, J. (1998). Cybernetic theory of stress, coping, and well-being: Review and extension to work and family. In C. L. Cooper (Ed.), *Theories of organizational stress* (pp. 122–152). New York, NY: Oxford University Press.

Edwards, J., Caplan, R., & Harrison, R. V. (1998). Person-environment fit theory: Conceptual foundations, empirical evidence, and directions for future research. In C. L. Cooper (Ed.), *Theories of organizational stress* (pp. 28–67). New York, NY: Oxford University Press.

Edwards, J., & Cooper, C. L. (1988). The impacts of positive psychological states on physical health: A review and theoretical framework. *Social Science Medicine, 27,* 1147–1159.

Evans, B., Crogan, N., & Shultz, J. (2004). Resident coping strategies in the nursing home: An indicator of the need for dietary services change. *Applied Nursing Research, 17*(2), 109–115.

Freudenberger, H., & Richelson, G. (1980). *Burnout: The high cost of high achievement. What it is and how to survive it.* New York, NY: Bantam Books.

Gabassi, P. G., Cervai, S., Rozbowsky, P., Semeraro, A., & Gregori, D. (2002, February). Burnout syndrome in the helping professions. *Psychological Report, 90*(1), 309–314.

Garrett, R. B. (2008). The effect of nurse staffing patterns on medical errors and nurse burnout. *AORN Journal, 87*(6), 1191–1204.

Gartner, F., Nieuwenhuijsen, K., van Dijk, F., & Sluiter, J. (2010). The impact of common mental health disorders on the work functioning of nurses and allied health professionals: A systematic review. *International Journal of Nursing Studies, 47*(8), 1047–1061.

Gilbody, S., Cahill, J., Barkham, M., Richards, D., Bee, P., & Glanville, J. (2006). Can we improve the morale of staff working in psychiatric units? A systematic review. *Journal of Mental Health, 15*(1), 7–17.

Gilligan, C. (1982). *In a different voice: Psychological theory and women's development.* Cambridge, MA: Harvard University Press.

Goetzel, R., Long, S., Ozminkowski, R., Hawkings, K., Wang, S., & Lynch, W. (2004). Health, absence, disability, and presenteeism cost estimates of certain physical and mental health conditions affecting U.S. employers. *Journal of Occupational and Environmental Medicine, 46*(4), 398–412.

Greco, P., Laschinger, H. K. S., & Wong, C. (2006). Leader empowering behaviours, staff nurse empowerment, and work engagement/ burnout. *Canadian Journal of Nursing Leadership, 19*(4), 42–57.

Gui, L., Barriball, K. L., While, A. E. (2009). Job satisfaction of nurse teachers: A literature review. Part II: Effects and related factors. *Nurse Education Today, 29*(5), 477–487.

Gutierrez, K. (2005). Critical care nurses' perceptions of and responses to moral distress. *Dimensions of Critical Care Nursing, 24,* 229–241.

Harrison, R. V. (1978). Person-environment fit and job stress. In C. L. Cooper & R. Payne (Eds.), *Stress at work* (pp. 175–205). New York, NY: Wiley.

Harrison, R. V. (1985). The person-environment fit model and the study of job stress. In T. A. Beehr & R. S. Bhagat (Eds.), *Human stress and cognition in organizations: An integrated perspective* (pp. 23–55). New York, NY: Wiley.

Hart, S. (2005). Hospital ethical climates and registered nurses' turnover intentions. *Journal of Nursing Scholarship, 37,* 173–177.

Johnson, C. (2001). *Meeting the ethical challenges of leadership: Casting light or shadow.* Thousand Oaks, CA: Sage.

Joseph, J., & Deshpande, S. (1997). The impact of ethical climate on job satisfaction of nurses. *Health Care Management Review, 22*(1), 76–81.

Karasek, R. (1979). Job demands, job decision latitude and mental strain: Implications for job redesign. *Administrative Science Quarterly, 24,* 285–308.

Kobasa, S. (1979). Stressful life events, personality and health: An inquiry into hardiness. *Journal of Personality and Social Psychology, 37,* 1–11.

Kohlberg, L. (1984). *The psychology of moral development.* New York, NY: Harper Row.

Lamontagne, A., Keegel, T., Louie, A., Ostry, A., & Landsbergis, P. (2007). A systematic review of the job-stress intervention evaluation literature, 1990–2005. *International Journal of Occupational Health, 13*(3), 268–280.

Lazarus, R. (1991). Psychological stress in the workplace. *Journal of Social Behavior and Personality, 6,* 1–13.

Lazarus, R., & Folkman, S. (1984). *Stress, appraisal, and coping.* New York, NY: Springer.

LeFevre, M. L., Kolt, G. S., & Matheny, J. (2006). Eustress, distress and their interpretation in primary and secondary occupational stress management interventions: Which way first? *Journal of Managerial Psychology, 21*(6), 547–565. doi:10.1108/02683940610684391

LeFevre, M. L., Matheny, J., & Kolt, G. S. (2003). Eustress, distress, and interpretation in occupational stress. *Journal of Managerial Psychology, 18*(7), 726–744. doi:10.1108/02683940310502412

Lerner, D., Adler, D. A., Rogers, W. H., Chang, H., Lapitsky, L., McLaughlin, T., & Reed, J. (2010). Work performance of employees with depression: The impact of work stressors.

American Journal of Health Promotion, 24(3), 205–213. doi:10.4278/ajhp.090313-QUAN-103

Levin-Epstein, J. (2005). *Presenteeism and paid sick days.* Retrieved September 19, 2010, from http://www.clasp.org/publications/files/0212.pdf

Little, L., Simmons, B. L., & Nelson, D. L. (2007). Health among leaders: Positive and negative affect, engagement and burnout, forgiveness and revenge. *Journal of Management Studies, 44*(2), 243–260.

Lu, H., While, A. E., & Barriball, K. L. (2005). A model of job satisfaction of nurses: A reflection of nurses' working lives in Mainland China. *Journal of Advanced Nursing, 58*(5), 468–479.

Luthans, F. (2002). The need for and meaning of positive organizational behavior. *Journal of Organizational Behavior, 23,* 695–706.

Lyons, J., & Schneider, T. (2008). The effects of leadership style on stress outcomes. *The Leadership Quarterly, 20,* 737–748.

Lyons, N. (1983). Two perspectives on self, relationship, and morality. *Harvard Educational Review, 53,* 125–145.

Malouf, A. (2003). *In the name of identity: Violence and the need to belong.* New York, NY: Penguin Books.

Maslach, C., & Goldberg, J. (1998). Prevention of burnout: New perspectives. *Applied and Preventive Psychology, 7,* 63–74.

Maslach, C., & Jackson, S. E. (1981a). *The Maslach Burnout Inventory.* Palo Alto, CA: Consulting Psychologists Press.

Maslach. C., & Jackson, S. E. (1981b). The measurement of experienced burnout. *Journal of Occupational Behaviour, 2,* 99–113.

May, D., Chan, A., Hodges, T., & Avolio, B. J. (2003). Developing the moral component of authentic leadership. *Organizational Dynamics, 32*(3), 247–260.

Nakakris, K., & Ouzouni, C. (2008). Factors influencing stress and job satisfaction of nurses working in psychiatric units: A research review. *Health Science Journal, 2*(4), 183–195.

Nelson, D. L., & Cooper, C. L. (2007). *Positive organizational behavior.* London, England: Sage.

Nelson, D. L., & Simmons, B. L. (2003). Health psychology and work stress: A more positive approach. In J. Quick & L. Tetrick (Eds.), *Handbook of occupational health psychology* (pp. 97–119). Washington, DC: American Psychological Association.

Nelson, D. L., & Simmons, B. L. (2004). Eustress: An elusive construct, an engaging pursuit. In P. L. Perrewé & D. C. Ganster (Eds.), *Research in occupational health and well being: Emotional and physiological processes and positive intervention strategies* (Vol. 3, pp. 265–322). Oxford, UK: Elsevier.

Palumbo, M., Rambur, B., McIntosh, B., & Naud, S. (2010). RN's perception of health and safety and intention to leave. *American Association of Occupational Health Nursing Journal, 58*(3), 95–103.

Park, N., & Peterson, C. (2003). Virtues and organizations. In K. Cameron, J. Dutton, & R. Quinn (Eds.), *Positive organizational scholarship* (pp. 33–47). San Francisco, CA: Berrett-Koehler.

Porter-O'Grady, T., Alexander, D. R., Blaylock, J., Minkara, N., & Surel, D. (2006). Constructing a team model: Creating a foundation for evidence-based teams. *Nursing Administration Quarterly, 30*(3), 211–220.

Price, S. L. (2009). Becoming a nurse: A meta-study of early professional socialization and career choice in nursing. *Journal of Advanced Nursing, 65*(1), 11–19.

Quick, J., & Macik-Frey, M. (2007). Healthy productive work: Positive strength through communication competence and interpersonal interdependence. In D. Nelson & C. L. Cooper (Eds.), *Positive organizational behavior* (pp. 25–39). Thousand Oaks, CA: Sage.

Quick, J., Nelson, D. L., & Quick, J. (1990). *Stress and challenge at the top: The paradox of the successful executive.* Chichester, UK: John Wiley and Sons.

Quick, J., Quick, J., & Nelson, D. (1998). The theory of preventive stress management in organizations. In C. L. Cooper (Ed.), *Theories of organizational stress* (pp. 246–268). Oxford, UK: University Press.

Rambur, B., Vallett, C., Cohen, J., & Tarule, J. (2010). The moral cascade: Distress, eustress, and the virtuous organization. *Journal of Organizational Moral Psychology, 1*(1), 1–14.

Redman, B., & Hill, M. (1997). Studies of ethical conflicts by nursing practice settings or roles. *Western Journal of Nursing Research, 19,* 243–250.

Rest, J., Narvacz, D., Bebeau, M., & Thoma, S. (1999). *Postconventional moral thinking: A neo-Kohlbergian approach.* Mahway, NJ: Erlbaum.

Rice, V. H. (Ed.). (2000). *Handbook of stress, coping, and health: Implications for nursing research, theory, and practice.* Thousand Oaks, CA: Sage.

Rosenman, R., Friedman, M., Straus, R., Wurm, M., Kositchek, R., Hahn, W., & Werthessen, M. (1964). A predictive study of coronary heart disease. *Journal of the American Medical Association, 189,* 15–22.

Rundqvist, E., Sivonen K., & Delmar, C. (2010). Sources of caring in professional nursing: A review of current nursing literature. *International Journal for Human Caring, 14*(1), 36–43.

Rushton, C. (1992). Care-giver suffering in critical care nursing. *Heart and Lung, 21,* 303–306.

Schluter, J., Winch, S., Holzhauser, K., & Henderson, A. (2008). Nurses' moral sensitivity and hospital ethical climate: A literature review. *Nursing Ethics, 15*(3), 304–321.

Seligman, M., & Csikszentmihalyi, M. (2000). Positive psychology. *American Psychologist, 55*(1), 5–14.

Selye, H. (1956). *The stress of life.* New York, NY: McGraw-Hill.

Selye, H. (1976). *Stress in health and disease.* Oxford, UK: Butterworths.

Selye, H. (1987). *Stress without distress.* London, England: Transworld.

Senge, P., Scharmer, C., Jaworski, J., & Flowers, B. (2004). *Presence: An exploration of profound change in people, organizations, and society.* New York, NY: Doubleday.

Sherman, A. C., Edwards, D., Simonton, S., & Mehta, P. (2006). Caregiver stress and burnout in an oncology unit. *Palliation Support Care, 4*(1), 65–80.

Simmons, B. L., Gooty, J., Nelson, D., & Little, L. (2009). Secure attachment: Implications for hope, trust, burnout, and performance. *Journal of Organizational Behavior, 30*(2), 233–247.

Simmons, B. L., & Nelson, D. L. (2001). Eustress at work: The relationship between hope and health in hospital nurses. *Health Care Management Review, 26,* 7–18.

Simmons, B. L., & Nelson, D. L. (2007). Eustress at work: Extending the holistic stress model. In D. L. Nelson & C. L. Cooper (Eds.), *Positive organizational behavior* (pp. 40–53). Thousand Oaks, CA: Sage.

Simmons, B. L., Nelson, D. L., & Neal, L. (2001). A comparison of positive and negative work attitudes of home healthcare and hospital nurses. *Health Care Management Review, 26,* 64–75.

Simmons, B. L., Nelson, D. L., & Quick, J. C. (2003). Health for the hopeful: A study of attachment behavior in home health care nurses. *International Journal of Stress Management, 10,* 361–371.

Skagert, K., Delive, L., Edlof, M., Pousetts, A., & Albourg, G. (2008). Leaders' strategies for dealing with own and their subordinates' stress in public human service organizations. *Applied Ergonomics, 39,* 803–811.

Spector, P. (1998). A control theory of the job stress process. In C. L. Cooper (Ed.), *Theories of organizational stress* (pp. 153–169). New York, NY: Oxford University Press.

Sporrong, S., Hoglund, A., & Arnetz, B. (2006). Measuring moral distress in pharmacy and clinical practice. *Nursing Ethics, 13*(4), 416–427.

Stewart, W., Matousek, D., & Verdon, C. (2003). *The American productivity audit and the campaign for work and health.* Hunt Valley, MD: The Center for Work and Health, Advanced PCS.

Sundin-Huard, D., & Fahy, K. (1999). Moral distress, advocacy, and burnout: Theorizing the relationships. *International Journal of Nursing Practice, 5,* 8–13.

Sutherland, V. J., & Cooper, C. L. (1990). *Understanding stress.* London, England: Chapman & Hall.

Szabo, S. (1998). Hans Selye and the development of the stress concept. Special reference to gastroduodenal ulcerogenesis. *Annals of the New York Academy of Sciences, 851,* 19–27.

Takase, M., Maude, P., & Manias, E. (2005). Comparison between nurses' professional needs and their perceptions of their jobs. *Australian Journal of Advanced Nursing, 23*(2) 28–33.

Trevino, L., & Brown, M. (2007). Ethical leadership: A developing construct. In D. L. Nelson & C. L. Cooper (Eds.), *Positive organizational behavior* (pp. 101–116). Thousand Oaks, CA: Sage.

Vallett, C. M. (2010). Organizational virtuousness and culture in continuing higher education. *Journal of Continuing Higher Education, 58,* 1–13.

van den Heuvel, S. G., Geuskens, G. A., Hooftman, W. E., Koppes, L. L., & van den Bossche, S. N. (2009). Productivity loss at work: Health-related and work-related factors. *Journal of Occupational Rehabilitation, 20*(3), 331–339. doi:10.1007/s10926–009–9219–7

Verhaeghe, R., Vlerick, P., Gemmel, P., Maele, G. V., & De Backer, G. D. (2006). Impact of recurrent changes in the work environment on nurses' psychological well-being and sickness absence. *Journal of Advanced Nursing, 56*(6), 646–656. doi:10.1111/j.1365–2648.2006.04058.x

Wang, J., Schmitz, N., Smailes, E., Sareen, J., & Patten, S. (2010). Workplace characteristics, depression, and health-related presenteeism in a general population sample. *Journal of Occupational and Environmental Medicine, 52*(8), 836–842. doi:10.1097/JOM.0b013e3181ed3d80

Weaver, G. (2006). Virtue in organizations: Moral identity as a foundation for moral agency. *Organization Studies, 27*(3), 341–368.

Weber, A., & Jaekel-Reinhard, A. (2000). Burnout syndrome: A disease of modern societies? *Occupational Medicine, 50*(7), 512–517.

Weberg, D. (2010, July–September). Transformational leadership and staff retention: An evidence review with implications for health care systems. *Nursing Administration Quarterly, 34*(3), 246–258.

Wilkinson, J. (1987). Moral distress in nursing practice: Experience and effect. *Nursing Forum, 23*(1), 16–29.

Williamson, G. J. (2000). The test of a nursing theory: A personal view. *Nursing Science Quarterly, 13,* 124–128.

Zander, M. A., Hutton, A. E., & King, L. A. (2010). Coping and resilience factors in pediatric oncology nurses CE. *Journal of Pediatric Oncology Nursing, 27*(2), 94–108.

PART V

STRESS, COPING, AND HEALTH: MEDIATING AND MODERATING FACTORS

13

Personality Constructs and the Stress Process

Matthew R. Sorenson and Barbara A. Harris

Patients with hypertension, gastrointestinal disease, or some other smooth muscle spasm . . . are likely to deny that they are nervous. This seems to be in part because these patients are universally afraid of their aggressive impulses. As already noted they are outstanding for the degree of their repressed or pent up hostility. (Dunbar, 1939)

Throughout history, personality has been considered a potential cause of illness. Certain personality types have been associated with the development of illness, conceivably through an inability to regulate emotion. In other words, some people are believed to be unable to cope effectively with negative emotions. The concept of personality is one that readily resonates in the study of stress and coping, and yet, the investigator is faced with a number of different conceptualizations and theoretical models. As well, the precise role of personality within investigations of stress and coping is oft debated.

Personality has been viewed as an intermediary factor located between stress appraisals and coping behaviors, a resistance factor influencing stress appraisal, or as a mediating influence impacting the selection and perceived effectiveness of coping styles. Regardless of the position that personality occupies within stress models, there are a number of related variables that

contribute to the relationship between personality and coping. Social, cultural, and biologic factors all contribute to the development of personality. Biological and genetic variables can affect the general responsiveness of the individual to environmental stimuli, and are considered by some to reflect temperament rather than personality (Connor-Smith & Flachsbart, 2007). A discussion of these influences is beyond the scope of this chapter, but demonstrates the potential influences on personality, and in turn, stress perceptions and coping responses.

The purpose of this chapter is to provide an overview of the personality constructs that play a role in investigations into stress and coping. Within this chapter, the phrase *stress process* will be used to describe the overall study of stress and coping and is used in reference to the multivariate nature of stress and coping. There are a number of theoretical approaches to personality constructs. For the purposes of this chapter, personality will be reviewed in its relationship to the main theories used in the study of stress and coping. They are psychodynamic approaches that include personality types and defense mechanisms and the cognitive–behavioral approach to stress and coping reflected in the transactional model (e.g., Lazarus & Folkman, 1984). Regardless of whether the world presents life events requiring a degree of adaption, stimuli necessitating a response or which forms part of a transactional relationship with the individual, personality dispositions play an important role in the stress process. A brief introduction to the major personality concepts involved in these processes follows.

Personality as Trait and State

Personality has primarily been studied within the field of stress and coping as either a trait or state. Trait elements are best considered as long-standing tendencies or predispositions. The individual who is quick to anger or to view events in a negative manner will most likely respond to life events with patterns of anger. A tendency to anger quickly (trait) could result in problems when confronted with an uncertain or novel situation (state). This approach is reflected in studies of personality and coping that investigate optimism, pessimism, narcissism, and other personality traits and patterns. While personality is most frequently considered a trait, there are situations that can influence aspects of the personality for only a brief period of time. Manifestations of anxiety or anger are emotional responses that can be considered as state elements of personality. Trait aspects of personality influence the rapidity with which such emotional states manifest themselves. A state could best be considered a temporary change or fluctuation in personality determined to some extent by underlying trait personality.

Trait dispositions then can be considered relatively stable factors influencing the likelihood of a particular personality state or emotional response appearing in a given situation. State personality factors may be viewed as those that arise from a particular situation. Coping studies investigating state dispositions often employ work settings, competitive challenges, testing situations, or emotional responses to a diagnostic finding.

State conceptualizations of personality are best viewed from the transactional perspective of stress. Elements of the environment interact with individual perceptions regarding factors within the environment, such as perceived controllability. The emotional and behavior responses of the individual are then, to a degree, dependent upon emerging perceptions of environmental stimuli. An example of how such elements are assessed in this research would be through the use of an instrument such as the State–Trait Personality Inventory. This well-known research tool examines for long-enduring dispositional personality traits, as well as transitory manifestations of anger, curiosity, anxiety, and depression. This provides information on the general approach an individual may take to life situations, and it also examines the manifestation of state responses to a particular environmental event.

Personality Constructs and the Stress Process

In general, personality can be defined as *an individualistic pattern of perception, emotion, and behavior that demonstrates temporal predictability.* In other words, personality could be considered the probability that a particular emotion or behavior occurs in response to stress-evoking stimuli. This pattern of perception, interpretation, and response influences the selection and utilization of select coping strategies and patterns. The exact role of personality within the stress process is debated. The differing theoretical approaches to the study of personality can locate personality in several places within coping models. It is then important to have a clear understanding of what personality constructs are being measured using a particular instrument or tool, and how the constructs are defined by the instrument.

Assumptions Underlying the Role of Personality

Several conceptual and theoretical assumptions underlie the perceived role of personality in the stress process. Psychodynamic models of personality emerged from psychoanalysis, with a different conceptualization of personality and its role in the process of stress and coping than cognitive–behavioral models. Such theoretical and conceptual differences become important in the attempt to locate personality within coping models and particularly in relation to measurement. One of the apparent difficulties investigating the role of personality in the stress process is the tendency for many personality and coping measures to focus on elements of psychopathology or negative health outcomes. Such investigative approaches neglect the potential positive role of dispositional traits in mediating or buffering stress appraisals.

A significant portion of daily cognition is pre-reflective, or occurring below the level of consciousness thought. The study of unconscious processes as aspects of personality is best reflected in the psychodynamic school. Psychodynamic theories evolved from psychoanalytic approaches and reflect elements of the self that occur reflexively. Using psychodynamic theories as concepts within the study of stress and coping that include investigation of defense mechanisms and dispositional elements of the personality that predispose one to behaving in a particular fashion. Type A through Type D personality types, or styles, would be an example of such baseline dispositions. One of the most frequently employed means of examining psychodynamic approaches is through a conceptual grouping of five personality styles referred to as the Big Five.

Assumptions underlying psychodynamic approaches include the belief that unconsciousness mechanisms mediate behavioral responses and actions. Another assumption would be one of causality. Psychodynamic theories place more weight on the conceptualization of psychic causality. In brief, the adage, "all behavior has meaning" would reflect this assumption. In short, behavioral responses are not random but reflect the underlying personality, motives, and desires of the individual. The cognitive–behavioral approach is perhaps best reflected in the study of stress and coping using the transactional model of Lazarus and Folkman (1984). The model presumes a base appraisal that is influenced by experiential factors and mediated by conscious cognition and decision making. A major assumption of this approach is the role of emotion in the selection of coping strategies. (See Chapter 9 in this text.)

As identified above, stress and coping have long been conceptualized as distinct human experiences and processes. Recent theorizing suggests that a fruitful direction for stress and coping investigations is to understand both stress and coping as integral aspects of the psychology of human behavior (Costa, Somerfield, & McCrae, 1996), specifically, how stable or enduring dimensions are an individual's way of perceiving and responding to the experience of stress and efforts to cope. Implicit in this perspective is that traits that are stable and enduring in one individual are different from those traits that are stable and enduring in another; the study of personality has been called the study of individual differences (Carver & Connor-Smith, 2010). This is fundamentally different from studies of stress and coping that focus on particular experiences or populations to determine sources of distress, mediators, and effective methods of coping across experiences and populations.

Hardiness and Resilience

The idea of personality variables that protect or buffer the individual from stress has often been investigated in the field of nursing and medicine. The general approach has been to examine whether a particular personality construct such as hardiness or resilience is associated with levels of stress or the development of adverse consequences. The concept of resilience implies experience with a stressor, to determine if an individual is resilient, there should be an outcome associated with the evaluation. Indeed, certain definitions of resilience see the concept more as an outcome itself, in that the individual who is able to weather a stressful situation in a more positive manner than others would be viewed as resilient (Zautra, Hall, & Murrary, 2010). The majority of current studies appear more focused on identifying factors associated with resilience, rather than determining end effects. An additional caveat is that the term *resilience* can refer to physiologic responsiveness as well as psychosocial. Here, the focus is on a discussion of psychosocial resilience.

While the physiologic vulnerability of the individual can play a role in terms of a propensity to develop stress, there are certain personality factors which also affect the stress process. A potential antecedent or moderating factor in the relationship between stress and physical health status is the possibility of dispositional personality aspects that may serve to protect the individual from the effects of stress (Kobasa, 1979). Such personality aspects are viewed as protecting the individual through the effects on cognitive appraisal processes of the individual, thus influencing event perception (Florian, Mikulincer, & Taubman, 1995; Ouellette, 1993).

Hardiness

The concept of hardiness has been referred to as "a constellation of personality characteristics that function as a resistance resource in the encounter with stressful life events" (Kobasa,

Maddi, & Kahn, 1982, p. 169). The personality characteristics referred to are the factors—or dimensions of—commitment, control, and challenge. *Commitment* was conceptualized as the tendency of the individual to become engaged or involved in an event and exhibiting a sense of purpose or of meaning. *Control* referred to an internal locus of control and the belief that the presenting stimulus event can be managed. *Challenge* is conceptually similar to the Lazarus and Folkman (1984) viewpoint of challenge as a belief that life presents certain opportunities and the event may be viewed as stimulating or exciting, rather than as a threat (Kobasa, 1979; Ouellette, 1993).

The original research of hardiness involved business executives. While certain subjects were found to experience a high degree of stress, they did not evidence a correspondingly high degree of illness, while other subjects did. The difference between those subjects experiencing the lower incidence of illness was the presence of a degree of hardiness that appeared to protect these individuals from illness (Kobasa, 1979). A follow-up study supported these findings, demonstrating that the presence of a high degree of hardiness, or a hardy personality, could decrease the likelihood of illness in relation to stressful life events (Kobasa, Maddi, & Puccetti, 1982). There have been critiques of the hardiness concept. Such dispositional aspects of personality

may be difficult to operationally define and measure (Benishek, 1997; Ouellette, 1993). Also, one variable may have more significance than another, particularly with study populations different from the original one of business executives. Commitment has been found positively related to control, even while challenge negatively correlated with both control and commitment (Hull, Van Treuren, & Virnelli, 1987). This led to a recommendation that investigators avoid investigation of challenge and instead focus on commitment and control (Hull et al., 1987). Levels of commitment and control alone have been found to predict mental health through influence upon appraisal and the selection of coping strategies (Florian et al., 1995).

Measuring Hardiness

There are several instruments available for the measurement of hardiness (see Table 13.1). Most of these measures have origins in the hardiness questionnaire initially developed by Kobasa (1979). That scale was a composite measure employing items derived from four other scales that evaluated the conceptual dimensions (challenge, control, commitment) of hardiness. In general, the various versions of the Hardiness Scale have demonstrated reliability within acceptable ranges. Factor analyses have generally supported the construct, although findings vary

Table 13.1 Recent Instruments Used in the Assessment of Hardiness

Instrument	Number of items	Format	Primary construct	Subscales/factors
Family Hardiness Index	20 items	Likert format with summation of scores	Family hardiness	1) Co-oriented commitment 2) Challenge 3) Control 4) Confidence
Health-Related Hardiness Scale	Several versions 34 items 40 items 42 items 48 items 50 items	Likert format (1–6)	Hardiness	1) Challenge/commitment 2) Control
Personal Views Survey	50 items	Likert format (1–6)	Hardiness	1) Challenge 2) Control 3) Commitment

between a two or three factor solution (Ouellette, 2003).

The Health-Related Hardiness (HRH) Scale was developed to measure the presence of hardiness in the chronically ill and is based on Pollock's theoretical definition of hardiness (Pollock, 1986, 1989). The scale built on the work of Maddi and Kobasa (1991) with the inclusion of additional items reflecting control (Wallston, Maides, & Wallston, 1978). While there are several versions of the HRH scale, each has demonstrated homogeneity and stable reliability. Support has been found for convergent validity (Pollock & Duffy, 1990).

One of the more common measures is the Personal Views Survey, derived from the original work of Kobasa and integrated with other work done by the research team of Maddi and Kobasa. The 50-item instrument has demonstrated homogeneity and stability reliability, with construct validity supported by factor analysis (Maddi, Harvey, Khoshaba, Fazel, & Resurreccion, 2009).

While it is has been speculated that the hardiness concept does not display the initial promise or robustness expected, the concept continues to hold appeal. Recent studies tend to investigate particular aspects of the concept, or see research with select populations. Research tools have been developed that examine specific aspects of the concept, or reformulate the concept of hardiness, such as with the Courage to Challenge Scale developed to study elements of personal hardiness within the gay and lesbian population (Smith & Gray, 2009). Such studies reformulated the concept and advanced research through research of specific personality elements that may contribute to stress resistance. It has also been speculated that early measures of hardiness were negatively worded, which could lead to conceptual confusion with elements of neuroticism. Modifying instrument items into positively worded items has been found to be helpful in distinguishing elements of hardiness from other personality constructs (Sinclair & Tetrick, 2000).

Resilience

Psychological resilience is a concept similar to hardiness, in that elements of personality work in concert to either buffer stress appraisal or lessen the occurrence of adverse consequences. Some of the initial work on resilience actually incorporated the hardiness concept. The construct appears to have grown from early work on the stress process that demonstrated that characteristics of stress-evoking situations alone are not sufficient to produce a state of illness or pathology. The search then began for elements of personality that either placed the individual at increased risk or served to protect individuals from adverse consequences of stress. Often conceptualizations of resilience include more physiologic variables or parameters than other personality approaches. Resilience has also been studied more extensively in child populations than many of the other personality constructs.

Measuring Resilience

While there are several tools available to measure resilience, the investigator needs to be aware of the apparent interdependency between many resilience measures and the concept of hardiness. Many of the existent resilience measures were based on the work of Kobasa on hardiness and reflect a potential confounding of concepts. For a list of recent measures, see Table 13.2. The Dispositional Resilience Scale reflects the original work of Kobasa on hardiness, but it is believed to represent a refinement of the concept. Three versions of the measure are available, the original 45-item version along with a 15- and 30-item version. Homogeneity reliability has been demonstrated and construct validity determined through principal components factor analysis (Bartone, Ursano, Wright, & Ingraham, 1989).

The Connor-Davidson Resilience Scale (CD-RISC) attempts to distinguish levels of resilience, providing a quantifiable measure of resilience. The scale comprises 25 items and uses a 5-point Likert scale. Homogeneity and stability reliability scores are appropriate and convergent validity established through comparison with other research instruments (Connor & Davidson, 2003). The Resilience Scale (RS) conceptualizes resilience as a positive personality characteristic enhancing adaptation. Originally derived from qualitative work, the instrument has 26 items. Homogeneity and stability reliability have been demonstrated, with convergent validity having been found with other measures of resilience (Wagnild & Young, 1993). The Baruth Protective Factors Inventory (BPFI) is a 16-item instrument designed to investigate elements of resilience within the individual. Unlike many of the other measures, it does not have origins within the

Table 13.2   Instruments Employed in Recent Investigations Into Resilience

Instrument	Number of items	Format	Primary construct	Subscales/factors
The Baruth Protective Factors Inventory	16 items	Likert 5 point	Resilience with four identified factors	1) Adaptable personality 2) Supportive environment 3) Fewer stressors 4) Compensating experiences
The Connor-Davidson Resilience Scale (2003)	10 items 25 items	Likert (0–4)	Hardiness with elements of goal setting and meaning	Five broadly defined factors
The Dispositional Resilience Scale	15 items 30 items 45 items	Likert	Hardiness	1) Challenge 2) Control 3) Commitment
The Resilience Scale	26 items	Likert (1–7)	Resilience	Personal competence and acceptance of self
The Resilience Scale for Adults	32 items	Likert 5 point	Adult resilience	1) Personal competence 2) Social competence 3) Personal structure 4) Family cohesion 5) Social resources

original work of Kobasa; instead, the instrument was based upon a review of the literature which identified four protective factors as being associated with resilience. These are the factors evaluated by the BPFI. Homogeneity reliability has been demonstrated and support found for construct validity (Baruth & Carroll, 2002).

The Resilience Scale for Adults (RSA) was developed to address perceived limitations in other instruments that the developers felt targeted more toward an adolescent population. The instrument was developed to provide appropriate questions for adults and to include elements of social support. As conceptualized, resilience is comprised of three major dimensions: dispositional attributes, family cohesion, and external support. Support has been found for homogeneity reliability and convergent validity (Friborg, Hjemdal, Rosenvinge, & Martinussen, 2003).

The concept of resiliency integrates other personality variables. The resilient individual is one more likely to engage in problem-oriented coping, exhibit higher levels of perceived control, and display higher levels of altruism along with increased positive emotionality (Southwick, Vythilingam, & Charney, 2005). These factors together appear to interact in such a way as to buffer the individual from stress. This demonstrates the multivariate nature of concepts such as resilience and hardiness, that the constructs are composed of several elements working synergistically to protect the individual. It is then important to investigate other personality constructs and biologic variables in concert in order to gain a complete picture of resilience.

PERSONALITY TRAIT AND TYPE MODELS

Five Factor Models

A trait can be defined as a distinguishing characteristic or quality. As early as the 1930s, researchers in psychology were identifying groups of characteristics in efforts to isolate factors, or traits, which accounted for individual differences in personality. One of the approaches used in studying personality was the lexical approach that assumes that important human phenomena are reflected in a language's frequently used words and, specifically, in adjectives. This approach provided the foundation for later factor analysis research that led to the emergence of factor models of personality.

The two predominant models of personality are referred to as the Big Five (BF) and the Five Factor Model (FFM). These models have considerable overlap and the five factors, or traits, are often used interchangeably in the psychological, sociological, and health care literature (Connor-Smith & Flachsbart, 2007). In this chapter, the phrase *Five Factor Model* will be used to reference both models. When discussing the model, the term *trait* is used, while *factor* is used to refer to a trait when discussing instruments used to measure them. It is noteworthy that the lexical approach to personality type and factor analysis has resulted in models grounded in empirics, not theory. This has been identified as a weakness of these models (Block, 2010) but progress has been made in extending the empirically based knowledge of the FFM to personality theory (McCrae & Costa, 1996). It has been suggested the FFM serves as the most generalizable and sound model of personality currently available (Gill & Hodgkinson, 2007).

The FFM includes the following traits: (a) *Neuroticism* reflecting the ease and frequency with which a person becomes upset or distressed. Experiences of anxiety or depressed mood are conceptualized to reflect higher levels of neuroticism (Carver & Connor-Smith, 2010); (b) *Extraversion,* defined as sociability, cheerfulness, or liveliness, is a concept frequently found in the psychological literature and other personality models; thus, it can be subject to differences in definition and measurement. Its counterpart in the Big Five model is *surgency;* (c) *Agreeableness* relates to trusting, altruistic, and empathic behavior and is considered to be the opposite of antagonistic, hostile, or oppositional behavior; (d) *Openness* to experience involves curiosity, imagination, and willingness to seek atypical experience. It is the trait over which there is the most disagreement. Because it can overlap with definitions of intellect, some feel that it belongs in the cognitive rather than psychological domain (Digman, 1996); and (e) *Conscientiousness* reflects valuation and use of purposeful activity, responsible and goal-directed behavior, as well as reliability and control of impulses (Carver & Connor-Smith). The traits are comprised of lower-order facet traits, which provide a more detailed picture of the trait (Bagby, Selby, Costa, & Widiger, 2008).

Measuring the Five Factor Model

The FFM was originally measured with the NEO-PI (Gill & Hodgkinson, 2007). Developed by Costa and McCrae (1985), the NEO-PI has been used extensively. NEO is an acronym for the three personality traits that Costa and McCrae originally identified: *Neuroticism, Extraversion,* and *Openness,* respectively. The NEO-PI was developed when the researchers added two factors, *Conscientiousness* and *Agreeableness,* where PI stands for Personality Inventory. There are multiple versions of the NEO-PI that are currently in use; choice of version depends on study population and study design. Both self-report and observer-report versions of the NEO-PI-3 are available. Empirical findings show that the personality constructs of the FFM are relatively stable within individuals over time and across cultures (Connor-Smith & Flachsbart, 2007).

The Five Factor Model and Coping

The FFM is often employed in stress and coping research. (See Table 13.3 for an overview of the research discussed here.) In some studies, specific subscales of the NEO-PI are used to tap one or two of the five traits. The traits most often studied in relation to stress and coping are neuroticism and extraversion. Neuroticism has long been considered to be a negative trait that, because of high emotionality and low tolerance for stimuli, will impact an individual's perceptions of stressors and choice of coping strategy or effectiveness of the strategy chosen. Another of the five factors, conscientiousness, has been thought to benefit efforts to cope with chronic illness because facets of the trait, such as purposeful and goal-directed behavior and low impulsivity, may foster adherence to treatment and active participation in care, with resulting improved health outcomes. Other studies cast a broader net, evaluating the association between coping and all five personality traits, looking for patterns of association between traits and coping

Table 13.3   Selected Studies Using the Five Factor Model and Three Factor Models in Relation to Stress and Coping Outcomes

Author	Construct/ instrument	Theoretical framework	Sample	Significant findings
O'Cleirigh, Ironson, Weiss, & Costa (2007)	Five Factor Model: conscientiousness/ NEO-FFI	Five Factor Model	HIV positive adults ($n = 119$)	Conscientiousness predicted significant increases in CD4 numbers and was related positively to medication adherence.
Robinson & Marwit (2006)	Three Factor Model/EPQ	Psychodynamic	138 women, after death of child	Neuroticism was a significant predictor of grief intensity.
Aarstad, Aarstad, & Olofsson (2008)	Three Factor Model/EPQ	Transactional model of stress and coping	Cancer patients ($n = 55$)	High neuroticism predicted lower quality of life.
Gunzerath, Connelly, Albert, & Knebel (2001)	NEO-FFI	No specific framework	Adults with α-1-antitrypsin deficiency ($n = 76$)	Less neuroticism and higher extraversion correlated with higher quality of life.
Burgess, Irvine, & Wallymahmed (2010)	NEO-PI-R	Transactional model of stress and coping	Critical care nurses ($n = 46$)	Conscientiousness negatively correlated with workload/ time pressure. Agreeableness was positively correlated with active coping.

styles. Others have focused on nurses, studying the relationship between personality traits and perceptions of stress in the workplace and related coping activities.

The FFM has also been useful in illuminating the stress and coping process related to transcultural experience, looking for ways to predict acculturative stress and ways to manage and prevent it (Mangold, Veraza, Kinkler, & Kinney, 2007). Interestingly, Duru and Poyrazli (2007) found that Openness to experience was unexpectedly found to be predictive of stress. The authors suggest that this may be because high levels of openness to experience can lead to increased encounters with non-native cultures, which can be a source of stress. This finding points out how much is still not known about the exact nature of personality traits and the complexity of their relationship with processes such as stress and coping and culture.

Some of the traits from the FFM have been linked to a newer concept in the psychosocial literature. Posttraumatic growth is a concept that focuses on the potential for positive growth as a result of trauma. Shiekh (2008) reviewed recent literature to illuminate variables associated with posttraumatic growth. She identified four of the five traits from the FFM to be consistently associated with posttraumatic growth: extraversion, openness to experience, agreeableness, and conscientiousness. Neuroticism is the only trait that has been negatively associated with posttraumatic growth, which is consistent with findings of other studies discussed above.

Three Factor Model

Eysenck and Eysenck's (1975) Three Factor Model is also a trait model of personality, although not used as frequently as the Five Factor Model. While there are parallels between this model and the Five Factor Model, there are principal differences that have maintained a conceptual separation between them. Possibly the biggest difference between the models is the issue of intellective and nonintellective traits; in the Three Factor Model, intellect-based traits are not considered personality traits. It has been argued that openness to experience in the FFM model does contain intellective dimensions (Carver & Connor-Smith, 2010). In addition, in the Three Factor Model, the FFM traits of Agreeableness and Conscientiousness are combined into one trait, (absence of) Psychoticism (Digman, 1996), so that the three factors are *Neuroticism, Extraversion,* and *Psychoticism.* The Eysenck Personality Questionnaire (EPQ) was the original measure of the Three Factor Model, consisting of 90 yes–no questions (Eysenck & Eysenck, 1975). A revised form, EPQR-S, can be found in some studies of personality and coping (Eysenck, Eysenck, & Barrett, 1985).

Temperament and Personality

Temperament is similar to personality and can be defined as *patterns of thoughts, feelings, and behaviors that persist over time and situations and is generally considered to apply to children and/or those whose behavioral repertoires have not yet been substantially shaped by interaction with environment* (Connor-Smith & Flachsbart, 2007). In contrast, the definition of personality contains these elements as well as characteristics, qualities, and traits that have developed over time and through experience. There are a number of constructs that describe temperament relevant to coping. Most can be classified as manifestations of the human need to self-regulate (Carver & Connor-Smith, 2010). These include approach-avoidance (Elliot & Thrash, 2010), positive and negative emotionality (Lengua & Long, 2002), and effortful control (Rothbart & Rueda, 2005). The majority of studies investigating temperament and coping involve child or adolescent populations.

Cloninger's (1987) model of personality focused on temperament and character, conceptualizing the two as contributing to personality, the former by being heritable, stable, and present in the young, the latter by contributing individual differences that develop through life experience (Fossati et al., 2007). Cloninger focused on the physiological bases of individual difference, generating a psychobiological theory of personality grounded in information from family studies and long-term developmental and neuroanatomical studies of learning. While Cloninger's original model contained three factors and was measured by the Tridimensional Personality Questionnaire (TPQ), Cloninger's (1994) revised model of personality contains seven domains of personality and is measured by the Temperament and Character Inventory (TCI) (see Table 13.4).

Table 13.4   Selected Studies Using Type D Personality and Stress and Coping Outcomes

Author	Construct/ instrument	Theoretical framework	Sample	Significant findings
Carless, Douglas, Fox, & McKenna (2006)	TCI	Psychobiological theory of personality	Cardiac patients ($n = 81$)	Those with low self-directed and high harm-avoidance domain scores were significantly more likely to report depression.
Gil & Caspi (2006)	TPQ	Transactional model of stress and coping	College undergraduates ($n = 180$)	Higher levels of harm avoidance significantly increased PTSD risk.
Mols, Holterhues, Nijsten, & van de Poll-Franse (2010)	Type D/DS14	Type D	Melanoma survivors ($n = 699$)	Type Ds reported significantly worse general health and mental health.
Williams, O'Carroll, & O'Connor (2009)	Type D/DS14	Type D; psychophysiology	Male adults ($n = 84$)	Significant effect of Type D on cardiac output in men.

Personality Types A and D

The Type A personality, or Type A Behavior Pattern (TABP), was the first composite of characteristics to be specifically developed as a pattern associated with risk for disease. Since then, the health care literature contains work related to Types B, C, D, R, and S. The TABP, characterized by urgency, hostility, impatience, time-consciousness, competitive attitude, and aggressive behavior, was empirically related to risk for cardiovascular disease, though recent studies have yielded inconsistent results, leading to decreased use of this construct (Spindler, Kruse, Zwisler, & Pedersen, 2009). The TABP can still be found in studies of coping-related topics, though its relevance in this area is not well established. See Alarcon, Eschleman & Bowling's (2009) meta-analysis of research on personality types and burn-out for further information and discussion.

Much of current research on personality types investigates a cluster of personality constructs referred to as Type D. Type D, the Distressed Personality, is defined as the interlocking effects of negative affectivity and high social inhibition (Mols, Holterhues, Nijsten, & van de Poll-Franse, 2010). Negative affectivity indicates a tendency to experience negative emotions; social inhibition refers to a pattern of not expressing emotion related to fears of others' disapproval. While Type D was developed to explore cardiovascular risk factors, it has been investigated in populations without cardiac disease. There is good evidence to suggest that Type D holds potential to inform the study of coping. A meta-analysis by Alarcon et al. (2009) found the negative affectivity dimension of Type D to explain significant variance in the relationship between personality and burn-out. Another systematic review (Mols & Denollett, 2010) highlighted the role of Type D as a vulnerability factor associated with poor mental and physical outcomes, and poor self-management of disease. Other studies, presented in Table 13.4, identify physical reactions to stress and behaviors related to negative coping associated with Type D.

Narcissism and Optimism

Narcissism

Narcissism is often defined as a personality trait or construct that involves self-centeredness, inflated sense of self, arrogance, entitlement, and hypersensitivity to criticism as well as difficulty empathizing with others (Kelsey, Ornduff, Reiff, & Arthur, 2002; Rhodewalt & Morf, 1995). While Kelsey et al. (2002) pointed out that narcissism can encompass positive personality dimensions such as assertiveness and self-sufficiency, it is most often conceptualized as a construct that carries significant potential for maladaptive behavior and psychopathology. However, it is considered a normally distributed personality trait (Cisek, Hart, & Sedikides, 2008) and may hold positive potential for an individual's general health (Sekides, Rudich, Gregg, Kumashiro, & Rusbult, 2004) and management of stress (Taylor, Lerner, Sherman, Sage, & McDowell, 2003).

Measurement of Narcissism

The Narcissistic Personality Inventory (NPI) (Raskin & Terry, 1988) is most often used in investigations in which narcissism is considered a personality dimension that may be impacting another psychosocial process such as coping. The NPI is based on the definition of narcissism in the Diagnostic and Statistical Manual of Mental Disorders, 3rd edition. Narcissism in the NPI is measured as a trait along a continuum so it is able to capture narcissistic traits that fall short of what could be identified as pathological expression (Sekides et al., 2004). There are several other instruments that have been used to measure narcissism, although they are grounded in the assumption that narcissism is pathological, including the O'Brien Multiphasic Narcissism Inventory, Narcissistic Personality Dimension, and others. (For more information, see Baron, Reznikoff, and Glenwick, 1992.) The usefulness of these instruments among nonclinical populations is limited.

Narcissism as a Stress Mediator

The role narcissism plays in the mediation of stressors is still unclear. Kelsey et al. (2001) found significant relationship between high scores on the NPI and biophysiologic indicators of stress. Sedikides et al. (2004) found relationships between narcissism and factors related to stress in a series of studies on normal narcissism and psychological variables. Of note is their finding that self-esteem fully mediated the relationship between narcissism and subjective well-being and other variables such as satisfaction with life and daily sadness, pointing out that it may be the self-esteem component of narcissism that is beneficial to psychological health.

Optimism

Dispositional optimism refers to an individual's tendency to expect that situations will result in positive outcomes. The tendency toward optimism is conceptualized as stable across both time and context, hence the use of the term, "dispositional" (Scheier & Carver, 1985). Optimism is considered an important personal difference prominent in the coping literature. It does not fit cleanly into factor models of personality, but it still reflects a general disposition, rather than a specific response to a situation (Carver & Connor-Smith, 2010).

An issue in the discussion of optimism and coping is the overlap between optimism and other psychological resources such as hope (Aspinwall & Leaf, 2002). Hope is addressed elsewhere in this text but is of interest here as it shares characteristics with dispositional optimism and, like that construct, can be described as an enduring pattern of identifiable behaviors accompanied by "trait-like emotional sets or moods" (Snyder, 2002, p. 253). Hope theory and the Dispositional Hope Scale are centered on motivation and beliefs about personal agency, while other conceptualizations of hope are anchored in affect or emotion (Roesch & Vaughn, 2006; Snyder, 2002). Both hope and optimism start with similar basic assumptions that human behavior is goal-directed and that the value of a goal and confidence about reaching it keep individuals motivated to move toward it. The point of departure lies in the source of motivation (Carver & Connor-Smith, 2010). For optimism, motivation can arise from confidence that an outcome will be attained one way or another, while motivation in hope theory is anchored more in belief that personal agency will facilitate goal attainment. It has been suggested that optimism is more reflective of actual human experience (Carver & Connor-Smith, 2010). A researcher working with personality dispositions and coping may need to determine which construct best fits his or her theoretical framework.

Measuring Optimism

The Life Orientation Test (LOT) is grounded in a goal-based model of human behavior, which is concerned with human approach and avoidance (Scheier & Carver, 1985). Understanding what individuals approach and avoid and why (values) is relevant to coping as there is usually a decision to be made regarding something unpleasant or harmful if there is a need to cope. Optimism, or how likely an individual believes a positive outcome will be, then, could be an influential shaper of actions in coping situations. The Attributional Style Questionnaire (ASQ) is an additional instrument available to measure optimism. It is grounded in the reformulated learned helplessness model and based upon the assumption that individuals make characteristic assessments of events that have three dimensions: stable–unstable, internal–external, global–local (Seligman, Abramson, Semmel, & von Baeyer, 1979). As the title of the instrument suggests, it is a measure of attributional style. While *attributions* imply cognitive processes, *style* implies behavior patterns or disposition toward behavior patterns. Gordon (2008) differentiated between the LOT and ASQ, suggesting the LOT measures expectations regarding likelihood of outcomes while the ASQ measures an individual's method of explaining outcomes. While optimism is not considered a personality trait from this perspective, it does reflect a stable style of explaining situations or a disposition to explain outcomes in a certain way.

Dispositional Optimism and Coping

There are multiple benefits of dispositional optimism to be accrued in coping according to recent conceptual and empirical work, such as greater resilience during stress experiences or a stress buffering effect. Majer, Jason, Ferrari, Olson, and North (2003) provided empirical confirmation of others' findings in the area of substance abuse recovery that optimism is positively related to a sense of abstinence self-efficacy, where abstinence self-efficacy is defined as confidence in one's ability to resist the urge to use drugs or alcohol. Others have studied the impact of dispositional optimism on experiences of specific disease states, including breast cancer, risk of cardiovascular death, and birth weight. Matthews and Cook's (2009) study of the impact of optimism and other variables on women's emotional well-being during treatment for breast cancer is notable as it is one of only a few that integrate nursing theory into the research; Reed's (1991) concept of self-transcendence is operationalized and studied to determine its impact on emotional well-being along with optimism.

Can Optimism Be Learned?

There is relatively little empirical study of the origins of optimism. In a review of existing research, Gillham and Reivich (2007) concluded a combination of genetics and environmental influences predispose an individual toward optimistic thinking. This conclusion led to an endorsement of future studies on means of cultivating optimism in children and young adults. Martin Seligman (1991) turned his theorizing away from learned helplessness and toward learned optimism, asserting that the understanding that has been gained by studying learned helplessness can be used to assist individuals to cultivate optimism. According to Seligman, optimistic people are better achievers, are better able to resist depression, and are often more physically healthy. While optimism and pessimism generally remain constant throughout a person's life, they can be changed enough so that individuals can reap more of the benefits of optimism. Key to this change is learning a new set of cognitive skills.

Optimistic Bias

The existence of optimistic bias is fairly well established. It is defined as a tendency to see others as more at risk than oneself and has also been called "unrealistic optimism" or "comparative optimism" (Harris, Griffin, & Murrary, 2008; Klein & Helweg-Larsen, 2002). Weinstein's work with unrealistic optimism is usually considered the starting point for studies of human tendencies to believe one to be less at risk than others in similar situations (Weinstein & Lachendro, 1982). It has been suggested that optimistic bias is an illusion that plays a role in psychological well-being, that all individuals hold illusions about events and situations that allow them to function or thrive (Harris et al.,

2008). Some findings suggest this can be protective (Gupta & Bonnano, 2010), in a manner similar to the self-enhancing cognitions common to narcissistic perspectives discussed above. On the other hand, unrealistic optimism can contribute to denial and defensiveness, which can be detrimental to effective problem solving, communication, and relationship building (Henselmens et al., 2009).

Optimistic bias itself is influenced by a number of factors, including degree of perceived controllability (Klein & Helweg-Larsen, 2002), the size of the target group the individual is comparing self with (Price, Smith, & Lench, 2006), and accountability demands, or how an individual believes he or she will be perceived on the basis of the optimistic estimates that he or she has made (Tyler & Rosier, 2009). The method of measuring optimistic bias can also influence the actual measurement. It is generally agreed that the direct method of measuring optimistic bias yields a greater degree of bias (Harris et al., 2008; Klein & Helweg-Larsen, 2002). Direct assessment occurs when an individual makes one comparative risk assessment of the likelihood she or he will experience a future event relative to someone else's likelihood of experiencing the same, whereas indirect assessment occurs when the individual makes two assessments: one regarding his or her likelihood of experiencing an event and separate estimate of another experiencing the same event in the future (Borkenau & Mauer, 2006). See selected studies that have measured optimism, stress, and coping outcomes in Table 13.5.

CONTROL CONSTRUCTS AND PERSONALITY

The multiplicity of theories, concepts, and instruments related to control attest to its centrality in human experience. Similarly, in the area of stress and coping, the use of multiple theoretical frameworks and instruments to study the mediating and moderating effects of control constructs on coping speaks to the importance of control in the coping process. In this section, the focus is narrowed to control constructs that can be conceptualized as dispositions or personality components and that have influence as mediators or moderators of stress and coping.

Table 13.5   Selected Studies Using Measures of Optimism and Stress and Coping Outcomes

Author	Construct/instrument	Theoretical framework	Sample	Significant findings
Baldwin, Kennedy, & Armata (2008)	Dispositional optimism/ LOT	Self-regulation	37 mothers	High optimists reported greater resiliency than low optimists.
Matthews & Cook (2009)	Dispositional optimism/ LOT	Self-regulation (Reed's theory of self-transcendence in nursing is used for one variable)	93 women receiving radiation therapy for breast cancer	Optimism related to emotional well-being.
Grote, Bledsoe, Larkin, Lemay, & Brown (2007)	Dispositional optimism/ LOT	Risk/protection framework	194 financially disadvantaged women	Optimism accounted for significant amount of variance in depressed mood.

Locus of Control

One of the first formal conceptualizations of control was the Locus of Control (LOC) Theory (Rotter, 1966), a concept that has displayed great heuristic value. Working within Social Learning Theory, a spotlight was placed on the importance of individuals' beliefs or expectations about the nature of control within the life context. Locus of control is a global construct focused on internal versus external control of reinforcement, or the degree to which individuals expect that an outcome or reinforcement of their behavior is contingent on personal characteristics or actions (internal) or the result of (external) forces outside of one's control (Rotter, 1966, 1990). What individuals believe and perceive about their own and others' abilities can be important predictors of behavior. To the extent that those beliefs are stable across situations and over time, sense of control is dispositional. What individuals believe or perceive about others in health care situations can likewise be important predictors of health outcome or coping style in health care situations. However, there is the question as to whether LOC related to health, or Health Locus of Control (HLOC), is dispositional or better conceptualized as a state construct.

Health Locus of Control

The construct of HLOC grew out of dual findings that perceptions of control were central to experience of illness, health care treatment, and patient response but that LOC was not a reliable predictor of health-related behavior and thus, that measurement of health LOC required more than a unidimensional scale (Wallston et al., 1978). The Multiple Health Locus of Control Scale (MHLC) developed by Wallston et al. is one of the most widely used measures of LOC in health care. The development of the MHLC-C and its subsequent popularity imply that HLOC may be better conceptualized as a state, not a trait, coping resource. The broad range of difference in illness manifestations and experiences indicated that individuals with a given condition might have different control beliefs than would individuals with another condition (Wallston et al., 1978). Further, as LOC is designed to be predictive and predictions are more useful at the level of specific situations, measures of control beliefs need to move from the general to the specific (Wallhagen, 1998). In addition, while studies using the MHLC-C may tap an individual's dispositional sense of control, that is usually not the information useful in health care situations; instead, the focus is on how an individual perceives a current health situation and how this can assist in predicting relevant health behaviors. As is the case with many of the personality constructs in this chapter, predictive ability is generally good, while usefulness in planning specific intervention or grounding research for evidence-based practice is more difficult.

Perceived Control

LOC, and subsequently HLOC, signaled the beginning of a trend to differentiate between actual control exerted and an individual's beliefs about the control one has. Many of the control-related concepts developed since then have made this focus explicit. Central to these concepts is the understanding that the perception of control can influence motivation, choice of behavior, and execution of behavior, and that these influences are distinct from actual control available to be exerted. Perceived control is also a global concept, backed by findings that an individual's sense of personal control can remain fairly steady through situations and across time (Steptoe & Wardle, 2001).

Other seminal sources of perceived control constructs include Ajzen's (2002) theory of planned behavior, in which perceived control is comprised of beliefs about an individual's control over behavior and their perceptions of what may help or hinder a desired behavior. According to the theory, perceived control contributes to the individual's intention to perform a behavior. Because Ajzen maps out the process of planned behavior from pre-execution beliefs through execution of behavior, the theory has been useful in health care as a way to predict behavior. It has been considered by some to be more effective than LOC or HLOC for this purpose because it can be easily applied to specific situations (Bodde & Van Puymbroeck, 2010). However, Jacelon (2007), in a theoretically based review of the literature on perceived control, notes that a number of studies using Ajzen's theory do not evidence a rationale for the instrument they use to measure perceived control; nor is there any trend or pattern in choice of instrument for use with this framework. A number of instruments have been used to measure perceived control.

Measures of Control

A search of the Health and Psychosocial Instruments database for 1997 to 2010, using the terms "perceived control" and "perceived controllability," yielded 13 different instruments, with no discernible trend among the more frequently used instruments in regard to compatibility with a theoretical framework. Many of the instruments were used only in one or two studies (Jacelon, 2007). The construct of perceived control is at times considered interchangeable with other concepts and is positioned differently from study to study in regard to relationship with other control constructs. For example, in a study of the predictive power of variables on level of distress in women undergoing treatment for breast cancer, personal control and mastery were used interchangeably with a conclusion that "personal control over life, or mastery, constitutes the belief that life is not ruled by fate but that one is personally able to influence the outcomes of important events or situations" (Henselmans et al., 2010, p. 161). There is also a degree of conceptual confusion among perceived control and related concepts. (See Jacelon, 2007, for further discussion.) Rodgers, Conner, and Murray (2008) also identified conceptual confusion and overlap between perceived control and self-efficacy. Girard and Murray (2010) suggest that this lack of conceptual clarity may be one of the reasons behind their finding that a small sample of nurses in a cardiac intervention unit were very open to using the concept of perceived control to guide patient education but had never done so and had little idea on how to do so.

Exploring the nature of the relationship of these constructs is potentially productive, as Mossbarger (2009) illustrated. He suggested that perceived control combined with desire for control gives rise to the construct of personal control. Perceived and desired control are orthogonal concepts, where the degree of congruence between them has more predictive power than either concept alone. Perceived control is defined by Mossbarger as a "cognitive interpretation that outcomes are contingent upon behavior" (p. 25) whereas desired control has been defined as an internal motivation to control one's environment.

Desire for Control

Desire for control (DC) is a construct researched in the social sciences and health care and reflects internal motivation in relation to the environment. It may derive conceptual roots from the work of Alfred Adler, who suggested that an individual's innate desire to demonstrate competency and superiority with and over life events is a primary motivational force (Mossbarger, 2009). The concept was first operationalized with the development of the Desirability of Control Scale (Burger & Cooper,

1979). Early findings using this scale suggested that DC might be innate and varies in intensity or degree from individual to individual, thus prompting social scientists to view DC as an individual difference, or dispositional variable (Mossbarger, 2009). Desire to control the environment is considered a cultural difference in some frameworks (Astin et al., 1999; Giger & Davidhizar, 2002).

Measuring Desire for Control

The Desire for Control Scale (DCS) was developed to measure the level of motivation individuals have to control the events in their lives (Burger & Cooper, 1979). A review of studies using the DCS noted there are few available measures to evaluate DC and most are adaptations of the DCS (Gebhardt & Brosschot, 2002). The review also noted there is a lack of conceptual clarity regarding components of desire for control. The items in the current DCS measure several domains: desire to make own decisions, avoiding situations where one is not in control, desire to act so that situations do not become out of control, and the desire to control others. However, Gebhardt and Brosschot noted that different samples yielded different solutions to factor analysis, leading them to conclude that more work is needed to determine the subdimensions of the DCS.

The Shapiro Control Inventory (SCI) (Shapiro, 1994) has also been used to measure desire for control. The SCI has been in use for over two decades and has been used on a variety of populations (Astin et al., 1999). Surgenor, Horn, and Hudson (2003), studying the relationship between control and anorexia nervosa, used the SCI because it has multiple scales. They note that the subscales measure several dimensions of desire for psychological control, including control over self, others, and environment. It also taps components of desire for control such as how important being in control is to the individual, how fearful one is of losing control, and how hard one will work to maintain control. Thus, the SCI may be a choice for researchers delving into phenomena where manifestations of control are complex and integral to the illness experience. Desire for control has been studied in other areas where control is a central component of an illness phenomenon, such as addictions (Fieulaine & Martinez, 2010). Other studies that measure DC tend to focus on psychosocial phenomena related to illness experiences, such as loss of control over quality of life or quality of experience. As with perceived control, some of the measures of desired control are specific to a health care setting or situation. This would be a state measure of desire for control, as opposed to a trait measure. For example, Logan, Baron, Keeley, Law, and Stein (1991) derived an instrument from the DCS that was specific to dental procedures and found that high desire for control exacerbated distress when low control was anticipated, suggesting that the health care practitioner's knowledge of the level of the patient's desire for control may help him or her anticipate specific needs in coping.

Mastery

Mastery is a construct often used interchangeably with perceived control. It is defined as a personal resource, or an aspect of self, that mediates or moderates the impact of stressors (Avison & Cairney, 2003; Turner & Lloyd, 1999). It involves a sense of personal control, or more specifically, a mental representation about one's ability to control and influence life events that protects against the stressful effects of such events (Hinnen, Ranchor, Baas, Sanderman, & Hagedoorn, 2009; Pearlin, 1989). By definition, mastery is a control construct more specific to stress and coping than other control constructs (Pearlin, Nguyen, Schieman, & Milkie, 2007). Mastery is not a fixed personality state, but rather it is a self-concept that implies a sense of constancy that can change in response to experience. It would follow, then, that an individual's sense of mastery may also change depending upon the coping context one is confronting and that it can develop and change over a lifetime (Pearlin et al., 2007). In addition, in a review of the literature, a theme emerged that was termed the "social malleability of mastery" (Avison & Cairney, 2003). That is, an individual's social position may "condition the development of psychosocial resources that enable individuals to cope with such stressors" (Avison & Cairney, 2003, p. 147). Thus, the construct of mastery is continuing to develop in response to knowledge generated.

Mastery Scale

There are few options for measuring mastery. Pearlin and Schooler's (1978) Mastery Scale has been the most often used tool in the psychological and health care literature. There are, however, a large number of studies of coping within health care settings that focus on the role of mastery; some use adaptations of the Mastery Scale. Rationale is often not given regarding instrument adaptation.

Mastery in Health Care

In the health care literature, mastery has been studied in regard to coping with the impact of various conditions and disease states. One theme in the research is understanding the protective effect that mastery, as a psychosocial resource, can provide in regard to stressors such as economic hardship (Caputo, 2003; Pudrovsa, Schieman, Pearlin, & Nguyen, 2005). Majer, Jason, Ferrari, Olson, and North (2003) raised an interesting issue in an exploration of the relationship between self-mastery, optimism, and abstinence self-efficacy (Majer et al., 2003). They found that their sample of recovering substance abusers showed a significant negative correlation between self-mastery and both optimism, and abstinence self-efficacy. They suggest that the Alcoholics Anonymous/12-step culture with principles of surrender and powerlessness may influence sense of or valuation of mastery in individuals in this sample. An area of recent research is the role of mastery in mediating the stress of partners and caregivers of individuals diagnosed with serious, life-threatening, or degenerative diseases. While Carter and Acton (2006) found that a caregiver's sense of mastery can influence their risk of depression, other work found breast cancer patients' sense of mastery can influence their perception of the helpfulness of spouse effort to assist with coping (Hinnen et al., 2009). Another research theme is looking at mastery as a mediator of pain/stress in serious illness such as cancer (Byma, Given, Given, & Mei, 2009). Mastery is also relevant in studies of coping needs related to normal, developmental stressors, such as aging, showing that mastery can impact levels of physical activity (Cairney, Faulkner, Veldhuizen, & Wade, 2009).

CONCLUSION

We know now that many physiologic processes which are of profound significance for health . . . can be controlled by the

emotions . . . yet, we have scarcely begun to use what we know. We lack perspective concerning our knowledge in this field and are confused in our concepts. (Dunbar, 1954, p. vii)

The above quote prefaced a text on psychosomatic changes, but it still relates to the study of personality, stress, and coping. Several personality concepts are interrelated and often indistinguishable from one another. Hardiness has been used a basis for the development of resilience measures, but it is currently considered a subconcept under resilience. For other personality constructs there may be several operational and theoretical definitions to choose from, and often one can find a lack of congruence in studies between the theoretical conceptualizations underlying an instrument and the intended theoretical perspective of the study. Parceling out the statistical influence of one particular construct from another can be difficult and, in the end, account for little variance.

In spite of these issues, the significance of personality constructs in the stress process is apparent, and studies incorporating personality constructs have made significant contributions in understanding the complex role of personality. Hope, perceived control, self-efficacy, and the like are all personality constructs that impact the study of stress process and have received recent attention. New conceptualizations of older concepts are emerging, and evidence is being found to support cross-cultural stability of personality constructs.

Future investigations would benefit from longitudinal designs and further investigation into the development of state personality. Much of the existent research on personality and coping has tended to examine aspects of personality or reactive coping strategies. Reactive strategies are those that occur in response to a particular situation. These strategies may be very different from those personality aspects that could activate anticipatory or proactive means of coping. Hardiness and resilience are comprised of several personality constructs that can aid in anticipatory/proactive coping. Many of these personality constructs have predictive value, and future research will hopefully shed greater light on the role personality has prior to encounters with stressful stimuli. This is an area in which nursing is well posed to make a contribution to the literature. Finding ways to assist patients to anticipate aspects of the stress response and to have coping strategies at the ready can be an effective way to promote self-care and enhance wellness. There is much potential to use the information in this chapter to inform nursing practice. However, there is little research that can readily be applied to evidence-based practice.

Evidence-Based Practice and Personality

Unfortunately, few interventional studies have been conducted using personality constructs in relation to the stress process. Clinical trials have begun investigating the effectiveness of interventions on personality constructs (Jain et al., 2007), but these are few and far between. The majority of the existent research demonstrates the predictive nature of personality constructs. Perhaps further examination of personality constructs can generate a set of characteristics that clinicians can use to aid patients as they negotiate the stress of illness, injury, or uncertainty.

References

Aarstad, K. H., Aarstad, H. J., & Olofsson, J. (2008). Personality and choice of coping predict quality of life in head and neck cancer patients during follow-up. *Acta Ontologica, 47,* 879–890.

Ajzen, I. (2002). Perceived behavioral control, self-efficacy, locus of control, and the theory of planned behavior. *Journal of Applied Social Psychology, 32*(4), 665–683.

Alarcon, G., Eschleman, K. J., & Bowling, N. A. (2009). Relationships between personality variables and burnout: A meta-analysis. *Work and Stress, 23*(3), 244–263.

Aspinwall, L. G., & Leaf, S. L. (2002). In search of the unique aspects of hope: Pinning our hopes on positive emotions, future-oriented thinking, hard times, and other people. *Psychology Inquiry, 13*(4), 276–321.

Astin, J. A., Anton-Culver, H., Schwartz, C. E., Shapiro, D. H., McQuade, J., Breuer, A., . . . Kurosaki, T. (1999). Sense of control and adjustment to breast cancer: The importance of balancing control coping styles. *Behavioral Medicine, 25*(3), 101–109.

Avison, W. R., & Cairney, J. (2003). Social structure, stress, and personal control. Personal control in social and life course contexts. In S. H. Zarit, L. I. Pearlin, & K. W. Schaie (Eds.), *Societal impact on aging* (pp. 127–164). New York, NY: Springer.

Bagby, M. R., Selby, M., Costa, P. T., & Widiger, T. A. (2008). Predicting Diagnostic and Statistical Manual of Mental Disorders-IV personality disorders with the five-factor model of personality and the personality psychopathology five. *Personality and Mental Health, 2,* 55–69.

Baldwin, D. R., Kennedy, D. L., & Armata, P. (2008). Short communication: De-stressing mommy: Ameliorative association with dispositional optimism and resiliency. *Stress and Health, 24,* 393–400.

Baron, L., Reznikoff, M., & Glenwick, D. S. (1992). Narcissism, interpersonal adjustment and coping in children of Holocaust survivors. *Journal of Psychology, 127,* 257–269.

Bartone, P. T., Ursano, R. J., Wright, K. M., & Ingraham, L. H. (1989). The impact of a military air disaster on the health of assistance workers. A prospective study. *Journal of Nervous and Mental Disease, 177*(6), 317–328.

Baruth, K. E., & Carroll, J. J. (2002). A formal assessment of resilience: The Baruth protective factors inventory. *The Journal of Individual Psychology, 58*(3), 235–244.

Benishek, L. A. (1997). Critical evaluation of hardiness theory: Gender differences, perception of life events, and neuroticism. *Work Stress, 11,* 33–45.

Block, J. (2010). The five-factor framing of personality and beyond: Some ruminations. *Psychological Inquiry, 21,* 2–25.

Bodde, A. E., & Van Puymbroeck, M. (2010). Reviewing theoretical foundations of perceived control: Application to health behaviors of adults with intellectual disabilities. *Annual in Therapeutic Recreation, 18,* 131–140.

Borkenau, P., & Mauer, N. (2006). Personality, emotionality, and risk prediction. *Journal of Individual Differences, 27*(3), 127–135.

Burger, J. M., & Cooper, H. M. (1979). The desirability of control. *Motivation and Emotion,* 381–393.

Burgess, L., Irvine, F., & Wallymahmed, A. (2010). Personality, stress, and coping in intensive care nurses: A descriptive, exploratory study. *Nursing in Critical Care, 15*(3), 129–140.

Byma, E. A., Given, B. A., Given, C. W., & Mei, Y. (2009). The effects of mastery on fatigue and pain resolution. *Oncology Nursing Forum, 36*(5), 544–552.

Cairney, J., Faulkner, G., Veldhuizen, S., & Wade, T. J. (2009). Changes over time in physical activity and psychological distress among older adults. *The Canadian Journal of Psychiatry, 54*(3), 160–169.

Caputo, R. K. (2003). The effects of socioeconomic status, perceived discrimination and mastery on health status in a youth cohort. *Social Work in Health Care, 37*(2), 17–42.

Carless, D., Douglas, K., Fox, K., & McKenna, J. (2006). An alternative view of psychological well-being in cardiac rehabilitation: Considering temperament and character. *European Journal of Cardiovascular Nursing, 5,* 237–243.

Carter, P. A., & Acton, G. J. (2006, February). Personality and coping: Predictors of depression and sleep problems among caregivers of individuals who have cancer. *Journal of Gerontological Nursing, 32*(2), 45–53.

Carver, C. S., & Connor-Smith, J. (2010). Personality and coping. *Annual Review of Psychology, 61,* 679–704.

Cloninger, C.R. (1987). A systematic method for clinical description and classification of personality variants. *Archives of General Psychiatry, 44,* 573–588.

Cloninger, C. R. (1994). *The Temperament and Character Inventory (TCI): A guide to its development and use.* St. Louis, MO: Center for Psychobiology of Personality.

Cisek, S. Z., Hart, C. M., & Sedikides, C. (2008). Do narcissists use material possessions as a primary buffer against pain? *Psychological Inquiry, 19,* 205–207.

Connor, K. M., & Davidson, J. R. (2003). Development of a new resilience scale: The Connor-Davidson Resilience Scale (CD-RISC). *Depression and Anxiety, 18*(2), 76–82.

Connor-Smith, J. K., & Flachsbart, C. (2007). Relations between personality and coping: A meta-analysis. *Journal of Personality and Social Psychology, 93*(6), 1080–1107.

Costa, P. T., & McCrae, R. R. (1985). *The NEO Personality Inventory Manual.* Odessa, FL: Psychological Assessment Resources, Inc.

Costa, P. T., Jr., Somerfield, M. R., & McCrae, R. R. (1996). Personality and coping: A reconceptualization. In M. Zeidner & N. S. Endler (Eds.), *Handbook of coping: Theory, research, applications* (pp. 44–61). New York, NY: Wiley.

Digman, J. M. (1996). The curious history of the five-factor model. In J. S. Wiggins (Ed.), *The five-factor model of personality* (pp. 1–20). New York, NY: Guilford.

Dunbar, F. (1939). Character and symptom formation—some preliminary notes with special reference to patients with hypertensive, rheumatic and coronary disease. *The Psychoanalytic Quarterly, 8,* 18–47.

Dunbar, F. (1954). *Emotions and bodily changes: Section One* (4th ed.). New York, NY: Columbia University.

Duru, E., &, Poyrazli, S. (2007). Personality dimensions, psychosocial-demographic variables, and English language competency in predicting level of acculturative stress among Turkish international students. *International Journal of Stress Management, 14*(1), 99–110.

Elliot, A. J., & Thrash, T. M. (2010). Approach and avoidance temperament as basic dimensions of personality. *Journal of Personality, 78*(3), 865–906.

Eysenck, H. J., & Eysenck, S. B. (1975). *Manul of the Eysenck Personality Questionnaire.* London, England: Hodder & Stoughton.

Eysenck, H. J., Eysenck, S. B., & Barrett, P. (1985). A revised version of the psychoticism scale. *Personality and Individual Differences, 6,* 21–29.

Fieulaine, N., & Martinez, F. (2010). Time under control: Time perspective and desire for control in substance abuse. *Addictive Behaviors, 35,* 799–802.

Florian, V., Mikulincer, M., & Taubman, O. (1995). Does hardiness contribute to mental health during a stressful real-life situation? The roles of appraisal and coping. *Journal of Personality and Social Psychology, 68,* 687–695.

Fossati, A., Cloninger, R. C., Villa, D., Borroni, S., Grazioli, F., Giarolli, L., . . . Maffei, C. (2007). Reliability and validity of the Italian version of the Temperament and Character Inventory–Revised in an outpatient sample. *Comprehensive Psychiatry, 48,* 330–387.

Friborg, O., Hjemdal, O., Rosenvinge, J. H., & Martinussen, M. (2003). A new rating scale for adult resilience: what are the central protective resources behind healthy adjustment? *International Journal of Methods in Psychiatric Research, 12*(2), 65–76.

Gebhardt, W. A., & Brosschot, J. F. (2002). Desirability of control: Psychometric properties and relationships with locus of control, personality, coping, and mental and somatic complains in three Dutch samples. *European Journal of Personality, 16,* 423–438.

Giger, J. N., & Davidhizar, R. (2002). The Giger and Davidhizar transcultural assessment model. *Journal of Transcultural Nursing, 13,* 185–188.

Gil, S., & Caspi, Y. (2006). Personality traits, coping style, and perceived threat as predictors of posttraumatic stress disorder after exposure to a terrorist attack: A prospective study. *Psychosomatic Medicine, 68,* 904–909.

Gill, C. M., & Hodgkinson, G. P. (2007). Development and validation of the five-factor model questionnaire (FFMQ): An adjectival-based personality inventory for use in occupational settings. *Personnel Psychology, 60*(3), 731–766.

Gillham, J., & Reivich, K. (2007). Cultivating optimism in childhood and adolescence. In A. Monat, R. S. Lazarus, & G. Reevy (Eds.),

The Praeger handbook on stress and coping (Vol. 2, pp. 309–326). Westport, CT: Praeger Publishers/Greenwood Publishing Group

Girard, B. R., & Murray, T. (2010). Perceived control: A construct to guide patient education. *Canadian Journal of Cardiovascular Nursing, 20*(3), 18–26.

Gordon, R. A. (2008). Attributional style and athletic performance: Strategic optimism and defensive pessimism. *Psychology of Sport and Exercise, 9,* 336–350.

Grote, N. K., Bledsoe, S. E., Larkin, J., Lemay, E. P. & Brown, C. (2007). Stress exposure and depression in disadvantaged women: The protective effects of optimism and perceived control. *Social Work Research 31*(1), 19–33.

Gunzerath, L., Connelly, B., Albert, P., & Knebel, A. (2001). Relationship of personality traits and coping strategies to quality of life in patients with alpha-1 antitrypsin deficiency. *Psychology, Health and Medicine, 6*(3), 335–341.

Gupta, S., & Bonnano, G. A. (2010). Trait self-enhancement as a buffer against potentially traumatic events: A prospective study. *Psychological Trauma: Theory, Research, Practice, and Policy, 2*(2), 83–92.

Harris, P. R., Griffin, D. W., & Murrary, S. (2008). Testing the limits of optimistic bias: Event and person moderators in a multilevel framework. *Journal of Personality and Social Psychology, 95*(5), 1225–1237.

Henselmans, I., Helgeson, V. S., Seltman, S., de Vries, J., Sanderman, R., & Ranchor, A. V. (2010). Identification and prediction of distress trajectories in the first year after a breast cancer diagnosis. *Health Psychology, 29*(2), 160–168.

Henselmens, I., Sanderman, R., Helgeson, V. S., de Vries, J., Smink, A., & Ranchor, A. V. (2009). Personal control over the cure of breast cancer: Adaptiveness, underlying beliefs and correlates. *Psycho-Oncology, 19,* 525–534.

Hinnen, C., Ranchor, A. V., Baas, P. C., Sanderman, R., & Hagedoorn, M. (2009). Partner support and distress in women with breast cancer: The role of patients' awareness of support and level of mastery. *Psychology and Health, 24*(4), 439–455.

Hull, J., Van Treuren, R., & Virnelli, S. (1987). Hardiness and health: A critique and alternative approach. *Journal of Personality and Social Psychology, 53*(3), 518–530.

Jacelon, C. S. (2007). Theoretical perspectives of perceived control in older adults: A selective review of the literature. *Journal of Advanced Nursing, 59*(1), 1–10.

Jain, S., Shapiro, S. L., Swanick, S., Roesch, S. C., Mills, P. J., Bell, I., & Schwartz, G. (2007). A randomized controlled trial of mindfulness meditation versus relaxation training: Effects on distress, positive states of mind, rumination, and distraction. *Annals of Behavioral Medicine, 33*(1), 11–21.

Kelsey, R. M., Ornduff, S. R., Reiff, S., & Arthur, C. M. (2002). Psychophysiological correlates of narcissistic traits in women during active coping. *Psychophysiology, 39,* 322–332.

Klein, C. T. F., & Helweg-Larsen, M. (2002). Perceived control and the optimistic bias: A meta-analytic review. *Psychology and Health, 17*(4), 437–446.

Kobasa, S. C. (1979). Stressful life events, personality, and health: An inquiry into hardiness. *Journal of Personality and Social Psychology, 37*(1), 1–11.

Kobasa, S. C., Maddi, S. R., & Kahn, S. (1982). Hardiness and health: A prospective study. *Journal of Personality and Social Psychology, 42*(1), 168–177.

Kobasa, S. C., Maddi, S. R., & Puccetti, M. C. (1982). Personality and exercise as buffers in the stress-illness relationship. *Journal of Behavioral Medicine, 5*(4), 391–404.

Lazarus, R. S., & Folkman, S. (1984). *Stress, appraisal, and coping.* New York, NY: Springer.

Lengua, L. J., & Long, A. C. (2002). The role of emotionality and self-regulation in the appraisal-coping process: Tests of direct and moderating effects. *Journal of Applied Developmental Psychology, 23*(4), 471–493.

Logan, H. L., Baron, R. S., Keeley, K., Law, A., & Stein, S. (1991). Desired control and felt control as mediators of Stress in a dental setting. *Health Psychology, 10*(5), 352–359.

Maddi, S. R., & Kobasa, S. C. (1991). The development of hardiness. In A. Monat & R. S. Lazarus (Eds.), *Stress and coping: An anthology* (pp. 245–257). New York, NY: Columbia University Press.

Maddi, S. R., Harvey, R. H., Khoshaba, D. M., Fazel, M., & Resurreccion, N. (2009). The Personality Construct of Hardiness–IV: Expressed in positive cognitions and emotions concerning oneself and developmentally relevant activities. *Journal of Humanistic Psychology, 49*(3), 292–305.

Majer, J. M., Jason, L. A., Ferrari, J. R., Olson, B. D., & North, C. S. (2003). Is self-mastery always a helpful resource? Coping with paradoxical findings in relation to optimism and abstinence self-efficacy. *The American Journal of Drug and Alcohol Abuse, 29*(2), 385–399.

Mangold, D. L., Veraza, R., Kinkler, L., & Kinney, N. A. (2007). Neuroticism predicts acculturative stress in Mexican American college students. *Hispanic Journal of Behavioral Sciences 29*(3), 366–379.

Matthews, E. E., & Cook, P. F. (2009). Relationships among optimism, well-being, self-transcendence, coping, and social support in women during treatment for breast cancer. *Psycho-Oncology, 18*, 716–726.

Mols, F., & Denollet, J. (2010). Type D personality among noncardiovascular patient populations: A systematic review. *General Hospital Psychiatry, 32*(1), 66–72.

Mols, F., Holterhues, C., Nijsten, T., & van de Poll-Franse, L. V. (2010). Personality is associated with health status and impact of cancer among melanoma survivors. *European Journal of Cancer, 46*(3), 573–580.

Mossbarger, R. (2009). The "fit" model of personal control and well-being in younger and older adults. *Journal of Adult Development, 16*, 25–30.

McCrae, R. R., & Costa, P. T. (1996). Social consequences of experiential openness. *Psychology Bulletin, 120*, 323–337.

O'Cleirigh, C., Ironson, G., Weiss, A., & Costa, P. T. (2007). Conscientiousness predicts disease progression (CD4 Number and Viral Load) in people living with HIV. *Health Psychology, 26*(4), 473–580.

Ouellette, S. C. (1993). Inquiries into hardiness. In L. Goldberg & S. Breznitz (Eds.), *Handbook of stess: Theoretical and clinical aspects* (2nd ed., pp. 77–100). New York, NY: Free Press.

Pearlin, L. I. (1989). The sociological study of stress. *Journal of Health and Social Behavior, 30*, 241–256.

Pearlin, L. I., Nguyen, K., Schieman, S., & Milkie, M. A. (2007). The life-course origins of mastery among older people. *Journal of Health and Social Behavior, 48*(2), 164–179.

Pearlin, L. I., & Schooler, C. (1978). The structure of coping. *Journal of Health and Social Behavior, 19*(1), 2–21.

Pollock, S. (1986). Human responses to chronic illness: Physiologic and psychosocial adaptation. *Nursing Research, 35*(2), 90–96.

Pollock, S. (1989). The hardiness characteristic: A motivating factor in adaptation. *Advances in Nursing Science, 11*(2), 53–62.

Pollock, S., & Duffy, M. E. (1990). The health-related hardiness scale: Development and psychometric analysis. *Nursing Research, 39*(4), 218–222.

Price, P. C., Smith, A. R., & Lench, H. C. (2006). The effect of target group size on risk judgements and comparative Optimism: The more, the riskier. *Journal of Personality and Social Psychology, 90*(3), 382–398.

Pudrovsa, T., Schieman, S., Pearlin, L. I., & Nguyen, K. (2005). The sense of mastery as a mediator and moderator in the association between economic hardship and health in late life. *Journal of Aging and Health, 17*, 634–660.

Raskin, R., & Terry, H. (1988). A principal-components analysis of the Narcissistic Personality Inventory and further evidence of its construct validity. *Journal of Personality and Social Psychology, 54*(5), 890–902.

Reed, P. (1991). Toward a nursing theory of self-transcendence: Deductive reformulation using developmental theories. *Advances in Nursing Science, 13*(4), 64–77.

Rhodewalt, F., & Morf, C. C. (1995). Self and interpersonal correlates of the Narcissistic Personality Inventory: A review and new findings [electronic version]. *Journal of Research in Personality, 29*(1), 1–23.

Robinson, T., & Marwit, S. J. (2006). An investigation of the relationship of personality, coping and grief intensity among bereaved mothers. *Death Studies, 30*, 677–696.

Rodgers, W. M., Conner, M., & Murray, T. C. (2008). Distinguishing among perceived control, perceived difficulty, and self-efficacy as determinants of intentions and behaviors. *British Journal of Social Psychology, 47*, 607–630. doi:10.1348/014466607X248903

Roesch, S. C., & Vaughn, A. A. (2006). Evidence for the factorial validity of the dispositional hope scale. *European Journal of Psychological Assessment, 22*(2), 78–84.

Rothbart, M. K., & Rueda, M. R. (2005). The development of effortful control. In M. Ulrich, E. Awh, & S. Keele (Eds.), *Developing individuality in the human brain: A tribute to Michael I. Posner* (pp. 167–188). Washington, DC: American Psychological Association.

Rotter, J. (1966). Generalized expectancies for internal versus external control of reinforcement. *Psychological Monographs, 80*(71), 1–28.

Rotter, J. (1990). Internal versus external control of reinforcement: A case history of a variable. *American Psychologist, 45*(4), 489–493.

Scheier, M. F., & Carver, C. S. (1985). Optimism, coping, and health: assessment and implications of generalized outcome expectancies. *Health Psychology, 4*(3), 219–247.

Sekides, C., Rudich, E. A., Gregg, A. P., Kumashiro, M., & Rusbult, C. (2004). Are normal narcissists psychologically healthy? Self-esteem matters. *Journal of Personality and Social Psychology, 87*(3), 400–416.

Seligman, M. E. (1991). *Learned optimism.* New York, NY: Alfred E. Knopf & Sons.

Seligman, M. E., Abramson, L. Y., Semmel, A., & von Baeyer, C. (1979). Depressive attributional style. *Journal of Abnormal Psychology, 88*(3), 242–247.

Shapiro, D. H. (1994). *Manual for the Shapiro Control Inventory* (SCI). Palo Alto, CA: Behaviordata.

Shiekh, A. (2008). Posttraumatic growth in trauma survivors: Implications for practice. *Counseling Psychology Quarterly, 2*(1), 85–97.

Sinclair, R. R., & Tetrick, L. E. (2000). Implications of item wording for hardiness structure, relation with neuroticism, and stress buffering. *Journal of Research in Personality, 43*(1), 1–25.

Smith, M. S., & Gray, S. W. (2009). The courage to challenge: A new measure of hardiness in LGBT adults. *Journal of Gay & Lesbian Social Services, 21*(1), 73–89.

Snyder, C. R. (2002). Hope theory: Rainbows in the mind. *Psychological Inquiry, 13*(4), 249–275.

Southwick, S., M., Vythilingam, M., & Charney, D. S. (2005). The psychobiology of depression and resilience to stress: Implications for prevention and treatment. *Annual Review of Clinical Psychology, 1*, 255–291.

Spindler, H., Kruse, C., Zwisler, A., & Pedersen, S. (2009). Increased anxiety and depression in Danish cardiac patients with a type D personality: Cross-validition of the type D scale (DS14). *International Journal of Behavioral Medicine, 16*, 98–107.

Steptoe, A., & Wardle, J. (2001). Locus of control and health behavior revisited: a multivariate analysis of young adults from 18 countries. *British Journal of Psychology, 92*, 659–672.

Surgenor, L. J., Horn, J., & Hudson, S. M. (2003). Empirical scrutiny of a familiar narrative: Sense of control in anorexia nervosa. *European Eating Disorders Review,11*, 291–305.

Taylor, S. E., Lerner, J. S., Sherman, D. K., Sage, R. M., & McDowell, N. K. (2003). Are self-enhancing cognitions associated with healthy or unhealthy biological profiles? *Journal of Personality and Social Psychology, 85*(4), 605–615.

Turner, R., & Lloyd, D. (1999). The stress process and the social distribution of depresson. *Journal of Health and Social Behavior, 40*(4), 374–404.

Tyler, J. M., & Rosier, J. G. (2009). Examining self-presentation as a motivation explanation for comparative optimism. *Journal of Personality and Social Psychology, 97*(4), 716–727.

Wagnild, G. M., & Young, H. M. (1993). Development and psychometric evaluation of the Resilience Scale. *Journal of Nursing Measurement, 1*, 165–178.

Wallhagen, M. I. (1998). Perceived control theory: A recontextualized perspective. *Journal of Clinical Geropsychology, 4*(2), 119–140.

Wallston, K., Maides, S., & Wallston, B. (1978). Health-related information seeking as a function of health-related locus of control and health value. *Journal of Research in Personality, 10*, 215–222.

Weinstein, N. D., & Lachendro, E. (1982). Egocentrism as a source of unrealistic optimism. *Personality and Social Psychology Bulletin, 8*(2), 195–200.

Williams, L., O'Carroll, R. E., & O'Connor, R. C. (2009). Type D personality and cardiac output in response to stress. *Psychology and Health, 24*(5), 489–500.

Zautra, A. J., Hall, J. S., & Murrary, K. E. (2010). Resilience: A new definition of health for people and communities. In J. W. Reich, A. J. Zautra, & J. S. Hall (Eds.), *Handbook of adult resilience* (pp. 3–29). New York, NY: Guilford.

14

SOCIAL SUPPORT

The Promise and the Reality

PATRICIA W. UNDERWOOD

Social support continues to be widely researched as both a moderator and mediator of stress. The inconsistencies in evidence supporting either mechanism are largely due to variability in both conceptualization and measurement. Nevertheless, both professional and lay groups continue to use support as part of interventions to enhance coping with stressful life events and health challenges. To further the science in this area, greater consistency in use of measurement tools and recognition of a broader framework in which social support may operate is necessary.

This chapter includes a discussion of the historical development of the conceptualization of social support and an examination of different models explaining the effect of the construct. Major tools to measure social support are compared, and selected research in nursing and related disciplines is reviewed. A model of the effect of social support components within the stress and coping framework is proposed.

HISTORICAL DEVELOPMENT

The attention to the role of social integration in health and well-being began as early as 1897 with Durkheim's (1938, 1897/1951) study linking suicide rates to decreased social ties. As a result of increasing industrialization and urbanization in the 1920s, attention was drawn to the negative effects of disruption of social networks and the loss of social integration (McKenzie, 1926; Park & Burgess, 1926; Thomas & Znaniecki, 1920). The concept of social support began to receive major attention in the 1970s, principally through the work of Antonovsky (1974, 1979); Caplan (1974); Cassel (1974, 1976); Cobb (1976); Kaplan, Cassel, and Gore (1977); and Weiss (1974) as they began to examine factors that could ameliorate the effects of negative life events.

In the 1980s, many researchers turned their attention to the conceptualization of social support and examination of the aspects that made a difference in coping with stress. Kahn and Antonucci (1980) were particularly interested in the role of social networks, whereas House (1981) examined the role of social support in coping with work stress and the saliency of various forms of support. Wortman (1984) was also interested in the components of social support that made a difference, particularly in coping with stressors such as cancer. In this regard, she built on earlier work focusing on the role of support groups for cancer patients (Dunkel-Schetter & Wortman, 1982). An inherent belief in the efficacy of support groups rather than a strong research base spurred their proliferation by both professionals and the public through-out the 1980s—a trend that has continued. Some researchers have examined the role of support groups more systematically for natu-rally occurring events such as bereavement (Stroebe, Stroebe, Abakoumkin, & Schut, 1996) and unnatural events such as rape (Coates & Winston, 1983).

Although nursing scientists were also inter-ested in the potential of social support to pro-mote postoperative recovery (Eisler, Wolfer, & Diers, 1972) and coping with birth complications (Nuckolls, Cassel, & Caplan, 1972), it was not until the 1980s that programs of research began, most notably with Brandt and Weinert (Brandt & Weinert 1981; Weinert, 1984, 1987, 1988; Weinert & Brandt, 1987), Norbeck (Norbeck & Anderson, 1989; Norbeck, Lindsey, & Carrieri, 1981, 1983), and Tilden (1983, 1984; Tilden & Gaylen, 1987), leading to the development of instruments to measure social support.

In the 1990s, Artinian (1991, 1992, 1993a), Graydon (Lee, Graydon, & Ross, 1991; Small & Graydon, 1993), and Stewart (Hirth & Stewart, 1994; Stewart, Hart, & Mann, 1995; Stewart, Ritchie, McGrath, Thompson, & Bruce, 1994) evidenced sustained research in the area of social support. The majority of researchers, however, incorporated social support as a critical variable in isolated studies examining health outcomes (Coffman, Levitt, & Deets, 1990; Ferketich & Mercer, 1990; McColl & Frieland; 1994; Willey & Silliman, 1990).

Major tool development was limited with two exceptions. Jalowiec (1993) included social support as a component of her studies that focused on the development of an instrument to assess coping. She suggested that the type of support used might affect the outcomes. Other researchers began to examine the type of sup-port needed in different situations and how needs might change during the course of an ill-ness. A study in the late 1980s (Nyamathi, 1987) had found that emotional support was needed in dealing with the diagnosis of a chronic illness, whereas more tangible help was important as the illness progressed. The other major tool development was associated with a large national study to investigate the effects of psychosocial intervention for cardiac patients. The ENRICHD Social Support Instrument (ESSI) was a short tool developed for use in the Enhancing Recovery in Coronary Heart Disease (ENRICHD) study.

CONCEPTUALIZATION AND MODEL DEVELOPMENT

Critical to any discussion of social support are the issues of conceptualization of the construct and consideration of the possible ways in which positive influence is exerted. Conceptualizations of social support have variously focused on the sources of support, the nature of what was pro-vided or available, and whether it functioned in a unidirectional or reciprocal manner. Conceptualizations have also varied according to whether social support is viewed as an objective quantity or more as a function of individual per-ception. Functional elements have included the perceived availability of support, what is received (perceived or observed), how much is provided, satisfaction with specific forms of support, or all these. Theoretical considerations have focused on mechanisms of influence, whether through the direct effect on an outcome or via moderating or mediating influences on other variables. These propositions have not always been clearly identi-fied nor consistently or appropriately evaluated from a statistical standpoint. The reciprocal nature of support and the cost incurred to obtain support are recent considerations in the social support literature.

Social support has been the primary focus in some studies but often is examined as one factor within a larger framework examining stress and coping. Within this context, it is frequently iden-tified as a resource for coping. If clinicians are to fully exploit the potential benefit of social sup-port as either a buffer from stress or a resource for coping with threatening or challenging phe-nomena, they must understand what social sup-port is and how it works. As has been amply demonstrated, simply increasing the number of studies that include social support is insufficient to provide the strong base needed for research-derived clinical interventions. Conceptual clar-ity is at the heart of the issue, and systematic testing of explicated components and their influence on other variables within a stress and coping framework is essential. Both the form and the source of social support should be included in any conceptualization.

Forms of Support

Lack of consistency and clarity of view has been the single greatest problem in advancing the development of social support as a coping resource. Numerous views have been advanced throughout the years, although most include components that reflect both physical and emotional assistance. A notable exception was that of Weiss (1974), who specified five dimensions: *attachment, social integration, nurturance, reassurance of worth,* and *reliable alliance with kin.* This conceptualization focused exclusively on emotional aspects of important relationships. Early on, Gottlieb (1978) added elements of physical intervention to the conceptualization of social support. His inductively derived categorization of the forms of support included emotionally sustaining behaviors, problem-solving behaviors, indirect personal influence, and environmental action.

Kahn (1979) and Kahn and Antonucci (1980) delineated three forms of social support: *aid* (direct assistance—things, money, and information), *affect* (expression of caring, respect, and love), and *affirmation* (acknowledgment of the appropriateness or rightness of acts or statements). Norbeck (1981, 1984) built on these dimensions in her research. House (1981) divided the dimension of aid into two components: instrumental or direct help and informational support. Affect and affirmation were labeled emotional and appraisal support, but they were conceptually the same. Wortman (1984) and Underwood (1986) added the form of listening. Barrera (1981) built on the work of Gottlieb and proposed a conceptualization that incorporated six elements with notable similarities to those of House (1981): material aid, physical assistance, intimate interaction, guidance, feedback, and social participation. Although the preponderance of conceptualizations has evolved deductively, inductive approaches have gained recent recognition. Gottlieb used qualitative methods to better understand support from the experiences of both cancer patients who were undergoing radiotherapy and their families (Hinds & Moyer, 1997). Three forms of social support were identified: being there (physically, emotionally, and spiritually), giving help, and giving information and advice. These findings helped confirm deductively derived conceptualizations.

Lugton (1997) also used qualitative approaches to examine the meaning of social support to women treated for breast cancer. The women needed support to make the diagnosis appear less threatening and to assist in maintaining or changing their identities. Humor, defining abnormality, companionship, and peer comparison were forms of support designed to decrease perception of threat. Six forms of support were important to maintaining or changing identity: emotional support, companionship, practical help, opportunity for confiding, experiential support, and sexual identity support. Previously proposed elements of emotional, affirmational, and informational support and direct help were reflected in this conceptualization. Within these conceptualizations of social support, forms were not tied to sources. Diamond (1979) stressed the importance of differentiating forms and sources of support to increase the consistency of findings across studies. Delineation of forms of support and their differentiation from sources is also important to answering the question of whether social support is a unidimensional or multidimensional resource. The more specific question, however, is whether certain forms of support are more important for coping in specific situations (Cobb, 1976). Blended conceptualizations such as that of Wandersman, Wandersman, and Kahn (1980), who described support as including group support, marital emotional support, network instrumental support, and marital instrumental support, make it more difficult to test the saliency of specific forms of support in specific situations.

Funch and Mettlin (1982) found forms of support to be differentially effective. In their study, only financial support was related to recovery among breast cancer patients. Other researchers have not found one form of support to be more effective than another (M. A. Brown, 1986; Meister, 1982; Underwood, 1986). Mitchell and Trickett (1980) suggested that the specific question is, "What types of social support are most useful for which individuals in terms of what particular issues and under what environmental conditions?" Carefully and systematically planned research is needed to answer this question.

Sources of Support

Conceptualizations of social support have varied with respect to their specification of sources of support. Differentiations have been made on the basis of individual, aggregate, or network providers; support from individuals with similar experiences; and lay versus professional sources of support. Definitions of social support have ranged from the availability of a confidant (Lowenthal & Haven, 1968) to network comprehensiveness (Berkman & Syme, 1979).

Qualitative and quantitative studies, however, have found no evidence that the size of the social network is related to satisfaction with social support or to enhanced outcomes (Elmore, 1984; Lambert, Lambert, Klipple, & Mewshaw, 1989; Powers, 1988).

There is evidence that differences in the benefit of social support are perceived on the basis of provider category (Carveth & Gottlieb, 1979; Dunkel-Schetter, 1981; Galvan, Davis, Banks, & Bing, 2008; Lederman, 1984; Lederman, Lederman, Work, & McCann, 1979; Peck & Boland, 1977; Underwood, 1986). Sources of support, however, may be viewed differentially with respect to the forms of support they are able to provide. Support from family and friends may be valued, but they may not be the best resources for information needed to facilitate effective coping in a given situation. Therefore, professional sources may at times play a more prominent role. The degree to which professional support is valued, sought out, and used may also be a function of culture. For example, middle-class Euro/Caucasian American childbearing women frequently turn to professional and semiprofessional sources of support in dealing with the challenges of childbearing (Underwood, 1986), whereas Latinos may prefer family and lay sources of support. Vaux and Harrison (1985) noted that social support varied across subgroups of the population. To date, the sociocultural and socioeconomic influences on preferred sources of support have received insufficient attention.

Some conceptualizations of sources of social support have reflected a strong focus on the quality of relationships between providers and recipients (Brown & Harris, 1978; Qureshi & Walker, 1989; Weiss, 1975). The quality of social ties (Berkman & Syme, 1979; Shoenbach, Kaplan, Fredman, & Kleinbaum, 1986) has been studied as well. Such a focus is often directed toward the examination of social networks. Networks have been described as convoys across the life span or as existing within the context of a specific situation that is identified or perceived to be stressful. Conceptualizations of social support that incorporate the dimension of network more frequently reflect their structural as opposed to functional properties. Neither structural nor functional network components were found to influence self-care practices of HIV-positive African American women (Hurst, Montgomery, Davis, Killion, & Baker, 2005).

Valence, Cost, and Reciprocity

Historically, social support has been viewed as having a positive valence; however, social support is not a fixed commodity. It is a dynamic process that may change with circumstances. The form that social support takes and by whom it is provided may be perceived as more or less helpful in different situations (Norwood, 1996). Hinds and Moyer (1997) strongly concur that "how actions are perceived determines whether or not they are felt to be supportive" (p. 375). This conclusion was reached through the qualitative study of cancer patients undergoing radiotherapy treatments. The researchers found that even acts not intended to be supportive could be perceived as such. Conceptualizing social support as perceived satisfaction with what is given by whom provides for the recommended differentiation of forms and sources but also gives appropriate weight to individual variations in need for support, expectations of receiving it, and the relative costs of obtaining it.

Social support has generally been conceptualized as positive and cost-free. Stewart and Tilden (1995) systematically explored the cost to the recipient of obtaining support and suggested the regular consideration of this element within conceptualizations of social support. Without consideration of the demands on the recipient of support, those with close-knit networks may be viewed as the automatic recipients of more support. In such networks, the positive effects of support may be ameliorated by the cost of obtaining it (Gottlieb, 1981; Norwood, 1996). Researchers and clinicians should be cautioned not to assume that support from professionals is cost-free. Any social or professional relationship is open to conflict and negative interaction. Stewart and Tilden support this contention.

The importance of a reciprocal element in the conceptualization of social support is another consideration. It addresses the question of whether outcomes are enhanced when persons are able to give and receive support. It implies a burden of guilt and obligation when support is received but not returned. Thus, the cost of obtaining support may be increased.

Riegel and Gocka (1995) conducted a longitudinal study of myocardial infarction patients and found that reciprocity in providing support was an important issue—but only for women. As their ability to give support decreased, stress in their supportive relationships increased. The possibility that reciprocity is a gender-specific issue warrants further investigation.

Future Conceptualizations

Greater consistency in conceptualization of social support across studies is a challenge that must be met. Research has supported the attempt to delineate forms and sources of support within any conceptualization. Although specific choices in concept labels may vary, emotional, informational, instrumental, and affirmational support appear to be common threads. Both subjective and objective elements seem desirable. Thus, conceptualizations might focus on perceptions about the support received, its availability, and a more objective assessment of network properties. Consideration of social support in terms of its cost also seems justified.

Barrera (1986) made an interesting proposal in an attempt to organize disparate elements within the definition of social support. It was suggested that social support be divided into the following categories: social embeddedness, enacted support, perceived availability, and satisfaction. Social embeddedness refers to the structural elements of support and the connections that individuals have within their social environment. Enacted support includes those actions that are performed to provide help to someone else. Perceived availability is the individual's sense that assistance is available if needed. Satisfaction refers to an assessment about the adequacy of social ties.

Enacted support seems to reflect two dimensions, whereas satisfaction as described appears to relate to social embeddedness. An alternative format might contain two categories: (a) Social currency, which would focus on the support network, including structural elements, quality of social ties, and perceived availability of general support and (b) perceived enacted support. The latter would reflect satisfaction with what was provided by whom and the cost of obtaining support in a specific situation perceived as threatening or challenging. Net satisfaction with enacted support would factor in cost.

The elements of social currency and perceived enacted support might be modified by personal resources, cultural expectations, and the need for reciprocity.

MECHANISMS OF EFFECT

The ability to examine the models or mechanisms whereby social support exerts a positive influence on health is predicated on both clarity of conceptualization of social support and clarity in explication of the models. It is generally accepted that social support works through main, mediating, and moderating mechanisms. Inconsistencies in the application of the terms mediating and moderating or buffering, as well as inappropriate selection of statistical tests of these relationships, have increased confusion regarding the efficacy of social support. It also must be considered that a particular aspect of social support may be more relevant to one model versus another.

Main Effects

Models that hypothesize and test the main effect of social support propose that there is a direct relationship between social support and outcome variables such as well-being. The main effects of social support have been supported in many studies. For example, Hatchett, Friend, Symister, and Wadhua (1997) studied 42 end-stage renal disease patients. The Inventory of Socially Supportive Behaviors (Barrera, Sandler, & Ramsey, 1981) was used to measure the exchange of four forms of social support (emotional, instrumental, appraisal, and informational). They found that increased perceived social support from family correlated with decreased hopelessness ($r = -.25$, $p < .05$). Increased perceived support from the medical staff was correlated with increases in optimism ($r = .27$, $p < .05$). In a study of 31 mothers who delivered premature infants (Younger, Kendell, & Pickler, 1997), ratings of the helpfulness of others in providing emotional, informational, tangible, and general support (Account of Social Resources Inventory) were positively correlated with mastery ($r = .35$, $p < .05$) and negatively correlated with depression ($r = .35$, $p < .05$). Frey (1989) found significant main effects for perceived availability of social support (Norbeck

Social Support Questionnaire 84) and family health among parents of diabetic children. Similar effects were not found for children's health. Chang and Krantz (1996) set out to test the mediating effect of social support on adjustment among adult children of alcoholics. Instead, they found a main effect for social support that supported findings of Billings and Moss (1986).

Moderating or Buffering Effects

Moderating effects are at times the most misunderstood of the effects models. Antonovsky (1979) suggested that resources such as social support can increase a person's resistance to stress. A moderating effect is achieved (Figure 14.1) when a "third variable affects the zero-order correlation between two other variables" (Hurley-Wilson, 1993, p. 137). Moderators are antecedent conditions that interact with a stressor to affect the outcome. The moderating effect is best tested through an analysis of variance (ANOVA). In this model, social support is thought to protect the individual from the potentially harmful effects of exposure to a stressor. It is unclear whether it works through influencing the individual's appraisal of a potential stressor. It might be fruitful to study whether having a strong support network would act as a moderator by producing a healthier environment, by decreasing events appraised as threatening or harmful, or both. Pearlin (1989) supported the idea that social support forms a shield that insulates the individual from stress exposure. Chan and Ward (1993) suggested that social support acts to reduce the risk of illness by reducing harmful stress appraisal.

The moderating or buffering effect has been supported by several researchers (Alloway &

Bebbington, 1987; Cadzow & Servoss, 2009; Cassel, 1976; Cobb, 1976; Cohen, 1988; Cohen & Willis, 1985; Dean & Lin, 1977; Kaplan et al., 1977; Krause, 2006; Russell & Taylor, 2009). Using the Norbeck Social Support Questionnaire (NSSQ) as the measure of social support, Kang, Coe, Karaszewski, and McCarthy (1998) found that social support buffered stress among 133 well-managed, middle-class asthmatic teens. When social support was measured on the basis of perceived support from spouse/partner, family, and friends, Russell and Taylor (2009) found that support buffered the relationship between living alone and depression for 947 Hispanic and non-Hispanic older adults in an urban setting. Also, in an urban free clinic setting, Cadzow and Servoss (2009) found evidence to suggest that perceived social support may buffer mental health disorders associated with stressful living conditions. Krause (2006) used data from a national study of older Americans ($N = 538$, 56% African American) who attend church more than twice a year to examine the role of secular and church-based emotional support. Support provided outside the church did not appear to positively influence health, while the frequent provision of emotional support by people within the church buffered the effects of financial strain on self-rated health for African Americans but not for Caucasians.

Other researchers have not found support for the moderating or buffering hypothesis (Gluhoski, Fishman, & Perry, 1997) or have found varied support (Preston, 1995). For example, a study of the effect of social support in buffering the distress of bereavement among 598 gay men found that ANOVA supported only main rather than buffering effects of social support (Gluhoski et al., 1997).

Figure 14.1 Moderating or Buffering Effect of Social Support

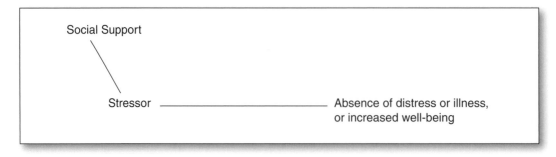

Social Support

Stressor ———————————— Absence of distress or illness, or increased well-being

Some researchers have found moderating or buffering effects in the context of studying other models. For example, Preston (1995) found that social support measured as the number of confidants had a buffering effect on health for married, elderly men. No such protective effect was found for women, however.

Sansom and Farnill (1997) did not test the buffering hypothesis but found direct, inverse relationships between network dimensions such as social integration and perceived everyday stress among recently divorced persons.

Mediating Effects

A third role for social support is that of mediator of the relationship between stress and health or coping outcomes (Figure 14.2). Baron and Kenny (1986, p. 1178) noted that the mediator effect occurs when

- there is a significant relationship between the independent and dependent variables (Path C);

- variations in levels of the independent variable significantly account for variations in the presumed mediator (Path A);

- variations in the mediator significantly account for variations in the dependent variable (Path B); and

- and when Paths A and B are controlled, a previously significant relationship between the independent and dependent variables is no longer significant (Path C).

Multiple regression is the appropriate statistical test for this model. Eckenrode and Gore

(1990) expanded on the discussion of these models in the context of their examination of work and family stress. One of the clearest tests of the mediation effect was conducted by Murrock and Madigan (2008) in examining the mediating effect of social support on the relationship between participating in a culturally specific dance and lifestyle physical activity among 126 African American women. The control group received only mailed health promotion information. Findings revealed that social support (measured by the Social Support for Exercise Scale [Sallis, Grossman, Pinski, Patterson, & Nader, 1987]) from friends mediated the relationship between dance and lifestyle physical activity. In other words, the support of friends played a critical role in the continued participation in the dance activity.

Several other examples of mediating effects were found. O'Brien, Wineman, and Nealon (1995) evaluated variables that mediated the relationship between the objective and subjective burden of caring for someone with multiple sclerosis and caregiver health and life satisfaction. Social support and family coping were evaluated as mediators of this relationship. The Social Network List and Support System Scale (Fiore, Becker, & Coppel, 1983; Hirsch, 1979) was used as the measure of social support. Although social support related to family coping ($r = .30$, $p < .05$), it did not mediate the relationship between burden and coping or life satisfaction. Social support did explain 7% unique variance in family satisfaction. The authors suggested that the failure to support the hypothesized relationships may have been a function of the social support measure used. This study was problematic in that

Figure 14.2   The Mediating Effect of Social Support

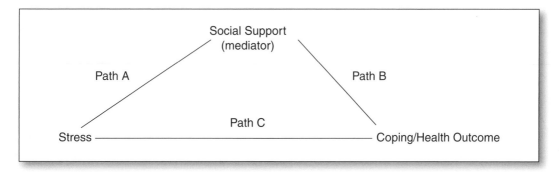

the terms "mediator" and "moderator" were used interchangeably.

Kim and Knight (2008) studied the effects of social support and coping styles on the physical health of 87 Korean American caregivers and a matched sample of noncaregivers. Social support included measurement of the quantity and quality of instrumental and emotional helpers. Path model analysis was used to examine the multiple relationships. Quantity of social support did not mediate the relationship between caregiver status and health outcomes; however, caregivers who reported a lower quality of instrumental support experienced greater physiologic stress (higher cortisol levels). Another study of 1,149 older Americans followed longitudinally found that the perceived availability of a confidant mediated the effects of disability on depression (Yang, 2006).

Oxman and Hull (1997) examined the ability of social support to mediate the relationships between activities of daily living and depression before and after heart surgery. Three measures of social support were used: the Social Network Questionnaire (SNQ; Seeman & Berkman, 1988), the Inventory of Socially Supportive Behaviors (ISSB; Barrera & Ainsley, 1983), and the Multidimensional Scale of Perceived Social Support (MSPSS; Zimet, Dahlem, Zimet, & Farley, 1988). The importance of the perceived adequacy of social support (MSPSS) was supported. The number of close network members seen (SNQ) had mediating and direct effects on activities of daily living and depression 6 months after surgery. In another study that used the MSPSS, Galvan et al. (2008) examined the stigma encountered by a group of 283 HIV-positive African Americans (70% male). Multivariate analysis revealed that only perceived support from friends mediated the relationship between negative self-image and depression.

Runtz and Schallow (1997) used structural equation modeling to examine the role of social support in mediating the relationship between maltreatment as a child and adult adjustment. Social support was measured by the Provisions of Social Relations Scale (PSR; Turner, Frankel, & Levin, [1983]). This 15-item instrument measures perceived support from family and friends. The role of social support as a mediator was confirmed. Social support explained 55% of the variance in adjustment. It is of concern that in

their conclusions the authors stated that these findings supported the contentions of others that social support acts as a buffer of stress.

Future Testing of Effects

Although clarity and consistency in the conceptualization of social support are a necessary first step in building evidence of its role within the stress and coping framework, a clear understanding of the nature of effects is an immediate second step. Conceptual and statistical models must be congruent, and labels for the nature of these models must be consistently applied. Only in this way will the role of social support in relation to stress and health outcomes be explicated. Clarity in conceptualization of social support and consistency in operationalization of the concept will help determine the specific aspects of social support that produce main, moderating, or mediating effects or all three.

Measures of Social Support

The variations in the conceptualization of social support are reflected in the operationalization of this construct. Artinian (1993b) found that more than 30 different instruments were used to measure social support in nursing research published between 1980 and 1990. Ducharme, Stevens, and Rowat (1994) suggest that four elements of measurement should be specified: the components being measured, whether the measures are objective, the unit of measurement, and validity and reliability. A frequent criticism is that many of the instruments have not been subjected to rigorous psychometric testing (Stewart, 1989). Notable exceptions are Norbeck's SSQ (Norbeck et al., 1981, 1983), Brandt and Weinert's (1981; Wienert & Brandt, 1987) Personal Relationships Questionnaire (PRQ), Tilden's (Tilden & Gaylen, 1987; Tilden, Nelson, & May, 1990b) Interpersonal Relationships Inventory (IPR), and the Enhancing Recovery in Coronary Heart Disease Social Support (ESSI) Instrument (Vaglio et al., 2004). These instruments are compared in Table 14.1. In addition to these more widely tested instruments, four other instruments are described here because of their varied conceptualizations of social support: Barrera and Ainsley's (1983) ISSB, Norwood's (1996) Social Support Apgar (SSA), Seeman and Berkman's (1988) SNQ, and

Zimet el al.'s (1988) Multidimensional Scale of Perceived Social Support (MSPSS).

Norbeck Social Support Questionnaire (NSSQ)

This instrument was based on attachment theory. The NSSQ (Norbeck et al., 1981, 1983) provides subjects with an opportunity to list members of their support network (up to 24) and to categorize them on the basis of their relationship to the individual (e.g., "spouse," "health care provider," and "friend"). It also provides an opportunity to indicate recent losses (number lost from the network and level of support lost in the past year). Sources of support are further rated on a 5-point scale in relation to the amount (none to a great deal) of aid, affect, or affirmational support provided. Two measures are obtained for each of the forms of support. Total scores reflect functional support and network properties. Internal consistency has been reported as .89 (Norbeck & Anderson, 1989) and .78 to .84 (Frey, 1989). Test-retest reliability ranged from .85 to .92 for the subscales (Norbeck & Anderson, 1989).

Personal Relationships Questionnaire (PRQ)

The PRQ85 was built on Weiss's (1974) conceptualization of social relations (Weinert & Brandt, 1987) and has two parts. Part 1 measures support needs for the past six months, including who was contacted for the support and how satisfied the individual was with the support they received. Satisfaction is rated on a 6-point scale, from very satisfied to very dissatisfied. Part 2 assesses five dimensions of social support—intimacy, social integration, nurturance, worth, and assistance—rated on a 7-point scale, from strongly disagree to strongly agree. Items vary according to whether they measure support needs, perceived availability of support, received support, and ability to provide support. Internal consistency has ranged from .87 to .91 (Gibson, Cheavens, & Warren, 1998; Weinert & Tilden, 1990). A factor analysis of Part 2 revealed three factors: intimacy/assistance, integration/affirmation, and reciprocity (Weinert & Tilden, 1990).

Interpersonal Relationships Inventory (IPR)

Social exchange theory (Cook, 1987) and equity theory (Messick & Cook, 1983) served as the basis for the IPR (Tilden et al., 1990b). This instrument is unique in acknowledging both the costs and the benefits of social support. The IPR consists of 39 items measured on a 5-point scale. For items measuring perceived states, the response options range from "strongly agree" to "strongly disagree." Enacted behaviors are measured with respect to frequency, from "never" to "very often." The following subscales are scored separately: social support, reciprocity, and conflict (Tilden et al., 1990b). The internal consistency and construct validity of the scales have been widely supported through quantitative (Tilden, Hirsch, & Nelson, 1994) and qualitative research (Tilden, Nelson, & May, 1990a).

ENRICHD Social Support Instrument (ESSI)

The ESSI was originally developed to provide a short but valid measure of social support for the multisite study to enhance outcomes following myocardial infarction by increasing social support and decreasing depression. It is a 7-item scale that measures emotional, instrumental, informational, and appraisal forms of support. Six items are rated on a 5-point scale indicating the frequency of someone being available to provide a particular form of social support (responses range from "none of the time" to "all of the time"). A seventh item is a "yes/no" response to whether the individual lives with a spouse. Sometimes this item is eliminated because it is considered redundant with questions asked elsewhere. Adequate internal consistency (.86–.90) has been reported in studies of cardiac patients (Trivedi et al., 2009; Vaglio et al., 2004). The instrument also has concurrent (Cowan et al., 2008; Vaglio et al., 2004), predictive (Vaglio et al., 2004), and discriminant (Camara, Lukas, Begre, Pettel, and von Kanel, 2010) validity.

Additional Instruments

Inventory of Socially Supportive Behaviors (ISSB)

The ISSB is a 40-item measure of support received during the preceding month in relation to three subscales: emotional support, guidance, and tangible support. The frequency with which each item has been received in the recent past is rated on a 5-point scale from "not at all" to "about every day." Concurrent validity was supported

Table 14.1 Comparison of More Consistently Tested Measures of Social Support in Nursing Research

Measure and Author	Variables Measured	Description	Reliability	Validity	Populations Studied
Norbeck Social Support Questionnaire (Norbeck, Lindsey, & Carrieri, 1981, 1983)	Network properties Functional support	Listing of support network and relationship; number lost from network in past year; rating of sources on aid, affect, and affirmation	Internal consistency = .69–.97 (Norbeck et al., 1983), .89 (Kang, Coe, Karaszewski, & McCarthy, 1998; Norbeck & Anderson, 1989), .78–.84 (Frey, 1989) Test-retest = .85–.92 (Norbeck & Anderson, 1989)	Content validity via experts Construct validity	Diabetic children and parents (Frey, 1989) Families of disabled preschoolers (Failla & Jones, 1991) Families of children with disabilities (Snowdon, Cameron, & Dunham, 1994) Asthmatic teens (Kang et al., 1998) Families (Norbeck, 1981) American women (Norbeck, DeJoseph, & Smith, 1996) Widows (Robinson, 1995) Prospective heart transplant patients (Hirth & Stewart, 1994)
Personal Relationships Questionnaire 85 (Weinert & Brandt, 1987)	Support needs Dimensions of social support	Part 1: Who was contacted for support and rating of satisfaction Part 2: Five dimensions (intimacy, social integration, nurturance, worth, and assistance)	Internal consistency = .87–.91 (Gibson, Cheavens, & Warren, 1998; Graydon & Ross, 1995; Weinert & Tilden, 1990)	Part 2 factor analysis revealed three factors: intimacy/assistance, integration/ affirmation, and reciprocity Convergent validity	Chronic obstructive pulmonary disease patients (Graydon & Ross, 1995; Lee, Graydon, & Ross, 1991) Diabetics (White, Richter, & Fry, 1992) Multiple chemical sensitivity (Gibson et al., 1998)

Measure and Author	Variables Measured	Description	Reliability	Validity	Populations Studied
Interpersonal Relationships Inventory (Tilden, 1991)	Costs and benefits of social support	39 items; three subscales (social support, reciprocity, and conflict)	Internal consistency = .83–.92 (Tilden et al., 1990b) Test-retest = .81–.91 (Tilden et al., 1990b)	Construct validity supported through factor analysis (Tilden et al., 1990b; Tilden, Hirsch, & Nelson, 1994)	Family caregivers (Hansell et al., 1998; Hughes & Caliandro, 1996; Vrabec, 1995) Males on hemodialysis (Cormier-Daigle & Stewart, 1997) Cancer patients (Douglass, 1997) Infertile couples (Jirka, Schuett, & Foxall, 1996)
Inventory of Socially Supportive Behaviors (Barrera, Sandler, & Ramsey, 1981)	Support received	40 items; three subscales (emotional support, guidance, and tangible support); 5-point rating of frequency during the preceding month	Internal consistency = .67–.94 Test-retest = .62–.88 (Barrera & Ainsley, 1983; Barrera et al., 1981; Friedman, 1997; Grossman & Rowat, 1995; Oxman, Freeman, Manheimer, & Stukel, 1994)	Concurrent validity (Barrera et al., 1981)	End-stage renal disease patients (Barrera et al., 1981; Hatchet, Friend, Symister, & Wadhua, 1997) Adolescents (Grossman & Rowat, 1995) Women and elderly with heart failure (Friedman, 1993, 1997; Friedman & King, 1994) Open-heart surgery patients (Oxman & Hull, 1997)
Multidimensional Scale of Perceived Social Support (Zimet, Dahlem, Zimet, & Farley, 1988)	Perceived adequacy of social support	12 items rated on 7-point agreement regarding adequacy of support from a significant other, family, and friends	High internal consistency and test-retest reliability (Blumenthal, Barefoot, Burg, & Williams, 1987)	Content validity (Blumenthal et al., 1987; Zimet et al., 1988)	Angiography patients (Blumenthal et al., 1987) Open-heart surgery patients (Oxman et al., 1994; Oxman & Hull, 1997) Cancer patients (Hann et al., 1995)

(*Continued*)

Table 14.1 (Continued)

Measure and Author	Variables Measured	Description	Reliability	Validity	Populations Studied
Social Network Questionnaire (Seeman & Berkman, 1983)	Number of close network members seen regularly	Number of children, relatives, and friends seen at least one time per month			Open-heart surgery patients (Oxman & Hull, 1997) Elderly (Seeman & Berkman, 1983)
Social Support Apgar (Norwood, 1996)	Perceived satisfaction with social support	25-items; 5 forms (adaptation, partnership, growth, affection, and commitment); 5 sources (partner, parents, friends, and other acquaintances)	Internal consistency = .88–.93 (Norwood, 1996)	Content validity with experts related to NSSQ and PRQ dimensions (Norwood, 1996) Factor analysis separated on source (Norwood, 1996)	Pregnant women (Norwood, 1996)
ENRICHD Social Support Instrument (Mitchell, et al., 2003.)	Forms of support	6 items measuring availability of someone to provide emotional, instrumental, informational, & appraisal support (5 pt. scale) + yes/no whether the supporter lives with the person.	Internal consistency = (.86–.90) (Trivedi et al., 2009; Vaglio et al., 2004)	Concurrent (Cowan et al., 2008; Vaglio et al., 2004) Predictive (Vaglio et al., 2004) Discriminant (Camara et al., 2010)	Recovering coronary heart disease patients; used in the national ENRIHD studies (Cowan, et al., 2008; Vaglio, et al., 2004; Mitchell, et al., 2003)

366

through correlations with the Arizona Support Interview Schedule and the Moos' Family Environment Scale (Barrera et al., 1981). Internal consistency and test-retest reliability have been supported (Barrera, 1981; Barrera & Ainsley, 1983; Oxman, Freeman, Manheimer, & Stukel, 1994).

Social Support Apgar (SSA)

The SSA (Norwood, 1996) is a 25-item instrument developed to be an easy-to-use tool to assess perceived satisfaction with five forms of support (adaptation, partnership, growth, affection, and commitment) from five sources (partner, parents, other family members, friends, and other acquaintances). Each item is rated on a 3-point scale from "hardly ever" to "almost always." Content validity was established, and items were linked to dimensions of social support assessed by the NSSQ and the PRQ. Factor analysis separated items on the basis of source rather than form of support, adding to the evidence supporting the unidimensionality of social support as it related to forms. Cronbach's alpha ratings ranged from .88 to .93 across three studies by Norwood (1996). A study of pregnancy outcome variables (birth weight, weeks of gestation, and number of prenatal visits) according to level of support among a sample of 220 postpartum patients revealed no differences (Norwood, 1996). The majority of women in this study were White, nonmarried, and had just delivered their second baby. In another study of 52 White, low-income, unmarried maternity patients with less than a high school education, Norwood (1996) did find that women with higher support had lower levels of perceived life stress, supporting a buffering hypothesis. As this instrument is tested further, its sensitivity might be evaluated. A 5-point rating might increase the ability to discriminate among subjects.

Multidimensional Scale of Perceived Social Support (MSPSS)

Twelve items of perceived adequacy of social support from significant others, family, and friends are rated on a 7-point scale from "very strongly disagree" to "very strongly agree" in the MSPSS (Zimet et al., 1988) Reliability and validity have been supported in studies of patients with angiography (Blumenthal, Barefoot, Burg, & Williams, 1987), open-heart surgery (Oxman

et al., 1994), and metastatic carcinoma (Hann, Oxman, Ahles, Furstenburg, & Stukel, 1995). Alpha ratings were .93 and .94.

Summary

Significant challenges remain in the measurement of social support. First, theoretical underpinnings need to be explicated. These are clear for the NSSQ, PRQ85, and IPR Inventory but are less so for other instruments. Second, the conceptualization of social support must be specified, even if the researchers choose to measure only a component of social support rather than attempting to capture the full dimensions of the construct. Such clarification is necessary if the process by which social support positively affects outcomes is to be revealed.

The instruments have varied in their inclusion of network components and evaluation of support received. It may be useful to distinguish between reference to network, meaning a general support convoy that goes along with the person, and sources of support when dealing with a specific situation. Evidence supports the importance of perceptions of social support available or received. Network elements appear to be less relevant.

Researchers should be encouraged to use well-established instruments—or components of them—to build evidence. If new instruments are developed, their rationale should be made clear. For example, the Social Support Apgar was developed to provide a quickly administered screening tool. More is not necessarily better with regard to the number of social support instruments. The challenge is to find those measures that match accepted conceptualizations and then to use these tools more consistently to build the science.

RESEARCH IN NURSING AND RELATED DISCIPLINES

Social support continues to be the most widely researched coping resource both in nursing and in related disciplines. Overall, positive influences on health outcomes and protective functioning with respect to stress have been observed but with some inconsistency due to variations in conceptualization, measurement, and effects modeling. It is not the intent here to offer a complete synthesis of social support research but rather to note a few promising trends and examples.

The bulk of the researchers studying social support used descriptive or correlational designs. Few researchers attempted to manipulate social support. Researchers in social support studies also tended to examine concepts in a cross-sectional dimension. It is encouraging to note, however, that sample sizes are increasing. This is particularly critical to increasing the power of research to detect the effects of subtle differences in social support.

Roberts et al.'s (1995) study is an example of the manipulation of social support as an intervention. A randomized clinical trial compared the effectiveness of phone-call support, support through face-to-face problem-solving counseling, and routine care for 293 adults who were not well adjusted to a chronic illness. The interventions were delivered by masters-prepared nurses and measurements taken at 6 and 12 months. Main effects for social support on life satisfaction were found for both intervention groups. The phone-call group experienced the greatest improvement. Interactive effects with demographic characteristics were also found. Problem-solving counseling was most effective for those who lived alone and frequently used avoidance as opposed to problem-solving coping.

Two more recent studies manipulated social support via electronic means (Dilorio et al., 2008; Scharer et al., 2009). Scharer et al. provided web-based ($n = 7$) or telephone ($n = 4$) support to mothers of children aged 5 to 12 years who had been hospitalized for mental illness. Transcripts from every 2-week telephone session and instances where the mother was alone in the chat room with a mother were qualitatively analyzed and compared. Mothers in both groups described similar issues and challenges, and the nurses provided informational, emotional, and appraisal support to both groups. The major difference was that telephone mothers could receive support whether they actively sought it or not. The Internet mothers, however, had to actively seek the support. The researchers determined that both mediums were effective for transmitting support.

The study by Dilorio et al. (2008) provided web-based self-management support to 29 individuals with epilepsy, with the intent of helping them to engage in strategies to reduce stress and to achieve medication adherence and adequate sleep. The participants valued this strategy, and 59% rated the program as good to excellent. The program was differentially effective with 59% stating that it helped to improve sleep, but only 41% indicated that it helped them to take medications more regularly or manage stress. Conceptualizing support in this manner appears more limited.

Social support researchers have tended to focus on patients or population groups coping with identified problems. The assessment of modifiers and mediators of burnout among nurses is one area in which there is considerable research focused on professionals as they carry out their roles. Duquette, Kerouac, Sandhu, and Beaudet (1994) conducted a thorough review of the literature in relation to burnout among nurses. They located eight studies that focused on the influence of social support (Constable & Russell, 1986; Dick, 1986; Duxbury, Armstrong, Drew, & Henly, 1984; Haley, 1986; Hare, Pratt, & Andrews, 1988; Mallett, 1988; Mickschl, 1984; Paredes, 1982). It was found that these studies used a consistent measure of burnout, the Maslach Burnout Index developed by Maslach and Jackson (1981). The same was not true for social support. Again, different tools were used. All studies consistently found a negative relationship between social support and burnout.

Ihlenfeld (1996) examined the support that staff nurses ($n = 24$), nursing faculty ($n = 107$), and home health nurses ($n = 128$) received from their administrators within the previous month. Both home health nurses and staff nurses wanted more support. Faculty members reported receiving little support from their deans or chairpersons but did not state that they wanted more support. In all the studies, statistically significant negative relationships were found between social support and burnout. The consistency of this finding suggests that it may be very cost-effective for nursing administrators to give conscious attention to provision of support to decrease burnout among staff. A growing number of studies focusing on social support and work-force variables have been conducted on Middle Eastern populations. For example, Abualrub, Omari, and Abu Al Rub (2009) examined the moderating effect of social support from coworkers on the relationship between stress and job satisfaction. Social support was measured with the Social Support Scale (Sargent & Terry, 2000) that measures social support from coworkers and supervisors (6 items each) rated on a 4-point scale, from "very much" to "not at all." Support from both co-workers and supervisors had an inverse relationship to perceived work stress. Perceived support from supervisors demonstrated a stronger relationship to job satisfaction ($r = .46$, $p < .01$) than did coworker support ($r = .19$, $p < .01$).

GENDER AND CULTURAL DIFFERENCES IN SOCIAL SUPPORT

The trend for social support researchers to focus on white, middle-class, adult samples was noted in reviews of nursing research (Artinian, 1993b; Ruiz-Bueno & Underwood, 1999). These samples almost exclusively are selected by convenience. It is encouraging to note an increasing interest in examining the contributions of age, gender, and ethnicity to the process of social support.

Gender-Focused Studies

There is increasing evidence that social support operates differentially within the context of gender. Two studies examined the continuity of support over time for spouses whose mates experienced coronary bypass surgery (Artinian, 1992) or chemotherapy (Dodd, Dibble, & Thomas, 1993). Researchers consistently reported a decrease in support over time for men, whereas support for women was maintained.

Riegel and Gocka (1995) examined social support needs of subjects one month following myocardial infarction. No differences were found in support needed. Women, however, received significantly more emotional support than men. Gibson et al. (1998) and Turner (1994) confirmed the higher levels of support received by women. Allen and Stoltenberg (1995) found that college freshmen women were more supported and better satisfied with that support than were their male counterparts. Similarly, Potts (1997) reported that among 151 members of a retirement village, women had higher levels of confidant relationships than

men. In contrast, Gulick (1992) found higher perceived social support in men than in women with multiple sclerosis.

In a study of 289 persons who attended an urban free clinic (Cadzow & Servoss, 2009), a relationship between available support in the past four weeks and cardiac health was found for women but not for men. There was an association between social support and anxiety in men. The fact that social support was measured in relation to the past month calls into question the direction of effect, however.

In a study of patients one or two years after experiencing a myocardial infarction (Conn, Taylor, & Abel, 1991), researchers reported a negative correlation between age and social support for men ($n = 117$, $r = -.31$) but not for women ($n = 80$, $r = -.08$). Preston (1995) studied 900 persons aged 65 or older and found a positive correlation between the number of confidants and health for married men. Married women had the poorest health regardless of social support. McColl and Frieland (1994) and Willey and Silliman (1990) found gender unrelated to social support. Although these findings were not uniformly consistent, women did seem to receive more support than did men, and gender did seem to have some differential relationship with selected variables.

In two studies, samples were limited to women. In the first study, the researchers found a relationship between form of support and outcome (Friedman, 1997). Older women with heart failure were studied to examine the relationship between support source loss, perceived enacted support, and psychological well-being. Emotional and tangible support sources were found to be stable over time for the 57 subjects. Emotional support and loss of tangible support measured by the ISSB were related to positive affect ($r = .36$ and $-.34$, respectively; $p < .01$). Stability of social relationships was also found by Kendler (1997) in a 5-year longitudinal study of female twins. In this study, social support was operationalized as relative problems, friend problems, relative support, confidants, friend support, and social integration. Kendler suggested that social support has a genetic component and that it is not just an environmental issue. Thus, women seem to have more support than men, and this support is relatively stable.

A study of 30 young men with testicular cancer used the Importance of Social Support instrument to examine social support in relation to mood (Davidson, Degner, & Morgan, 1995). No relationship was found between these two variables. The men in this study reported that they were well supported. These findings suggested that support needs to be evaluated within the context of the individuals' requirements and their perceptions of whether it does or does not meet their needs.

Cultural Implications

Fewer investigators have examined social support within ethnically diverse populations. When they have, social support appears to have differential effects. Cetingok, Winsett, Russell, and Hathaway (2008) sought to describe the social networks of 258 conveniently selected transplant recipients who were part of a larger NINR-funded study. The sample was 62% Caucasian and 33% African American and 60% male and 40% female. The researchers found that African Americans had higher frequency of support and duration than Caucasian subjects. While there were no differences for gender, it might have been interesting to examine a potential interactive effect between race and gender for social support.

Sammarco and Konecny (2010) compared the perceived social support and uncertainty of Caucasian and Latina breast cancer survivors with their quality of life. The sample included 280 survivors, 65% Caucasian and 35% Latina. The Northouse Social Support Questionnaire (Northouse, 1988) was used to measure total support. They found that Caucasians had significantly higher perceived social support and quality of life (QOL), although there were no differences on the SSQ subscales. Latinas had higher levels of uncertainty. Unfortunately interactive effects were not examined. It would also be useful to attempt to tease out cultural values. This study added to previous work (Sammarco & Konecny, 2008) that looked at an exclusively Latina sample ($N = 89$). The same instruments were used. In the earlier study it was found that social support was related to quality of life ($r = .39$, $p < .001$) and predicted 15% of the variance in QOL.

Rees, Karter, and Young (2010) examined race/ethnicity and social support in relation to self-care by diabetics. Social support was measured by looking at the presence/absence of emotional and financial support. Network dimensions of marital status, number of close friends, and number of times attending church was also measured. Of the 171 subjects, 39.5% were White, 34.6% Black, and 25.9% Latino. No associations between social support dimensions and outcome variables were found for Latinos. Whites has a positive association between social support and LDL levels, while social support for Blacks was associated with controlling weight, engaging in exercise, and controlling caloric intake.

A growing number of studies have focused exclusively on specific minority populations. A study by Norbeck, DeJoseph, and Smith (1996) examined the effect of a culturally relevant intervention on the birth weight of infants born to low-income African American women ($N = 319$). Focus groups suggested the potential efficacy of provision of support by nurses following a standard protocol in the subjects' homes. An experimental design was used to test a main effect for social support. Subjects identified as higher risk due to inadequate support (lacking support from mothers or male partners) were randomly placed in experimental and control groups. The intervention consisted of four face-to-face sessions, in which the nurses also tried to help subjects mobilize additional support from their networks. The intervention group also received follow-up phone calls in the two-week interval between sessions. The rate of low birth weight was significantly less ($p = .045$) in the experimental group (9.1% compared to 22.4% for the control group). The effectiveness of social support in this study was consistent with the findings of Edwards et al. (1994) and Heins, Nance, and Levey-Mickens (1988) but inconsistent with those of several other studies (Bryce, Stanley, & Garner, 1991; Oakley, Rajan, & Grant, 1990; Rothberg & Lits, 1991; Spencer, Thomas, & Morris, 1989; Villar, Farnot, Barros, Victoria, & Langer, 1992). An explanation may lie in the attempt to maximize the cultural relevance of the intervention.

Linn, Poku, Cain, Holzapfel, and Crawford (1995) studied an adult African American population ($N = 255$) infected with HIV.

A correlational design was used to examine the relationship between HIV symptoms and depression and anxiety. It was hypothesized that higher levels of social support would be related to lower anxiety and depression. Unfortunately, social support was measured by asking subjects if there was anyone they could talk to or count on for understanding and support and then counting the available number of confidants. Picot (1995) also focused on an African American population. A positive but weak correlation ($r = .29$, $p < .01$) was found between social support and confrontational coping in African American women who were caring for relatives with Alzheimer's disease. The association of social support and depressive symptoms in 159 urban African American females was studied by Wu, Prosser, and Taylor (2010). The MSPSS was used to measure social support and a negative correlation between social support and depressive symptoms was found ($r = -.44$, $p < .001$)

Abramowitz et al. (2009) had a diverse sample (72% Black, 20% Hispanic, 8% White) but did not examine social support in a differential way. They looked at the relationship between social support and depression in a sample of HIV-infected adolescents aged 13 to 21. Social support was measured using the HIV Specific Social Support Scale where source (family or friends) was examined in relation to components of structure, perceived instrumental, and satisfaction. The Medical Outcomes Social Support Survey was also used to measure general support. There were significant differences in perceived social support between youth who had been infected perinatally and those who were infected due to their behavior. Correlations with depression for specific and general support were very weak even if significant. Youth were significantly more satisfied with support from family than friends.

Nursing research in Korea (Choi, 1994) was reviewed in relation to social support, and 11 studies were found. These studies tended to use univariate analysis techniques and different measures of social support in addition to small sample sizes, thus making it difficult to generalize across studies. Two studies examined the supportive interventions provided by nurses. M. J. Kim (1985) found that sodium excretion was lower in experimental versus control groups

of hospitalized patients ($N = 66$) following a nursing intervention, although anxiety scores were not significantly different. J. A. Kim (1990), however, found that military patients ($N = 150$) with lower back pain experienced increased satisfaction, an increase in positive mood, and a decrease in depression following supportive nursing care. Choi suggests that in studying social support in Korean families, attention needs to be paid to variations in philosophy among family members and the differential effects that conflicts regarding philosophical outlook may have on the appraisal of support provided. This advice appears to be well founded. Regardless of the extent of research within a culture, it appears wise to check with members of that culture to determine the meaning and value that they as individuals ascribe to social support.

When J.-H. Kim and Knight (2008) studied the relationships among coping styles and quantity and quality of perceived social support and the physical health of Korean American caregivers, they found that decreased quality of social support was associated with increased stress. They also seem to suggest that the efficacy of social support may depend on congruence with cultural expectations and preferences more than any specific quantitative measures.

FUTURE DIRECTIONS FOR THEORY DEVELOPMENT

In the past decade (2000–2010) more than 420 nursing research studies that included social support have been published. Research on psychosocial factors mediating stress has continued to examine social support for its value as both a component of interventions that incorporate direct and technological modes. There has also been increased attention to evaluating the moderating (buffering) and/or mediating role of social support. The role of social support in ameliorating negative sequela associated with chronic illnesses such as HIV/AIDS (Galvan et al., 2008), depression (Yang, 2006), diabetes (Coffman, 2008; Rees et al., 2010; Zhang, Norris, Gregg, & Beckles, 2007), chronic leg ulcers (Edwards, Courtney, Finlayson, Shuter, &

Lindsay, 2009), sickle cell disease (Jenerette, 2008) and Crohn's disease (Camara et al., 2010). There has been less attention to acute illnesses and to a primary focus on social support. Ways of conceptualizing and measuring this variable continue to abound but less attention seems to be paid to the construct itself, that is, systematic investigation and evaluation of components for model and theory building.

Conceptualizations of social support have varied widely, inconsistent measures have been used, research designs and statistical models have occasionally lacked conceptual consistency, and support interventions have not been investigated extensively. Nevertheless, studies of social support continue to yield findings sufficient to validate the belief that mobilization or proffering of support will produce positive gains in coping and health. More collaborative approaches to the systematic investigation of social support are needed. A model of social support designed by this author is suggested to guide this research (Figure 14.3).

The proposed model draws from the work of Lazarus (Lazarus, 1990; Lazarus & Folkman, 1984), House (1981), Benner and Wrubel (1989), and Lyon (1990). Objective conditions refer to those events, phenomena, or potential stressors that may produce stress if they are viewed as threatening or exceeding an individual's resources to deal with them. The key is how these conditions are perceived by the individual. The initial evaluation of the potential stressor is labeled *primary appraisal* by Lazarus. It might be helpful to attempt to categorize situations that are perceived as stressful to determine whether certain forms of support are more relevant to coping in specific situations. The individual's perceptions may be modified by both individual and situational factors. It is at this point that network variables may play a role. The ongoing presence of at least one confidant may help the individual to perceive the potential stressor as less threatening. Although *network* is a commonly misunderstood term, there may be some advantage to retaining it as a reference to structural components and labeling the broader concept *social currency* to connote a resource that may be spent. This may be especially appropriate if the definition includes perceived availability of network support and some measure of the quality of social ties. Social currency may play

a greater role in the moderation or buffering of social support (Figure 14.3, Path A) than in affecting the health outcome.

The primary appraisal of an event as a threat or a challenge can trigger secondary appraisal—an assessment of the resources available to address the threat or challenge. Perception of available support may include an assessment of the form of support needed, who is available to provide it, and the cost of obtaining it. These situational variables might in turn be influenced by personal factors, such as personality, preferred coping style, personal resources, cultural expectations, need for reciprocity, and gender-specific socialization (see Figure 14.3, Path B).

A third component that is critical to measure is perceived satisfaction with social support (perceived enacted support) (see Figure 14.3, Path C). Theoretically, to make this judgment, people would consider their needs, what they received to address those needs, and what it cost them to get the needed help. In this model, perceived satisfaction with social support would mediate the relationship between perceived stress and health outcome (Figure 14.3, Path D). Current measures of social support would need slight modification and reassembly to capture the new conceptualization of social support. Path analysis might be used in addition to ANOYA and multiple regression techniques to test these relationships.

Summary

Social support continues to hold promise as a resource to protect against stress or to facilitate coping. To critically manipulate it in clinical situations and expect predictable outcomes, we must clearly understand how it works. Such understanding will evolve from our shared conceptualizations and the application of consistent and congruent measures within the context of research designs that maintain the integrity of the conceptualization. It is imperative that propositions such as those proposed in the suggested model of social support be systematically tested with diverse populations in varied and potentially stress-producing situations. In this way, we can identify those effects that will make the promise of social support a reality.

Figure 14.3 Proposed Model for the Examination of the Influence of Social Support: Path A, Buffering or Moderating Effect; Paths B and C, Mediating Effect; Path D, Direct Effect of Appraisal on Outcome

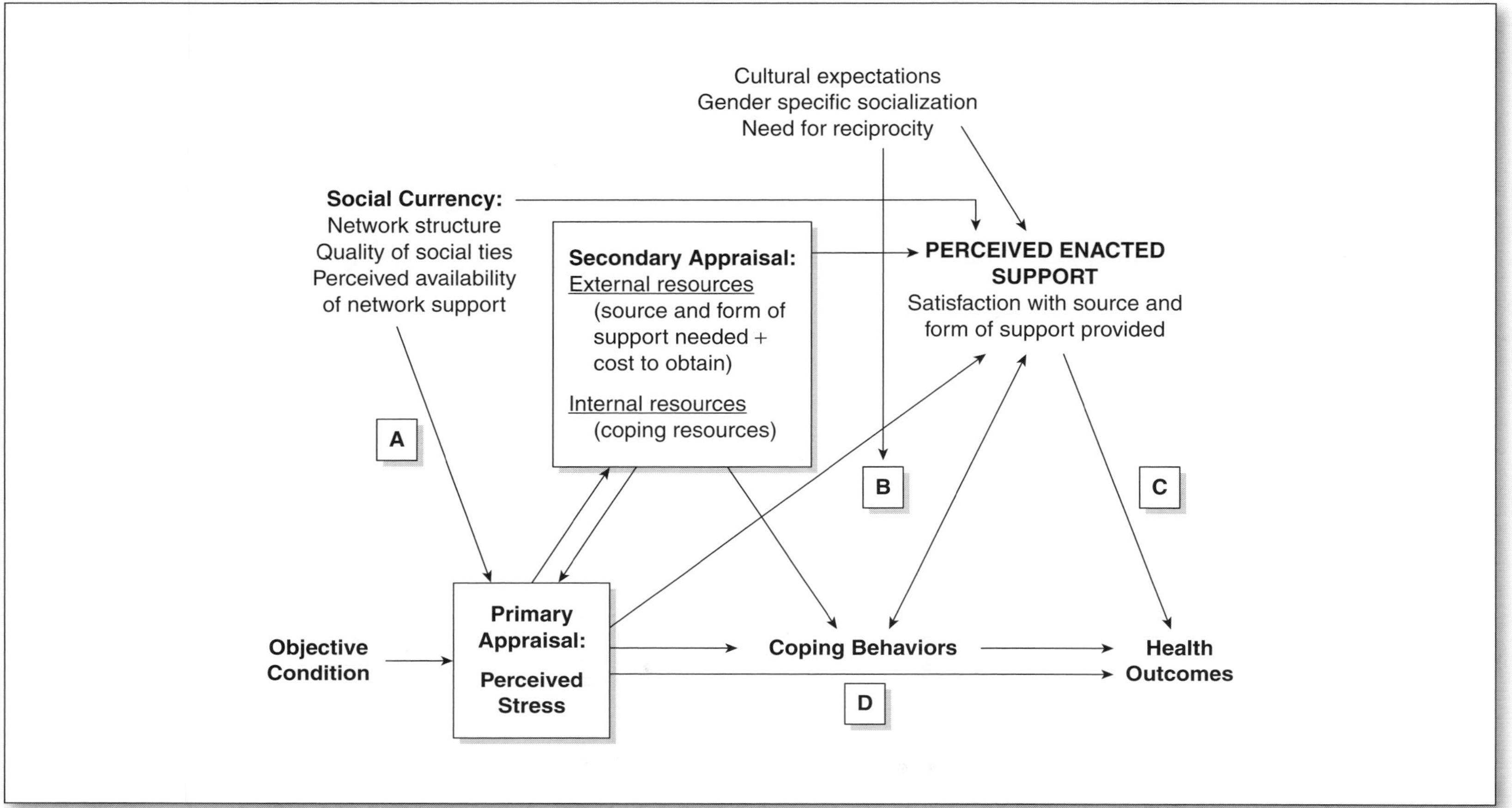

Social Currency:
Network structure
Quality of social ties
Perceived availability
of network support

Cultural expectations
Gender specific socialization
Need for reciprocity

PERCEIVED ENACTED SUPPORT
Satisfaction with source and
form of support provided

Secondary Appraisal:
External resources
(source and form of
support needed +
cost to obtain)

Internal resources
(coping resources)

A

B

C

D

Primary Appraisal: Perceived Stress

Objective Condition

Coping Behaviors

Health Outcomes

REFERENCES

Abramowitz, S., Koenig, L. J., Chandwani, S., Orban, L., Stein, R., LaGrange, R., & Barnes, W. (2009). Characterizing social support: Global and specific social support experiences of HIV-infected youth. *AIDS Patient Care and STDs, 23,* 323–330.

Abualrub, R. F., Omari, F. H., & Abu Al Rub, A. F. (2009). The moderating effect of social support on the stress-satisfaction relationship among Jordanian hospital nurses. *Journal of Nursing Management, 17,* 870–878.

Allen, S., & Stoltenberg, C. (1995). Psychological separation of older adolescents and young adults from their parents: An investigation of gender differences. *Journal of Counseling and Development 73,* 542–546.

Alloway, R., & Bebbington, P. (1987). The buffer theory of social support: A review of the literature. *Psychological Medicine, 17,* 91.

Antonovsky, A. (1974). Conceptual and methodological problems in the study of resistance resources and stressful life events. In B. Dohrenwend & B. Dohrenwend (Eds.), *Stressful life events: Their nature and effects* (pp. 245–258). New York, NY: John Wiley.

Antonovsky, A. (1979). *Health, stress, and coping.* San Francisco, CA: Jossey-Bass.

Artinian, N. T. (1991). Stress experience of spouses of patients having coronary artery bypass during hospitalization and 6 weeks after discharge. *Heart & Lung—Journal of Critical Care, 20,* 52–59.

Artinian, N. T. (1992). Spouse adaptation to mate's CA BG surgery: 1-year follow-up. *American Journal of Critical Care, 1,* 36–42.

Artinian, N. T. (1993a). Spouses' perceptions of readiness for discharge after cardiac surgery. *Applied Nursing Research, 6,* 80–88.

Artinian, N. T. (1993b). Resources: Factors that mediate the stress-health-outcome relationship. In J. S. Barnfather & B. L. Lyon (Eds.), *Stress and coping: State of the science and implications in nursing theory, research and practice.* Indianapolis, IN: Sigma Theta Tau International.

Baron, R. M., & Kenny, D. A. (1986). The moderator mediator variable distinction in social psychological research: Conceptual, strategic and statistical considerations. *Journal of Personality and Social Psychology, 51,* 1173–1182.

Barrera, M. (1981). Social support in the adjustment of pregnant adolescents: Assessment issues. In B. Gottlieb (Ed.), *Social networks and social support* (pp. 69–96). Beverly Hills, CA: Sage.

Barrera, M. (1986). Distinctions between social support concepts, measures, and models. *American Journal of Community Psychology, 14,* 413–445.

Barrera, M., & Ainsley, S. (1983). The structure of social support: A conceptual and empirical analysis. *Journal of Community Psychology, 11,* 133–143.

Barrera, M., Sandler, I., & Ramsey, T. (1981). Preliminary development of a scale of social support: Studies on college students. *American Journal of Community Psychology, 9,* 435–447.

Benner, P., & Wrubel, J. (1989). *The primacy of caring: Stress and coping in health and illness.* Reading, MA: Addison Wesley.

Berkman, L., & Syme, L. (1979). Social networks, host resistance, and mortality: A nine year follow-up study of Alameda County residents. *American Journal of Epidemiology, 109,* 186–204.

Billings, A., & Moss, R. (1986). Children of parents with unipolar depression: A controlled 1-year follow-up. *Journal of Abnormal Child Psychology, 14,* 149–166.

Blumenthal, J., Barefoot, J., Burg, M., & Williams, R. B., Jr. (1987). Psychological correlates of hostility among patients undergoing coronary angiography. *British Journal of Medical Psychology, 60,* 149–355.

Brandt, P., & Weinert, C. (1981). The PRQ-A social support measure. *Nursing Research, 30,* 277–280.

Brown, G., & Harris, T. (1978). *Social origins of depression.* New York, NY: Free Press.

Brown, M. A. (1986). Social support during pregnancy: A unidirectional or multidirectional construct? *Nursing Research, 35,* 4–9.

Bryce, R., Stanley, E., & Garner, J. (1991). Randomized controlled trial of antenatal social support to prevent preterm birth. *British Journal of Obstetrics and Gynecology, 98,* 1001–1008.

Cadzow, R. B., & Servoss, T. J. (2009). The association between perceived social support and health among patients at a free urban clinic. *Journal of the National Medical Association, 101,* 243–250.

Camara, R. J. A., Lukas, P. S., Begre, S., Pittet, V., & von Kanel, R. (2010). *Effects of social support on the clinical course of Crohn's disease.* Obtained online at http://onlinelibrary.Wiley.com/doi/10.1002/ibd.28481/pdf

Caplan, G. (1974). *Support systems and community mental health.* New York, NY: Behavioral Publications.

Carveth, W., & Gottlieb, B. (1979). The measurement of social support and its relation to stress. *Canadian Journal of Behavioral Science, 11,* 179–387.

Cassel, J. (1974). Psychosocial processes and stress: Theoretical foundations. *International Journal of Health Services, 3,* 471–482.

Cassel, J. (1976). The contribution of the social environment to host resistance. *American Journal of Epidemiology, 104,* 107–123.

Cetingok, M., Winsett, R. P., Russell, C. L., & Hathaway, D. K. (2008). Relationships between sex, race, and social class and social support networks in kidney, liver, and pancreas transplant recipients. *Progress in Transplantation, 18*(2), 80–88.

Chan, T., & Ward, S. (1993). A tool to reduce stress and cardiovascular disease. *AAOHN Journal, 41*, 499–503.

Chang, J., & Krantz, M. (1996). Personal and environmental factors in relation to adjustment of offspring of alcoholics. *Substance Use & Misuse, 31*, 1401–1412.

Choi, E. C. (1994). Nursing research in Korea. *Annual Review of Nursing Research, 12*, 215–229.

Coates, D., & Winston, T. (1983). Counteracting the deviance of depression: Peer support groups for victims. *Journal of Social Issues, 39*, 169–194.

Cobb, S. (1976). Social support as a moderator of life stress. *Psychosomatic Medicine. 38*, 100–314.

Coffman, M. (2008). Effects of tangible social support and depression on diabetes self-efficacy. *Journal of Gerontological Nursing, 34*, 32–39.

Coffman, S., Levitt, M., & Deets, C. (1990). Personal and professional support for mothers of NICU and healthy newborns. *Journal of Obstetrics, Gynecologic, and Neonatal Nursing, 20*, 406–415.

Cohen, S. (1988). Psychosocial models of the role of social support in the etiology of physical disease. *Health Psychology, 7*, 269–297.

Cohen, S., & Willis, T. (1985). Stress, social support and the buffering hypothesis. *Psychological Bulletin, 98*, 310–357.

Conn, V. S., Taylor, S. G., & Abel, P. H. (1991). Myocardial infarction survivors: Age and gender differences in physical health, psychosocial state and regimen adherence. *Journal of Advanced Nursing, 16*, 1026–1034.

Constable, J. F., & Russell. D. W (1986). The effect of social support and the work environment upon burnout among nurses. *Journal of Human Stress,12*, 20–26.

Cook, K. S. (1987). *Social exchange theory.* Newbury Park, CA: Sage.

Cormier-Daigle, M., & Sewart, M. (1997). Support and coping of male hemodialysis-dependent patients. *International Journal of Nursing Studies, 34*, 420–430.

Cowan, M. J., Freedland, K. E., Burg, M. M., Saab, P. G., Youngblood, M. E., Cornell, C. E., . . . Czajkowski, S. M. (2008). Predictors of treatment response for depression and inadequate social support—The ENRICHD randomized clinical trial. *Psychotherapy and Psychosomatics, 77*, 27–37.

Davidson, L., Degner, L., & Morgan, T. (1995). Information and decision-making preferences of men with prostate cancer. *Oncology Nurse Forum, 22*, 1401–1408.

Dean, A., & Lin, N. (1977). The stress-buffering role of social support. *Journal of Nervous and Mental Diseases, 165*, 403.

Diamond, M. (1979). Social support and adaptation to chronic illness: The case of maintenance hemorialysis. *Research in Nursing & Health, 2*, 101–108.

Dick, M. (1986). Burnout in nurse faculty: Relationships with management style, collegial support, and work load in collegiate programs. *Journal of Professional Nursing, 2*, 252–260.

Dilorio, C., Escoffery, C., McCarty, F., Yeager, K. A., Henry, T. R., Koganti, A., . . . Wexler, B. (2008). Evaluation of WebEase: An epilepsy self-management web site. *Health Education Research*, 185–197.

Dodd, M. J., Dibble, S. L., & Thomas, M. L. (1993). Predictors of concerns and coping strategies of cancer chemotherapy outpatients. *Applied Nursing Research, 6*, 2–7.

Douglas, L. (1997). Reciprocal support in the context of cancer: Perspectives of the patient and spouse. *Oncology Nursing Forum, 24*, 1529–1536.

Ducharme, E., Stevens, B., & Rowat, K. (1994). Social support: Conceptual and methodological issues for research in mental health nursing. *Issues in Mental Health Nursing, 15*, 373–392.

Dunkel-Schetter, C. (1981). *Social support and coping with* cancer (Unpublished doctoral dissertation). University of Michigan, Ann Arbor.

Dunkel-Schetter, C., & Wortman, C. (1982). The role of social support in adaptation and recovery from physical illness. In S. Cohen & S. Syme (Eds.), *Social support and health* (pp. 281–302). Orlando, FL: Academic Press.

Duquette, A., Kerouac, S., Sandhu, B., & Beaudet, L. (1994). Factors related to nursing burnout: A review of empirical knowledge. *Issues in Mental Health Nursing, 15*, 337–358.

Durkheim, E. (1938). *The rules of sociological method.* New York, NY: Free Press.

Durkheim, E. (1951). *Suicide: A study in sociology.* New York, NY: Free Press. (Original work published 1897).

Duxbury, M., Armstrong, G., Drew, D., & Henly, S. (1984). Head nurse leadership style with staff burnout and job satisfaction in neonatal intensive care units. *Nursing Research, 33*, 97–101.

Eckenrode, J., & Gore, S. (1990). *Stress between work and family.* New York, NY: Plenum.

Edwards, C., Cole, O., Oyemade, U., Knight, E., Johnson, A., Westney, O., . . . Westney, L. (1994). Maternal stress and pregnancy outcomes in a prenatal clinic population. *Journal of Nutrition, 124*, 10065–10215.

Edwards, H., Courtney, M., Finlayson, K., Shuter, P., & Lindsay, E. (2009). A randomized controlled trial of a community nursing intervention: Improved quality of life and healing for clients with chronic leg ulcers. *Journal of Clinical Nursing, 18,* 1541–1549.

Eisler, J., Wolfer, J., & Diers, D. (1972). Relationship between need for social approval and postoperative recovery and welfare. *Nursing Research, 21,* 520–525.

Elmore, S. (1984). The moderating effect of social support upon depression. *Communicating Nursing Research, 17,* 17–22.

Failla, S., & Jones, L. C. (1991). Families of children with developmental disabilities: An examination of family hardiness. *Research in Nursing & Health, 14,* 41–50.

Ferketich, S., & Mercer, R., (1990). Effects of antepartal stress on health status during early motherhood. *Scholarly Inquiry in Nursing Practice International Journal, 4,* 127–149.

Fink, S. (1995). The influence of family demands on the strains and well-being of caregiving families. *Nursing Research, 44,* 139–146.

Fiore, J., Becker, J., & Coppel, D. B. (1983). Social network interactions: A buffer or a stress. *American Journal of Community Psychology, 11,* 423–439.

Frey, M. (1989). Social support and health: A theoretical formulation derived from King's conceptual framework. *Nursing Science Quarterly, 2,* 138–148.

Friedman, M. (1993). Social support sources and psychological well-being in older women with heart disease. *Research in Nursing & Health, 16,* 405–413.

Friedman, M. (1997). Social support sources among older women with heart failure: Continuity versus loss over time. *Research in Nursing & Health, 2,* 319–327.

Friedman, M., & King, K. (1994). The relationship of emotional and tangible support to psychological well-being among older women with heart failure. *Research in Nursing & Health, 17,* 433–440.

Funch, D. P., & Mettlin, C. (1982). The role of support in relation to recovery from breast surgery. *Social Science and Medicine,16,* 91–98.

Galvan, F. H., Davis, E. M., Banks, D., & Bing, E. G. (2008). HIV stigma and social support among African Americans. *AIDS Patient Care and STDs, 22,* 423–436.

Gibson, P., Cheavens, I., & Warren, M. (1998). Social support in persons with self-reported sensitivity to chemicals. *Research in Nursing & Health, 21,* 103–115.

Gluhoski, V., Fishman, B., & Perry, S. (1997). Moderators of bereavement distress in a gay male sample. *Personality and Individual Differences, 23,* 761–767.

Gottlieb, B. (1978). The development and application of a classification scheme of informal helping behaviors. *Canadian Journal of Behavioral Sciences, 10,* 105–115.

Gottlieb, B. (1981). *Social networks and social support.* Beverly Hills, CA: Sage.

Graydon, J., & Ross, E. (1995). Influence of symptoms, lung function, mood, and social support on level of functioning of patients with COPD. *Research in Nursing & Health, 18,* 52.

Gulick, E. E. (1992). Model for predicting work performance among persons with multiple sclerosis. *Nursing Research, 41,* 266–272.

Haley, D. J., (1986). *The relationship among social support, alienation, religiosity, length of service and the burnout experienced by nurses' aides and licensed practical nurses employed in skilled care nursing homes.* Unpublished doctoral dissertation, Loyola University of Chicago, Chicago.

Hann, D., Oxman, T., Ahles, T., Furstenburg, C., & Stukel, T. (1995). Social support adequacy and depression in older patients with metastatic cancer. *Psycho-Oncology, 4,* 213–221.

Hansell, P., Hughes, C., Caliandro, G., Russo, P., Budin, W., Hartman, B., & Hernandez, O. (1998). The effect of a social support boosting intervention on stress, coping, and social support in caregivers of children with HIV/AIDS. *Nursing Research, 47*(2), 79–86.

Hare, J., Pratt, C. C., & Andrews, D. (1988). Predictors of burnout in professional and paraprofessional nurses working in hospitals and nursing homes. *International Journal of Nursing Studies. 25*(2), 105–115.

Hatchett, L., Friend, R., Symister, P., & Wadhua, N. (1997). Interpersonal expectations, social support, and adjustment to chronic illness. *Journal of Personality and Social Psychology, 73,* 560–573.

Heins, H., Nance, N., & Levey-Mickens, G. (1988). The resource mom—A program of social support for pregnant teens. *Journal of the South Carolina Medical Association. 84,* 361–363.

Hinds, C., & Moyer, A. (1997). Support as experienced by patients with cancer during radiotherapy treatments. *Journal of Advanced Nursing, 26,* 371–379.

Hirsch, B. J. (1979). Psychological dimensions of social networks: A multimethod analysis. *American Journal of Community Psychology, 7,* 263–277.

Hirth, A., & Stewart, M. (1994). Hope and social support as coping resources for adults waiting for cardiac transplantation. *Canadian Journal of Nursing Research, 26*(3), 30–47.

House, J. (1981). *Work stress and social support.* Englewood Cliffs, NJ: Prentice-Hall.

Hughes, C., & Caliandro, G. (1996). Effects of social support, stress, and level of illness on caregiving of children with AIDS. *Journal of Pediatric*

Nursing: Nursing Care of Children and Families, 11, 347–358.

Hurley-Wilson, A. (1993). Perception, appraisal and meaning as mediators of the stress-health linkage. In J. S. Barnfather & B. L. Lyon (Eds.), *Stress and coping: Slate of the science and implications for nursing theory, research and practice* (pp. 129–149). Indianapolis, IN: Sigma Theta Tau International.

Hurst, C., Montgomery, A.J., Davis, B., Killion, C., & Baker, S. (2005). The relationship between social support, self-care agency, and self-care practices of African American women who are HIV-positive. *Journal of Multicultural Nursing & Health, 11*(3), 11–22.

Ihlenfeld, J. (1996). Nurses' perceptions of administrative social support. *Issues in Mental Health Nursing, 17,* 469–477.

Jalowiec, A. (1993). Coping with illness: Synthesis and critique of the nursing coping literature from 1980–1990. In J. Barnfather & B. Lyon (Eds.), *Stress and coping: State of the science and implications for nursing theory, research and practice* (pp. 65–83). Indianapolis, IN: Sigma Theta Tau International.

Jenerette, C. (2008). Relationships among types of social support and QOL in adults with sickle cell disease. *Southern Online Journal of Nursing Research, 8.* Retrieved from http://www.snrs.org/publications/SOJNR_articles2/Vol08Num03Main.html

Jirka, J., Schuett, S., & Foxall, M. (1996). Loneliness and social support in infertile couples. *Journal of Obstetrics, Gynecologic, and Neonatal Nursing, 25,* 55–60.

Kahn, R. (1979). Aging and social support. In M. Riley (Ed,), *Aging from birth to death.* Washington, DC: American Association for the Advancement of Science.

Kahn, R., & Antonucci, T. (1980). Convoys over the life course: Attachment, roles and social support. In P. B. Baltes & O. Brim (Eds.), *Life-span development and behavior* (Vol. 3, pp. 253–286). New York, NY: Academic Press.

Kang, D.-H., Coe, C. L., Karaszewski, J., & McCarthy, D. O. (1998). Relationship of social support to stress responses and immune function in healthy and asthmatic adolescents. *Research in Nursing & Health, 21,* 117–128.

Kaplan, B., Cassel, J., & Gore, S. (1977). Social support and health. *Medical Care, 15*(5 Suppl), 47–58.

Kendler, K. (1997). Social support: A genetic-epidemiologic analysis. *American Journal of Psychiatry, 154,* 1398–1404.

Kim, J.-H., & Knight, B. G. (2008). Effects of caregiver status, coping styles, and social support on the physical health of Korean American caregivers. *The Gerontologist, 48,* 287–299.

Kim. J. A. (1990). *The effect of supportive nursing care on depression, mood and satisfaction in military patients with low back pain.* Unpublished doctoral dissertation, The Graduate School of Yonsei University, Seoul, South Korea.

Kim, M. J. (1985). *An experimental study of the effects of supportive nursing care on stress relief for hospitalized patients.* Unpublished doctoral dissertation, The Graduate School of Yonsei University, Seoul, South Korea.

Krause, N. (2006). Exploring the stress-buffering effects of church-based and secular social support on self-rated health in late life. *The Journals of Gerontology, 61B,* 1, S35–S43.

Lambert, V. A., Lambert, C. E., Klipple, G. L., & Mewshaw, E. A. (1989). Social support, hardiness and psychological well-being in women with arthritis. *Image: The Journal of Nursing Science, 21,* 128–131.

Lazarus, R. (1990). Theory-based stress measurement. *Psychological Inquiry, 1,* 3–13.

Lazarus, R. S., & Folkman, S. (1984). *Stress, appraisal, and coping.* New York, NY: Springer.

Lederman, R. (1984). Anxiety and conflict in pregnancy: Relationship to maternal health status. In H. Werley & J. Fitzpatrick (Eds.), *Annual review of nursing research. (Vol. 2,* pp. 27–62). New York, NY: Springer.

Lederman, R., Lederman. E., Work, B., & McCann, D. (1979). Relationship of maternal anxiety, plasma catecholamines and plasma cortisol to progress in labor. *American Journal of Obstetrics and Gynecology, 132,* 495–500.

Lee, R. N., Graydon, J. E., & Ross, E. (1991). Effects of psychological well-being, physical status, and social support on oxygen-dependent COPD patients' level of functioning. *Research in Nursing & Health, 14,* 323–328.

Linn, J., Poku, K., Cain, Y., Holzapfel, K., & Crawford, D. (1995). Psychosocial outcomes of HIV illness in male and female African American clients. *Social Work in Health Care, 21*(3), 43–60.

Lowenthal, M., & Haven, C. (1968). Interaction and adaptation: Intimacy as a critical variable. *American Sociological Review, 33,* 20–30.

Lugton, J. (1997). The nature of social support as experienced by women treated for breast cancer. *Journal of Advanced Nursing, 25,* 1181–1191.

Lyon, B. (1990). Getting back on track: Nursing's autonomous scope of practice. In N. Chaska (Ed.), *The nursing profession: Turning points.* St. Louis, MO: C. V. Mosby.

Mallett, K. (1988). *The relationship between burnout, death anxiety and social support in hospice and critical care nurses.* Doctoral dissertation, University of Toledo, Toledo, OH.

Maslach, C., & Jackson, S. (1981). *Maslach burnout inventory research edition.* Palo Alto, CA: Consulting Psychologists Press.

McColl, M., & Frieland, J. (1994). Social support, aging, and disability. *Topics in Geriatric Rehabilitation, 9*(3), 54–71.

McKenzie, R. (1926). The ecological approach to the study of the human community. In R. Park & C. Burgess (Eds.), *The city.* Chicago, IL: University of Chicago Press.

Meister, S. (1982). *Perceived social support, subnetworks and well-being at life change.* Doctoral dissertation, University of Michigan, Ann Arbor.

Messick, D., & Cook, M. (1983). *Equity theory.* New York, NY: Praeger.

Mickschl, D. (1984). *A study of critical care nurses: The relationship among needs fulfillment discrepancy, attitudes and feelings of burnout, and unit leadership style.* Unpublished doctoral dissertation, Gonzaga University, Spokane, WA.

Mitchell, R., & Trickett, E. (1980). Social networks as mediators of social support: An analysis of the effects and determinants of social networks. *Community Mental Health Journal, 16*, 27–44.

Murrock, C. J., & Madigan, E. (2008). Self-efficacy and social support as mediators between culturally specific dance and lifestyle physical activity. *Research and Theory for Nursing Practice: An International Journal, 22*, 192–204.

Norbeck, J. (1981). Social support: A model for clinical research and application. *Advances in Nursing Science, 3*(4), 43–59.

Norbeck, J. (1984). The Norbeck Social Support Questionnaire. *Birth Defects: Original Article Series, 20*(5), 45–55.

Norbeck, J. (1991). Social support needs of family caregivers of psychiatric patients from three age groups. *Nursing Research, 40*, 208–213.

Norbeck, J., & Anderson, N. (1989). Psychosocial predictors of pregnancy outcomes in low-income Black, Hispanic and White women. *Nursing Research, 38*, 204–209.

Norbeck, J., DeJoseph, J., & Smith, R. (1996). A randomized trial of an empirically derived social support intervention to prevent low birth weight among African American women. *Social Science & Medicine, 43*, 947–954.

Norbeck, J. S., Lindsey, A. M., & Carrieri, V. L. (1981). The development of an instrument to measure social support. *Nursing Research. 30*(5), 264–269.

Norbeck, J. S., Lindsey, A. M., & Carrieri, V. L. (1983). Further development of the Norbeck Social Support Questionnaire: Normative data and validity testing. *Nursing Research, 32*(1), 4–9.

Northouse, L. L. (1988). Social support in patients' and husbands' adjustment to breast cancer. *Nursing Research, 37*, 91–95.

Norwood, S. (1996). The Social Support Apgar: Instrument development and testing. *Research in Nursing & Health, 19*, 143–152.

Nuckolls, K., Cassel, J., & Kaplan, B. (1972). Psychosocial assets, life crisis and the prognosis of pregnancy. *American Journal of Epidemiology, 95*, 431–441.

Nyamathi, A. M. (1987). The coping responses of female spouses of patients with myocardial infarction. *Heart and Lung, 16*, 86–92.

Oakley, A., Rajan, T., & Grant, A. (1990). Social support and pregnancy outcome. *British Journal of Obstetrics and Gynecology, 97*, 155–162.

O'Brien, R., Wineman, N., & Nealon, N. (1995). Correlates of the caregiving process in multiple sclerosis. *Scholarly Inquiry for Nursing Practice, 9*, 323–342.

Oxman, T., Freeman, D., Manheimer, E., & Stukel, T. (1994). Social support and depression after cardiac surgery in elderly patients. *American Journal of Geriatric Psychiatry, 2*, 309–323.

Oxman, T., & Hull, J. (1997). Social support, depression, and activities of daily living in older heart surgery patients. *Journal of Gerontology, 52B*, 1–14.

Paredes, F. (1982). *The relationship of psychological resources and social support, occupational stress and burnout in hospital nurses* Unpublished doctoral dissertation, University of Houston, Houston, TX.

Park, R., & Burgess, E. (Eds.) (1926). *The city.* Chicago, IL: University of Chicago Press.

Pearlin, L. (1989). The sociological study of stress. *Journal Health and Social Behavior, 30*, 241–256.

Peck, A., & Boland, J. (1977). Emotional reactions to radiation treatment. *Cancer, 40*, 180–184.

Picot, S. (1995). Rewards, costs, and coping of African American caregivers. *Nursing Research, 44*, 147–152.

Potts, M. (1997). Social support and depression among older adults living alone: The importance of friends within and outside of a retirement community. *Social Work, 42*, 348–362.

Powers, B. (1988). Social networks, social support, and elderly institutionalized people. *Advances in Nursing Science, 10*(2), 40–58.

Preston, D. (1995). Marital status, gender roles, stress and health in the elderly. *Health Care for Women International, 16*, 149–165.

Qureshi, H., & Walker, A. (1989). *The caring relationship: Elderly people and their families.* New York, NY: Macmillan.

Rees, C. A., Karter, A. J., & Young, B. A. (2010). Race/ethnicity, social support, and associations with diabetes self-care and clinical outcomes in NHANES. *The Diabetes Educator, 36*, 435–445.

Riegel, B. J., & Gocka, I. (1995). Gender differences in adjustment to acute myocardial infarction. *Heart & Lung, 24*, 457–466.

Roberts, J., Browne, G., Streiner, D., Gafni, A., Pallister, R., Hoxby, H., . . . Meichenbaum, D. (1995). Problem-solving counseling or phone-call support for outpatients with chronic illness:

Effective for whom? *Canadian Journal of Nursing Research, 27,* 111–137.

Robinson, J. (1995). Grief responses, coping processes, and social support of widows: Research with Roy's model. *Nursing Science Quarterly, 8,* 158–164.

Rothberg, A., & Lits, B. (1991). Psychosocial support for maternal stress during pregnancy: Effect on birth weight. *American Journal of Obstetrics and Gynecology, 165,* 403–407.

Ruiz-Bueno, J. B., & Underwood, P. (1999). Resources as moderators/mediators of the stress-health outcome linkage. In J.S. Werner (Ed.), *Stress and coping: State of the science and implications for nursing theory, research and practice.* Chicago, IL: Midwest Nursing Research Society.

Runtz, M., & Schallow, J. (1997). Social support and coping strategies as mediators of adult adjustment following childhood maltreatment. *Child Abuse and Neglect, 21,* 211–226.

Russell, D., & Taylor, J. (2009). Living alone and depressive symptoms: The influence of gender, physical disability, and social support among Hispanic and non-Hispanic older adults. *The Journals of Gerontology, 64B,* 95–104.

Sallis, J., Grossman, R. M., Pinski, R. B., Patterson, T. L., & Nader, P. R. (1987). The development of scales to measure social support for diet and exercise behaviors. *Predictive Medicine, 16,* 825–836.

Sammarco, A., & Konecny, L. M. (2008). Quality of life, social support, and uncertainty among Latina breast cancer survivors. *Oncology Nursing Forum, 35,* 844–849.

Sammarco, A., & Konecny, L. M. (2010). Quality of life, social support, and uncertainty among Latina and Caucasian breast cancer survivors: A comparative study. *Oncology Nursing Forum, 37,* 93–99.

Sansom, D., & Farnill, D. (1997). Stress following marriage breakdown: Does social support play role. *Journal of Divorce & Remarriage, 26*(3/4), 39–49.

Sargent, L., & Terry, D. (2000). The moderating role of social support in Karasek's job strain model. *Work & Stress, 14,* 245–261.

Scharer, K., Colon, E., Moneyham, L., Hussey, J., Tavakoli, A., & Shugart, M. (2009). A comparison of two types of social support for mothers of mentally ill children. *Journal of Child and Adolescent Psychiatric Nursing, 22,* 86–98.

Seeman, T., & Berkman, L. (1988). Structural characteristics of social networks and their relationship with social support in the elderly: Who provides support. *Social Science and Medicine, 26,* 737–749.

Shoenbach, V., Kaplan, B., Fredman, L., & Kleinbaum, D. (1986). Social ties and mortality in Evans County, Georgia. *American Journal of Epidemiology, 123,* 577–591.

Small, S., & Graydon, J. (1993). Uncertainty in hospitalized patients with chronic obstructive pulmonary disease. *International Journal of Nursing Studies, 30,* 239–246.

Snowdon, A., Canmeron, S., & Dunham. K. (1994). Relationships between stress, coping resources and satisfaction with family functioning in families of children with disabilities. *Canadian Journal of Nursing Research, 26*(3), 63–76.

Spencer, B., Thomas, H., & Morris, J. (1989). A randomized controlled trial of the provision of a social support service during pregnancy: The South Manchester Family Worker Project. *British Journal of Obstetrics and Gynecology, 96,* 281–288.

Stewart, M. (1989). Social support instruments created by nurse investigators. *Nursing Research, 38,* 268–275.

Stewart, M., Hart, G., & Mann, K. (1995). Living with haemophilia and HIV/AIDS: Support and coping. *Journal of Advanced Nursing, 22,* 1101–1111.

Stewart, M., Ritchie, J., McGrath, P., Thompson, D., & Bruce, B. (1994). Mothers of children with chronic conditions: Supportive and stressful interactions with partners and professionals regarding caregiving burdens. *Canadian Journal of Nursing Research, 26*(4), 61–81.

Stewart, M., & Tilden, V. (1995). The contributions of nursing science to social support. *International Journal of Nursing Studies, 32,* 535–544.

Stroebe, W., Stroebe, M., Abakoumkin, G., & Schut, H. (1996). The role of loneliness and social support in adjustment to loss: A test of attachment versus stress theory. *Journal of Personality and Social Psychology, 70,* 1241–1249.

Thomas, W., & Znaniecki, F (1920). *The Polish peasant in Europe and America.* New York, NY: Knopf.

Tilden, V. P. (1983). The relation of selected psychosocial variables to emotional disequilibrium during pregnancy. *Research in Nursing & Health, 6,* 167–174.

Tilden, V. P. (1984). The relation of selected psychosocial variables to single status of adult women during pregnancy. *Nursing Research, 33,* 102–107.

Tilden, V. P. (1991). *The Interpersonal Relationship Inventory (IPRI): Instrument development summary.* Portland: Oregon Health Science University, School of Nursing.

Tilden, V. P., & Gaylen, R. D. (1987). Cost and conflict: The darker side of social support. *Western Journal of Nursing Research, 9,* 9–18.

Tilden, V. P., Hirsch, A., & Nelson, C. (1994). The Interpersonal Relationship Inventory: Continued psychometric evaluation. *Journal of Nursing Measurement, 2,* 63–78.

Tilden, V. P, Nelson, C, & May, B. (1990a). Use of qualitative methods to enhance content validity. *Nursing Research, 39,* 172–175.

Tilden, V. P., Nelson, C., & May, B. (1990b). The IPR inventory: Development and psychometric characteristics. *Nursing Research, 39,* 337–343.

Trivedi, R. B., Blumenthal, J. A., O'Connor, C., Adams, K., Hinderliter, A., Sueta-Dupree, C., . . . Sherwood, A. (2009). Coping styles in heart failure patients with depressive symptoms. *Journal of Psychosomatic Research, 67,* 339–346.

Turner, H. (1994). Gender and social support: Taking the bad with the good? *Sex Roles, 30,* 521–540.

Turner, R., Frankel, B., & Levin, D. (1983). Social support: Conceptualization, measurement, and implications for mental health. *Research in Community and Mental Health, 3,* 67–111.

Underwood, P. W. (1986). *Psychosocial variables: Their prediction of birth complications and relationship to perception of childbirth.* Ann Arbor, MI: University Microfilms, International.

Vaglio, J., Conrad, M., Poston, W. S., O'Keefe, J., Haddock, K., House, J., & Spertus, J.A. (2004). Testing the performance of the ENRICHD Social Support Instrument in cardiac patients. *Health and Quality of Life Outcomes, 2,* 2. Retrieved June 24, 2010, from http://www.hqlo .com/content

Vaux, A., & Harrison, D. (1985). Support network characteristics associated with support satisfaction and perceived support. *American Journal of Community Psychology, 13,* 245–267.

Villar, J., Farnot, U., Barros, F., Victoria, C., & Langer, A. (1992). A randomized clinical trial of psychosocial support during high-risk pregnancies. *New England Journal of Medicine, 327,* 1266–1271.

Vrabec, N. (1995). *Burden in rural versus urban family caregivers.* Unpublished doctoral dissertation, University of Wisconsin-Milwaukee.

Wandersman, L., Wandersman, A., & Kahn, S. (1980). Social support in the transition to parenthood. *Journal of Community Psychology, 8,* 332–342.

Weinert, C. (1984). Evaluation of the PRQ: A social support measure. In K. Barnard, P. Brandt, & B. Raff (Eds.), *Social support and families of vulnerable infants* (Birth Defects, Original Article Series No. 20, pp. 59–97). White Plains, NY: March of Dimes Defects Foundation.

Weinert, C. (1987). A social support measure: PRQ8S. *Nursing Research, 36,* 273–277.

Weinert, C. (1988). Measuring social support: Revision and further development of the Personal Resource Questionnaire. In C. Waltz & O. Strictland (Eds.), *Measurement of nursing outcomes.* (Vol. I, pp. 309–327). New York, NY: Springer.

Weinert, C., & Brandt, P. (1987). Measuring social support with the Personal Resources Questionnaire. *Western Journal of Nursing Research, 9,* 589–602.

Weinert, C., & Tilden, V. P. (1990). Measures of social support: Assessment of validity. *Nursing Research, 39,* 212–216.

Weiss, R. (1974). The provisions of social relationships. In Z. Ruhin (Ed.), *Doing unto others.* Englewood Cliffs, NJ: Prentice-Hall.

Weiss, R. (1975). *Marital separation.* New York, NY: Basic Books.

White, N., Richter, J., & Fry, C. (1992). Coping, social support, and adaptation to chronic illness. *Western Journal of Nursing Research, 14,* 211–224.

Willey, C., & Silliman, R. (1990). The impact of disease on the social support experiences of cancer patients. *Journal of Psychosocial Oncology, 8,* 79–95.

Wortman, C. (1984). Social support and cancer. Conceptual and methodological issues. *Cancer, 53,* 2339–2160.

Wu, C. Y., Prosser, R. A., & Taylor, J. Y. (2010). Association of depressive symptoms and social support on blood pressure among urban African American women and girls. *Journal of the American Academy of Nurse Practitioners, 22,* 694–704.

Yang, Y. (2006). How does functional disability affect depressive symptoms in late life? The role of perceived social support and psychological resources. *Journal of Health and Social Behavior, 47,* 355–372.

Younger, L. Kendell, M., & Pickler, R. (1997). Mastery of stress in mothers of preterm infants. *Journal of the Society of Pediatric Nurses, 2,* 29–35.

Zhang, X., Norris, S. L., Gregg, E. W., & Beckles, G. (2007). Social support and mortality among older persons with diabetes. *The Diabetes Educator, 33,* 273–281.

Zimet, G. D., Dahlem, N. W., Zimet, S. G., & Farley, G. K. (1988). The Multidimensional Scale of Perceived Social Support. *Journal of Personality Assessment, 52,* 30–41.

15

Psychosocial and Biological Stressors and the Pathogenesis of Cardiovascular Disease

Holli A. DeVon and Karen L. Saban

In most cases stress is the root cause of death; illnesses are just the wrap up.

Yordan Yordanov

The relationship between psychosocial stress, risk for cardiovascular disease (CVD), and patient outcomes has been extensively studied. However, the relationships between stress, physiological responses, and the mechanisms leading to CVD continue to mystify researchers. Explaining these relationships is imperative for several reasons. First, CVD remains the number one killer of American women and men despite advances in technology and science that have significantly reduced mortality and morbidity (American Heart Association [AHA], 2010). Second, traditional risk factors of CVD, such as smoking, obesity, and diabetes, account for 58% to 75% of the incidence of heart disease; consequently, a significant portion of disease causation remains unexplained (Gallo, Ghaed, & Bracken, 2004). Third, some of the causal mechanisms of CVD, including inflammation and coagulation, have been well established but mediating and moderating factors have not been. Fourth, advances in acute care and primary prevention strategies have led to improved survival rates and resulted in a significant number of patients with chronic disease (AHA, 2010). Finally, the identification of mechanisms and determinants of CVD may open a new line of inquiry focused on the design and testing of interventions.

Brief Background

Cardiovascular disease refers to diseases of the heart and blood vessels. The four most common types of CVD are coronary heart disease (CHD), ischemic stroke, hypertension, and heart failure (AHA, 2010). The most common mechanism for the development of CVD is atherogenesis, a complex process by which the artery becomes obstructed with plaque. The process appears to begin early in life with the deposit of small lipoprotein particles in the intima and progresses with leukocyte recruitment, formation of lipid-laden macrophages, and foam cells. Foam cells serve as a reservoir for excess lipids and serve as a rich source for pro-inflammatory mediators, leading to the development of fatty streaks, plaque build-up, and rupture (Libby, 2005). Identification of the psychosocial and biobehavioral mechanisms of CVD development and progression holds great promise for the design of new primary and secondary prevention strategies.

PURPOSE AND RATIONALE

The purpose of this chapter is to elucidate the relationship between psychosocial and biobehavioral stressors, physiological responses, inflammation, and the development of CVD and to propose a new model to examine these relationships. We are taking a disease-oriented approach in which we evaluate the impact of upstream stimuli (stressors) on downstream outcomes (development of disease). Miller, Chen, and Cole (2009) proposed that identifying psychobiologic interactions relevant to health should begin with the identification of biologic processes involved in the development of the disease. Then, the biological and behavioral factors modulated by those same processes should be ascertained. Finally, an analysis of those factors should be conducted to determine which are amenable to regulation in the social world. This disease-centric approach could be construed as a myopic view based on the medical model of disease, but that view is shortsighted. Identification of psychobiological determinants of disease acknowledges the individual as the center of a dynamic environment where multiple social, psychological, biological, behavioral, and cultural factors mediate and moderate disease progression and outcomes. Such a view is related to the phenomena of allostatic load (McEwen & Seeman, 2009), a concept derived from the term *allostasis* (Sterling & Eyer, 1988), *meaning the maintenance of stability* or "homeostasis." Since the human condition is dynamic, the term allostatic load was coined to express the fluctuations in health status based on response to stressors. One can think of *allostatic load* as the wear and tear on the body that results from acute and chronic stressors. B. S. McEwen (1998) conceptualized a model of the relationship between perceived stress and physiologic responses and the resulting allostatic load on the individual (Figure 15.1).

Our approach to developing a new model of stress in CVD is grounded in the concept of allostatic load. Stress is a nebulous term that encompasses emotional, psychological, social,

Figure 15.1   The Stress Response and Development of Allostatic Load

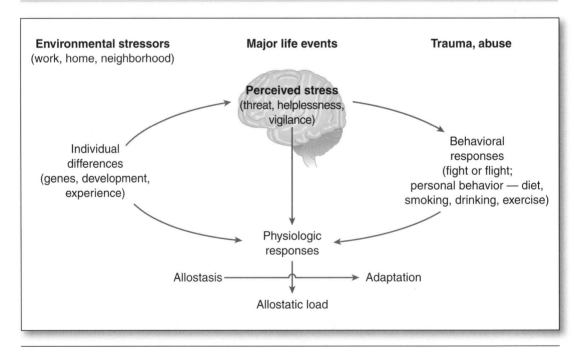

SOURCE: Reprinted from B. S. McEwen (1998) by permission from the *New England Journal of Medicine*.

biological, and physiological phenomena. Each of these components is influenced by individual and environmental characteristics. Stress also has temporal (acute and chronic) qualities. For our model, we define *stress as a complex psychobiological state that occurs when there is a threat to homeostasis.* Table 15.1 presents a list of definitions of the concepts used in this chapter.

Table 15.1   Definition of Key Concepts in This Chapter

Term	Definition
allostasis	Maintaining stability or homeostasis (B. McEwen & Seeman, 2009).
allostatic load	Wear and tear on the body due to repeated cycles of allostasis as well as the inefficient turning on or shutting off of these responses (B. S. McEwen, 1998).
cardiovascular disease	Cardiovascular disease refers to diseases of the heart and blood vessels most often caused by atherosclerosis. The four most common types of CVD are coronary heart disease, ischemic stroke, hypertension, and heart failure (American Heart Association, 2010).
culture	The totality of socially transmitted behavioral patterns, arts, beliefs, values, customs, and lifeways and all other products of human work and characteristics of a population of people that guide their worldview and decision-making (Purnell & Paulanka, 2005).
epigenetics	Changes in gene expression without alterations in DNA sequencing in response to environment. Involve modifications to chromatin, such as DNA methylation (Veenema, 2009).
inflammatory response	The physiological response to a physical or psychological stressor involving complex coordination of the brain and the immune system aimed at protecting the organism from harm (Ferencik, Stvrtinova, Hulin, & Novak, 2007).
mind	Ability to form neural representations that can become images, be manipulated in a process called thought, and eventually influence behavior. A conscious or unconscious thought process (Damasio, 1994; Taylor, Goehler, Galper, Innes, & Bourguignon, 2010).
mind–body connection	The capacity for an individual's thought to affect physiological processes and symptoms (Astin, Shapiro, Eisenberg, & Forys, 2003).
top-down and bottom-up mechanism	Top-down mechanisms begin with mental processing at the level of the cerebral cortex, particularly conscious and intentional mental activities. Bottom-up mechanisms are initiated by stimulation of various somatic, visceral, and chemical/sensory receptors (Taylor et al., 2010).
physiological	Characteristic of or appropriate to an organism's healthy or normal functioning (Guyton & Hall, 2000).
psychobiological	An association between a psychosocial characteristic and changes in biological processes that drive disease progression (G. Miller, Chen, & Cole, 2009).
psychological	Relating to behavior (e.g., actions, feelings, and biological states) and mental processes (e.g., problem solving, intelligence, and memory) (Pastorino & Doyle-Portillo, 2009).
social	Existence, structure, regulation, quantity, and quality of interpersonal relationships (House, Umberson, & Landis, 1988).
stress	The nonspecific response to noxious stimuli. Includes both the initial impact of the stressor (alarm system) on tissues and the adaptive mechanisms that result from the stressor (Selye, 1956).
upstream/ downstream	Upstream variables are those that effect the development of chronic disease, and downstream variables are those that speed disease progression and affect outcomes (Sindall, 2001).

Contemporary Models of Stress and Cardiovascular Disease

It's not stress that kills us, it is our reaction to it.

Hans Selye, 1937

Psychosocial stress has typically been viewed as a stimulus in the cardiovascular literature. Decades of research have provided evidence of the influence of psychosocial stress on the development and progression of CVD. Several contemporary authors have conceptualized these relationships as well. G. Miller et al. (2009) present a graphic representation of the relationship between chronic stress and biological and physiological dysfunction that leads to disease (Figure 15.2). These stressors have been shown to be both antecedent and a consequence of CVD.

The model contains examples of social stressors, but other psychological stressors and individual characteristics are not included. Brotman, Golden, and Wittstein (2007) designed a model of the cardiovascular effects of the stress response (Figure 15.3). It depicts the upstream impact of social and physical stressors on the cardiovascular system by means of the hypothalamic-pituitary-adrenal (HPA) axis and the sympathetic nervous system, but it also lacks psychological, environmental, and personal stressors.

Finally, Steptoe and Brydon (2007) developed a model illustrating the hypothesized role of psychosocial and biological stressors at various stages of CHD (Figure 15.4). This comprehensive view of stress and CVD also includes cardiac outcomes. Environmental and individual stressors are subsumed under *chronic stressors* and acute stressors are called *acute triggers*. According to these authors, there is strong evidence that the initiation, progression, and complications of atherosclerosis leading to CVD are due to inflammation and thrombotic activity. Other possible causal pathways by which psychosocial and biological processes impact the development of inflammation and lead to atherosclerosis, including immune dysregulation, autonomic nervous system dysfunction, neuroendocrine processes, infection, genetic mutations, or epigenetic changes, have not been identified (Steptoe et al., 2002; Steptoe & Brydon, 2007).

Toward a Causal Model of Stress and CVD Development

The models presented thus far provide excellent direction for examining specific stressor hypotheses. However, gaps remain in the identification of stressors that are independent predictors or that moderate or mediate the development and progression of CVD. Therefore, a synthesis of the literature linking stress and the development of CVD is necessary and follows. The first section addresses individual and environmental characteristics and the second presents current thoughts on biological responses and indicators of stress. Finally, we propose a new model representing the relationship among the respective characteristics, biological responses, and CVD for testing by researchers.

Individual Characteristics

Psychological stress is a nonspecific term that encompasses sadness, frustration, anxiety, and a number of other negative mood states. It includes both mild and severe forms of these mood states, as well as both transient and persistent ones. It also refers both to the symptoms of psychiatric disorders and to normal emotional responses to adversity. Researchers in the United Kingdom enrolled 6,576 healthy women and men to test for an association between psychological distress and cardiovascular events. Cardiovascular events were measured over an average of 7.2 years. Risk was more than 50% higher for those reporting greater psychological distress after adjusting for age and sex (Hazard Ratio [HR] = 1.54, 95% confidence interval [CI] = 1.09–2.18, $p = 0.013$). Psychological distress was examined in a Finnish cohort to determine if there was a gender-specific association with cardiovascular risk scores. Participants were stratified into three groups according to distress scores. Men with the highest distress scores had significantly higher mean CVD risk scores (3.6, ±3.3) compared to men with the lowest distress scores (2.5, ±2.6). No association was found between psychological distress and cardiovascular risk scores in women (Puustinen, Koponen, Kautiainen, Mantyselka, & Vanhala, 2010).

Psychological distress was associated with a higher prevalence of CVD in both women and men in a cohort of adult Croatians ($N = 9,070$).

Figure 15.2   The Influence of the Social World on Disease Pathogenesis

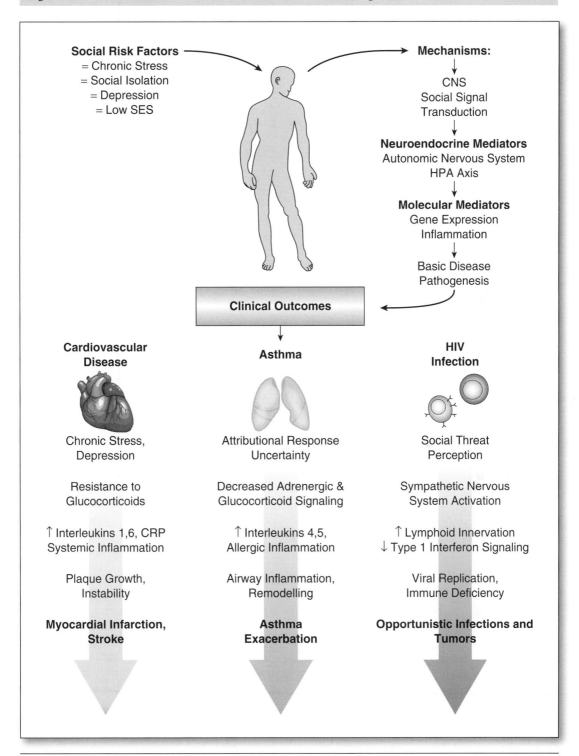

SOURCE: Miller, G., Chen, E., Cole, S.E., Health Psychology: Developing Biologically Plausible Models Linking the Social World and Physical Health (2009) *Annual Review of Psychology, Volume 60.* Reprinted by permission.

Figure 15.3   The Cardiovascular Toll of Stress

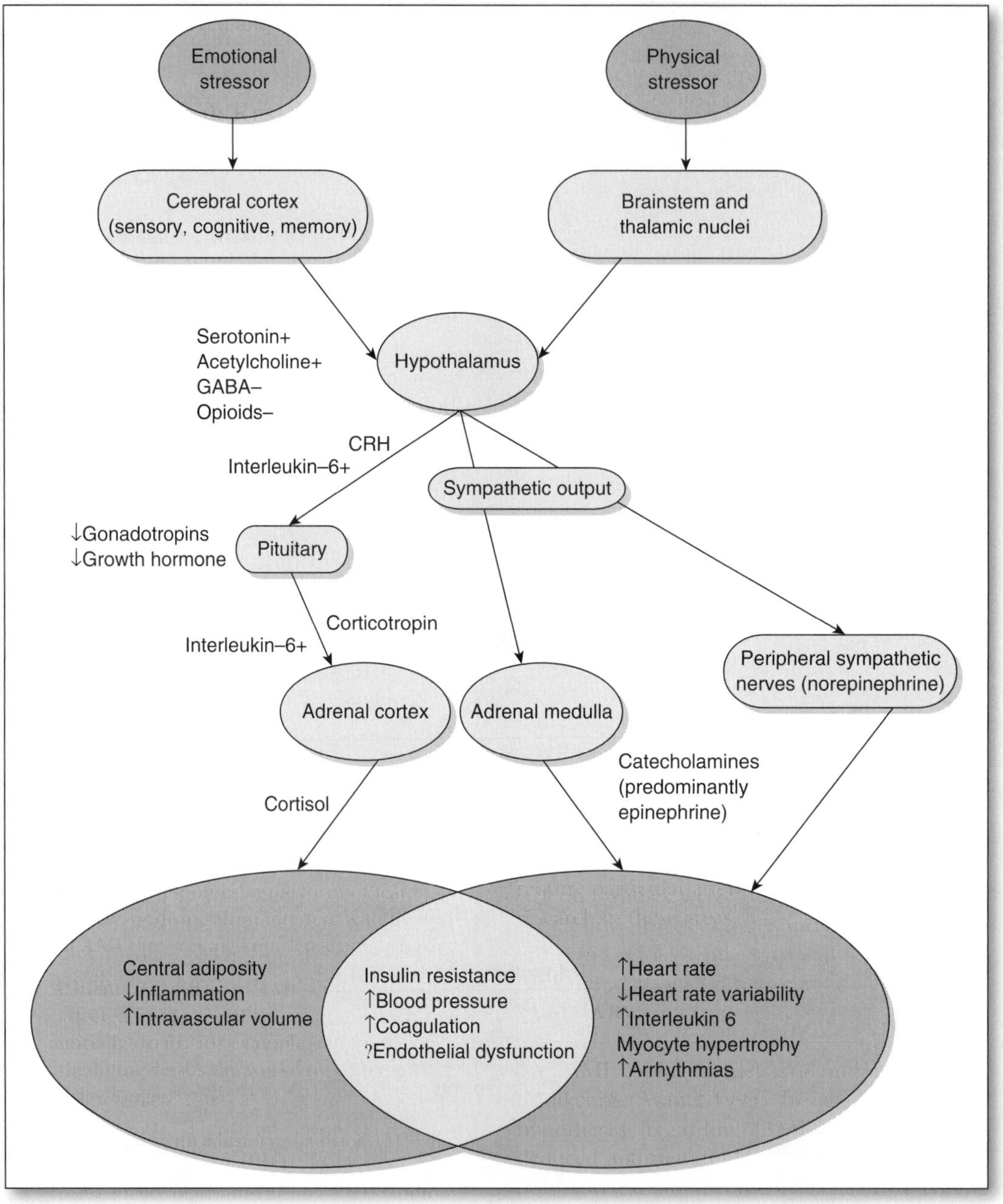

SOURCE: Brotman, D. J., Golden, S. H., & Wittstein, I. S. (2007). The cardiovascular toll of stress. *The Lancet*, 370, 1089–1100. Reprinted with permission.

NOTE: GABA = y-aminobutric acid, CRH = corticotrophin-releasing hormone.

Women also had higher levels of psychological distress compared to men (Brborović et al., 2009).

Perceived stress is a measure of the degree to which situations in one's life are appraised as disturbing. Functional independence, depression, and emotions predicted 45% of the variance in scores on the Perceived Stress Scale in stroke survivors immediately following hospital

Figure 15.4   Psychosocial Factors and Coronary Heart Disease: The Role of
Psychoneuroimmunological Processes

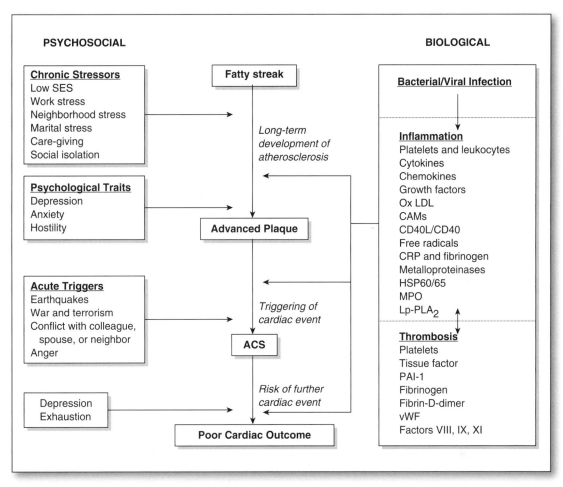

SOURCE: In R. Ader (Ed.), *Psychoneuroimmunology* (4th ed., pp. 945-974). New York: Elsevier. Reprinted with permission.

discharge, which suggests perceived stress impacted recovery from stroke (Dodd et al., 2001). In the Copenhagen City Heart Study (N = 7,066), investigators evaluated the long-term effects of perceived stress on health behaviors and cardiac risk profiles in women and men. After 10 years of follow-up, those with high levels of perceived stress were less likely to have quit smoking (OR = 0.58, 95% CI = 0.4–0.83), more likely to be inactive (OR = 1.90, 95% CI = 1.41–2.55), and less likely to have stopped drinking (OR = 0.43, 95% CI = 0.24–0.79) compared to those with low stress. High perceived stress was related to a higher risk of death from ischemic heart disease for younger, but not older, men

(HR = +2.59, 95% CI = 1.20–5.61). There was no association between high stress and CVD mortality in women (N. T. Nielsen, Kristensen, Schnohr, & Gronbaek, 2008). Women reporting high stress were more likely to have become overweight (OR = 1.55, 95% CI = 1.12–2.15) (Rod, Grønbæk, Schnohr, Prescott, & Kristensen, 2009).

Personality Characteristics and Mood States

A number of personality characteristics and mood states have been found to be related to the development and progression of CVD. Included are Type A Behavior Pattern (TABP), anger, anxiety, hostility, depression, low self-esteem, high stress reactivity, and Type D personality. Early literature tied anger to a configuration of personality characteristics known as the Type A Behavior Pattern (TABP) that was hypothesized to contribute to the development of CVD. Friedman and Rosenman (1974) described Type A persons as hard-driving, competitive, ambitious, impatient, quick-tempered, and time urgent. In addition, Type As have a strong desire to achieve recognition and advancement. People exhibiting Type A behavior have a hyper awareness of time and thus walk, eat, and perform most activities rapidly and perfunctorily. Studies of middle-aged men suggested that TABP was an independent risk factor for CHD (Rosenman et al., 1975); it was one of the first psychosocial stressors implicated in the cause of CHD. However, subsequent research did not unequivocally support the early findings (e.g., Schwalbe, 1990) and investigators attempted to isolate the factors in the pattern that were truly affecting disease development. *Anger* and *hostility* were identified as culprit variables.

Anger, *an emotion characterized by irritation or annoyance, reflects a reaction to a threat.* Hostility, *considered a trait rather than a state, is characterized by a suspicious or mistrustful attitude toward others signaled by aggressive behavior.* How individuals express anger has also been linked to CVD. Those who internalize anger and tend to ruminate have been shown to be at higher risk for CVD than those who express their anger. In a study of 200 healthy postmenopausal women, high hostility, trait anger, and internalized anger scores were associated with carotid atherosclerosis at 10-year follow-up (Mathews, Owens, Kuller, Sutton-Tyrrell, & Jansen-McWilliams, 1998). In 1996, T. Q. Miller, Smith, Turner, Guijarro, and Hallet conducted a meta-analysis of 45 studies and concluded that hostility was an independent risk factor for CHD. In the Multiple Risk Factor Intervention Trial (MRFIT), men at high risk for CVD, who also scored high on ratings of hostility, were more likely to die from CVD (OR = 1.61, 95% CI = 1.09–2.39) (Matthews, Gump, Harris, Haney, & Barefoot, 2004). Anxiety, another factor in the development of CVD, is not as well understood yet; however, evidence points to it as a predictor of adverse outcomes in patients with CHD. *Anxiety has been defined as an unpleasant feeling that is typically associated with uneasiness, apprehension, and worry. It is a generalized mood condition that most often occurs without an identifiable stimulus and is distinguishable from fear, which occurs in the presence of an observed threat. Anxiety has been conceptualized as both an emotional state and a character trait* (Schocken, Greene, Worden, Harrison & Spielberger, 1987). Shibeshi, Young-Xu, and Blatt (2007) measured anxiety for up to 3.4 years in a study of 516 outpatients (82% male) with coronary artery disease (CAD). A high anxiety score was associated with an increased risk of nonfatal myocardial infarction (MI) or death (HR = 1.06, 95% CI = 1.01–1.12, $p = .02$). Additionally, the odds of an adverse outcome were nearly twice as high for patients in the top tertile compared to those in the lowest tertile of anxiety (HR = 1.97, 95% CI = 1.03–3.78). Investigators followed a cohort of 49,321 young Swedish men for 37 years who were initially examined for medical service in 1969 and 1970. Anxiety was an independent predictor of acute myocardial infarctions (HR = 2.51, 95% CI = 1.38–4.55) and subsequent CHD events (HR = 2.17, 95% CI = 1.28–3.67) (Janszky, Ahnve, Lundberg, & Hemmingsson, 2010). Moser and others (2007) found that anxiety in inpatients, following myocardial infarction, was associated with increased risk of arrhythmia and ischemic events (OR = 1.5, 95% CI = 1.1–2.0, $p = .01$).

Depression, *a mental and mood state characterized by a pessimistic sense of inadequacy and a despondent lack of activity characterized by feelings of doom and gloom*, may be the single most investigated stress-related phenomenon in the cardiovascular literature. Depression, alone or as part of a general psychological stress picture including anxiety, anger, hostility, and negative affect, has been shown to trigger acute coronary syndromes and strokes (Arbelaez, Ariyo, Crum, Fried, & Ford, 2007; Bhattacharyya, Perkins-Porras, Wikman, & Steptoe, 2010; Garcia-Vera, Sanz, Espiosa, Fortun, & Magan, 2010). See Table 15.2 for hypotheses tested related to moods and psychological distress and CVD. Results have been equivocal with some studies showing an association between depression and other psychological stressors and CVD and some showing no association.

Research examining the link between depression and biological processes has also been equivocal. Depression and psychological distress have been related to impaired baroreflex sensitivity (Watkins, Blumenthal, & Carney, 2002), autonomic control of the heart (Pitzalis et al., 2001), and decreased heart rate variability (Pieper, Brosscholt, Van der Leeden, & Thayer, 2007). However, Carroll, Phillips, Hunt, and Der (2007) found an inverse relationship between depression, systolic blood pressure, and heart rate. There is some evidence to suggest that depression may lead to inflammation that ultimately contributes to the development of CVD (Stewart, Rand, Muldoon, & Kamarck, 2009). Table 15.2 presents studies of the relationships between psychological stressors, moods, and physiological processes.

Other individual characteristics include self-esteem, stress reactivity, and Type D personality. *Self-esteem is a subjective judgment of personal worth or adequacy and self-acceptance.* It is partially dependent on approval early in life occurring through social interaction with family and others (Baumeister, Campbell, Krueger, & Vohs, 2003). Prior studies have established relationships between low self-esteem and coronary risk

(e.g., Stamatakis et al., 2004). The mechanism of action may be related to stimulation of the neuroendocrine system including cortisol responses. In a study of 101 healthy students, O'Donnell, Brydon, Wright, and Steptoe (2008) tested the hypothesis that lower levels of self-esteem would lead to increased cardiovascular and inflammatory responses following exposure to mentally stressful tasks. Researchers found that greater self-esteem was associated with lower levels of tumor necrosis factor-α (TNF-α) and interleukin-1 receptor antagonist (IL-1ra) immediately following acute stress and smaller IL-1ra responses at 45 minutes post-stress event. There were no differences in levels of interleukin-6 (IL-6). Higher self-esteem was also associated with lower heart rates. The authors concluded that high self-esteem may protect against the development of CVD.

Stress reactivity, characterized by a heightened cardiovascular response to acute mental stress as well as a prolonged recovery to the stressor, may be

Table 15.2   The Relationship Between Mood and Psychological Processes: Hypotheses Tested

Author	Hypothesis	Stressor	Sample	Result
Bleil, Gianaros, Jennings, Flory, & Manuck (2008)	Depression, anxiety, anger, or negative affect related to variations in parasympathetic cardiac autonomic function	Depression Anxiety Anger Negative affect	Community volunteers	Depression, anxiety, and negative affect were inversely related to high frequency heart rate variability
Carroll, Phillips, Hunt, & Der (2007)	Depression alters autonomic nervous system function	Depression	3 healthy age cohorts	Inverse relationship between depression, systolic blood pressure, and heart rate
Pitzalis et al. (2001)	Mood causes an imbalance in autonomic nervous system activity	Depression Anxiety	Myocardial infarction	Depression but not anxiety negatively influenced autonomic control of heart rate
Schott, Kamarck, Matthews, Frockwell, & Sutton-Tyrell (2009)	Trait anger, hostility, depression, and anxiety are associated with endothelial dysfunction	Anger Hostility Depression Anxiety	Healthy elders	Endothelial dysfunction was associated with hostility in women only There were no differences in other variables
Watkins, Blumenthal, & Carney (2002)	Mood has no effect on the autonomic nervous system	Depression Anxiety	Myocardial infarction	Depression unrelated to baroreflex sensitivity (BRS) Anxiety associated with impaired BRS

influential in the development of CVD. In a meta-analysis, Chida and Steptoe (2009) found that stress reactivity and poor stress recovery (characterized by a sustained cardiovascular response including increased heart rate and blood pressure, heart rate variability, and increased cardiac output in response to an acute mental stressor) significantly predicted CVD occurrence and the progression of CVD. These findings reflect the concept of allostatic load in that CVD develops when the balance of homeostasis is tipped by either a heightened response to a stressor or a prolonged recovery from a stressor.

Type D individuals have the tendency to experience increased negative emotions across time and situations and tend not to share these emotions with others because of fear of rejection or disapproval. (The D stands for distressful.) Denollet (2005) described the construct based on clinical observations of cardiac patients, empirical evidence, and existing theories of personality. The characteristics can be assessed by means of a reliable and valid 14-item questionnaire (DS14 Scale). Seven items refer to negative affectivity, and seven items refer to social inhibition. People who score 10 points or more on both dimensions are classified as Type D. The DS14 can be used in clinical practice to stratify risk in cardiac patients.

It has been postulated that the Type D personality is linked to physiological changes that would explain increased risk for poor CVD outcomes (Denollet & Kupper, 2007). Conraads and colleagues (2006) found study patients with a Type D personality had increased levels of TNF-α, indicating that increased inflammation may be one mechanism of action for the development of CVD. Similarly, Molloy, Perkins-Porras, Strike, and Steptoe (2008) tested the hypothesis that Type D personality was associated with elevated cortisol levels in patients following an episode of acute coronary syndrome. After adjusting for age, gender, hypertension, risk score, recurrence of cardiac symptoms, previous MI, body mass index, and depressed mood, the Type D patients had significantly higher levels of salivary cortisol during daytime measures ($\beta = 8.03$, 95% CI = 0.23–15.82, $p = .044$) but not on awakening. The authors surmised that those with Type D personality have disruption of the HPA axis that may lead to disturbances in

metabolism, abdominal obesity, insulin resistance, pro-thrombotic responses, and vascular inflammation.

Environmental Characteristics

A number of environmental conditions increase one's risk for CVD. Factors include living conditions, infectious agents, racism, social class, available social support, and one's work environment. As with individual characteristics, many of these factors can exist alone or overlap with others at the same time.

An association was found between neighborhood psychosocial hazards and *living conditions* and CVD in a random sample of participants in the Baltimore Memory Study ($N = 1,140$). After adjusting for individual risk factors, residents who scored in the highest quartile on the Neighborhood Psychosocial Hazards scale were more than three times as likely to have experienced MI, stroke, transient ischemic attack, or intermittent claudication compared to residents scoring in the lowest quartile (Augustin, Glass, James, & Schwartz, 2008). Researchers in Denmark sought to determine if environmental factors were related to high levels of perceived stress. Living in a neighborhood with low average education was associated with higher levels of perceived stress for women (OR = 1.29, 95% CI = 1.01–1.52) but not men. For men, living in a neighborhood with high crime (OR = 1.45; 95% CI = 1.17–1.80) was associated with higher perceived stress. Also, neighborhoods with higher ethnic diversity were associated with less perceived stress in men (OR = 0.80; 95% CI = 0.65–0.99). The authors indicated that perceived stress, an unhealthy lifestyle, and low socioeconomic status (SES) are accumulated stressors that can be used to identify a high-risk group (L. Nielsen, Curtis, Kristensen, & Nielsen, 2008). *Accumulated stressors* could be another way of saying allostatic load.

Atherosclerosis is an inflammatory process that may be triggered by infectious pathogens or agents. A variety of mechanisms linking infectious pathogens to atherosclerosis have been proposed. It has been hypothesized that the immune response against heat shock proteins, such as heat shock protein 60 (hsp60) derived from pathogens causing chronic infection, may trigger or exacerbate atherosclerosis

(Ayada et al., 2009). Others have proposed that infectious pathogens may directly induce endothelial wall dysfunction (Oshima et al., 2005). Studies have demonstrated that pathogens such as cytomegalovirus (Stassen, Vega-Cordova, Vliegen, & Bruggeman, 2006), helicobacter pylori (Fagoonee et al., 2010; Niccoli et al., 2010), and periodontal-related pathogens (Higashi et al., 2009), have been associated with atherosclerosis. In addition, researchers have demonstrated that humans may be more susceptible to a CAD event or ischemic stroke after experiencing an infection. For example, acute respiratory infections have been shown to increase the risk of acute coronary syndrome up to two weeks after the infection (Harskamp & van Ginkel, 2008). In a study of 999 multi-ethnic adults, it was found that low education and high levels of chronic stress were significant predictors of seroprevalence of helicobacter pylori, cytomegalovirus, herpes simplex virus-1, and chlamydia pneumonia suggesting that infection may play a role in explaining the link between chronic stress, low socioeconomic status, and CVD (Aiello et al., 2009). Epstein, Zhu, Najafi, and Burnett (2009) have suggested that complex interactions between pathogens and a person's genetic makeup may influence the initiation and progression of atherosclerosis.

Most of the studies cited above have been cross-sectional and cause and effect have yet to be established. In addition, large randomized clinical trials have failed to demonstrate that antibiotics, even if administered for a full year, prevent secondary coronary artery events (Grayston et al., 2005; O'Connor et al., 2003), questioning the link between infection and CVD (Stassen, Vega-Cordova, Vliegen, & Bruggeman, 2006). The potential role of infectious pathogens in the development of atherosclerosis is an important area for future research since it may help to identify potential prevention and treatment methods.

We have combined the terms *racial discrimination* and *racism* because researchers have used both in studies of associations with CVD. Some studies have also used the terms *race* and *ethnicity* interchangeably even though little biological evidence exists for distinct races (Brondolo et al., 2008). Researchers have hypothesized that psychosocial stress, particularly perceived racism, may account for racial differences in prevalence of CVD. Cooper (2001) reported that income inequalities were correlated with heart disease in the 47 largest American cities ($r = -0.4$, $p = .006$). Racial segregation (geographic separation) was also found to be correlated with heart disease independent of income.

Studies have consistently revealed that minorities report a higher degree of stress than nonminorities. Oppression, racism, discrimination, and socioeconomic marginalization have been suggested as possible explanations for these disparities (Gehlert et al., 2008). Researchers have also found associations between racism and increased risk of CVD. In a study of 357 Blacks and Latinos, Brondolo et al. (2008) reported a significant relationship between perceived racism and nocturnal ambulatory blood pressures ($t = 2.64$, $p < .01$). Lewis and others (2006) found that Black women reporting higher levels of perceived chronic discrimination had increased coronary artery calcification. Researchers found that relative to White women, Black women have significantly higher mean diastolic blood pressure reactivity in response to a racial stressor compared to a nonracial stressor (Lepore et al., 2006). Albert and researchers (2010) reported that perceived racism did not increase the relative risk of mortality from CVD or cancer in a large cohort ($n = 48,924$) of Black women participating in the Black Women's Health Study. Mean age of participants (40.5 years) may have been a confounding factor since mortality rates are low in younger populations.

Low social and economic status has been found to be associated with a higher incidence of CHD. Part of the effect is the correlation of SES with traditional risk factors such as smoking and obesity and the stress of limited income and education is also hypothesized to mediate traditional risk. Hemingway and others (2005) theorized that autonomic impairment, manifested as low heart rate variability, may help to explain the relationship between low SES and risk of CHD. A cohort of 2,197 male civil servants completed measures of heart rate variability, risk behaviors, and psychosocial stress in the Whitehall II study. Low employment grade ($p < .02$) and adverse behavioral factors ($p < .03$) were associated with low heart rate variability. There was also a strong association between lower heart rate variability and the presence of metabolic syndrome ($p < .001$).

In a study of 92 middle-aged women, community SES was inversely related to pessimism, stress, and ambulatory diastolic blood pressure and exhibited moderate to large effect sizes (Appel et al., 2005). Socioeconomic status was also associated with a less healthy diet and exercise behaviors. Studies have consistently demonstrated that subjective social status is more strongly associated with health than objective measures of SES when objective indicators are controlled for statistically (Adler & Stewart, 2007; Wright & Steptoe, 2005). This suggests that subjective social status may better represent social status across the lifespan than traditional objective measures of SES. Of note, in the Coronary Artery Risk Development in Young Adults study (Adler & Stewart) predictors of subjective social status differed between Black and White participants. Although financial security, material deprivation, and education were found to be significant predictors of subjective social status for both Blacks and Whites, household income and wealth predicted subjective social status only for Whites, indicating that perception of social status varies for Blacks compared to Whites.

Social support has been conceptualized as a sense of belonging or attachment (Pierce, 1997). It has been consistently linked to positive health outcomes in patients with MI and stroke (Welin, Lappas, & Wilhelmsen, 2000). Social networks and social interactions that provide emotional and psychological support may help mitigate exposure to chronic stress (Rutledge et al., 2008). Lett and others (2005) reviewed the evidence for the role of social support in the development and progression of CHD. Social support was defined using two broad domains. Structural support referred to the size, type, density, and frequency of contact with people, and functional support described the perceived support provided by the social structure. Studies of healthy individuals as well as those with existing CHD were included to evaluate social support as a predictor of CHD. Results indicated that low social support increased risk of CHD or complications by 50% to 100%. In some cases, odds ratios were as high as 4.26. Explanations for the mechanism by which social support improves health outcomes include reduction of stress and improved adherence to treatment regimens (Ikeda & Iso, 2008).

Evidence has emerged suggesting that stressors in the work environment are independent risk factors for the development of atherosclerosis and ischemic heart disease (Eller et al., 2009). Eller and colleagues conducted a review of 33 studies of workplace stress, many including women. It is noteworthy that 20 of the studies were conducted in Nordic countries and only 7 in the United States. Twenty-three studies were guided by the Demand-Control Model, which describes two dimensions of work life: demands of the work environment and control over work. This model is grounded on the premise that demands are not inherently stressful, but stress occurs if there is low control over the work environment as well. The authors concluded that there was moderate evidence that high psychological demands and lack of social support are risk factors for ischemic heart disease among men. The most recent studies in the review did not show a link between lack of control and risk for heart disease. There were no associations between work demands, control, or effort and reward and the development of heart disease in women. The authors noted numerous limitations to the studies reviewed including inadequate power, lack of standardized measures, varying definitions of endpoints, and no evaluation of women or gender differences.

The effect of job strain on the development of CHD was evaluated in the Framingham Offspring Study. Contrary to other studies, there was no association between job strain and CHD in men. Surprisingly, women with active job strain (high demands, high control) were nearly 3 times as likely (OR = 2.8, 95% CI = 1.1–7.2) as women with high job strain (high demands, low control) to develop CHD (Eaker, Sullivan, Kelly-Hayes, D'Agostino, & Benjamin, 2003). In an examination of 10,308 London-based civil servants, with an average follow-up of 12 years, investigators found associations between work stress and poor diet, metabolic syndrome, higher morning rise in cortisol levels, and lower heart rate variability. Chronic work stress was associated with CHD, and the association was stronger in those under age 50 (RR = 1.68, 95% CI = 1.17–2.42) (Chandola et al., 2008). Similarly, Aboa-Éboulé and others (2007) found a link between job strain after MI and a recurrent risk of CHD (HR = 2.0, 95% CI = 1.08–3.66) in a sample of Canadian patients under age 60.

The Intersection of Individual and Environmental Characteristics

Several factors cannot be categorized as only individual or only environmental because they are influenced to a large degree by one another. They are discussed here in terms of their interactions.

Caregiver Burden

The impact of caring for others who are ill or disabled has been labeled *a psychological stressor and a strain* (Aggarwal, Liao, Christian, & Mosca, 2009). Despite the fact that caregiver burden may actually represent a syndrome of distress, it is included here because it has been studied from the perspective of many psychological variables including depression, anxiety, and social support (Cacioppo, Poehlmann, Kiecolt-Glaser, & Malarkey, 1998). Aggarwal and others (2009) examined primary caregivers of cardiac patients. The caregivers had more CVD risk factors, including less physical activity ($p < .01$) and higher waist circumference ($p < .01$). Mean caregiver strain was significantly higher in those reporting low social support ($p < .01$) and more depressive symptoms ($p < .01$). Lee, Colditz, Berkman, and Kawachi (2003) reported that caregiving to ill or disabled spouses was predictive of an increased risk for personal development of CHD in a cohort of women in the Nurses' Health Study (RR = 1.82; 95% CI = 1.08–3.05). Interestingly, increased risk for CHD was not present for nonspouse caregivers, suggesting that stress in the marital relationship, rather than caregiving alone, led to increased risk. In a review of measures of psychological and physical health in family caregivers of stroke survivors, Saban, Sherwood, DeVon, and Hynes (2010) found family caregivers were at increased risk for developing depression, anxiety, sleep disturbances, poor quality of life, and CHD.

Epigenetics

Traditional risk factors of CVD, such as genetics, diet, and lifestyle, do not fully explain CVD or CVD morbidity (Turunen, Aavik, & Yla-Herttuala, 2009). In addition, rapid increases and decreases in the incidence of CVD globally cannot be accounted for by the genetic mutations, which tend to occur slowly across many generations (Turunen et al., 2009). *Epigenetic processes are the changes in gene expression without alterations in DNA sequencing and involve modifications to chromatin, such as DNA methylation* (Veenema, 2009). Epigenetic changes may be temporary or may last through several generations. The interaction between environment and genetic makeup may be an important factor in the development of CVD. This will only be discussed briefly here as Chapter 4 in this text focuses on epigenetics, stress, and health.

Although the study of epigenetics as it relates to CVD is in its infancy, evidence points to the role of epigenetics in the development of atherosclerosis. Animal studies have demonstrated that in utero vessel walls may be primed to develop atherosclerosis later in life by exposure of the fetus to maternal hypercholesterolemia and associated risk factors (Alkemade et al., 2007). Only a few human studies have been conducted. In a study of 718 elderly participants, exposure to ambient particulate traffic pollutants was related to decreased blood leukocyte DNA methylation, an epigenetic marker (Baccarelli et al., 2009). Loss of DNA methylation has been linked to the development of health problems, including CVD (Jirtle & Skinner, 2007). Other factors, such as early life adverse events (Roth, Lubin, Funk, & Sweatt, 2009), perinatal stress (Champagne, 2008; Darnaudery & Maccari, 2008; Roth et al., 2009), adverse social environment (Champagne, 2010), and stressful life events (Reul & Chandramohan, 2007; Roth et al., 2009) all influence the pathogenesis of inflammatory diseases, such as atherosclerosis, through epigenetic mechanisms.

Sleep Deprivation

Poor sleep has been linked with high blood pressure, atherosclerosis, heart failure, heart attack and stroke, diabetes, and obesity. The thread that ties these together may be inflammation, the body's response to injury, infection, irritation, or disease. Poor sleep increases levels of C-reactive protein and other substances that reflect active inflammation. It also revs up the body's sympathetic nervous system, which is activated by fright or stress (Zisapel, 2007). Sleep is a biologically driven restorative process fundamental to health as well as a health behavior (Steptoe, Dockray, &

Wardle, 2009). It is also affected by environmental factors such as temperature or noise and internal factors such as worry and anxiety. In a study of 495 healthy middle-aged adults, calcium deposits in the coronary arteries were linked to insufficient sleep (King et al., 2008). After adjusting for multiple possible covariates, longer sleep duration was significantly associated with reduced calcium calcification incidence (OR = 0.67 per hour, 95% CI = 0.64–0.68, p = .02).

The relationship between sleep apnea and heart disease has been topic of interest as well. The objective of a recent study (Gottlieb et al., 2010) was to assess the relationship of obstructive sleep apnea and the prevalence of coronary heart disease and heart failure in a general community sample of 1,927 adult men and 2,495 adult women who were free of CHD and heart failure on study intake. On average, participants were followed for 8.7 years. Findings showed that among men 40 to 70 years old, those with an apnea-hypopnea index (AHI) of 30 or higher were 68% more likely to develop coronary heart disease than those with AHI of less than 5. Obstructive sleep apnea predicted incidental heart failure in men (per 10-unit increases in AHI), but not in women (adjusted hazard ratio 1.13 [95% CI = 1.02 to 1.26]). Obstructive sleep apnea was associated with an increased risk of heart failure in community-dwelling middle-aged and older men; its association with coronary heart disease in this sample is equivocal. Many more studies are needed to determine the incidence and the predictors of this relationship.

In summary, a number of personality patterns (i.e., Types A and D) and moods (anger, hostility, anxiety), job stressors, social support, social factors, and environmental factors including lack of sleep have all been found to increase the risk for CVD and subsequently poorer patient outcomes. Limited research on caregiving has found an increase in CVD development for spouses of caregivers, but not for nonspousal caregivers. Depression has been shown to be an independent risk factor for the development of CVD in numerous studies, but not all. Results for racism/discrimination, work strain, environmental stress, and general psychological stress are mixed. These variables increased the risk of CVD in some populations, but not others. There is insufficient evidence addressing the impact of environmental stressors on the development of CVD. Type D personality has been associated with a

disruption in hypothalamic-pituitary-adrenal (HPA) axis functioning, leading to increased inflammation and thrombotic events. Finally, many of the stress variables discussed here were linked to other stressors, such as poor lifestyle, and are unlikely to have a direct effect on atherogenesis or disease development. As with many of the stress variables discussed here, it is nearly impossible to determine which stressors have a direct link to CVD, which may moderate or mediate other stressors, or which may be latent variables that remain unidentified, hence the need to examine the physiological stress factors further.

PHYSIOLOGICAL STRESS RESPONSE

Neuroendocrine System

The body responds to acute stress with a multifaceted, complex array of interactions coordinated between the neuroendocrine and immune system designed to fight off or avoid the stressor, traditionally known as the "fight or flight" response (Selye, 1956). Both physical and psychological stressors can trigger the physiological stress response.

Aldosterone

Researchers have focused on the link between chronic stress, CVD, and aldosterone (Kubzansky & Adler, 2010). The levels of aldosterone are increased in response to activation of the HPA axis and the renin-angiotensin system, which plays a pivotal role in maintaining fluid and sodium balance as well as blood pressure (Kubzansky & Adler, 2010). Evidence demonstrates that aldosterone activates the type 1 glucocorticoid receptor, leading to cardiovascular injury including inflammation and vascular dysfunction (Kubzansky & Adler , 2010). In addition, it has been suggested that aldosterone may be the primary corticosteroid activating the type 1 glucocorticoid receptor system in response to stress, thereby mediating blood pressure and salt appetite (Carey, 2010; Geerling, Engeland, Kawata, & Loewy, 2006).

Cortisol

In response to stress, the HPA axis system is activated and cortisol is released (McEwen

& Wingfield, 2003). During acute stress, cortisol serves to attenuate and contain stress-induced inflammation (Munck & Naray-Fejes-Toth, 1994; Sapolsky, Romero, & Munck, 2000). However, chronic stress can lead to dysregulation of cortisol secretion, thereby reducing the effectiveness of cortisol in dampening inflammation. As a result, cortisol resistance promotes an increase in inflammatory cytokines and may explain the greater inflammatory disease risk in those with chronic stress. In healthy persons, cortisol levels are highest in the morning about 30 minutes after awakening, then decrease during the day and rise again during the night just before awakening. However in individuals with chronic stress, the diurnal cortisol pattern may be altered (Chrousos & Gold, 1998; Gallagher-Thompson et al., 2006). Individuals with depression exhibit loss of evening suppression of cortisol levels, producing a dampening of the cortisol diurnal slope (Deuschle et al.,1997). Other studies have found cynical hostility to be related to a declining phase of the awakening cortisol response (Ranjit et al., 2009). In addition, cortisol response to chronic stress may shift over time, with elevated levels during the early phase of the stressor and lower levels as time passes (Dickerson & Kemeny, 2004).

Several researchers have demonstrated a link between cortisol levels and CVD. They found that total cortisol levels, while awake, were positively and independently associated with the amount of atherosclerosis in the carotid arteries (Dekker et al., 2008). Similarly, Matthews, Schwartz, Cohen, and Seeman (2006) found flatter slopes of cortisol levels (resulting from higher afternoon and evening cortisol levels) were associated with a greater degree of coronary calcification. Although the specific mechanisms for how cortisol is related to CVD are unclear, it is thought that psychological distress resulting from anxiety and/or depression activates the HPA axis, stimulating corticotrophin-releasing hormone (CRH) which, in turn, increases serum cortisol. Increased levels of catecholamines act to stimulate platelet activity resulting in changes in the endothelium of the circulatory system (Born, 1991; Cottone et al., 1998). In addition, pro-inflammatory cytokines promote destruction of the endothelium, resulting in the formation of atherosclerotic plaques (Viles-Gonzalez, Fuster, & Badimon, 2006). This theory is indirectly corroborated by studies where patients with depression were at a significantly higher risk of CVD after controlling for traditional risk factors such as hypercholesteremia, hypertension, obesity, and personal history of CHD (Grippo & Johnson, 2009).

Sympathetic Nervous System

The sympathetic nervous system (SNS) reacts quickly to stressors with the release of catecholamines, increasing heart rate and blood pressure. As a result, oxygen to the muscle tissues and brain readies the body for an increase in physical and mental activity. Within minutes of a perceived stressor, the hypothalamus secretes corticotrophin-releasing factor (CRF) that triggers the pituitary to activate the release of adrenocorticotrophic hormone (ACTH) (Denollet & Kupper, 2007). During acute stress, changes in metabolism, including increased availability of glucose, are mediated by the HPA axis. In addition, the HPA axis coordinates and directs interactions among the hypothalamus, pituitary gland, and adrenal gland, regulating the body's response to stress via an exquisite, intricate system affecting energy expenditure, digestion, mood, and the immune system (Darnaudery & Maccari, 2008)—all designed to protect the human body from harm. Figure 15.5 depicts the biological response to stressors.

BIOMARKERS OF INFLAMMATION AND IMMUNE RESPONSE

It is becoming increasingly evident that chronic stress can influence the immune system, promoting inflammatory-based diseases, such as CVD (Black, 2002). Elevations of inflammatory cytokines, an integral component of the immune system, have been associated with socioeconomic position, depressive symptoms, and stress of a breast cancer diagnosis (Kiecolt-Glaser et al., 2003; Loucks et al., 2010; Raison, Capuron, & Miller, 2006; Witek-Janusek, Gabram, & Mathews, 2007). Key markers related to chronic inflammation and the development of CVD, such as cortisol, aldosterone, c-reactive protein (CRP), cytokines, and heat shock proteins will be discussed. Novel markers, such as cd40-ligand, will also be addressed.

Figure 15.5   Biological Response to Stress

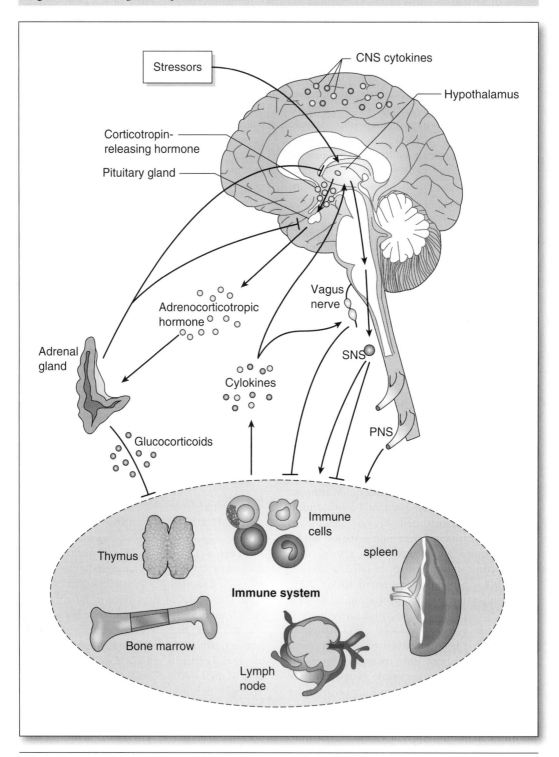

SOURCE: National Institute of Mental Health http://www.nimh.nih.gov/science-news/2008/errant-stress-immune-indicators-detected-in-depression-prone-womens-sweat.shtml

C-Reactive Protein (CRP)

C-reactive protein, a marker of inflammation, has been widely studied in relation to CVD. It is secreted by the liver in response to pro-inflammatory cytokines such as interleukin-6 and TNF-α (Ballou & Kushner, 1992). Several researchers have demonstrated that high sensitivity (hs) CRP is a strong independent predictor of CVD in healthy individuals (Ridker, Hennekens, Buring, & Rifai, 2000; Steptoe & Brydon, 2007). Furthermore, evidence suggests that high levels of CRP are associated with low SES, offering a partial explanation for the increased risk of CVD and higher mortality in persons of lower SES (Muennig, Sohler, & Mahato, 2007). Whether CRP is a causal link to CVD or a marker of it is an ongoing debate (Davey, Timpson, & Lawlor, 2006). In addition, since CRP is related to several other risk factors, such as obesity, fasting triglycerides, and smoking, its true independent relationship with CVD is unclear (Poledne et al., 2009). Increased levels of CRP may also be found in other inflammatory disease states, such as chronic obstructive pulmonary disease, making it difficult to interpret relative risk for CVD (Emerging Risk Factors Collaboration et al., 2010).

Cytokines

Cytokines are key regulators of inflammation with pro- and anti-inflammatory functions (Lin & Karin, 2007; Smyth, Cretney, Kershaw, & Hayakawa, 2004). Uncontrolled and sustained generation of cytokines, as found in chronic stress, can lead to inflammatory disease. Pro-inflammatory cytokines, such as IL-6, TNF-α (Dranoff, 2004; Smyth et al., 2004), IL-1ra (Bartolomucci et al., 2003), and interleukin-8 (IL-8) (Weik, Herforth, Kolb-Bachofen, & Deinzer, 2008) have been found to play a role in chronic inflammation.

IL-6 influences the development of CVD by regulating fibrinogen synthesis (Carty et al., 2010). Researchers have found that IL-6 is a predictor of acute stroke survival (Shenhar-Tsarfaty et al., 2010) as well as CVD (Patterson et al., 2010). In addition, increased IL-6 levels preoperatively predict early graft occlusion 3 months following coronary artery bypass (Hedman et al., 2007). There is evidence to suggest that patients with depression who are treated with antidepressants have lower levels of circulating cytokines (Kenis & Maes, 2002) and lower risk of CVD compared to untreated depressed patients (Kitzlerova & Anders, 2007). However, in a large study of women with suspected coronary ischemia, inflammatory biomarkers explained only a small portion of the variance between depression and CVD (Vaccarino et al., 2007). Evidence suggests that genetics may play a significant role in individual cytokine levels (Berrahmoune, Lamont, Fitzgerald, & Visvikis-Siest, 2005). For example, MI survivors with specific polymorphisms on the IL-6 gene had higher IL-6 concentrations (Ljungman et al., 2009).

Interleukin-18 is an inflammatory cytokine secreted by adipose tissue and represents a link between obesity and CVD (Prasad & Tsimikas, 2008) through the metabolic syndrome (Corson, 2009). Animal studies have suggested that IL-18 plays a role in the development of atherosclerosis as well as destabilizing advanced plaques (de Nooijer et al., 2004). However, findings from human studies have been inconsistent. One study found that high levels of serum IL-18 were associated with intima media thickness of the carotid artery after controlling for traditional risk factors (Yamagami et al., 2005), while another found a strong association between baseline IL-18 in healthy men and subsequent CAD events (Blankenberg et al., 2003). Other studies have not found significant associations between IL-18 and CVD after adjusting for other risk factors (Zirlik et al., 2007).

Heat Shock Proteins (hsp)

Heat shock proteins (hsp), found in a variety of tissues, are a family of proteins that act as molecular chaperones in the coordination and transport of intracellular proteins (Dreiza et al., 2010). Heat shock proteins are categorized by their molecular weight. For example, hsp 60 refers to a hsp weighing 60 kilodaltons (Li & Srivastava, 2004). They are found in every living organism, and increased production of the protein is triggered by a variety of stressors including psychological stress, infection, inflammation, exercise, and hypoxia (Ghayour-Mobarhan, Rahsepar, Tavallaie, Rahsepar, & Ferns, 2009). Several heat shock proteins, including hsp 65 and hsp 70 have been associated with CVD, and their levels have been found to predict the development of CVD in persons with hypertension (Pockley, Georgiades, Thulin, de Faire, & Frostegard, 2003; Pockley et al., 2002).

Lipoprotein Phospholipase A₂ (Lp-PLA₂)

Lipoprotein phospholipase A_2 (Lp-PLA$_2$) is an enzyme that circulates through binding apolipoprotein B to low-density lipoprotein (LDL) and is believed to influence atherogenesis (Hatoum, Hu, Nelson, & Rimm, 2010). Several prospective studies have demonstrated a statistically significant association between Lp-PLA$_2$ and cardiovascular risk after adjusting for level of LDL cholesterol (Koenig & Khuseyinova, 2009). In a large prospective study of both men and women enrolled in the Health Professionals Follow-Up Study and the Nurses' Health Study, Lp-PLA$_2$ levels were significantly associated with CVD in men and women with type 2 diabetes after controlling for traditional risk factors (Hatoum et al., 2010). In a study comparing the association of Lp-PLA$_2$ and CAD in Blacks and Whites undergoing coronary angiography, it was found that, although the Lp-PLA$_2$ mass and activity were higher in Whites, the Lp-PLA$_2$ index (an integrated measure of mass Lp-PLA$_2$ and activity) was similar between the two groups (Anuurad, Ozturk, Enkhmaa, Pearson, & Berglund, 2010). However, among those subjects diagnosed with CAD, Lp-PLA$_2$ was independently associated with disease among Blacks, but not Whites, suggesting an independent impact on inflammation in Blacks (Anuurad et al., 2010). Despite associations found between CAD and Lp-PLA$_2$ levels, a large collaborative analysis of 32 prospective studies found reduced associations between CAD and Lp-PLA$_2$ after adjusting for baseline concentrations of lipids and apolipoproteins, questioning a unique link between CAD and Lp-PLA$_2$ (Thompson et al., 2010).

Monocyte Chemotactic Protein (MCP-1)

Monocyte chemotactic protein (MCP-1) is a chemokine involved in the initiation and development of atherosclerosis. It is believed to play a role in inflammation related to adipose tissue (Gustafson, 2010). In addition, macrophages within atherosclerotic plaques are capable of expressing MCP-1, which recruit monocytes that have been observed in the early formation of atheromas (Gerszten et al., 1999). Increased levels of MCP-1 have been found to be predictive of higher mortality in persons with coronary artery syndromes (Amasyali, Kose, Kursaklioglu, Barcin, & Kilic, 2009; Gustafson, 2010; Piemonti

et al., 2009). Therefore, high levels of MCP-1 may be an early biomarker of atheroma and cardiovascular outcomes.

Myeloperoxidase (MPO)

Myeloperoxidase (MPO) is an enzyme that is released by leukocytes during inflammation and is believed to play a role in defending the body against infection (Schindhelm, van der Zwan, Teerlink, & Scheffer, 2009). It also has been implicated in the initiation and progression of atherosclerosis. As several studies have demonstrated, higher levels of MPO are associated with increased CVD risk after controlling for other cardiac risk factors (Kals et al., 2008; Schindhelm, van der Zwan, Teerlink, & Scheffer, 2009). MPO may be a promising biomarker for risk stratification in CVD.

Soluble CD-40 Ligand (sCD-40L)

Soluble CD-40 Ligand (sCD-40L) and its receptors CD40 and CD40L are pro-inflammatory cytokines and members of the tumor necrosing family. They contribute to atherogenesis and promote coagulation (Schonbeck & Libby, 2001). Several cell types have been shown to express CD-40L. T-lymphocytes promote coagulation through the expression of CD-40L, which stimulates tissue factor production by macrophages (Ferencik et al., 2007). Freedman (2003) suggests that inflammation and thrombosis are a result of the formation of platelet aggregates in association with monocytes. These have been shown to be an early marker of acute myocardial infarction and contribute to atherosclerosis. As CD-40L is involved in both activation of platelets and lymphocytes, reflecting both inflammation and platelet activation, it has the potential to be a useful biomarker of thrombus formation in atherosclerosis.

In normal, healthy women, sCD-40L has been shown to be associated with an increase of cardiovascular events (Schonbeck, Varo, Libby, Buring, & Ridker, 2001). Heeschen and colleagues (2003) have also shown that elevated levels of sCD-40L correlated with an increased risk of acute coronary syndrome. Some studies have shown that increased levels of sCD-40L are linked to a high risk for developing thrombosis (e.g., Heeschen et al., 2003; Schonbeck et al., 2001). However, other studies have not found an association between sCD40-L and risk for CVD (e.g., Olenchock et al., 2008). In a sample of low risk for CVD participants derived from the Framingham Offspring Study, sCD40-L levels were independently predictive of CVD, demonstrating that sCD-40 may have the potential to be a valuable predictive biomarker for CVD (Keaney et al., 2008).

THE EIRENE MODEL OF STRESS AND CARDIOVASCULAR DISEASE

We have proposed a new model of stress and CVD based on Steptoe & Brydon's (2007) work and the literature reviewed in this chapter. The Eirene (named for the Greek goddess of peace) Model of Stress and CVD addresses the importance of what Sindall (2001) referred to as upstream and downstream factors affecting the occurrence and progression of chronic disease,

in this case CVD. Upstream factors are those factors that influence development and early progression of disease. Primary prevention would moderate these influences to prevent CVD. Downstream factors are those which speed the progression of disease and affect disease outcomes. Intervening to change these factors includes secondary prevention strategies. As Sindall (2001) noted, the new prevention paradigm supports the need to move beyond previous "static" models of disease prevention based on traditional risk factors.

This model postulates that atherosclerosis proceeds in a progressive manner that leads to an acute event and consequently puts patients at high risk for poor outcomes such as ACS, stroke, rehospitalization, or death (Figure 15.6).

Items in the light boxes running down the middle of the model represent the stressor variables and the individual's appraisal of the stressors that have been implicated in the development

Figure 15.6   Eirene Model of Stress and Cardiovascular Disease

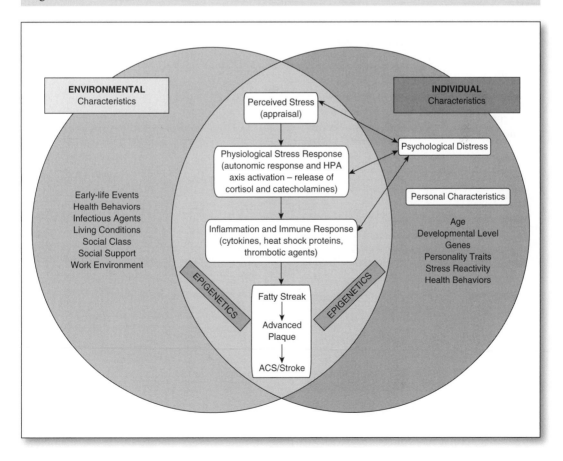

of CVD. These variables are all influenced by epigenetics. Additionally, psychological stress, which may be acute or chronic, results from both an appraisal of stress and from physiological stress responses. For example, a heightened immune response to stressors may further stimulate the HPA and/or neuroendocrine system, resulting in additional psychological stress. Both psychosocial and biological stressors and responses are impacted by individual and environmental characteristics, which appear on the right and the left on the model. Relationships among the variables are represented with arrows running in both directions so that future studies can test causal relationships rather than simple correlations.

Conclusions

Psychosocial stressors have been linked to increased risk factors, atherogenesis, development and progression of CVD, poorer outcomes following acute CVD events, and activation of neuroendocrine and immunologic dynamics (G. Miller et al., 2009). Our efforts and the efforts of other researchers to construct a model of stress and CVD is complicated by the numerous conceptualizations and operational definitions of stressors, study methods, identification of independent and latent variables, and outcome measures. The lack of standardization in definitions and measures make it challenging for researchers to compare results across studies and to determine clinical utility of the findings. Measurement issues are another limitation in studies reviewed here. The psychosocial variables related here were measured using a wide variety of instruments. Hence, direct comparison of findings is impossible. Many investigators used generic forms, such as the SF-36 mental component, to measure "psychological distress." Outcome variables differed and included CVD risk factors, diagnosis of CVD, and "CVD lifestyle." Use of terms "primary" or "independent" risk factor is tenuous. It can be reasonably inferred from the evidence presented here that there are few "independent" risk factors for CVD. Psychosocial and biologic stressors often interact and lead to disease. There can be additive as well as multiplicative effects.

Of interest, many of the studies were international, including data from Canada, Croatia, Britain, Denmark, Finland, Japan, Sweden, and the United Kingdom. American investigators are less likely to examine psychosocial variables. Why is this? It is possible that many American patients prefer the convenience of a drug or device to manage their risk factors or chronic disease as opposed to interventions designed to reduce psychosocial stress or specific behavior-modification techniques. Or is it that the drug and device companies are funding the research in the United States? Funding priorities and reimbursement for care directly affects the conduct of research and it is not known whether or not findings from international studies are generalizable to the American population.

Weak links have been reported between psychosocial distress, CVD occurrence, and CVD outcomes. A slightly stronger association between biological processes and CVD has been identified. Therefore, there is a need for large-scale studies in which causal pathways and moderator and mediator variables can be tested using statistical methods such as structural equation modeling. For example, SES, gender, and ethnicity have been described as moderators of social support and heart disease (Lett et al., 2005). More research is needed to better elucidate the role of cortisol and stress in the development of metabolic syndrome as these insights may lead to the development of interventions for metabolic syndrome, an antecedent to the occurrence of CVD.

Evidence-Informed and Evidence-Based Practice Interventions

While there is extensive research demonstrating the effectiveness of behavioral change on stress reduction, there is limited evidence to support stress reduction for reducing inflammation in CVD (Hamer, Molloy, & Stamatakis, 2008). In a study of 2,481 persons with MI suffering from depression, cognitive–behavioral therapy had no effect on the number of cardiac events and survival during a 29-month follow-up period, despite significant reductions in the levels of depression (Berkman et al., 2003). However, there is evidence that changes in lifestyle may reduce cardiac risk. In a pilot study of 27 persons with existing CAD or significant cardiovascular risk factors, it was found that a 12-week cardiac lifestyle intervention program that involved a 10% reduction of fat in the diet, 3 hours of moderate exercise per week, and the practice of stress management 1 hour a day significantly improved endothelium brachial artery flow, CRP, and IL-6 levels when compared to an age, gender, and CAD matched control group (Dod et al., 2010). However, since there were multiple lifestyle changes included in this program, it is not known which lifestyle change—or combination of changes—influenced the cardiac profiles of these participants. Clearly, more research is needed on multiple levels from basic animal research and epidemiological research to human clinical studies, prior to the confident translation of research into practice in order to reduce stress and, therefore, CVD.

Summary of Key Points

1. Some psychosocial stressors are upstream determinants of atherogenesis and the development of CVD.

2. Psychosocial stressors activate the neuroendocrine and sympathetic nervous systems, leading to atherogenesis and CVD.

3. The direct and indirect impact of psychosocial stressors is difficult to determine due to varying conceptualizations of stress, study design, and methods.

4. CVD is an inflammatory process driven by the immune system.

5. The role of epigenetics in the development of CVD is not yet well understood.

References

Aboa-Éboulé, C. C., Maunsell, E., Masse, B., Bourbonnais, R., Vézina, M., Milot, A., . . . Dagenais, G. R. (2007). Job strain and risk of acute recurrent coronary heart disease events. *Journal of the American Medical Association, 298*(14), 1652–1660.

Ader, R. (Ed.). (2007). *Psychoneuroimmunology* (4th ed., pp. 945–974). New York, NY: Elsevier.

Adler, N. E., & Stewart, J. (2007). Research network on socioeconomic status and health. Retrieved from http://www.macses.ucsf.edu/Research/Psychosocial/notebook/subjective.html

Aggarwal, B., Liao, M., Christian, A., & Mosca, L. (2009). Influence of caregiving on lifestyle and psychosocial risk factors among family members of patients hospitalized with cardiovascular disease. *Journal of General Internal Medicine, 24*(1), 93–98.

Aiello, A. E., Diez-Roux, A., Noone, A. M., Ranjit, N., Cushman, M., Tsai, M. Y., & Szklo, M. (2009). Socioeconomic and psychosocial gradients in cardiovascular pathogen burden and immune response: The multi-ethnic study of atherosclerosis. *Brain, Behavior, & Immunity, 23*(5), 663–671.

Albert, M. A., Cozier, Y., Ridker, P. M., Palmer, J. R., Glynn, R. J., Rose, R. J., . . . Rosenberg, L. (2010). Perceptions of race/ethnic discrimination in relation to mortality among Black women: Results from the Black Women's Health Study. *Archives of Internal Medicine, 170*(10), 896–904.

Alkemade, F. E., Gittenberger-de Groot, A. C., Schiel, A. E., VanMunsteren, J. C., Hogers, B., van Vliet, L. S., . . . DeRuiter, M. C. (2007). Intrauterine exposure to maternal atherosclerotic risk factors increases the susceptibility to atherosclerosis in adult life. *Arteriosclerosis, Thrombosis & Vascular Biology, 27*(10), 2228–2235.

Amasyali, B., Kose, S., Kursaklioglu, H., Barcin, C., & Kilic, A. (2009). Monocyte chemoattractant protein-1 in acute coronary syndromes: Complex vicious interaction. *International Journal of Cardiology, 136*(3), 356–357.

American Heart Association (AHA). (2010). Heart disease and stroke statistics—2010 update. Dallas, TX: Author. Retrieved from http://www.americanheart.org/downloadable/heart/1265665152970DS-3241%20HeartStrokeUpdate_2010.pdf

Anuurad, E., Ozturk, Z., Enkhmaa, B., Pearson, T. A., & Berglund, L. (2010). Association of lipoprotein-associated phospholipase A2 with coronary artery disease in African-Americans and Caucasians. *Journal of Clinical Endocrinology & Metabolism, 95*(5), 2376–2383.

Appel, S. J., Floyd, N. A., Giger, J. N., Weaver, M. T., Luo, H., Hannah, T., & Ovalle, F. (2005). African-American women, metabolic syndrome, and National Cholesterol Education Program criteria. *Nursing Research, 54*(5), 339–346.

Arbelaez, J. J., Ariyo, A. A., Crum, R. M., Fried, L. P., & Ford, D. E. (2007). Depressive symptoms, inflammation, and ischemic stroke in older adults: A prospective analysis in the cardiovascular health study. *Journal of the American Geriatrics Society, 55*(11), 1825–1830.

Astin, J. A., Shapiro, S. L., Eisenberg, D. M., & Forys, K. L. (2003). Mind-body medicine: State of the science, implications for practice. *Journal of the American Board of Family Practitioners, 16,* 131–147.

Augustin, T., Glass, T. A., James, B. D., & Schwartz, B. S. (2008). Neighborhood psychosocial hazards and cardiovascular disease: The Baltimore Memory Study. *American Journal of Public Health, 98*(9), 1664–1670.

Ayada, K., Yokota, K., Kobayashi, K., Shoenfeld, Y., Matsuura, E., & Oguma, K. (2009). Chronic infections and atherosclerosis. *Clinical Reviews in Allergy & Immunology, 37*(1), 44–48.

Baccarelli, A., Wright, R. O., Bollati, V., Tarantini, L., Litonjua, A. A., Suh, H. H., . . . Schwartz, J. (2009). Rapid DNA methylation changes after exposure to traffic particles. *American Journal of Respiratory & Critical Care Medicine, 179*(7), 572–578.

Ballou, S. P., & Kushner, I. (1992). C-reactive protein and the acute phase response. *Advances in Internal Medicine, 37,* 313–336.

Bartolomucci, A., Palanza, P., Parmigiani, S., Pederzani, T., Merlot, E., Neveu, P. J., . . . Dantzer, R. (2003). Chronic psychosocial stress down-regulates central cytokines mRNA. *Brain Research Bulletin, 62*(3), 173–178.

Baumeister, R. F., Campbell, J. D., Krueger, J. I., Vohs, K. D. (2003). Does high self-esteem cause better performance, interpersonal success, happiness, or healthier lifestyles? *Psychological Science in the Public Interest, 4,* 1–24.

Berkman, L. F., Blumenthal, J., Burg, M., Carney, R. M., Catellier, D., Cowan, M. J., . . . Schneiderman, N. (2003). Effects of treating depression and low perceived social support on clinical events after myocardial infarction: The Enhancing Recovery in Coronary Heart Disease Patients (ENRICHD) Randomized Trial. *Journal of the American Medical Association, 289*(23), 3106–3116.

Berrahmoune, H., Lamont, J., Fitzgerald, P., & Visvikis-Siest, S. (2005). Inter-individual variation of inflammatory markers of cardiovascular risks and diseases. *Clinical Chemistry & Laboratory Medicine, 43*(7), 671–684.

Bhattacharyya, M. R., Perkins-Porras, L., Wikman, A., & Steptoe, A. (2010). The long-term effects of acute triggers of acute coronary syndromes on adaptation and quality of life. *International Journal of Cardiology, 138*(3), 246–252.

Black, P. H. (2002). Stress and the inflammatory response: A review of neurogenic inflammation. *Brain, Behavior, & Immunity, 16*(6), 622–653.

Blankenberg, S., Luc, G., Ducimetiere, P., Arveiler, D., Ferrieres, J., Amouyel, P., . . . Tiret, L. (2003). Interleukin-18 and the risk of coronary heart disease in European men: The Prospective Epidemiological Study of Myocardial Infarction (PRIME). *Circulation, 108*(20), 2453–2459.

Bleil, M. E., Gianaros, P. J., Jennings, J. R., Flory, J. D., & Manuck, S. B. (2008). Trait negative affect: Toward an integrated model of understanding psychological risk for impairment in cardiac autonomic function. *Psychosomatic Medicine, 70,* 328–337.

Born, G. V. (1991). Recent evidence for the involvement of catecholamines and of macrophages in atherosclerotic processes. *Annals of Medicine, 23*(5), 569–572.

Brborovic´, O., Rukavina, T., Pavlekovic´, G., Džakula, A., Šogoric´, S., & Vuletic´, S. (2009). Psychological distress within cardiovascular risks behaviors, condition and diseases conceptual framework. *Collegium Antropologicum, 1,* Suppl-3.

Brondolo, W., Libby, D. J., Denton, E., Thompson, S., Beatty, D. L., Schwartz, J., . . . Gerin, W. (2008). Racism and ambulatory blood pressure in a community sample. *Pscyhosomatic Medicine, 70,* 49–56.

Brotman, D. J., Golden, S. H., & Wittstein, I. S. (2007). The cardiovascular toll of stress. *The Lancet, 370,* 1089–1100.

Cacioppo, J. T., Poehlmann, K. M., Kiecolt-Glaser, J. K., & Malarkey, W. B. (1998). Cellular immune responses to acute stress in female caregivers of dementia patients and matched controls. *Health Psychology, 17*(2), 182–189.

Carey, R. M. (2010). Aldosterone and cardiovascular disease. *Current Opinion in Endocrinology, Diabetes & Obesity, 17*(3), 194–198.

Carroll, D., Phillips, A. C., Hunt, K., & Der, G. (2007). Symptoms of depression and cardiovascular reactions to acute psychological stress: Evidence from a population study. *Biological Psychology, 75*(1), 68–74.

Carty, C. L., Heagerty, P., Heckbert, S. R., Jarvik, G. P., Lange, L. A., Cushman, M., . . . Reiner, A. P. (2010). Interaction between fibrinogen and IL-6 genetic variants and associations with cardiovascular disease risk in the Cardiovascular Health Study. *Annals of Human Genetics, 74*(1), 1–10.

Champagne, F. A. (2008). Epigenetic mechanisms and the transgenerational effects of maternal care. *Frontiers in Neuroendocrinology, 29*(3), 386–397.

Champagne, F. A. (2010). Epigenetic influence of social experiences across the lifespan. *Developmental Psychobiology, 52*(4), 299–311.

Chandola, T., Britton, A., Brunner, E., Hemingway, H., Malik, M., Kumari, M., . . . Marmot, M. (2008). Work stress and coronary heart disease: What are the mechanisms? *European Heart Journal, 29,* 640–648.

Chida, Y., & Steptoe, A. (2009). The association of anger and hostility with future coronary heart disease: A meta-analytic review of prospective evidence. *Journal of the American College of Cardiology, 53,* 936–946. doi:10.1016/j.jacc.2008.11.044

Chrousos, G. P., & Gold, P. W. (1998). A healthy body in a healthy mind—and vice versa—the damaging power of "uncontrollable" stress. *Journal of Clinical Endocrinology & Metabolism, 83*(6), 1842–1845.

Conraads, V., Denollet, J., Clerck, L. S. de, Stevens, W. J., Bridts, C., & Vrints, C. J. (2006). Type D personality is associated with increased levels of tumour necrosis factor (TNF)-α and TNF-α receptors in chronic heart failure. *International Journal of Cardiology, 113*(1), 34–38.

Cooper, R. S. (2001). Social inequality, ethnicity, and cardiovascular disease. *International Journal of Epidemiology, 30,* Suppl-1.

Corson, M. A. (2009). Emerging inflammatory markers for assessing coronary heart disease risk. *Current Cardiology Reports, 11*(6), 452–459.

Cottone, S., Vella, M. C., Vadala, A., Neri, A. L., Riccobene, R., & Cerasola, G. (1998). Influence of vascular load on plasma endothelin-1, cytokines and catecholamine levels in essential hypertensives. *Blood Pressure, 7*(3), 144–148.

Damasio, A. R. (1994). *Descartes' error: Emotion, reason, and the human brain.* New York, NY: Putnam.

Darnaudery, M., & Maccari, S. (2008). Epigenetic programming of the stress response in male and female rats by prenatal restraint stress. *Brain Research Reviews, 57*(2), 571–585.

Davey, S. G., Timpson, N., & Lawlor, D. A. (2006). C-reactive protein and cardiovascular disease risk: Still an unknown quantity? *Annals of Internal Medicine, 145*(1), 70–72.

de Nooijer, R., von der Thusen, J. H., Verkleij, C. J., Kuiper, J., Jukema, J. W., van der Wall, E. E., . . . Biessen, E. A. (2004). Overexpression of IL-18 decreases intimal collagen content and promotes a vulnerable plaque phenotype in apolipoprotein-E-deficient mice. *Arteriosclerosis, Thrombosis & Vascular Biology, 24*(12), 2313–2319.

Dekker, M. J., Koper, J. W., van Aken, M. O., Pols, H. A., Hofman, A., de Jong, F. H., & Tiemeier, H. (2008). Salivary cortisol is related to atherosclerosis of carotid arteries. *Journal of Clinical Endocrinology & Metabolism, 93*(10), 3741–3747.

Denollet, J. (2005). DS14: Standard assessment of negative affectivity, social inhibition, and Type D personality. *Psychosomatic Medicine, 67,* 89–97.

Denollet, J., & Kupper, N. (2007). Type-D personality, depression, and cardiac prognosis: Cortisol dysregulation as a mediating mechanism. *Journal of Psychosomatic Research, 62*(6), 607–609.

Deuschle, M., Schweiger, U., Weber, B., Gotthardt, U., Korner, A., Schmider, J. et al. (1997). Diurnal activity and pulsatility of the hypothalamus-pituitary-adrenal system in male depressed patients and healthy controls. *Journal of Clinical Endocrinology & Metabolism, 82*(1), 234–238.

Dickerson, S. S., & Kemeny, M. E. (2004). Acute stressors and cortisol responses: A theoretical integration and synthesis of laboratory research. *Psychological Bulletin, 130*(3), 355–391.

Dod, H. S., Bhardwaj, R., Sajja, V., Weidner, G., Hobbs, G. R., Konat, G. W., . . . Jain, A. C. (2010). Effect of intensive lifestyle changes on endothelial function and on inflammatory markers of atherosclerosis. *American Journal of Cardiology, 105*(3), 362–367.

Dodd, M., Janson, S., Facione, N., Faucett, J., Froelicher, E. S., Humphreys, J., . . . Taylor, D. (2001). Advancing the science of symptom management. *Journal of Advanced Nursing, 33*(5), 668–676.

Dranoff, G. (2004, January). Cytokines in cancer pathogenesis and cancer therapy. [Review] [136 refs] *Nature Reviews Cancer, 4*(1), 11–22.

Dreiza, C. M., Komalavilas, P., Furnish, E. J., Flynn, C. R., Sheller, M. R., Smoke, C. C., . . . Brophy, C. M. (2010). The small heat shock protein, HSPB6, in muscle function and disease. *Cell Stress & Chaperones, 15*(1), 1–11.

Eaker, E. D., Sullivan, L. M., Kelly-Hayes, M., D'Agostino, R. B., & Benjamin, E. J. (2003). Does job strain increase the risk for coronary heart disease or death in men and women? *American Journal of Epidemiology, 159*(10), 950–958.

Eller, N. H., Netterstrøm, B., Gyntelber, F., Kristensen, T. S., Nielsen, F., Steptoe, A., & Theorell, T. S. (2009). Work-related psychosocial factors and the development of ischemic heart disease. *Cardiology in Review, 17,* 83–97.

Emerging Risk Factors Collaboration (Kaptoge, S., Di Angelantonio, E., Lowe, G., Pepys, M. B., Thompson, S. G. et al.). (2010). C-reactive protein concentration and risk of coronary heart disease, stroke, and mortality: An individual participant meta-analysis. *Lancet, 375*(9709), 132–140.

Epstein, S. E., Zhu, J., Najafi, A. H., & Burnett, M. S. (2009). Insights into the role of infection in atherogenesis and in plaque rupture. *Circulation, 119*(24), 3133–3141.

Fagoonee, S., De Angelis, C., Elia, C., Silvano, S., Oliaro, E., Rizzetto, M., & Pellicano, R. (2010). Potential link between Helicobacter pylori and ischemic heart disease: Does the bacterium elicit thrombosis? *Minerva Medica, 101*(2), 121–125.

Ferencik, M., Stvrtinova, V., Hulin, I., & Novak, M. (2007). Inflammation—a lifelong companion. Attempt at a non-analytical holistic view. *Folia Microbiologica, 52*(2), 159–173.

Freedman, J. E. (2003). CD40 ligand—assessing risk instead of damage? *New England Journal of Medicine, 348*(12), 1163–1165.

Friedman, M., & Rosenman, R. H. (1974). Type A behavior pattern: Its association with coronary heart disease. *Annuals of Clinical Research, 3,* 300–312.

Gallagher-Thompson, D., Shurgot, G. R., Rider, K., Gray, H. L., McKibbin, C. L., Kraemer, H. C. et al. (2006). Ethnicity, stress, and cortisol function in Hispanic and non-Hispanic white women: A preliminary study of family dementia caregivers and noncaregivers. *American Journal of Geriatric Psychiatry, 14*(4), 334–342.

Gallo, L. C., Ghaed, S. G., & Bracken, W. S. (2004). Emotions and cognitions in coronary heart disease: Risk, resilience, and social context. *Cognitive Therapy & Research, 28*(5), 669–694.

Garcia-Vera, M. P., Sanz, J., Espiosa, R., Fortun, M., & Magan, I. (2010). Differences in emotional personality traits and stress between sustained hypertension and normotension. *Hypertension Research, 33*(3), 203–208.

Geerling, J. C., Engeland, W. C., Kawata, M., & Loewy, A. D. (2006). Aldosterone target neurons in the nucleus tractus solitarius drive sodium appetite. *Journal of Neuroscience, 26*(2), 411–417.

Gehlert, S., Sohmer, D., Sacks, T., Mininger, C., McClintock, M., & Olopade, O. (2008). Targeting health disparities: A model linking upstream determinants to downstream interventions. *Health Affairs, 27*(2), 339.

Gerszten, R. E., Garcia-Zepeda, E. A., Lim, Y. C., Yoshida, M., Ding, H. A., Gimbrone, M. A., Jr. et al. (1999). MCP-1 and IL-8 trigger firm adhesion of monocytes to vascular endothelium under flow conditions. *Nature, 398*(6729), 718–723.

Ghayour-Mobarhan, M., Rahsepar, A. A., Tavallaie, S., Rahsepar, S., & Ferns, G. A. (2009). The potential role of heat shock proteins in cardiovascular disease: Evidence from in vitro and in vivo studies. *Advances in Clinical Chemistry, 48*, 27–72.

Gottlieb, D. J., Yenokyan, G., Newman, A. B., O'Connor, G., Punjabi, N. M., Quan, S., . . . Shahar, E. (2010). Prospective study of obstructive sleep apnea and incident coronary heart disease and heart failure. The Sleep Heart Health Study. *Circulation, 122*(4), 352–360.

Grayston, J. T., Kronmal, R. A., Jackson, L. A., Parisi, A. F., Muhlestein, J. B., Cohen, J. D., . . . Knirsch, D. (2005). Azithromycin for the secondary prevention of coronary events. *New England Journal of Medicine, 352*(16), 1637–1645.

Grippo, A. J., & Johnson, A. K. (2009). Stress, depression and cardiovascular dysregulation: A review of neurobiological mechanisms and the integration of research from preclinical disease models. *Stress, 12*(1), 1–21.

Gustafson, B. (2010). Adipose tissue, inflammation and atherosclerosis. *Journal of Atherosclerosis & Thrombosis, 17*(4), 332–341.

Guyton, A. C., & Hall, J. E. (2000). *Textbook of medical physiology* (10th ed.). Philadelphia, PA: W. B. Sanders.

Hamer, M., Molloy, G. J., & Stamatakis, E. (2008). Psychological distress as a risk factor for cardiovascular events: Pathophysiological and behavioral mechanisms. *Journal of the American College of Cardiology, 52*(25), 2156–2162.

Harskamp, R. E., & van Ginkel, M. W. (2008). Acute respiratory tract infections: A potential trigger for the acute coronary syndrome. *Annals of Medicine, 40*(2), 121–128.

Hatoum, I. J., Hu, F. B., Nelson, J. J., & Rimm, E. B. (2010). Lipoprotein-associated phospholipase A2 activity and incident coronary heart disease among men and women with type 2 diabetes. *Diabetes, 59*(5), 1239–1243.

Hedman, A., Larsson, P. T., Alam, M., Wallen, N. H., Nordlander, R., & Samad, B. A. (2007). CRP, IL-6 and endothelin-1 levels in patients undergoing coronary artery bypass grafting. Do preoperative inflammatory parameters predict early graft occlusion and late cardiovascular events? *International Journal of Cardiology, 120*(1), 108–114.

Heeschen, C., Dimmeler, S., Hamm, C. W., van den Brand, M. J., Boersma, E., Zeiher, A. M., . . . Simoons, M. L. (2003). Soluble CD40 ligand in acute coronary syndromes. *New England Journal of Medicine, 348*(12), 1104–1111.

Hemingway, H., Shipley, M., Brunner, E., Britton, A., Malik, M., & Marmot, M. (2005). Does autonomic function link social position to coronary risk? The Whitehall II Study. *Circulation, 111*, 3071–3077.

Higashi, Y., Goto, C., Hidaka, T., Soga, J., Nakamura, S., Fujii, Y., . . . Taguchi, A. (2009). Oral infection-inflammatory pathway, periodontitis, is a risk factor for endothelial dysfunction in patients with coronary artery disease. *Atherosclerosis, 206*(2), 604–610.

House, J. S., Umberson, D., & Landis, K. R. (1988). Structures and processes of social support. *Annual Review of Sociology, 14*, 293–318.

Ikeda, A., & Iso, H. (2008). Social support and stroke and coronary heart disease: The JPHC study cohorts II. *Stroke, 39*(3), 768–775.

Janszky, I., Ahnve, S., Lundberg, I., & Hemmingsson, T. (2010). Early-onset depression, anxiety, and risk of subsequent coronary heart disease: 37-year follow-up of 49,321 young Swedish men. *Journal of the American College of Cardiology, 56*(1), 31–37.

Jirtle, R. L., & Skinner, M. K. (2007). Environmental epigenomics and disease susceptibility. *Nature Reviews Genetics, 8*(4), 253–262.

Kals, J., Kampus, P., Kals, M., Pulges, A., Teesalu, R., Zilmer, K., . . . Zilmer, M. (2008). Inflammation and oxidative stress are associated differently with endothelial function and arterial stiffness in healthy subjects and in patients with atherosclerosis. *Scandinavian Journal of Clinical & Laboratory Investigation, 68*(7), 594–601.

Keaney, J. F., Jr., Lipinska, I., Larson, M. G., Dupuis, J., Freedman, J. E., Hamburg, N. M., . . . Benjamin, E. J. (2008). Clinical correlates, heritability, and genetic linkage of circulating CD40 ligand in the Framingham Offspring Study. *American Heart Journal, 156*(5), 1003–1009.

Kenis, G., & Maes, M. (2002). Effects of antidepressants on the production of cytokines. *International Journal of Neuropsychopharmacology, 5*(4), 401–412.

Kiecolt-Glaser, J. K., Preacher, K. J., MacCallum, R. C., Atkinson, C., Malarkey, W. B., & Glaser, R. (2003). Chronic stress and age-related increases in the proinflammatory cytokine IL-6. *Proceedings of the National Academy of Sciences of the United States of America, 100*(15), 9090–9095.

King, C. R., Knutson, K. L., Rathouz, P. J., Sidney, S., Liu, K., & Lauderdale, D. S. (2008). Short sleep duration and incident coronary artery calcification. *Journal of the American Medical Association, 300*(24), 2859–2866.

Kitzlerova, E., & Anders, M. (2007). The role of some new factors in the pathophysiology of depression and cardiovascular disease: Overview of recent research. *Neuroendocrinology Letters, 28*(6), 832–840.

Koenig, W., & Khuseyinova, N. (2009). Lipoprotein-associated and secretory phospholipase A2 in cardiovascular disease: The epidemiological evidence. *Cardiovascular Drugs & Therapy, 23*(1), 85–92.

Kubzansky, L. D., & Adler, G. K. (2010). Aldosterone: A forgotten mediator of the relationship between psychological stress and heart disease. *Neuroscience & Biobehavioral Reviews, 34*(1), 80–86.

Lee, S., Colditz, G. A., Berkman, L. F., & Kawachi, I. (2003). Caregiving and risk of coronary heart disease in U.S. women: A prospective study. *American Journal of Preventive Medicine, 24*(2), 113–119.

Lepore, S. J., Revenson, T. A., Weinberger, S. L. et al. (2006). Effects of social stressors on cardiovascular reactivity in Black and White women. *Annals of Behavioral Medicine, 31*(2), 120–127.

Lett, H. S., Blumenthal, J. A., Babyak, M. A., Strauman, T. J., Robins, C., & Sherwood, A. (2005). Social support and coronary heart disease: Epidemiologic evidence and implications for treatment. *Psychosomatic Medicine, 67,* 869–878.

Lewis, T. T, Everson-Rose, S. A., Powell, L. H. et al. (2006). Chronic exposure to everyday discrimination and coronary artery calcification in African-American women: The SWAN Heart Study. *Psychosomatic Medicine, 68*(3), 362–368.

Li, Z., & Srivastava, P. (2004). Heat-shock proteins. *Current Protocols in Immunology.* Appendix 1: Appendix 1T.

Libby, P. (2005). The vascular biology of atherosclerosis. In P. Zipes, P. Libby, R. O. Bonow, & E. Braunwald (eds.), *Braunwald's heart disease: A textbook of cardiovascular medicine* (7th ed., pp. 921–958). Philadelphia, PA: Saunders.

Lin, W. W., & Karin, M. (2007). A cytokine-mediated link between innate immunity, inflammation, and cancer. *Journal of Clinical Investigation, 117*(5), 1175–1183.

Ljungman, P., Bellander, T., Nyberg, F., Lampa, E., Jacquemin, B., Kolz, M. et al. (2009). DNA variants, plasma levels and variability of interleukin-6 in myocardial infarction survivors: Results from the AIRGENE study. *Thrombosis Research, 124*(1), 57–64.

Loucks, E. B., Pilote, L., Lynch, J. W., Richard, H., Almeida, N. D., Benjamin, E. J., . . . Murabito, J. M. (2010). Life course socioeconomic position is associated with inflammatory markers: The Framingham Offspring Study. *Social Science & Medicine, 71*(1), 187–195.

Mathews, K. A., Owens, J. F., Kuller, L. H., Sutton-Tyrrell, K., & Jansen-McWilliams, L. (1998). Are hostility and anxiety associated with carotid atherosclerosis in healthy postmenopausal women? *Psychosomatic Medicine, 60,* 633–638.

Matthews, K. A., Gump, B. B., Harris, K. F., Haney, T. L., & Barefoot, J. C. (2004). Hostile behaviors predict cardiovascular mortality among men enrolled in the multiple risk factor intervention trial. *Circulation, 109,* 66–70.

Matthews, K. A., Schwartz, J., Cohen, S., & Seeman, T. (2006). Diurnal cortisol decline is related to coronary calcification: CARDIA Study. *Psychosomatic Medicine, 68,* 657–661.

McEwen, B. S. (1998). Protective and damaging effects of stress mediators. *New England Journal of Medicine, 338,* 171–179.

McEwen, B., & Seeman, T. (2009). Allostatic load and allostasis. Retrieved from http://www.macses .ucsf.edu/research/allostatic/allostatic.php

McEwen, B. S., & Wingfield, J. C. (2003). The concept of allostasis in biology and biomedicine. *Hormones & Behavior, 43*(1), 2–15.

Miller, G., Chen, E., & Cole S. W. (2009). Health psychology: Developing biologically plausible models linking the social world and physical health, *Annual Review of Psychology, 60,* 501–524.

Miller, T. Q., Smith, T. W., Turner, C. W., Guijarro, M. L., & Hallet A. J. (1996). A meta-analytic review of research on hostility and physical health. *Psychological Bulletin, 119,* 322–348.

Molloy, G. J., Perkins-Porras, L., Strike, P. C., & Steptoe, A. (2008). Type-D personality and cortisol in survivors of acute coronary syndrome. *Psychosomatic Medicine, 70,* 863–868.

Moser, D. K., Riegel, B., McKinley, S., Doering, L. V., An, K., & Sheahan, S. (2007). Impact of anxiety and perceived control on in-hospital complications after acute myocardial infarction. *Psychosomatic Medicine, 69,* 10–16.

Muennig, P., Sohler, N., & Mahato, B. (2007). Socioeconomic status as an independent predictor of physiological biomarkers of cardiovascular disease: Evidence from NHANES. *Preventive Medicine, 45*(1), 35–40.

Munck, A., & Naray-Fejes-Toth, A. (1994). Glucocorticoids and stress: Permissive and suppressive actions. *Annals of the New York Academy of Sciences, 746,* 115–130.

National Institute of Mental Health. (2008). Errant stress/immune indicators detected in depression-prone women's sweat. Retrieved from http://www.nimh.nih.gov/science-news/2008/errant-stress-immune-indicators-detected-in-depression-prone-womens-sweat.shtm

Niccoli, G., Franceschi, F., Cosentino, N., Giupponi, B., De, M. G., Merra, G., . . . Crea, F. (2010). Coronary atherosclerotic burden in patients with infection by CagA-positive strains of Helicobacter pylori. *Coronary Artery Disease, 21*(4), 217–221.

Nielsen, L., Curtis, T., Kristensen, T. S., & Nielsen, N. R. (2008). What characterizes persons with high levels of perceived stress in Denmark? A national representative study. *Scandanavian Journal of Public Health, 36,* 369–379.

Nielsen, N. T., Kristensen, T. S., Schnor, P., & Gronbaek, M. (2008). Perceived stress and cause-specific mortality among men and women: Results from a prospective cohort study. *American Journal of Epidemiology, I*(5), 481–491.

O'Connor, C. M., Dunne, M. W., Pfeffer, M. A., Muhlestein, J. B., Yao, L., Gupta, S., . . . Cook, T. D. (2003). Azithromycin for the secondary prevention of coronary heart disease events: The WIZARD study—a randomized controlled trial. *Journal of the American Medical Association, 290*(11), 1459–1466.

O'Donnell, K., Brydon, L., Wright, C. E., & Steptoe, A. (2008). Self-esteem levels and cardiovascular and inflammatory responses to acute stress. *Brain, Behavior, and Immunity, 22,* 1241–1247.

Olenchock, B. A., Wiviott, S. D., Murphy, S. A., Cannon, C. P., Rifai, N., Braunwald, E., . . . Morrow, P. A. (2008). Lack of association between soluble CD40L and risk in a large cohort of patients with acute coronary syndrome in OPUS TIMI-16. *Journal of Thrombosis & Thrombolysis, 26*(2), 79–84.

Oshima, T., Ozono, R., Yano, Y., Oishi, Y., Teragawa, H., Higashi, Y., . . . Kambe, M. (2005). Association of Helicobacter pylori infection with systemic inflammation and endothelial dysfunction in healthy male subjects. *Journal of the American College of Cardiology, 45*(8), 1219–1222.

Pastorino, E. E., & Doyle-Portillo, S. M. (2009). *What is psychology* (2nd ed.). Florence, KY: Cengage Learning.

Patterson, C. C., Smith, A. E., Yarnell, J. W., Rumley, A., Ben-Shlomo, Y., & Lowe, G. D. (2010). The associations of interleukin-6 (IL-6) and downstream inflammatory markers with risk of cardiovascular disease: The Caerphilly Study. *Atherosclerosis, 209*(2), 551–557.

Piemonti, L., Calori, G., Lattuada, G., Mercalli, A., Ragogna, F., Garancini, M. P., . . . Perseghin, G. (2009). Association between plasma monocyte chemoattractant protein-1 concentration and cardiovascular disease mortality in middle-aged diabetic and nondiabetic individuals. *Diabetes Care, 32*(11), 2105–2110.

Pieper, S., Brosscholt, J. F., Van der Leeden, R., & Thayer, J. F. (2007). Cardiac effects of momentary assessed worry epidsodes and stressful events. *Psychosomatic Medicine, 69,* 901–909.

Pierce, G. R. (1997). Personality and social support processes: A conceptual overview. In G. R. Pience, B. Lakey, B. R. Sarason, and I. G. Sarason (Eds.), *Sourcebook of social support and personality* (pp. 3–18). New York, NY: Plenum Press.

Pitzalis, M. B., Iacoviello, M., Todarello, O., Fioretti, A., Guida, P., Massarti, F., . . . Rizzon, P. (2001). Depression but not anxiety influences the autonomic control of heart rate after myocardial infarction. *American Heart Journal, 141*(5), 765-771.

Pockley, A. G., DeFaire, U., Kiessling, R., Lemne, C., Thulin, T., & Frostegard, J. (2002). Circulating heat shock protein and heat shock protein antibody levels in established hypertension. *Journal of Hypertension, 20*(9), 1815–1820.

Pockley, A. G., Georgiades, A., Thulin, T., de Faire, U., & Frostegard, J. (2003). Serum heat shock protein 70 levels predict the development of atherosclerosis in subjects with established hypertension. *Hypertension, 42*(3), 235–238.

Poledne, R., Lorenzova, A., Stavek, P., Valenta, Z., Hubacek, J., Suchanek, P., & Pitha, J. (2009). Proinflammatory status, genetics and atherosclerosis. *Physiological Research, 58,* Suppl-8.

Prasad, A., & Tsimikas, S. (2008). Candidate biomarkers for the detection of coronary plaque destabilization and rupture. *Current Atherosclerosis Reports, 10*(4), 309–317.

Purnell, L. D., & Paulanka, B. J. (2005). *Guide to culturally competent health care.* Philadelphia, PA: F. A. Davis.

Puustinen, P. J., Koponen, H., Kautiainen, H., Mantyselka, P., & Vanhala, M. (2010). Gender-specific association of psychological distress with cardiovascular risk scores. *Scandinavian Journal of Primary Health Care, 28*(1), 36–40.

Raison, C. L., Capuron, L., & Miller, A. H. (2006). Cytokines sing the blues: Inflammation and the pathogenesis of depression. *Trends in Immunology, 27*(1), 24–31.

Ranjit, N., Diez-Roux, A. V., Sanchez, B., Seeman, T., Shea, S., Shrager, S., & Watson, K. (2009). Association of salivary cortisol circadian pattern with cynical hostility: Multi-ethnic study of atherosclerosis. *Psychosomatic Medicine, 71*(7), 748–755.

Reul, J. M., & Chandramohan, Y. (2007). Epigenetic mechanisms in stress-related memory formation. *Psychoneuroendocrinology, 32,* Suppl-5.

Ridker, P. M., Hennekens, C. H., Buring, J. E., & Rifai, N. (2000). C-reactive protein and other markers of inflammation in the prediction of cardiovascular disease in women. *New England Journal of Medicine, 342*(12), 836–843.

Rod, N. H., Grønbæk, M., Schnohr, P., Prescott, E., & Kristensen, T. S. (2009). Perceived stress as a risk factor or changes in health behaviour and cardiac risk profile: A longitudinal study. *Journal of Internal Medicine, 266,* 467–475.

Rosenman, R. H., Brand, J. H., Jenkins, C. D., Friedman, M., Straus, R., & Wurm, M. (1975). Coronary heart disease in the Western Collaborative Group Study: Final follow-up experience of 8.5 years. *Journal of the American Medical Association, 233,* 872–877.

Roth, T. L., Lubin, F. D., Funk, A. J., & Sweatt, J. D. (2009). Lasting epigenetic influence of early-life adversity on the BDNF gene. *Biological Psychiatry, 65*(9), 760–769.

Rutledge, T., Linke, S. E., Olson, M. B., Francis, J, Johnson, B. D., Bittner, V., . . . Merz, C. N. (2008). Social networks and incident stroke among women with suspected myocardial ischemia. *Psychosomatic Medicine, 70*(3), 282–287.

Saban, K. L., Sherwood, P. R., DeVon, H. A., & Hynes, D. M. (2010). Measures of psychological stress and physical health in family caregivers of stroke survivors: A literature review. *Journal of Neuroscience Nursing, 42*(3), 128–138.

Sapolsky, R. M., Romero, L. M., & Munck, A. U. (2000). How do glucocorticoids influence stress responses? Integrating permissive, suppressive, stimulatory, and preparative actions. *Endocrine Reviews, 21*(1), 55–89.

Schindhelm, R. K., van der Zwan, L. P., Teerlink, T., & Scheffer, P. G. (2009). Myeloperoxidase: A useful biomarker for cardiovascular disease risk stratification? *Clinical Chemistry, 55*(8), 1462–1470.

Schocken, D. D., Greene, A. F., Worden, T. J., Harrison, E. E., & Spielberger, C. D. (1987). Effects of age and gender on the relationship between anxiety and coronary artery disease. *Psychosomatic Medicine, 49*(2), 118–126.

Schonbeck, U., & Libby, P. (2001). The CD40/CD154 receptor/ligand dyad. *Cellular & Molecular Life Sciences, 58*(1), 4–43.

Schonbeck, U., Varo, N., Libby, P., Buring, J., & Ridker, P. M. (2001). Soluble CD40L and cardiovascular risk in women. *Circulation, 104*(19), 2266–2268.

Schott, L. L., Kamarck, T. W., Matthews, K. A., Frockwell, S. E., & Sutton-Tyrell, K. (2009). Is brachial artery flow-mediated dilation associated with negative affect? *International Journal of Behavioral Medicine, 16*(3), 241–247.

Schwalbe, F. (1990) Relationship between Type A personality and coronary heart disease. Analysis of five cohort studies. *Journal of Florida Medical Association, 77*(9), 803–805.

Selye, H. (1956). *The stress of life.* New York, NY: McGraw-Hill.

Shenhar-Tsarfaty, S., Ben, A. E., Bova, I., Shopin, L., Fried, M., Berliner, S., . . . Bornstein, N. M. (2010). Interleukin-6 as an early predictor for one-year survival following an ischaemic stroke/transient ischaemic attack. *International Journal of Stroke, 5*(1), 16–20.

Shibeshi, W. A., Young-Xu, Y., & Blatt, C. M. (2007). Anxiety worsens prognosis in patients with coronary artery disease. *Journal of the American College of Cardiology, 49,* 2021–2027.

Sindall, C. (2001). Health promotion and chronic disease: Building on the Ottawa Charter, not betraying it? *Health Promotion International, 16*(3), 215–17.

Smyth, M. J., Cretney, E., Kershaw, M. H., & Hayakawa, Y. (2004). Cytokines in cancer immunity and immunotherapy. *Immunological Reviews, 202,* 275–293.

Stamatakis, K. A., Lynch, J., Everson, S. A., Raghunathan, T., Salonen, J. T., & Kaplan, G. A. (2004). Positive affect and psychobiological processes relevant to health. *Journal of Personality, 77*(6), 1747–1776.

Stassen, F. R., Vega-Cordova, X., Vliegen, I., & Bruggeman, C. A. (2006). Immune activation following cytomegalovirus infection: More important than direct viral effects in cardiovascular disease? *Journal of Clinical Virology, 35*(3), 349–353.

Steptoe, A., & Brydon, L. (2007). Psychosocial factors and coronary heart disease: The role of psychoneuroimmunological processes. In R. Ader (Ed.), *Psychoneuroimmunology* (4th ed., pp. 945–974). New York, NY: Elsevier.

Steptoe, A., Dockray, S., & Wardle, J. (2009). Positive affect and psychobiological processes relevant to health. *Journal of Personality, 77*(6), 1747–1776.

Steptoe, A., Feldman, P. J., Kunz, S., Owen, N., Willemsen, G., & Marmot, M. (2002). Stress responsivity and socioeconomic status: A mechanism for increased cardiovascular disease risk? *European Heart Journal, 23*(22),1757–1763.

Sterling, P., & Eyer, J. (1988). Allostasis: A new paradigm to explain arousal pathology. In S. Fisher & J. Reason (Ed.), *Handbook of Life Stress, Cognition and Health.* Hoboken, N.J.: J. Wiley & Sons.

Stewart, J. C., Rand, K. L., Muldoon, M. F., & Kamarck, T. W. (2009). A prospective evaluation of the directionality of the depression-inflammation relationship. *Brain, Behavior, & Immunology, 23*(7), 936–944.

Taylor, A. G., Goehler, L. E., Galper, D. I., Innes, K. E., & Bourguignon, C. (2010). Top-down and bottom-up mechanisms in mind-body medicine: Development of an integrative framework for psychophysiological research. *Explore, 6,* 29–41.

Thompson, A., Gao, P., Orfei, L., Watson, S., Di Angelantonio, E. et al. (2010). Lipoprotein-associated phospholipase A(2) and risk of coronary disease, stroke, and mortality: Collaborative analysis of 32 prospective studies. *Lancet, 375*(9725), 1536–1544.

Turunen, M. P., Aavik, E., & Yla-Herttuala, S. (2009). Epigenetics and atherosclerosis. *Biochimica et Biophysica Acta, 1790*(9), 886–891.

Vaccarino, V., Johnson, B. D., Sheps, D. S., Reis, S. E., Kelsey, S. F., Bittner, V., . . . Bairey Merz, C. N. (2007). Depression, inflammation, and incident cardiovascular disease in women with suspected coronary ischemia: The National Heart, Lung, and Blood Institute–sponsored WISE study.

Journal of the American College of Cardiology, 50(21), 2044–2050.

Veenema, A. H. (2009). Early life stress, the development of aggression and neuroendocrine and neurobiological correlates: What can we learn from animal models? *Frontiers in Neuroendocrinology, 30*(4), 497–518.

Viles-Gonzalez, J. F., Fuster, V., & Badimon, J. J. (2006). Links between inflammation and thrombogenicity in atherosclerosis. *Current Molecular Medicine, 6*(5), 489–499.

Watkins, L. L., Blumenthal, J. A., & Carney, R. M. (2002). Association of anxiety with reduced baroreflex cardiac control in patients after acute myocardial infarction. *American Heart Journal, 143*(3), 460–466.

Weik, U., Herforth, A., Kolb-Bachofen, V., & Deinzer, R. (2008). Acute stress induces proinflammatory signaling at chronic inflammation sites. *Psychosomatic Medicine, 70*(8), 906–912.

Welin, C., Lappas, G., & Wilhelmsen, L. (2000). Independent importance of psychosocial factors for prognosis after myocardial infarction. *Journal of Internal Medicine, 247*(6), 629–639.

Witek-Janusek, L., Gabram, S., & Mathews, H. L. (2007). Psychologic stress, reduced NK cell activity, and cytokine dysregulation in women experiencing diagnostic breast biopsy. *Psychoneuroendocrinology, 32*(1), 22–35.

Wright, C. E., & Steptoe, A. (2005). Subjective socioeconomic position, gender and cortisol responses to waking in an elderly population. *Psychoneuroendocrinology, 30*(6), 582–590.

Yamagami, H., Kitagawa, K., Hoshi, T., Furukado, S., Hougaku, H., Nagai, Y., & Hori, M. (2005). Associations of serum IL-18 levels with carotid intima-media thickness. *Arteriosclerosis, Thrombosis & Vascular Biology, 25*(7), 1458–1462.

Zirlik, A., Abdullah, S. M., Gerdes, N., MacFarlane, L., Schonbeck, U., Khera, A., . . . de Lemos, J. A. (2007). Interleukin-18, the metabolic syndrome, and subclinical atherosclerosis: Results from the Dallas Heart Study. *Arteriosclerosis, Thrombosis & Vascular Biology, 27*(9), 2043–2049.

Zisapel, N. (2007). Sleep and sleep disturbances: biological basis and clinical implication. *Cellular and Molecular Life Sciences, 64*(10), 1174–1186.

16

The Acute Myocardial Infarction Coping Model

A Midrange Theory

Elizabeth Roe, Alissa L. Firmage, Angelo A. Alonzo, and Nancy R. Reynolds

The Acute Myocardial Infarction Coping Model (Alonzo & Reynolds, 1996a, 1996b, 1997, 1998) provides a framework for understanding acute myocardial infarction (AMI) care-seeking behavior. In this model, it is proposed that the relatively neglected areas of social situation and emotional response are key elements in understanding why individuals may delay seeking definitive health care services following the onset of life-threatening AMI symptoms. This chapter provides an overview of the origins and key elements of the model and an analysis of its utility for nursing research and practice. In addition, related research and implications for evidence-based practice will be discussed.

Origins

It has been well established that to receive maximal benefit from reperfusion therapies, individuals who are experiencing an AMI must obtain treatment as quickly as possible. The timeliness of reperfusion is very important because the benefits of these therapies diminish over time (Masoudi et al., 2008). There is evidence that early restoration of coronary blood flow in patients with AMI is key to short- and long-term health outcomes regardless of whether the reperfusion is by fibronolysis or percutaneous coronary intervention (PCI) (De Luca, Suryapranata, Ottervanger, & Antman, 2004; De Luca et al., 2003). Even though the advantages of rapid AMI treatment are clear, the time from the onset of acute symptoms of AMI to definitive care is often protracted, and some studies have shown that individuals with a prior history of AMI or coronary artery disease (CAD) or both are particularly prone to delaying care seeking (Bleeker et al., 1995; Saczynski et al., 2008). Despite decades of study, delay in seeking treatment in this population remains a major problem (Moser et al., 2006). Rather than examining the prehospital period as a time when the individual must actively cope with a difficult-to-assess acute health care crisis that is occurring in the midst of many interacting social, psychological, and cultural processes, researchers have often taken a more narrow clinical approach (Alonzo & Reynolds, 1998).

Research completed in nursing thus far demonstrates how difficult it may be for patients to accurately interpret their AMI symptoms and determine whether to seek care. For example, atypical presentation of cardiac symptoms (Lee, Bahler, Taylor, Alonzo, & Zeller, 1998; Morgan, 2005; Moser et al., 2006; Roe, 2006), a mismatch between symptom expectations and actual symptoms experienced (Carney, Fitzsimmons, & Dempsey, 2002; King & McGuire, 2007; Lee, Bahler, Chung, Alonzo, & Zeller, 2000), and failure to experience or appraise symptoms as serious (Dracup & Moser, 1997; McKinley, Moser, & Dracup, 2000; Quinn, 2005) have all been found to delay AMI care seeking. Although this research provides important insight, there have been only a few studies that have considered how social situational and emotional processes may influence AMI symptom interpretation and care-seeking behavior (Moser et al., 2006; Walsh, Lynch, Murphy, & Daly, 2004).

In the AMI model of coping (Figure 16.1), the problem of extended care seeking during AMI is conceptualized within a broad inclusive theoretical framework that considers the multidimensional features of care seeking and coping and focuses specifically on the importance of the social situation and emotions. The four-phase model was inductively and deductively derived (Alonzo & Reynolds, 1996a, 1996b) from an analysis of empiric and theoretic literature and is driven mainly by self-regulation theory (Leventhal, 1980; Leventhal & Cameron, 1987) and Mead's (1938) conceptualization of the "act." The phases of the AMI coping model are in essence a synthesis of these two conceptualizations as applied to AMI coping. The *act* is a way of analytically conceptualizing the primary structure of our ongoing, emergent social behavior (Mead, 1938). In the Self-Regulation Model, Leventhal and colleagues (Leventhal, 1980; Leventhal & Cameron, 1987) suggested a conceptualization similar to Mead's in which individuals cope with symptoms of illness within a self-regulative systems model. Both conceptualizations emphasize that relevant self-monitoring information is processed over time.

Since its initial development (Alonzo & Reynolds, 1996a, 1996b), the AMI coping model has been further refined to consider in more detail the role of emotions and coping, the potential of posttraumatic stress disorder (PTSD) (Alonzo, 1999), and related problems in response to the experience of AMI (Alonzo & Reynolds, 1997, 1998), and the influence of cumulative adversity (Alonzo, 1999, 2000). Although only one research study has been

identified that explicitly tested the AMI coping model (Roe, 2006), there have been several other studies that have examined the AMI care-seeking process using variables that are consistent with the AMI coping model (King & McGuire, 2007; Lee et al., 2000; Morgan, 2005; Nymark, Mattiasson, Henriksson, & Kiessling, 2009; Quinn, 2005; Rosenfeld, 2004; Walsh et al., 2004).

ELEMENTS OF THE AMI COPING MODEL

Coping

In the AMI coping model, the individual is viewed as an active problem solver who engages in conscious, and intentional, cognitive and behavioral efforts to manage specific external or internal demands or both that are appraised as taxing or exceeding the resources of the individual. This view is consistent with conceptions of coping described by Leventhal and Cameron (1987), Lazarus and Folkman (1984), and Mead (1938). In the AMI coping model, particular emphasis is placed on the relationship that the individual has with both internal and external environments, namely, his or her body and the surrounding socially defined situation as described by Ball (1972). Coping efforts are regarded as either problem focused or focused on emotional regulation (Leventhal & Cameron, 1987), where problem-solving efforts are viewed as attempts to do something constructive about stressful conditions and emotion-focused coping is viewed as an effort to regulate the emotional consequences of the stressful event. In both coping circumstances, internal biophysiological and emotional stressors produced by the experience of symptoms have exceeded the resources of the individual (Lazarus & Folkman, 1984) and become a taxing and potentially traumatic experience (Goldberger, 1983). The process of attempting to restore balance in the situation of an impending AMI is conceptualized in terms of four phases of coping (Figure 16.1): impulse and cognitive recognition, perception and covert action plan, overt manipulation, and assessment and consummation. We will review these four phases and provide recent findings in care-seeking delay that support the model.

Figure 16.1   Phases of the Acute Myocardial Infarction (AMI) Coping Model

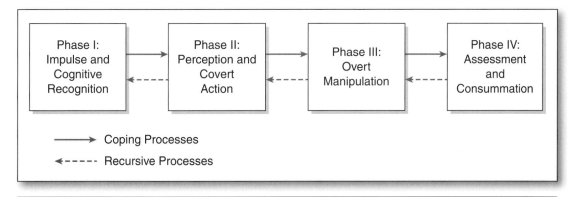

SOURCE: Alonzo, A. A., & Reynolds, N. R. (1998).

Phases of Coping

Phase I: Impulse and Cognitive Recognition

The primary substantive process of Phase I is symptom recognition and labeling. Phase I begins when the individual experiences a symptomatic impulse or stimuli that distinguishes itself from background expectancies (Alonzo, 1979) and that exceeds normal expectations in a manner compelling enough that it is not easily ignored. The labeling process requires that symptoms are placed within an understandable framework or, as Leventhal (Leventhal, 1980; Leventhal & Cameron, 1987) suggests, an illness representation—the cognitive structure by which individuals organize, analyze, and interpret information.

Memories are thought to be a significant aspect of illness representations. Memories reflect the individual's past experiences and include affective, emotional responses, such as those associated with AMI, and the more common abstract and conceptual information about symptoms and signs provided by health care professionals or associations (e.g., the American Heart Association's [2007] warning signs of a heart attack). Illness representations involve beliefs about possible associated symptoms, the cause of the disease, how long it lasts, how it might be treated and cured, and likely sequelae (see Chapter 19, this volume).

Phase I ends when the individual has a tentative label or a hypothesis regarding the meaning of the symptoms and proceeds to address the demands of the symptom representation in terms of developing a coping strategy. Central to developing a strategy are knowledge, behaviors, and efforts to regulate emotional arousal (Alonzo & Reynolds, 1998).

Related Research

Retrospective research studies show that individuals with AMI do label their symptomatic experiences in terms of classic chest pain, abdominal pain, nausea, or fatigue (Grossman et al., 2003; Lee et al., 2000; Perkins-Porras, Whitehead, Strike, & Steptoe, 2008; Rosenfeld, 2004). The labeling of symptoms has been found to differ by gender (King & McGuire, 2007) and race (Lee et al., 2000). Furthermore, research has also shown that the symptoms experienced by AMI patients are often not what they expected for a heart attack (King & McGuire, 2007; Morgan, 2005), thus making identification difficult. Uncertainty in terms of labeling symptoms as related to a heart attack delays treatment seeking (Carney et al., 2002; Fox-Wasylyshyn, El-Masari, & Artinian, 2010; Henriksson, Lindahl, & Larsson, 2007; Leslie, Urie, Hooper, & Morrison, 2000). However, in general, studies have shown that attribution of the symptoms to a cardiac cause resulted in shorter delay (Carney et al., 2002; Fox-Wasylyshyn et al., 2010; Moser, McKinley, Dracup, & Chung, 2005; Moser et al., 2006; Quinn, 2005).

Phase II: Perception and Covert Action Plan

The primary process in the second phase is covert construction, manipulation, and assessment of strategies to cope with symptoms. Covert coping means constructing a "line of action" (Blumer, 1969) directed toward establishing a stable relationship with symptoms and what Mead (1938) referred to as the "collapsed act," meaning that the individual engages in covert reflective analysis to determine how to achieve restoration of equilibrium.

In the case of symptoms, the individual examines his or her environment for possible causes, explanations, consequences, remedies, strategies, or all of these to make them stable and predictable. In this context, predictable and stable mean that symptoms will be lessened in intensity or frequency, made predictable in terms of their reoccurrence or being associated with a treatment regimen, brought below an acceptable threshold of attention or emotional arousal, or all of these. For Mead (1938), the collapsed act is a "subjective substitute for an objective reality" (p. 122) with which one anticipates having contact. In the current context, if the individual perceives signs and symptoms to be of a noncardiac, respiratory problem, his or her covert coping activities could include thinking about using an inhaler (if he or she is an asthma patient) or possibly calling a friend who sometimes complains of shortness of breath for information. Alternatively, if the individual is a cardiac patient, he or she may try to recall a prior cardiac event and mentally run through his or her past symptoms, problem solving, and resources, whether lay or medical.

As a result of symptoms and covert coping, the individual is now in a new and more sensitive relationship with his or her environments (biophysical, social situational, psychological or cognitive, and emotional). Covert action requires the use of knowledge and perceived behavioral resources immediately available to the individual, more distant resources possessed by lay others, and the medical resources of physicians and other health care providers such as nurses.

Related Research

In patients with AMI, misattribution of their symptoms to a less serious cause, such as GI disturbances, is typical and suggests a sense of self-care or efficacy is initially a reasonable line of action. However, this misattribution can lead to increased delays in seeking treatment

(Carney et al., 2002; Dracup et al., 2003; Henriksson et al., 2007; Khraim, Schere, Dorn, & Carey, 2009; Moser et al., 2005; Nymark et al., 2009).

Phase III: Overt Manipulation

Phase III is characterized by overt behavior, manipulation, and recursive reassessment. Manipulation is the locus of reality for Mead (Natanson, 1956) and can prove to be extremely time-consuming (Alonzo, 1980; Hartford, Karlson, Sjölin, Holmberg, & Herlitz, 1993). In essence, the covertly constructed line of action is now implemented, and in so doing the individual is constantly testing, revising, and reconstructing lines of action. As symptoms evolve, change, or reoccur, and if overt manipulation is not effective, the processes of impulse relabeling and covert actions are revisited and can occur simultaneously as the individual and lay others attempt to manipulate the environment to cope with the stressful event of symptoms and emotional arousal.

Covertly constructed behavioral strategies are overtly implemented to establish a predictable and stable relationship with the symptoms. As overt coping develops, the individual and lay others are constantly evaluating whether instrumental efforts and resources are effective, whether available information is accurate and consistent with their ongoing experiences and representations, and whether emotional and affective responses to symptoms and the emerging coping efforts are under control and, particularly for lay others, not blocking instrumental coping and assessment. If, in the course of behavioral coping, problems or additional impulses occur, the individual may return recursively to Phases I and II to modify his or her illness representations, behavior, knowledge, or emotional regulation so that consummation can occur.

Following up on the prior respiratory example of Phase II, if the signs and symptoms are not responding to a respiratory regimen, the individual and those around him or her will return to Phases I and II to relabel signs and symptoms and to construct a new or modified strategy for coping with the signs and symptoms. The process is recursive in that it continues until some sense of stability or equilibrium is reached, whether clinically appropriate or not.

Related Research

Studies have examined the coping strategies used by individuals experiencing AMI. As previous described in Phase II, the symptoms experienced are often attributed to less serious disorders, and therefore the self-management strategies used are initially directed at those causes. Only when treatment for these less serious disorders was not effective did they seek treatment. However, studies demonstrate that even when attributing the symptoms to a heart attack, most individuals do not call emergency medical services (Carney et al., 2002; Dracup et al., 2003; Leslie et al., 2000; Moser et al., 2005; Roe, 2006). Instead, studies show that patients, as part of their overt action, contact family or friends (Dracup et al., 2003; Henriksson et al., 2007; King & McGuire, 2007; MacInnes, 2006; Nymark et al., 2009) or medical professionals (Carney et al., 2002; King & McGuire, 2007; Leslie et al., 2000). Contacting medical professionals has been found to increase delay (Leslie et al., 2000; Moser et al., 2006). Resting and waiting to see what would happen is a common management strategy (Khraim et al., 2009; King & McGuire, 2007; McKinley et al., 2000; Moser et al., 2005; Moser et al., 2006; Roe, 2006). Use of emotion-focused coping strategies is also common during the symptomatic experience (Khraim et al., 2009; MacInnes, 2006; Moser et al., 2005; Nymark et al., 2009; Roe, 2006). In addition, self-medication to relieve the perceived cause has also been found to be a common coping strategy (Dracup et al., 2003; King & McGuire, 2007; Leslie et al., 2000; Moser et al., 2005; Moser et al., 2006).

Phase IV: Assessment and Consummation

In Phase IV, or the consummatory phase, the primary process is the experience of fulfillment or restored equilibrium, fulfillment of covertly constructed strategies, and reduced emotional and affective arousal. Although the assessment and consummation phase conceptualizes the process of restored equilibrium, in a real sense it is an analytic point that is used to highlight the outcome of coping with a single discrete illness event that has occurred within the life course and flow of life course events (Alonzo, 1999). On consummation, the AMI event has been contained by available resources (e.g., stabilizing care obtained in the emergency department) and a measure of equilibrium achieved. In actuality, the individual and others will continue to cope with the consequences of an AMI for a considerable time.

Emotions and Coping

Each of the phases described previously combines the Meadian and Leventhal conceptions of how individuals cope with a traumatic, turbulent experience in a self-regulatory action scheme. Emotions are thought to have a particularly profound influence on AMI care-seeking behavior. Emotions are regarded as having an involuntary, compelling quality that is mediated through the individual's perception and the situational response to emotions (Safran & Greenberg, 1991). Emotions can be a product of genetically programmed states of arousal and socialized sentiments (Gordon, 1981) that are situationally connected and biophysically independent. At the fundamental organismic and biopsychological level of processing, there is a very basic primary, even primal, response to symptoms normally associated with AMI (e.g., chest pressure, discomfort or pain, left arm pain and tingling, gastrointestinal distress, shortness of breath, lightheadedness and dizziness, perspiration, and overwhelming dread). This may arouse fear, anxiety, or helplessness in the individual that can be quite independent of the socially defined situation. Thus, at an organismic or autonomic and hormonal level (Izard, 1993), symptoms of AMI have the potential to provide a turbulent, traumatic stimuli independent of the individual's constructive propensities. It is these independent stimuli and the arousal produced that are addressed by the AMI coping model. A fundamental assumption is that emotional arousal becomes objectified from the flow of ongoing experience and action. In this sense, the affect control theory (Heise, 1989; MacKinnon, 1994; Smith-Lovin, 1990) is consistent with what is proposed in the context of AMI. Emotional states are the product of the interaction between physiological arousal and cognition about the cause of the arousal. Leventhal (1980) argues, "The problem of the relationship of cognition to emotion should not be reduced to the issue of who is to rule, but how the pair interact to govern" (p. 193).

If we view individuals as being in social situations and assume they desire a stable social identity (Robinson & Smith-Lovin, 1992), then we can understand individuals' cognitive response to symptoms, especially if we assume the primacy of desiring to maintain social situational engagement and participation. MacKinnon (1994) aptly summarizes an appropriate basic understanding of responses to AMI: "[E]motions are episodic, situationally instigated, ephemeral affective experiences with physiological and cognitive components. . . . [Emotions] are cognitive signals, rich in affective meaning, that inform people how they are doing in establishing and validating situated identities in social interaction" (p. 31).

Integrating the strands of emotional conceptualizations from symbolic interaction inspired affect control theory, and Leventhal's (1980) emotion component of self-regulation theory, the convergent point appears to be that emotions are a consequence of a discrepancy between what the individual expects to occur, to experience, to be perceived as, or to engage in and what is actually experienced. In a sense, experiencing symptoms of AMI is a discrepancy in bodily and health expectations in situationally meaningful settings. In Leventhal's conceptualization, the violation of social and emotional schematic expectations is a "critical source of affective experiences and reactions" (p. 187). Emotions come from both the deviation from expectation and the specific meaning of the stimulus. Emotions are thus an evaluation of some part of the world in relation to oneself (Franks & McCarthy, 1989) or, as Hochschild (1990) suggests, in relation to bodily sensations.

In a very real sense, symptoms of an AMI and their potential meaning and consequences represent a turbulent, traumatic stimuli that arouses in the individual, and those around him or her, a level of emotional responsiveness requiring an adaptive coping strategy to regain a sense of comfort, normality, or restored situational sentiments regarding the self. Studies have found that emotional arousal is often present at least during the initial AMI symptom experience (Moser et al., 2005; Nymark et al., 2009; Roe, 2006; Walsh et al., 2004).

Prior History of AMI and Emotional Coping

Individuals with a prior history of AMI and CHD are a unique group that experience an aftermath of increased morbidity and mortality compared to the general population. The American Heart Association's 2010 statistics show that within 1 year after a first AMI for individuals age 40 and older, 18% of men and 23% of women will die (Lloyd-Jones et al., 2010). One would expect that prior knowledge and emotional and behavioral experiences would enhance sensitivity and responsiveness to recurrent AMI symptoms, but there is a dearth of support for such a relationship. Studies have been inconsistent thus far, confirming that this subset of the population requires special attention in AMI research. Interestingly, although some studies have shown that individuals with a history of AMI are more likely to attribute their symptoms to the heart (Fox-Wasylyshyn et al., 2010; Leslie et al., 2000), compared to those with no cardiac history, there is no difference in prehospital delay time or reasons for delaying (Leslie et al., 2000). Further, in studies examining gender differences in treatment-seeking delay, women with a previous AMI have been found to have both longer (Moser et al., 2005) and shorter (Lefler & Bondy, 2004) delay time, with men showing a completely reverse relationship (Moser et al., 2005) or no difference at all (King & McGuire, 2007). Although these results seem to elicit many questions, such research only demonstrates and reinforces the need for further investigation of gender in care-seeking delay (Fox-Wasylyshyn et al., 2010).

Other research has shown that individuals with a prior history of AMI and coronary heart disease (CHD) do not tend to seek time-dependent medical care during subsequent episodes of acute coronary disease faster (and frequently do so more slowly) (Carney et al., 2002; Perkins-Porras et al., 2008; Saczynski et al., 2008). This is problematic because, dependent upon gender and clinical outcome, individuals with a history of AMI have a 1.5 to 15 times greater risk for death and increased morbidity than the general population (Lloyd-Jones et al., 2010). When this phenomenon of potential care-seeking delay is considered within the framework described previously, a possible explanation can be derived.

Individuals with a history of ischemic heart disease have episodic or autobiographical memories (Leventhal & Cameron, 1987) of prior responses to and experiences with symptoms of AMI and CHD diagnostic procedures and their potential meanings and consequences. These experiences may interfere with and preclude expedient care seeking for the following reasons. First, individuals with preexistent disease may have an idiosyncratic illness representation. Research has revealed that symptoms of a recurrent AMI can present differently than in previous ones (Pattenden, Watt, Lewin, & Stanford, 2002) and that this unique population is less likely to have classic AMI symptoms, resulting in delayed care seeking (Saczynski et al., 2008). They may therefore mislabel symptoms and signs of subsequent AMIs (Carney et al., 2002) and find difficulty seeking time-dependent care (Carney et al., 2002; McKinley et al., 2000; Perkins-Porras et al., 2008; Saczynski et al., 2008), especially if new symptoms are not similar enough to previous ones (Morgan, 2005; Zerwic, Ryan, DeVon, & Drell, 2003).

Second, those who have had an AMI and who have participated in cardiac rehabilitation may engage in longer periods of evaluation because the rehabilitation process may encourage a sense of optimism, efficacy, and invulnerability (Wielgosz, Nolan, Earp, Biro, & Wielgosz, 1988). Rehabilitation may contribute to what Weinstein (1988) terms an "optimistic bias," wherein cardiac patients erroneously believe that their own risk is less than that of others because of their participation. Weinstein further indicates that the source of this optimism could also be incorrect information, a need to sustain self-esteem and, as noted previously, to sustain situational participation, or both.

Third, some individuals (as many as 31%; Chung, Berger, & Rudd, 2008) may experience a form of post-traumatic stress disorder (PTSD) (Gander & von Kanel, 2006; Guler et al., 2009; Jones, Chung, Berger, & Campbell, 2007; Pedersen, Middel, & Larsen, 2003; Rocha et al., 2008; Spindler & Pedersen, 2005; Wiedemar et al., 2008) and/or dissociative tendencies (Ginzburg, Solomon, Dekel, & Bleich, 2006). When study parameters are expanded to include diagnostic PTSD or PTSD symptoms, the number reaches as high as 33.8% (Ayers, Copland, & Dunmore, 2009). Post-AMI PTSD has been shown to increase morbidity and mortality one year post-AMI (Shemesh et al., 2004). In addition, the experience of an AMI may be similar in many respects to the reported experiences of assault, domestic abuse, combat survivors, and so on (Mundy & Baum, 2004). Post-AMI individuals with PTSD demonstrate intrusion of past experiences, a desire to avoid stimuli associated with past experiences, increased psychological arousal or hypervigilance, and psychic numbing or ideational constriction consistent with PTSD clinical

diagnoses (Bennett & Brooke, 1999; Chung, Berger, & Rudd, 2007; Ginzburg, 2006; Rocha et al., 2008; Wiedemar et al., 2008).

Though the prevalence rates of post-AMI PTSD are relatively lower than victims of violence, recent literature has postulated that post-AMI PTSD may be a "common, persistent, and overlooked cause of psychological morbidity" (Jones et al., 2007). Ayers et al. (2009) found that participants with PTSD and PTSD symptoms post-AMI had a concurrent increase in somatic symptoms, anxiety, depression, and social dysfunction, similar to the results found in violence-associated PTSD. In addition, Ginzburg (2006) supported those findings, showing that 7 months post-AMI, 16% of post-AMI participants were identified with PTSD, 8% with comorbid PTSD and depression, and 14% with high levels of depression without full PTSD. Post-AMI PTSD can persist over time if left untreated (Abbas et al., 2009).

Further, there are three traumas of AMI that may contribute to PTSD-like symptoms, dissociative tendencies, or both. First is the primary trauma of the insult to the myocardium or heart muscle and related symptoms and signs. Sociopsychologically, there is the fright and overwhelming dread of the potential loss of life and of social control, of the breakdown of social situations, of a diminished continuity of life, and of future expectations and the assault on ones' social identity across many domains. The outcome of an AMI may leave the individual with angina pectoris, or chest pain with exertion, and other disabilities. In addition, and a very significant part of medical treatment, are the relatively invasive experiences of coronary bypass surgery, angioplasty, angiography, pacemaker implantation, stress testing, and the numerous side effects of cardiac medications. One study found that individuals who underwent such procedures tended to report more PTSD symptoms (Chung et al., 2008). In essence, the individual is now clinically diagnosed as having a potentially fatal and life-threatening, possibly terminal, chronic disease (American Psychological Association [APA], 2000).

Next, there are secondary traumas of experiences in accessing and using emergency medical services (EMS) or dialing 911, calling a physician, entering the emergency department (ED), and experiencing hospitalization. Over the long term, becoming a cardiac patient, going through cardiac rehabilitation, changing work and lifestyles, and experiencing repeated physician consultations and medical regimens can become part of the secondary trauma of AMI.

Last, at the tertiary level, there are many stressful mini-events of being a patient in the modern health care system. These small but cumulative traumas are the administrative hassles associated with health insurance, workers' compensation and other disability insurance, hospital and physician billing services, and, if eligible, Medicare and Medicaid.

Individuals who experience repeated traumas are particularly apt to demonstrate a range of maladaptive coping. Chung et al. (2008) found that following AMI, individuals who utilized emotion-focused or avoidant coping strategies were more likely to report comorbid symptoms such as somatic problems, anxiety, social dysfunction, and depression. Similarly, Turner and Lloyd (1995) demonstrated that individuals who experienced the "cumulative adversity" of lifetime traumas are at risk for manifesting psychopathologies that, in the context of AMI, could interfere with effective coping. There is an increasing body of evidence linking AMI and depression (Ayers et al., 2009; Bush et al., 2005; Ginzburg, 2006; Ginzburg et al., 2003). In a systematic review of 20 studies, Barth, Schumacherm, & Herrmann-Lingen (2004) found that depressive symptoms increased the risk of mortality in patients with CHD. Other links uncovered in the literature include anxiety and acute stress disorder (ASD) as risk factors for PTSD development (Ginzburg et al., 2003). Ginzburg et al. (2003) shows that the rates of PTSD among post-AMI patients who had ASD were three times higher than among those without ASD. Geyer, Broer, Haltenhof, Buhler, and Merschbacher (1994) also found data to support the connection between adverse event frequency and severity and subsequent depressive disorders.

Considered within the AMI model of coping, it can be seen that emotion-focused coping impaired by PTSD-like symptomatology or dissociative tendencies could inhibit a timely response to symptoms of AMI within a self-regulatory process. Whether the individual experiences the avoidance of PTSD or the numbness of dissociation, the result is a maladaptive coping response that obstructs the application of knowledge or the use of problem-focused coping that might facilitate expeditious arrival at the emergency department (ED) during subsequent AMIs or other cardiac events. Fox-Wasylyshyn et al. (2010) found that emotion-focused coping was associated with prolonged AMI care-seeking delay. Overall, the traumatogenic potential of AMI may have implications for maladaptive coping during subsequent ischemic events and for other comorbidities over the life course (Alonzo, 1998, 1999).

IMPLICATIONS FOR PRACTICE

Consistent with the emphasis of nursing, the AMI coping model stresses the client perspective and the importance of the social situation. The model suggests that an understanding of the clients' response to the threat of AMI is ascertained by understanding their perceptions or implicit models of the threat that may be particularly influenced by prior experiences with the threat of AMI or other chronic health problems or both, priorities strongly influenced by the home context, and untoward emotional reaction.

As represented in Figure 16.2, this framework provides guidance for the development of intervention strategies to reduce care-seeking delay. This conceptualization suggests that if individuals in the midst of the potentially traumatic experience of AMI (particularly those with histories of AMI and CHD) are to call the EMS or arrive at hospital EDs sooner, interventions, whether at the individual or community level, should take into consideration three elements derived from self-regulation theory and the Meadian conceptualization of the act (Leventhal, 1980; Leventhal & Cameron, 1987; Mead, 1938). First, knowledge is needed by the individual and lay others to correctly label symptoms (typical and atypical) as indicative of an AMI. A study by Buckley et al. (2007) found that an education and counseling intervention on AMI symptoms resulted in improved knowledge of AMI symptoms and that was sustained at 12 months. In a systematic review of interventions to reduce delay in patients with suspected heart attack, Kainth et al. (2004) stated "there is limited evidence that community wide media based or one on one education interventions were successful in reducing delay time" (p. 508). Second, it is necessary to provide feasible behaviors that individuals and lay others can engage in to access definitive medical care (e.g., dialing 911). Last, and perhaps most important, it is necessary to provide an understanding of, and skills to cope with, the primary emotional arousal in regard to the traumatic experience of AMI symptoms. It must be understood that the knowledge and behaviors necessary to obtain effective care may contribute to emotional arousal and paralyze timely action. Thus, the secondary and tertiary arousal engendered by knowledge and behaviors necessary to construct a strategy to cope with the acute AMI illness experience and potential consequences need to be addressed.

Issues discussed previously are also relevant to the clinical setting in the early phases of clinical assessment. Although a certain amount of dissociative behavior may be beneficial in the early phases of AMI hospitalization (Croyle & Ditto, 1990; Esteve, Valdes, Riesco, Jodar, & de Flores, 1992; Flowers, 1992; Kenyon, Ketterer, Gheorghiade, & Goldstein, 1991), continued anxiousness, depersonalization, and dissociation could be considered indicative of a form of reactive posttraumatic stress syndrome and cumulative adversity syndromes. This assessment would be especially appropriate among patients with a history of cardiovascular disease or other chronic diseases and those with comorbid psychosocial life course experiences. The pursuit of an agenda of systematic patient assessment or screening,

and a logical extension into research, could be facilitated by the use of available and validated instruments designed to measure PTSD. Small preliminary studies have agreed, suggesting the prospect of clinical screening tools to help identify post-AMI patients at risk for PTSD (Wiedemar et al., 2008). There are 47 accepted screening tools listed on the National Center for PTSD website (National Center for PTSD, 2009), but only a handful appear in the research literature. First, studies have used the Posttraumatic Diagnostic Scale, or PDS (Bennett & Brooke, 1999; Chung et al., 2007), a structured interview that can be administered in 10 to 15 minutes and is based on *DSM-IV-TR* diagnostic criteria for PTSD diagnosis. Second, Ginzburg and others (2006) used the PTSD Inventory Scale, also based on the *DSM-IV* criteria for PTSD. Other tools utilized have been the Structured Clinical Interview for DSM-IV (SCID) and the Impact of Events Scale–Revised (IES–R), a self-report screening (Rocha et al., 2008). All are accepted by the National Center for PTSD, but the PDS and IES–R do not allow for multiple traumas. Assessing

Figure 16.2   Phases of AMI Coping and Interventions

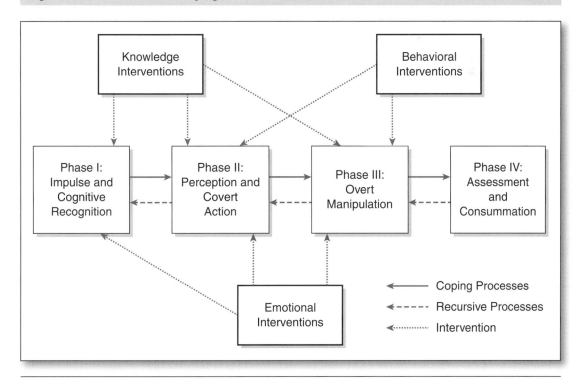

SOURCE: Alonzo, A. A., & Reynolds, N. R. (1998).

cumulative adversity can be accomplished by using Turner and Lloyd's (1995) scale of adverse events. These instruments are relatively short and easily administered and scored.

IMPLICATIONS FOR RESEARCH

The scope of this model extends beyond a United States–only utility. Prehospital delay holds true across continents, highlighting the potential universality of the Acute Myocardial Infarction Coping Model and further confirming the importance of continued research in the area (Dracup et al., 2003). To date, review of the literature has indicated that the model has only been tested by one American researcher who tested the model with a sample of women who had experienced AMI (Roe, 2006). Original support has been derived by systematic review of extant literature and empirical studies supporting self-regulation theory and the Meadian conception of the act (Alonzo & Reynolds, 1996a, 1996b, 1997, 1998). From the basic set of conceptualizations, the following propositions are derived:

1. The decision to seek AMI care is a process that occurs over time.

2. Patients and lay others are aware of and can recall their problem-solving and decision-making activities that contributed to their delayed or expeditious AMI care seeking.

3. Emotional responses in the form of fear, anxiety, or dissociation interfere with the use of AMI care-seeking knowledge and behavior.

4. Patients' responses to AMI symptoms will be affected by the social situation in which they initially occur. For example, individuals in the home versus the work environment will delay longer.

5. Individuals with a history of a prior AMI will be more likely to delay AMI care seeking as a consequence of (a) mislabeling AMI symptoms, (b) optimistic bias (if they participated in cardiac rehabilitation), or (c) AMI-related trauma and PTSD/PTSD-like syndromes.

6. Individuals with a history of comorbidities or cumulative adversity or both will be more likely to delay AMI care seeking as a consequence of (a) mislabeling AMI symptoms, (b) emotional arousal (in the form of fear, anxiety, or dread), (c) PTSD, or (d) all of these.

7. Knowledge, behaviors, and emotional interventions applied to strategic points in the care-seeking process will be more effective than general educational strategies.

The Acute Myocardial Infarction Coping Model lends itself to both qualitative and quantitative approaches to understanding the care-seeking behavior of individuals experiencing an AMI as demonstrated by Roe (2006). Its usefulness extends to approaches that focus on the phenomenological experience of the individual client as well as ones that focus on understanding responses across individuals. In a scientific statement from the American Heart Association, Moser et al. (2006) state that in order to advance knowledge in this area, four challenges need to be addressed. First, move beyond examining sociodemographic and health history factors, thereby allowing a fuller understanding of the social, cognitive, and emotional factors contributing to delay. Second, test new interventions that target high-risk populations and that move beyond providing information about symptoms to formulating recommendations for action that address social, cognitive, and emotional reasons for delay. Third, incorporate evidence-based practice by applying what is known from research to date to the education of at-risk patients. Lastly, focus on previously understudied, underserved, and special populations. As previously noted, individuals with a prior history of AMI and possible "post-AMI PTSD/PTSD symptomatology" require particular attention due to the scarcity of research in these areas.

SUMMARY

The AMI coping model is a midrange theory (Walker & Avant, 1995) from which testable hypotheses regarding AMI coping can be deduced and new findings can be used to support and extend the theory. The AMI coping model was inductively and deductively derived from extant empiric and theoretic literature. The following are key assumptions of the model: (a) The individual is an active problem solver who engages in conscious, intentional cognitive and behavioral effort to manage specific external or internal demands or both that are appraised as taxing or exceeding the resources of the individual; (b) individuals desire a stable social situational identity; (c) emotions have an involuntary, compelling quality that is mediated through the individual's perception and situational responses; and (d) emotional arousal becomes objectified from the flow of ongoing experience and action.

Key concepts in the model are coping, emotions, cumulative stress, and the phases of AMI coping—impulse and cognitive recognition, perception and covert action plan, overt manipulation, and assessment and consummation. These concepts are defined theoretically and to date have been operationalized by one study (Roe, 2006). Relational statements are described but have not been tested. The theory has fairly broad boundaries that have recently been expanded to consider the effects of cumulative adversity on AMI coping processes. The model is complex, yet it has the potential to be useful to nursing research and practice. Although aspects of the model are abstract and difficult to operationalize at this point, several components are testable.

Individuals experiencing symptoms of AMI are in the midst of a potentially traumatic, turbulent emotional experience. Although the advantages of rapid AMI treatment are clear, time from the onset of acute AMI symptoms to definitive emergency care is often protracted, and individuals with a prior history of AMI or CAD or both may be particularly apt to delay care seeking. In specifying emotional response and social reality as key elements, the AMI model of coping provides a health care framework for broadening our understanding of AMI care-seeking behavior.

REFERENCES

Abbas, C., Schmid, J., Guler, E., Wiedemar, L., Begre, S., Saner, H., . . . vonKanel, R. (2009). Trajectory of posttraumatic stress disorder caused by myocardial infarction: A two-year follow-up study. *International Journal of Psychiatry in Medicine, 39*(4), 359–376.

Alonzo, A. A. (1979). Everyday illness behavior: A situational approach to health status deviations. *Social Science and Medicine, 13A*, 397–402.

Alonzo, A. A. (1980). Acute illness behavior: A conceptual exploration and specification. *Social Science and Medicine, 14A*, 515–526.

Alonzo, A. A. (1998, April). The experience of chronic illness and post-traumatic stress disorder: Understanding coping behavior. Paper presented at the annual meeting of the Pacific Sociological Association, San Francisco, CA.

Alonzo, A. A. (1999). Acute myocardial infarction and post-traumatic stress disorder: The consequences of cumulative adversity. *Journal of Cardiovascular Nursing, 13*, 33–45.

Alonzo, A. A. (2000). The experience of chronic illness and post-traumatic stress disorder: The consequences of cumulative adversity. *Social Science & Medicine, 50*, 1475–1484.

Alonzo, A. A., & Reynolds, N. R. (1996a). Emotions and care-seeking during acute myocardial infarction: A model for intervention. *International Journal of Sociology and Social Policy, 16*, 97–122.

Alonzo, A. A., & Reynolds, N. R. (1996b). Care-seeking during acute myocardial infarction: A model for intervention. *Research in the Sociology of Health Care, 13B*, 393–409.

Alonzo, A. A., & Reynolds, N. R. (1997). Responding to symptoms and signs of acute myocardial infarction: How do you educate the public? *Heart & Lung, 26*, 263–272.

Alonzo, A. A., & Reynolds, N. R. (1998). The structure of emotions during acute myocardial infarction. *Social Science & Medicine, 46*, 1099–1110.

American Heart Association. (2007). What are the warning signs of heart attack [Fact Sheet]. Dallas, TX: Author.

American Psychiatric Association (APA). (2000). *Diagnostic and statistical manual of mental disorders, fourth edition, text revision (DSM-IV-TR)*. doi:10.1176/appi.books.9780890423349

Ayers, S., Copland, C., & Dunmore, E. (2009). A preliminary study of negative appraisals and dysfunctional coping associated with post-traumatic stress disorder symptoms following myocardial infarction. *British Journal of Health Psychology, 14(Pt 3)*, 459–471.

Ball, D. W. (1972). The definition of the situation: Some theoretical and methodological consequences of taking W. I. Thomas seriously. *Journal for the Theory of Social Behavior, 2*, 61–82.

Barth, J., Schumacherm, M., & Herrmann-Lingen, C. (2004). Depression as a risk factor for mortality in patients with CHD—a meta-analysis. *Psychosomatic Medicine, 66*, 802–813.

Bennett, P., & Brooke, S. (1999). Brief report: Intrusive memories, post-traumatic stress disorder and myocardial infarction. *British Journal of Clinical Psychology, 38*, 411–416.

Bleeker, J. K., Simons, M. L., Erdman, R. A. M., Leenders, C. M., Kruyssen, H. A. C. M., Lamers, L. M., & Van Der Does, E. (1995). Patient and doctor delay in acute myocardial infarction: A study of Rotterdam, the Netherlands. *British Journal of General Practice, 45*, 181–184.

Blumer, H. (1969). *Symbolic interaction: Perspective and method.* Englewood Cliffs, NJ: Prentice Hall.

Buckley, T., McKinley, S., Gallagher, R., Dracup, K., Moser, D. K., & Aitken, L. M. (2007). The effect of education and counseling on knowledge, attitudes and beliefs about responses to acute myocardial infarction symptoms. *European Journal of Cardiovascular Nursing, 6,* 105–111.

Bush, D., Ziegelstein, R., Patel, U., Thombs, B., Ford, D., Fauerbach, J., & Bass, E. (2005). *Post myocardial infarction depression.* U.S. Department of Health & Human Services: Agency for Healthcare Research and Quality.

Carney, R., Fitzsimmons, D., & Dempsey, M. (2002). Why people experiencing acute myocardial infarction delay seeking medical assistance. *European Journal of Cardiovascular Nursing, 1,* 237–242.

Chung, M. C., Berger, Z., & Rudd, H. (2007). Comorbidity and personality traits in patients with different levels of posttraumatic stress disorder following myocardial infarction. *Psychiatry Research, 152*(2–3), 243–252.

Chung, M. C., Berger, Z., & Rudd, H. (2008). Coping with posttraumatic stress disorder and comorbidity after myocardial infarction. *Comprehensive Psychiatry, 49*(1), 55–64.

Croyle, R., & Ditto, P. H. (1990). Illness cognition and behavior: An experimental approach. *Journal of Behavioral Medicine, 13,* 31–52.

De Luca, G., Suryapranata, H., Ottervanger, J. P., & Antman, E. M. (2004). Time to delay to treatment and mortality in primary angioplasty for acute myocardial infarction: Every minute of delay counts. *Circulation, 109,* 1223–1225.

De Luca, G., Suryapranata, H., Zijlstra, F., et al., for the ZWOLLE Myocardial Infarction Study Group. (2003). Symptom-onset-to-balloon time and mortality in patients with acute myocardial infarction treated by primary angioplasty. *Journal of American College of Cardiology, 42,* 991–997.

Dracup, K., & Moser, D. K. (1997). Beyond sociodemographics: Factors influencing the decision to seek treatment for symptoms of acute myocardial infarction. *Heart & Lung: The Journal of Acute and Critical Care, 26,* 253–262.

Dracup, K., Moser, D. K., McKinley, S., Ball, C., Yamasaki, K., Kim, C., . . . Caldwell, M. A. (2003). An international perspective on the time to treatment for acute myocardial infarction. *Journal of Nursing Scholarship, 35*(4), 317–323.

Esteve, L. G., Valdes, M., Riesco, N., Jodar, I., & de Flores, T. (1992). Denial mechanisms in myocardial infarction: Their relations with psychological variables and short-term

outcome. *Journal of Psychosomatic Research, 36,* 491–496.

Flowers, B. J. (1992). The cardiac denial of impact scale: A brief, self-report research measure. *Journal of Psychosomatic Research, 36,* 469–475.

Fox-Wasylyshyn, S. M., El-Masri, M., & Artinian, N. T. (2010). Testing a model of delayed care-seeking for acute myocardial infarction. *Clinical Nursing Research, 19*(1), 38–54.

Franks, D. D., & McCarthy, E. D. (Eds.). (1989). *The sociology of emotions: Original essays and research papers.* Greenwich, CT: JAI.

Gander, M. L., & von Kanel, R. (2006). Myocardial infarction and post-traumatic stress disorder: Frequency, outcome, and atherosclerotic mechanisms. *European Journal of Cardiovascular Prevention & Rehabilitation, 13*(2), 165–172.

Geyer, S., Broer, M., Haltenhof, H., Buhler, K. E., & Merschbacher, U. (1994). The evaluation of life event data. *Journal of Psychosomatic Research, 38,* 823–835.

Ginzburg, K. (2006). Comorbidity of PTSD and depression following myocardial infarction. *Journal of Affective Disorders, 94*(1–3), 135–143.

Ginzburg, K., Solomon, Z., Dekel, R., & Bleich, A. (2006). Longitudinal study of acute stress disorder, posttraumatic stress disorder and dissociation following myocardial infarction. *Journal of Nervous & Mental Disease, 194*(12), 945–950.

Ginzburg, K., Solomon, Z., Koifman, B., Keren, G., Roth, A., Kriwisky, M., & Bleich, A. (2003). Trajectories of posttraumatic stress disorder following myocardial infarction: A prospective study. *Journal of Clinical Psychiatry, 64*(10), 1217–1223.

Goldberger, L. (1983). The concept and mechanisms of denial: A selective overview. In S. Breznitz (Ed.), *The denial of stress.* New York, NY: International University Press.

Gordon, S. L. (1981). Sociology of sentiments and emotion. In M. Rosenberg & R. H. Turner (Eds.), *Social psychology sociological perspectives* (pp. 562–592). New York, NY: Basic Books.

Grossman, S., Brown, D., Chang, Y., Chung, W., Cranmer, H., Dan, L., Fisher, J., et al. (2003). Predictors of delay in presentation to the ED in patients with suspected acute coronary syndromes. *American Journal of Emergency Medicine, 21*(5), 425–427.

Guler, E., Schmid, J. P., Wiedemar, L., Saner, H., Schnyder, U., & von Kanel, R. (2009). Clinical diagnosis of posttraumatic stress disorder after myocardial infarction. *Clinical Cardiology, 32*(3), 125–129.

Hartford, M., Karlson, B. W., Sjölin, M., Holmberg, S., & Herlitz, J. (1993). Symptoms, thoughts, and environmental factors in suspected acute myocardial infarction. *Heart and Lung, 22,* 64–70.

Heise, D. (1989). Effects of emotion displays on social identification. *Social Psychology Quarterly, 52,* 10–21.

Henriksson, C., Lindahl, B., & Larsson, M. (2007). Patients' and relatives' thoughts and actions during and after symptom presentation for an acute myocardial infarction. *European Journal of Cardiovascular Nursing, 6,* 280–286.

Hochschild, A. R. (1990). Ideology and emotion management: A perspective and path for future research. In T. Kemper (Ed.), *Research agendas in the sociology of emotions.* Albany: State University of New York Press.

Izard, C. (1993). Four systems for emotional activation: Cognitive and noncognitive processes. *Psychological Review, 100,* 68–90.

Jones, R. C., Chung, M. C., Berger, Z., & Campbell, J. L. (2007). Prevalence of post-traumatic stress disorder in patients with previous myocardial infarction consulting in general practice. *British Journal of General Practice, 57*(543), 808–810.

Kainth, A., Hewitt, A., Pattenden, J., Sowden, A., Duffy, S., Watt, I., & Lewin, R. (2004). Systematic review of interventions to reduce delay in patients with suspected heart attack. *Emergency Medicine Journal, 21,* 506–508.

Kenyon, L. W., Ketterer, M. W., Gheorghiade, M., & Goldstein, S. (1991). Psychological factors related to prehospital delay during acute myocardial infarction. *Circulation, 84,* 1969–1976.

Khraim, F. D., Schere, Y. K., Dorn, J. M. & Carey, M. G. (2009). Predictors of decision delay to seeking care among Jordanians with acute myocardial infarction. *Journal of Nursing Scholarship, 41*(3), 260–267.

King, K., & McGuire, M. A., (2007). Symptom presentation and time to seek care in women and men with acute myocardial infarction. *Heart and Lung, 36,* 235–243.

Lazarus, R. S., & Folkman, S. (1984). *Stress, appraisal, and coping.* New York, NY: Springer.

Lee, H., Bahler, R., Chung, C., Alonzo, A., & Zeller, R. (2000). Prehospital delay with myocardial infarction: The interactive effect of clinical symptoms and race. *Applied Nursing Research, 13*(3), 125–133.

Lee, H., Bahler, R., Taylor, A., Alonzo, A., & Zeller, R. A. (1998). Clinical symptoms of myocardial infarction and delayed treatment-seeking behavior in blacks and whites. *Journal of Applied Biobehavioral Research, 3,* 135–159.

Lefler, L. L., & Bondy, K. N. (2004). Women's delay in seeking treatment with myocardial infarction a meta-synthesis. *Journal of Cardiovascular Nursing, 19*(4), 251–268.

Leslie, W. S., Urie, A., Hooper, J., & Morrison, C. E. (2000). Delay in calling for help during myocardial infarction: reasons for the delay and subsequent pattern of accessing care. *Heart, 84*(2), 137–141.

Leventhal, H. (1980). Toward a comprehensive theory of emotion. *Advances in Experimental Social Psychology, 13,* 139–207.

Leventhal, H., & Cameron, L. (1987). Behavioral theories and the problem of compliance. *Patient Education and Counseling, 10,* 117–138.

Lloyd-Jones, D., Adams, R. J., Brown, T. M., Carnethon, M., Dai, S., et al. (2010). Heart disease and stroke statistics—2010 update: A report from the American Heart Association. *Circulation, 121*(7), e89–91. doi:10.1161/CIRCULATIONAHA.109.192667

MacInnes, J. D. (2006). The illness perceptions of women following symptoms of acute myocardial infarction. *European Journal of Cardiovascular Nursing, 5,* 280–288.

MacKinnon, N. J. (1994). *Symbolic interactionism as affect control.* Albany: State University of New York Press.

Masoudi, F. A., Bonow, R. O., Brindis, R. G., Cannon, C. P., DeBuhr, J., Fitzgerald, S., . . . Wharton, T. P. (2008). ACC/AHA 2008 statement on performance measurement and reperfusion therapy: A report of the ACC/AHA Task Force on Performance Measures (Work Group to Address the Challenges of Performance Measurement and Reperfusion Therapy). *Circulation, 118,* 2649–2661.

McKinley, S., Moser, D. K., & Dracup, K. (2000). Treatment-seeking behavior for acute myocardial symptoms in North America and Australia. *Heart and Lung, 29*(4), 237–247.

Mead, G. H. (1938). *The philosophy of the act.* Chicago, IL: University of Chicago Press.

Morgan, D. M. (2005). Effect of incongruence of acute myocardial infarction symptoms on the decision to seek treatment in a rural population. *Journal of Cardiovascular Nursing, 20*(5), 365–371.

Moser, D. K., Kimble, L. P., Alberts, M. J., Alonzo, A., Croft, J. B., Dracup, K., . . . Zerwic, J. J. (2006). Reducing delay in seeking treatment by patients with acute coronary syndrome and stroke: A scientific statement from the American Heart Association Council on Cardiovascular Nursing and Stroke Council. *Circulation, 114,* 168–182.

Moser, D. K., McKinley, S., Dracup, K., & Chung, M. L. (2005). Gender differences in reasons patients delay seeking treatment for acute myocardial infarction symptoms. *Patient Education and Counseling, 56,* 45–54.

Mundy, E., & Baum, A. (2004). Medical disorders as a cause of psychological trauma and PTSD:

How are medical stressors different? *Current Opinion in Psychiatry, 17*(2), 123–127.

Natanson, M. (1956). *The social dynamics of George H. Mead.* Washington, DC: Public Affairs Press.

National Center for PTSD. (2009). PTSD checklist. Retrieved May 2, 2010, from http://www.ptsd.va.gov/professional/pages/assessments/ptsd-checklist.asp

Nymark, C., Mattiasson, A., Henriksson, P., & Kiessling, A. (2009). The turning point: From self-regulative illness behaviour to care-seeking in patients with an acute myocardial infarction. *Journal of Clinical Nursing, 18,* 3358–3365.

Pattenden, J., Watt, I., Lewin, R. J., & Stanford, N. (2002). Decision making processes in people with symptoms of acute myocardial infarction: Qualitative study. *British Medical Journal, 324,* 1006–1009.

Pedersen, S. S., Middel, B., & Larsen, M. L. (2003). Posttraumatic stress disorder in first-time myocardial infarction patients. *Heart & Lung, 32*(5), 300–307.

Perkins-Porras, L. P, Whitehead, D. L., Strike, P. C., Steptoe, A. (2008). Prehospital delay in patients with acute coronary syndrome: Factors associated with patient decision time and home-to-hospital delay. *European Journal of Cardiovascular Nursing, 8,* 26–33.

Quinn, J. R. (2005). Delay in seeking care for symptoms of acute myocardial infarction: Applying a theoretical model. *Research in Nursing and Health, 28,* 283–294.

Robinson, D. T., & Smith-Lovin, L. (1992). Selective interaction as a strategy for identity maintenance: An affect control model. *Social Psychology Quarterly, 55,* 12–28.

Rocha, L. P., Peterson, J. C., Meyers, B., Boutin-Foster, C., Charlson, M. E., Jayasinghe, N., et al. (2008). Incidence of posttraumatic stress disorder (PTSD) after myocardial infarction (MI) and predictors of PTSD symptoms post-MI—a brief report. *International Journal of Psychiatry in Medicine, 38*(3), 297–306.

Roe, E. (2006). *Treatment seeking in women with myocardial infarction.* Unpublished Doctoral Dissertation, Wayne State University.

Rosenfeld, A. G. (2004). Treatment-seeking delay among women with acute myocardial infarction. *Nursing Research, 53*(4), 225–236.

Saczynski, J. S., Yarzebski, J., Lessard, D., Spencer, F. A., Gurwitz, J. H., Gore, J. M., & Goldberg, R. J. (2008).

Trends in prehospital delay in patients with acute myocardial infarction (from the Worcester heart attack study). *The American Journal of Cardiology, 102,* 1589–1594.

Safran, J., & Greenberg, L. (1991). *Emotion, psychotherapy, and change.* New York, NY: Guilford.

Shemesh, E., Yehuda, R., Milo, O., Dinur, I., Rudnick, A., Vered, Z., & Cotter, G. (2004). Posttraumatic stress, nonadherence, and adverse outcome in survivors of a myocardial infarction. *Psychosomatic Medicine, 66,* 521–526.

Smith-Lovin, L. (1990). Emotion as the confirmation and disconfirmation of identity: An affect control model. In T. Kemper (Ed.), *Research agendas in the sociology of emotions.* Albany: State University of New York Press.

Spindler, H., & Pedersen, S. S. (2005). Posttraumatic stress disorder in the wake of heart disease: Prevalence, risk factors, and future research directions. *Psychosomatic Medicine, 67*(5), 715–723.

Turner, R. J., & Lloyd, D. A. (1995). Lifetime traumas and mental health: The significance of cumulative adversity. *Journal of Health and Social Behavior, 36,* 360–376.

Walker, L. O., & Avant, K. C. (1995). *Strategies for theory construction in nursing* (3rd ed.). Norwalk, CT: Appleton & Lange.

Walsh, J. C., Lynch, M., Murphy, A. W., & Daly, K. (2004). Factors influencing decision to seek treatment for symptoms of acute myocardial infarction an evaluation of the Self-Regulatory Model of Illness. *Journal of Psychosomatic Research, 56,* 67–73.

Weinstein, N. D. (1988). The precaution adoption process. *Health Psychology, 7,* 355–386.

Wiedemar, L., Schmid, J. P., Muller, J., Wittmann, L., Schnyder, U., Saner, H., et al. (2008). Prevalence and predictors of posttraumatic stress disorder in patients with acute myocardial infarction. *Heart & Lung, 37*(2), 113–121.

Wielgosz, A. T. J., Nolan, R. P., Earp, J. A., Biro, E., & Wielgosz, M. B. (1988). Reasons for patient's delay in response to symptoms of acute myocardial infarction. *Canadian Medical Association Journal, 139,* 853–857.

Zerwic, J. J., Ryan, C. J., DeVon, H. A., & Drell, M. J. (2003). Treatment seeking for acute myocardial infarction symptoms: Differences in delay across sex and race. *Nursing Research, 52,* 159–167.

17

Quality of Life in Relation to Stress and Coping

Anita E. Molzahn, Gail Low, and Marilyn Plummer

Quality of life (QOL) is a topic that has considerable relevance for nurses who are interested in stress and coping. In this chapter, we describe conceptualizations and theories of QOL (nonnursing and nursing), measurements of QOL, empirical adequacy of the QOL research, (including health, cognitive beliefs, external environment, active engagement, and social relationships), and briefly summarize the relationship of stress and coping and QOL. Since the goal of nursing is to maintain and improve QOL where possible, it is important to understand the history, the relationships, and the ways that QOL can be enhanced. Minimizing stress and assisting people to cope with their life situations are important nursing strategies to improve QOL.

Conceptualizations of Quality of Life

QOL, as a concept, has been considered important since the times of the early Greek philosophers. Aristotle wrote extensively on "the good life" (Adler, 1980) and the means to a life of quality. After World War II, use of the term "quality of life" appeared both in relation to societal well-being as well as to individual perceptions of their current life circumstances. In health care, there has been recognition that just measuring

morbidity and mortality rates is not sufficient; consideration must also be given to QOL. With the rapid advances in technology, it is critical to demonstrate that health care innovations improve quality as well as quantity of life. Use of the QOL construct has grown rapidly over the last three decades. However, there have been multiple definitions and interpretations of QOL. It has been described as experiences of life (Meeburg, 1993), satisfaction with life (Cummins, 2005), and well-being (Ferrans, 1996; Haas, 1999a, 1999b; Meeburg, 1993). It is generally agreed that QOL is inherently subjective in nature, relatively stable over time, and multidimensional. Although there is no single agreed-upon definition of the concept, most definitions and measures include physical, psychological, and social dimensions. However, consensus regarding a universal set of domains has yet to be obtained. Some scholars consider QOL to be intangible. For example, Rogers (1990) refers to it as "relative and infinite," and Peplau (1994) describes it as "a moving target."

The World Health Organization Quality of Life (WHOQOL) group defined QOL as "*individuals' perceptions of their position in life in the context of the culture and value systems in which they live and in relation to their goals, expectations, standards, and concerns*" (1998, p. 551). This definition emphasizes a holistic assessment that recognizes human tendencies to compare their situation with that of others, both on an individual and societal basis. This definition also reflects the broad nature of QOL that incorporates assessments of many aspects of an individual's life, including health, work, personal relationships, friendships, emotional state, and environment. Only the person can assess his or her own QOL.

Distinctions are usually made between QOL and health-related quality of life (HRQOL). The first is intended to be a broad encompassing concept; HRQOL is narrower in focus. Patrick and Erickson (1993) describe *HRQOL as "the value that an individual assigned to the duration of life as modified by impairments, functional states, perceptions and social opportunities that are influenced by disease, injury, treatment or policy"* (p. 22). Health care researchers often prefer to measure HRQOL because it is not always possible or realistic to expect that a health-related intervention will influence many of the broader aspects of QOL. On the other hand, with the importance of social determinants of health, there is an argument for health professionals to attend to QOL in its broadest definition. Consistency in the definition of QOL is important because "differences in meaning can lead to profound differences in outcomes for research, clinical practice, and allocation of health care resources" (Ferrans, 1996, p. 294). However, different disciplines think about QOL in various ways, and the specific use or application may warrant a specific approach that is not appropriate in another situation (Fayers & Machin, 2000).

THEORETICAL PERSPECTIVES ON QUALITY OF LIFE

Although much of the research on QOL is atheoretical, it is more common to find that a social science rather than nursing perspective has been used in the study of the construct. Many nurses conduct QOL studies, and both nonnursing and nursing perspectives inform their thinking about QOL. The models discussed in this chapter are theoretical frameworks or conceptual models wherein the elements of the model and the relationships among variables are considered, and QOL is formally defined (e.g., Halvorsrud & Kalfoss, 2007; Taillefer, Dupuis, Roberge, & LeMay, 2003). The need for more theory in relation to

QOL has been emphasized by a number of QOL scholars including Brown and Gordon (1994), Farquhar (1995), Bullinger (2002), and Low, Molzahn, and Kalfoss (2008). Although it is not possible to be exhaustive, we have described some guiding conceptual frameworks/theoretical models in which QOL is considered, initially from a nonnursing then a nursing perspective.

Nonnursing Theories Relating to Quality of Life

Early philosophers such as Aristotle theorized about QOL. Philosophical theory has been used to guide the study and understanding of QOL, or *the good life*. A good life refers to "a whole human life well lived, a life enriched by all real goods—all the possessions a human being should have, all the perfections that a human being should have, all the perfections a human being should attain" (Adler, 1984, p. 90). The Aristotelian-Thomistic (1225–1274) philosophical theory describes the seven real "goods" required to have a good life, specifically, goods of the body, mind, character, and personal association as well as social, political, and economic goods (Adler, 1980). The real goods are the constituents of a good life and are real goods in that they meet natural human needs. Goods are to be sought and enjoyed in proportion to their relative importance to the quality life (Adler, 1981). Assessment of an individual's attainment of real goods can be very useful in planning nursing interventions and has been used as a framework for nursing research (e.g., Molzahn, 1991a; Molzahn & Kikuchi, 1998). The following nonnursing theorists describe their perspective of QOL over the past 20 years.

Lawton (1991) conceived of QOL as evaluations of interrelated sectors of life (current physical, psychological, and time use and social behavior competence) from the perspective of the older person *and* others. Others' perceptions provide a point of comparison to ensure the intrusiveness of illness and disability is not underestimated because of personal compromise. Environments such as neighborhoods that provide outlets for socializing or dwellings that limit mobility are also appraised. Weighting of past and current competencies with expected or future competencies in each sector results in an appraisal of overall sense of well-being. QOL is thus a time-oriented, intersubjective, and environmentally conscious appraisal. Wilson and Cleary (1995) describe QOL as distinct from health; it represents the synthesis of life experienced with changing expectations and aspirations. Along with peoples' preferences or values, there appears a chain of causal effects beginning with physiological markers influencing felt psychophysical symptoms. In turn, the individual's ability to function is determined, in part, by his or her symptom status. General health perceptions represent an integrated appraisal of physiological factors, symptoms, and functioning. It is theorized that individual and environmental characteristics (though not defined) influence all factors beyond the physiological.

Leventhal and Colman (1997) defined QOL as a subjective judgment concerning physical and psychological function, symptoms, affect, economics, and relationships. Representations of illness establish a common-sense understanding about the symptoms of and dysfunction from illness and its treatment such as perceived causes and consequences, controllability, and the timing of symptoms. Contextual factors such as communications with practitioners, cultural beliefs, and illness-related discussions with close kin influence QOL. Representations also shape procedures ("if-then" rules) that, when enacted, confirm or contradict common-sense understandings. When procedural action leads to favorable outcomes such as greater perceived control, self-worth, and time gains, QOL changes for the better. Ormel, Lindenberg, Steverink, and Vonkorff (1997) equate QOL with an overall state of psychological well-being maintained by using resources. Psychological well-being is a cumulative appraisal of one's physical and social well-being. Peoples' resources are put to use so they can engage in activities that produce physical and social well-being. For example, close others and volunteer agencies bring a sense of intimacy and confirmation that enhance social well-being. When resources are scarce or lost, people turn to substitute resources to maintain well-being over the long term. When resource losses are severe, peoples' options are restricted. In essence, the greater the variety and amount of resources people have, the greater the likelihood of maintaining well-being (QOL) over time.

Albrecht and Devlieger (1999) define QOL as the ability of the self to build and manage balance between one's body, mind, and spirit. Spirit refers to one's belief in a higher order, being, and purpose. Balance is achieved through compensatory processes when loss and ambiguity imposed by physical disability threaten the individual. Compensatory mechanisms include engaging in rational thinking and regenerating one's spiritual energy to become resilient to bodily limitations. People with high QOL retain balance by learning about and making sense of their disability, conserving energy, and remaining engaged with social networks.

Michalos (2004) relates the quality (or values and good) of peoples' lives to net levels of satisfaction, for which happiness and life satisfaction are possible indicators (also see Michalos & Kahlke, 2010). In his work on Multiple Discrepancies Theory, Michalos (1983, 1985, 1986) focuses on peoples' happiness and satisfaction with life as a whole and with health, finances, family, job, friends, housing, area, recreation, religion, self-esteem, transit, and government services. Net satisfaction is theorized as being a function of multiple discrepancies or gaps between what people perceive they have in life compared to similar others; the best that people have had in the past versus what they expect, deserve, and need results in perceived gaps in achieving goals (what people have versus what they want in life). Felt discrepancies in relation to others and the past influence net satisfaction both directly and indirectly through goal achievement. Demographics (gender, age, education, ethnicity) and conditioners (self-esteem, income, social support) are related to net satisfaction and felt discrepancies.

For Cummins (2005), QOL is a global indicator of personal well-being or the satisfaction with life as a whole. Satisfaction is under homeostatic management and hovers around a positively biased and personality-driven set point. A hierarchy of life domains contribute to global life satisfaction, these being personal (achieving in life, one's standard of living, and personal relationships) and distal (the state of the environment, economic situation, and access to social support programs). As domains become less personal, satisfaction is under lesser homeostatic influence and prone to change. While decrements in one domain are typically compensated for by satisfaction in others, sudden or intense changes can create negative ripple effects, and thwart homeostatic influences. QOL also changes through response shifts (Rapkin & Schwartz, 2004; Schwartz & Sprangers, 1999).

Response shifts are changes in the way people understand and appraise QOL owing to the cognitive processes of reconceptualizing, reprioritizing, and recalibrating. Reconceptualizing refers to changes in one's frame of reference regarding life experiences to particular dimensions of life. Equally important are how people prioritize and recollect their life experiences, and the standards of comparison (calibrations) by which sampled life experiences are judged as relevant. Problem-focused coping produces indirect response shifts through buffering the disruptive effects of stressful life events, health states, and treatments on QOL. Emotion-focused coping directly changes the way QOL is understood.

For Devins, Bezjak, Mah, Loblaw, and Gotowiec (2006), QOL is the sense of well-being in relation to *intimacy, relationships and personal development*, and *instrumental life*. Illness-related symptoms, disabilities, and treatment-related lifestyle disruptions limit peoples' ability to engage in valued activities and interests in the four life domains. Other negative outcomes include a reduced sense of control in each life domain. Illness intrusions impact well-being differently depending on, for example, one's gender, culture, and illness consequences such as disfigurement.

From an economic perspective, Ferriss (2006) claims that the demographic base of a society and its institutional structures provide the conditions of living in which people derive satisfaction, purpose of life, and the fulfillment of aspirations or goals. Good QOL is a product of the way in which people respond to their living conditions and the social structures that create opportunities for supportive living conditions. For example, people need secure employment and income to satisfy the wants and enhance the QOL of oncoming generations. Membership in a faith-based organization provides an overarching set of beliefs and values, and enhances perceived satisfaction. Activity outlets for civic engagement promote social cooperation and QOL. The size of a community also affects the number of and access to institutions, and thus satisfaction and QOL.

Hajiran (2006) links QOL with life events in nine domains such as winning a lottery (economics) or losing a loved one (social relationships). Life events invoke feelings of happiness or sadness. The *gap* between how people expect to respond and actually do respond to these events represents overall happiness or QOL. Over time,

however, people become desensitized and adapt to life events which, in turn, hold less utility for happiness. Happiness is purported to be more reliably captured as the *monetary gap* or value difference between positive and negative life domain indicators of a nation's gross domestic product. For example, happiness could be quantified as the amount of income required to make unemployed people as happy as employed people. Within this context, QOL is defined as the net domestic product of happiness.

Bowling and Gabriel's (2007) work is unique as they offer a lay theory of QOL pertaining to key factors and why these are important in older age. Examples include health as an enabling activity, and accessible, friendly, and safe physical environments, each helping older people get pleasure and enjoyment out of life. Being independent fosters the ability to socialize and drive. Social relationships bring a sense of security and intimacy. Having a positive outlook brings mental harmony and overall satisfaction with life. From the perspective of older people themselves, QOL is both a personal and socio-environmental appraisal. Bishop, Stenhoff, and Shepard's (2007) Disability Central Model focuses on adaptation to chronic illness and disability. QOL is the overall sense of well-being arising from cumulative evaluations in key life domains: physical health, emotional health, social support, employment and productivity, and economic or material well-being. Illness and disability reduce domain satisfactions and personal control, and enhance negative emotions. People typically adapt by investing in resources to maintain a personally derived set point for well-being. However, when efforts to regain personal control are ineffective, domains become differentially important. In turn, efforts and resources are invested in domains of life wherein satisfaction is still attainable.

Gurland and Gurland (2009) believe that making informed choices that fit best with peoples' personal preferences (values) for ways of living improves QOL. People continuously gather information and reflect on what they have learned in the past, weigh long-term versus short-term gains or rewards, and anticipate consequences of their choices. When choices are restricted, people engage in compensatory mechanisms such as reducing the value attached to a preferred choice and exercising a substitute choice sparingly to preserve its longevity. Thus,

QOL improves through a process of acquiring and accepting potential choices and then choosing among them. McDougall, Wright, and Rosenbaum (2010) argue that all people develop some forms of disability. Disability hinders their functioning due to bodily impairment, activity limitations, and participation restrictions. Functional abilities constantly change in response to changes in, for example, one's age and health, and environmental factors such as the availability of support services. Over time, people are capable of adapting to disability. Adaptation enhances their capacity for participation and activity, and their growth and development. QOL is thus a composite appraisal with both functional and contextual facets, and intimately links to positive development.

Nonnursing theories represent several themes, including illness and disability and appraisal change. How QOL is defined varies considerably, as do the factors that influence its appraisal, for example, illness treatments or scarce resources. There is no single or "over-arching" theory of QOL. However, those above point to the sheer complexity of QOL and the range of factors affecting it. This diverse conceptualization of QOL is represented in the nursing theoretical frameworks that have evolved since the early 1950s as well.

Nursing Theorists and Their Consideration of Quality of Life

Plummer and Molzahn (2009) examined how nurse theorists defined and used the QOL concept. In a systematic review of the literature, they found several nursing theorists that have included the construct in their thinking to varying degrees. Hildegard Peplau (1952) was one of the early nurse scholars to develop a theoretical perspective for nursing. QOL is described in her nursing theory as *an intangible, all-encompassing phenomenon: it is the subjective perception of the condition of a person's life. It "is synonymous with well-being or psychological wellness"* (Peplau, 1994, p. 10) and it is often associated with health. QOL varies with changing circumstances, it is time and situation-dependent, and has an intangible quality. QOL, in Peplau's theory, is primarily influenced by health, personal relationships, and context.

Two decades later, Martha Rogers (1970), also a systems theorist, proposed her own nursing theory. Implicit in Rogers's theory is the notion of life satisfaction, a valuation of the life process (Leksell, Johansson, Wibell, & Wikblad, 2001; Lutjens, 1991). Life satisfaction or QOL fluctuates with interactions between individuals and their environments and is relative to one's circumstances. It also varies over the life course (Rogers, 1990, 1994). Like Rogers, Imogene King (1981) believes that human beings are open systems in constant interaction with each other and their environment to attain life satisfaction. QOL is implied in King's notion of life satisfaction. It is influenced by one's ability to set and attain goals and perceive a sense of accomplishment (I. King, 1994). Life satisfaction is also influenced by communication, interaction, and transaction between individuals. It is timeless and not bound by cultural norms (I. King, 1994). Madeline Leininger (1994) based her theory on culture care, that is, the learned values, beliefs, and patterned ways that assist, facilitate, or enable another individual or group to maintain their well-being (George, 2002; Leininger, 1978; Leininger, 1994). According to Leininger, QOL is culturally constructed, abstract, and represents the values, beliefs, symbols, and patterned expressions of a particular culture. QOL is considered to be a stimulus to achieve well-being rather than an outcome of health.

In Rosemarie Rizzo Parse's Human Becoming Theory (1981), human beings are considered unique individuals who are situated in the world and who act with intent and free will. QOL is explicitly described and used in Parse's theory; *it is a subjective, global perception of the meaning of one's lived experiences in the moment* (Parse, 1994, 1996). It fluctuates moment to moment in co-creation with the universe (Mitchell, 1995; Parse, 1994). The personal nuances of the nurse–person process enhance QOL (Mitchell, 1995). The concept of QOL has been well developed by Parse and Parse scholars (e.g., Hee, 2004; Pilkington & Mitchell, 2004). Through extensive research, Parse and colleagues have explicitly described QOL in its various subjective forms in different contexts. Parse clearly articulates that the goal of contemporary nursing practice is QOL.

All of the nurse theorists above consider QOL to be an overarching health outcome. This is consistent with the way the concept has been used since the 1980s in the social sciences as well (Meeburg, 1993). King and Leininger also perceive QOL to be a motivating force. Rogers and

King specifically refer to QOL as life satisfaction. While some QOL researchers concur with this perspective (Ferrans, 1996; Haas, 1999b; Kinney, Burfitt, Stullenbarger, Rees, & DeBolt, 1996; Moons, Budts, & De Geest, 2006), others consider life satisfaction to be a similar but related concept (C. R. King, 1998). The nursing theories identified are broad conceptual models rather than theories. They have not been tested and indeed are not at a level specific enough to test empirically. However, they do contribute to our understanding of the interconnectedness of the person, his or her relationships and environment, and QOL. More research is needed in this area to help nurses and others involved in health care delivery to develop greater understanding of the nature of QOL. A nursing lens on QOL research may help build further knowledge for the discipline. In the following sections are the measurements for quality of life and the empirical literature on the predictors of QOL, many of which are considered in the previously noted theories.

MEASUREMENT OF QUALITY OF LIFE

Measurement of QOL has shown to be a challenge partly because of the range of definitions and conceptualizations of the term. Numerous instruments have been developed and tested. Some are generic instruments that provide an overall summary of QOL and others are disease-specific measures that focus on problems associated with single disease states or patient populations. Selection of the most appropriate measure is very important. Ideally, a QOL measure should be easy to use, score, and interpret. Considerations in selection include the appropriateness of the measure for the population that uses it, the length of the instrument, the burden that it would create for the patient, the responsiveness to change and clinical sensitivity, the purpose of the study and/or measurement, and of course, the reliability and validity of the measure. The ProQOLID (n.d.) online database lists numerous patient reported outcome measures (see http://www.proqolid.org/proqolid) including generic and disease-specific QOL measures. Numerous resources are available to assist researchers and clinicians in their selection of the most appropriate measure (see Bowling, 1995, 1997; McDowell & Newell, 1996; Salek, 1999; Wilkin, Hallam, & Doggett, 1993).

In addition to psychometric assessment of measures of QOL, it is important to consider its responsiveness to change and the clinical sensitivity of the measure. A measure is responsive when it is able to capture changes in the patient's condition. Clinical sensitivity refers to "the smallest differences that are perceived as beneficial and which would mandate, in the absence of troublesome side effects and excessive cost, a change in the patient's management" (Jaeschke, Singer, & Guyatt, 1989). In recent years, QOL measures have been adopted in clinical practice settings and routine use has been found to improve physician–patient communication (Detmar, Muller, Schornagel, Wever, & Aaronson, 2002) and other patient outcomes (Velikova et al., 2004). These studies need to be extended to various clinical practice settings, and the potential utility for nursing assessment and practice needs further exploration.

QOL measurement can also be useful for quality assurance and policy purposes in clinical settings. Establishing goals for improvement of QOL of patient populations can result in significant improvements in quality of care. Reductions in QOL of a population/sample over time may suggest areas where care delivery needs to be improved. For instance, Edwards, Koehoorn, Boyd, and Levy (2010) noted a clinically significant reduction in QOL scores of people with strokes from 1996 to 2005 using data from two Canadian population surveys. They concluded that despite improvements in medical management, QOL after stroke was not improving in Canada. One of the issues in QOL assessment was whether proxies could assess QOL. Some of the early measures of "QOL," such as the Karnofsky scale (Karnofsky & Burchenal, 1949), involved physician ratings of the functional abilities of people, with a scale ranging from 0 (dead) to 100 (normal, no complaints, no evidence of disease).

Research has shown, however, that people have different assessments of their QOL than those of their health professionals, and there is a relatively low correlation between physician and patient measures and between nurse and patient ratings in adults with end-stage renal disease (Molzahn, Northcott, & Dossetor, 1997). Similarly, Harris et al. (2009) found in a study of five oncology centers worldwide that health care professionals' ratings of their patients' QOL were consistently higher than were their patients' (with bony metastases) own ratings. A substantial difference was found in relation to the perceived importance of psychosocial and somatic issues. Patients emphasized psychosocial issues while health care professionals rated symptoms as more important, particularly those related to pain. Bounthavong and Law (2008) found that patient and health care provider perspectives were similar in relation to emotional well-being, social functioning, medication, and diet, but they were quite different in how these factors were perceived in relation to QOL. While proxy measurements can be relatively accurate for some physical limitations, such as the ability to perform specific activities of daily living, they are less accurate where subjective assessments are considered (Hrisos et al., 2009).

One measure that is widely used and often described as a QOL measure, the Medical Outcomes Survey Short Form (SF-36), is actually a measure of health and functional status. It was developed for the Medical Outcomes Trust studies in the 1990s and has been extensively used and tested. As a result, norms are available for various populations. The SF-36 includes 36 items that measure physical function, role limitations due to physical problems, social functioning, bodily pain, general mental health, role limitation due to emotional problems, vitality, and general health perceptions (Ware, Kosinski, & Keller, 1994). Scores for each domain can range from 0 to 100; flooring effects are common and are a limitation of this measure. A shorter version, the SF-12, with 12 items, is also available and yields physical and mental but not domain scores.

Another instrument that is more appropriately labeled a generic measure of QOL is the WHOQOL-100. This 100-item inventory assesses physical, psychological, social, environment, level of independence, and spiritual aspects of QOL. There is also a shorter version with 26 items, the WHOQOL-BREF. Add-on modules are available for the study of older adults (WHOQOL-OLD; Power, Quinn, Schmidt, & WHOQOL-OLD Group, 2005); people with HIV/AIDS (WHOQOL-HIV Group, 2003) and spirituality (WHOQOL-SRPB Group, 2006). The WHOQOL instruments were designed to facilitate cross-cultural comparisons, and versions are available in many languages. They have been tested and validated and are available free of charge for the principal investigators of the country of interest.

Preference-based measures or utility scores are measured on a scale from 0 to 1.0 and integrate an assessment of health state preference over death. They are typically used in economic evaluations of treatments. Visual analogue scales can be used as direct preference-based measures, with death as the worst health state (at the bottom of the scale—0) and perfect health is at the top of the scale (100). The difference between the rating of various health states indicates differences in preferences. Standard "gamble" also measures preferences for health outcomes. In the standard gamble, the participant is offered two alternatives. In one option there is a lottery with two different outcomes; in the second, a chronic state for a specified period of time followed by death is offered. The time trade-off (TTO) method also measures cardinal preferences for health outcomes. In the TTO, the individual is posed with a choice of two alternatives, a current health state for a time followed by death or perfect health for less time followed by death. Time is varied until the respondent cannot decide between a briefer period in perfect health and a longer period in impaired health (Drummond, O'Brien, Stoddart, & Torrance, 1997; Santana & Feeny, 2008). The TTO score is calculated by dividing the trade-off point by normal remaining life expectancy.

One example of a disease-specific measure is the European Organization for Research and Treatment of Cancer (EORTC) instruments. The EORTC QLC-C30 is a cancer-specific questionnaire that is multidimensional, brief, and easy to complete. It includes physical, role, cognitive, emotional, and social subscales, a global health status/QOL scale, and a number of single items that relate to symptoms commonly experienced by cancer patients (Aaronson et al., 1993). There are additional modules that have been developed for specific forms of cancer and therapy. Other disease-specific measures include the Asthma Quality of Life Questionnaire (Juniper et al., 1992) and the Chronic Heart Failure Questionnaire (CHQ) (Guyatt et al., 1989). Some instruments that are called "disease-specific" actually measure other constructs such as depression or symptoms, for example, the Beck Depression Inventory (BDI) (Beck, Ward, & Mendelson, 1961). Disease-specific instruments are often useful in clinical trials or evaluative studies because they tend to be more sensitive to change. However, it may not be accurate to label them HRQOL measures.

EMPIRICAL ADEQUACY
OF QUALITY OF LIFE

There is a huge volume of empirical research on QOL, some of it relating to general populations, and some relating to specific illness populations and developmental phases, making it challenging to summarize key findings. Although it is not possible to be exhaustive, we will summarize some key findings pertaining to the relationship of QOL with physical health and functioning, cognitive beliefs, the external environment, active engagement, and social relationships.

Physical Health and Functioning

There is some conflation of the concepts health status and QOL in the literature. The terms and the measures are sometimes used interchangeably. However, as noted previously, these are different concepts. QOL is broader, and health is a predictor or correlate of QOL and not a component part of it. Health status is measured in many ways, ranging from subjective self-assessments to objective physical or biological indicators. There has been extensive research that demonstrates the relationship between subjective health status and QOL.

Health and functioning consistently impact QOL appraisals. There are consistent findings using various models that demonstrate the direct effects of health on QOL. For instance, Molzahn, Northcott, and Hayduk (1996) found that perceived health had direct effects on QOL of people with end-stage renal disease. Similarly, Low and Molzahn (2007) found health had direct effects on QOL of older adults as well as indirect effects through purpose in life. Further, it has been found that QOL is a predictor of mortality and hospitalization (Lowry, Curtin, LePain, & Schattel, 2003; Mapes et al., 2003) in people receiving dialysis therapy. Health-related QOL was also found to be prognostic of survival in critically ill patients (Iribarren-Diarasarri et al., 2009) and explained subsequent mortality among middle-age and older women (using the SF-36) (Kroenke, Kubzansky, Adler, & Kawachi, 2008).

For older adults, independence, also related to health, influences QOL (Bowling & Gabriel, 2007; T. W. Lee, Ko, & Lee, 2006; Puts et al., 2007). Physical mobility per se (Gabriel &

Bowling, 2004; Kostka & Jachimowicz, 2010; J. J. Lee, 2005) and the need for greater help with activities of daily living (ADL) (Hellstrom, Andersson, & Hallberg, 2004) significantly reduce QOL. Older adults who do not feel limited by health problems in relation to ADL capacity report a significantly higher QOL than do their counterparts (Bowling, Banister, Sutton, Evans, & Windsor, 2002; Fagerstrom, Holst, & Hallberg, 2007; Levasseur, Desrosiers, & Whiteneck, 2010; Netuveli, Wiggins, Hildon, Montgomery, & Blane, 2006). Being in poor health and losing one's physical independence has the potential to significantly reduce QOL among adults of all ages (Alvarez-Diaz, Gonzales, & Radcliff, 2010; Averina et al., 2005; Michalos & Kahlke, 2008; Schok & de Vries, 2005; Siegrist & Wahrendorf, 2009).

Changes in health status often result in impairments of QOL. For example, Cully, Phillips, Kunik, Stanley, and Deswal (2010) found that disease severity and depression significantly affected QOL of veterans with heart failure. Degenholz, Rosen, Castle, Mittal, and Liu (2008), in a longitudinal study of resident QOL in two nursing homes, found an association between physical health and self-reported QOL, and similar findings are noted by many other researchers. Similarly, the number of chronic illnesses affects QOL (Bowling, Seetai, Morris & Ebrahim, 2007; Hellstrom & Hallberg, 2001; Netuveli et al., 2006; Puts et al., 2007). Further research exploring the pattern of changes in various QOL dimensions in relation to specific clinical factors would be useful. Symptoms can be associated with decreases in QOL. For instance, sleep disturbances (Baldwin et al., 2010) are associated with reductions in QOL of adults over the age of 40 and people with many chronic illnesses (Krishnan et al., 2008). Fatigue has a negative correlation with QOL in women with chronic conditions (Khemthong, 2010), and the strength of the correlation was greater in a low (compared to a high) fatigue group. The mechanisms of the effects of symptoms on QOL can be highly varied. People having few physical health complaints such as pain and fatigue (Averina et al., 2005; Borglin, Jakobsson, Edberg, & Hallberg, 2006) report a significantly higher QOL.

Improvements in QOL have been associated with therapies that improve physical health. For instance, Ballan and Lee (2007) found SF-36 scores were significantly improved in three of the eight domains (physical functioning, general health perception, and energy/vitality) after coronary artery bypass surgery. Renal and cardiac transplantation have been found to improve QOL over pre-transplant states (Molzahn, 1991b). In other research, physical activity and/or exercise has been found to have significant positive effects on physical and psychological QOL relative to controls. Better overall QOL was reported for those people undertaking light-intensity exercise in a group setting with greater improvement in physical QOL after moderate-intensity exercise (Gillison, Skevington, Sato, Standage, & Evangelidou, 2009). Similarly, Ho et al. (2007) found that SF-36 scores were higher in a group of elderly practicing Tai Chi Chuan than in an age- and sex-matched control group.

In summary, although it is clear that there is a relationship between health and QOL, the distinctions between the concepts are not always clear. Exploration of QOL opens opportunities to address a wide range of human conditions and health challenges that are broader than traditional physical definitions of health might imply.

Cognitive Beliefs

Cognitive beliefs, such as sense of control, meaning and purpose in life, self-efficacy, satisfaction, and attitudes, can influence perceptions of QOL. A sense of control has been found to explain overall QOL (Bowling, Banister, Sutton, Evans, & Windsor, 2002; Bowling et al., 2007), as does the sense of meaning and purpose gained through opportunities to continue achieving in life (Cooney, Murphy, & O'Shea, 2009; Low & Molzahn, 2007). Similar findings were noted for the sense of self-efficacy (Bayliss, Ellis, & Steiner, 2007; Bowling et al., 2002), having a positive outlook for accepting circumstances which cannot be changed (Bowling & Gabriel, 2004; Bowling & Gabriel, 2007; Wilhelmson, Andersson, Waern, & Allebeck, 2005), particularly bodily changes (Borglin, Edberg, & Hallberg, 2005), and enjoyment in and the sense of control over one's life (Gabriel & Bowling, 2004; J. J. Lee, 2005; Warner, Schuez, Wurm, Ziegelmann, & Tesch-Roemer, 2010). Satisfaction with accomplishments in past life has also been found to positively predict QOL in older adults (Low et al., 2008). Older adults also link living each day in

its own right, viewing life positively (Borglin et al., 2005; Bowling & Gabriel, 2007), and being contented with one's existence (Wilhelmson et al., 2005) with positive QOL.

External Environment

Considerable research also supports the relationship between QOL and the environment. Paskulin and Molzahn (2007) found that a healthy physical environment contributed statistically to overall QOL in a Brazilian sample but not in a Canadian one. The Canadian finding was explained by the observation that Canadians take healthy physical environments for granted. Similarly, Paschoal (2005) found that good living conditions (water supply, discharging system, security, comfort) and a pollution-free physical environment were important contributors to perceptions of QOL in Brazil. Crime, graffiti, noise, and living in a deprived area have been found to negatively impact QOL (Bowling, Barber, Morris, & Ebrahim, 2006; Halvorsrud, Kirkevold, Diseth, & Kalfoss, 2010; Netuveli et al., 2006; Wiggins, Higgs, Hyde, & Blane, 2004), as opposed to living in a desirable and safe physical environment (Borglin et al., 2006; Bowling et al., 2003; Low & Molzahn, 2007) which has a positive effect on QOL. Having the positive effect on QOL are access to shops, leisure outlets, safe areas to walk (Bowling & Gabriel, 2004; Bowling & Iliffe, 2006; Puts et al., 2007); affordable transit (Bowling & Gabriel, 2007; Gabriel & Bowling, 2004); and few barriers to activity (Degenholtz, Kane, Kane, Bershadsky, & Kling, 2006; Levasseur et al., 2010; Low et al., 2008). Having good relationships with neighbors who provide practical help, a sense of reassurance, and look out for one another (Bowling & Gabriel, 2004; Wiggins et al., 2004) also fosters good QOL. Older adults receiving help at home report a far higher QOL than those residing in assisted-living residences (Hellstrom et al., 2004). Among adults of all ages, desirable housing, accessible physical amenities, parks and open spaces (Baker & Palmer, 2006; Williams, Kitchen, Randall, & Muhajarine, 2008), and greater area size of residence partly owing to better living conditions (Tokuda, Jimba, Yanai, Fujii, & Inoguchi, 2008) matter. It is apparent that multiple aspects of physical surroundings are important to QOL.

Active Engagement

As noted earlier, positive QOL is related to being independent and active (Cooney et al., 2009; Levasseur, Desrosiers & St-Cyr Tribble, 2008; World Health Organization [WHO], 2002). Indeed, having opportunities to continue achieving in life brings sense of meaning (Low & Molzahn, 2007), and reflecting on meaning in life and pursuing favorite activities (Cooney et al., 2009; Richard, LaForest, Dufresne, & Sapinski, 2004) have been found to enhance QOL. While higher physical activity frequency has also been associated with higher physical, psychological, and social QOL among adults 60 and older (Acree et al., 2006), physical health problems have been found to limit engagement in activities in general (Bayliss et al., 2007; Bukov, Maas, & Lampert, 2002; Puts et al., 2007) and volunteer work (Kloseck, Crilly, & Mannell, 2006; Netuveli et al., 2006).

In relation to other activities, among those living independently and in assisted-living settings, Jenkins, Pienta, and Horgas (2002) found HRQOL to be positively related to more active pursuits such as hobbies and recreation activities, particularly those outside of one's home. Iwasaki (2007) notes that leisure activities such as volunteering and hobbies give personal, social, cultural, spiritual, and altruistic meaning to life and promote QOL. Other positive activities include staying busy, learning and performing new activities, and being informed of what is happening in the world (Puts et al., 2007), as well as those pertaining to religion or gathering in a place of worship (Borglin et al., 2005; Bowling et al., 2003; Lin, Yen, & Fetzer, 2007; Wilhelmson et al., 2005). Overall, engaging in life intellectually, socially, and physically in a structured way gives meaning to life and fosters QOL (Borglin et al., 2005).

Social Relationships

A number of studies draw attention to the benefits of maintaining social activities and connections (Bayliss et al., 2007; Bowling et al., 2003; Bowling & Gabriel, 2004; Bowling et al., 2007; Mo & Winnie, 2010; Cooney et al., 2009; Degenholtz et al., 2006). In the QOL literature, sharing one's life with others has been described as enhancing QOL by offering a purpose and sharing a life history with others, and remaining with one's spouse well in to older age as love,

solidarity, and a strength to carry on living (Borglin et al., 2005). The value of social relationships within the context of QOL has also been linked to the prevention of loneliness, the sense of reciprocity and confidence, and having someone to confide in and for everyday and emergent help (Bowling & Gabriel, 2007; Bowling & Iliffe, 2006; Gabriel & Bowling, 2004). Social network quality is also important (Cooney et al., 2009; Wiggins et al., 2004). Having good social and trusting, close relationships in general (Bowling & Gabriel, 2004; Netuveli et al., 2006) and close and intimate ties (Low & Molzahn, 2007; Low et al., 2008; Warner et al., 2010) are reported to enhance QOL. Similar findings have been reported with respect to being connected with one's community and not feeling excluded from activities because of age (Levasseur et al., 2008; Low et al., 2008) and greater frequency of contact with friends (Netuveli et al., 2006). In adults of all ages, the sense of belonging and trust in people in one's community (Inoguchi & Fujii, 2009; Michalos & Kahlke, 2008; Tokuda et al., 2008), friendship ties (Bramston, Chipuer, & Pretty, 2005; Inoguchi & Fujii, 2009), and social relationships in general (Schok & de Vries, 2005) contribute to QOL.

Discussion about relational aspects of QOL is emerging in the nursing literature. For example, Scott, Setter-Kline, and Britton (2004) found that engaging in mutual goal setting between nurses and clients resulted in significantly improved QOL. Erci et al. (2003) used Watson's caring model to guide their inquiry into the impact of caring relationships on QOL of people with hypertension. More work in this area is needed to further develop how nurses can enhance QOL of people through their relationships with them.

STRESS, COPING, AND QUALITY OF LIFE

There is considerable research, both qualitative and quantitative, linking stress and coping with QOL. Illness is a stressor that often has a significant negative effect on QOL. Stressors such as a lack of sense of control, uncertainty (Puts et al., 2007), and financial worry/strain reduce QOL (Averina et al., 2005; Bayliss et al., 2007; Kostka & Jachimowicz, 2010; J. J. Lee, 2005; Levasseur et al., 2008; Mo & Winnie, 2010). Interpersonal stress related to worrying, coping, and relationships (Bramston et al., 2005) also results in lower QOL.

Coping strategies can buffer the effects of that stressor, and many qualitative studies have identified strategies that patients use to cope with their illness and enhance their QOL (e.g., Al-Arabi, 2006). Avoidance-focused coping strategies are associated with lower QOL in people with head and neck squamous cell carcinoma (Aarstad, Aarstad, & Olofsson, 2008). For some people, religious or spiritual support is helpful. Balboni et al. (2007) reported that 88% of their sample of people with advanced cancer found religion to be at least somewhat important, and interestingly, most (72%) did not believe that the health system helped them with their spiritual needs. In another study of people with cancer, perceptions that faith helped them enhanced their perceptions of QOL but where it was perceived that illness decreased their faith, there were lower ratings on QOL domains (Aukst-Margetic et al., 2009). Aarstad, Aarstad, Bru, and Oloffson (2005) found that avoidance-focused coping was associated with lower QOL in people with head and neck squamous-cell carcinoma patients. There have been numerous attempts to measure and model coping and QOL. In one study, coping had a variable influence across QOL domains, with little influence on domains that included symptoms and physical functioning but considerable influence on those with psychosocial domains (Abbott, Hart, Morton, Gee, & Conway, 2008). Over time, coping behaviors such as positive reframing and planning have significantly improved QOL, and avoidance markedly reduced psychological, but not physical QOL (Kershaw et al., 2008). Others have found task-oriented and emotional-focused coping and avoidance to matter little to global, physical, and psychosocial QOL (Masthoff et al., 2007).

A review of strategies to reduce stress and enhance coping is beyond the scope of this chapter; however, consideration of the factors described in relation to QOL—namely health, cognitive beliefs, environment, active engagement, and support—may offer direction for ways that health care professionals can intervene. Enhancing social support in general, as an instigator of active coping, and strengthening the sense of self-efficacy to lessen perceived illness threats and problems has been found to promote psychological QOL (Kershaw et al., 2008).

Exploring strategies for retaining paid work and involving an intimate partner in care planning could be beneficial to overall, physical, and environmental QOL (Masthoff et al., 2007). Stress, coping, and QOL are important concepts for nursing. There are many studies that demonstrate the interrelationships among these concepts. It is important for future empirical and theoretical work to address these interrelationships in the provision of nursing care to individuals, families, communities, and health care populations.

REFERENCES

Aaronson, N. K., Ahmedzai, S., Bergman, B., Bullinger, M., Cull, A., Duez, N. J., Filiberti, A., et al. (1993). The European Organization for Research and Treatment of Cancer QLQ-C30: A quality-of-life instrument for use in international clinical trials in oncology. *Journal of the National Cancer Institute, 85,* 365–376.

Aarstad, A. K., Aarstad, H. J., Bru, E., & Olofsson, J. (2005). Psychological coping style versus disease extent, tumour treatment and quality of life in successfully treated head and neck squamous cell carcinoma patients. *Clinical Otolaryngology, 30*(6), 530–538.

Aarstad, A. K., Aarstad, H. J., & Olofsson, J. (2008). Personality and choice of coping predict quality of life in health and neck cancer patients during follow-up. *Acta Oncologica, 47*(5), 879–890.

Abbott, J., Hart, A., Morton, A., Gee, L., & Conway, S. (2008). Health-related quality of life in adults with cystic fibrosis: The role of coping. *Journal of Psychosomatic Research, 64*(2), 149–157. doi:10.1016/jpsychores.2007.08.017 ER

Acree, L. S., Longfors, J., Fjeldstad, A. S., Fjeldstad, C., Schank, B., Nickel, K. J., & Gardner, A. W. (2006). Physical activity is related to quality of life in older adults. *Health and Quality of Life Outcomes, 4,* 1–6. doi:10.1186/1477–7525-4-37

Adler, M. J. (1980). *Aristotle for everybody.* Toronto, Canada: Bantam Books.

Adler, M. J. (1981). *Six great ideas.* New York, NY: Simon & Schuster.

Adler, M. J. (1984). *A vision of the future: Twelve ideas for a better life and a better society.* New York, NY: Simon & Schuster.

Al-Arabi, S. (2006). Quality of life: Subjective descriptions of challenges to patients with end stage renal disease. *Nephrology Nursing Journal, 33,* 285–292.

Albrecht, G. L., & Devlieger, P. J. (1999). The disability paradox: Quality of life against all odds. *Social Science & Medicine, 48,* 977–988.

Alvarez-Diaz, A., Gonzalez, L., & Radcliff, B. (2010). The politics of happiness: On the political determinants of quality of life in American states. *Journal of Politics, 72*(3), 894–905. doi:10.1017/S0022381610000241

Aukst-Margetic, B., Jakovljevic, M., Ivanec, D., Margetic, B., Ljubicic, D., & Samija, M. (2009). Religiosity and quality of life in breast cancer patients. *Collegium Antropologicum, 33,* 1265–1271.

Averina, M., Nilssen, O., Brenn, T., Brox, J., Arkhipovsky, V., & Kalinin, A. G. (2005). Social and lifestyle determinants of depression, anxiety, sleeping disorders, and self-evaluated quality of life in Russia. *Social Psychiatry and Psychiatric Epidemiology, 40*(7), 511–518. doi:10.1007/s00127–005–0918-x

Balboni, T. A., Vanderwerker, L. C., Block, S. D., Paulk, M. E., Lathan, C. S., Peteet, J., & Prigerson, H. G. (2007). Religiousness and spiritual support among advanced cancer patients and associations with end-of-life treatment preferences and quality of life. *Journal of Clinical Oncology, 25,* 555–560.

Baldwin, C. M., Ervin, A. M., Mays, M. Z., Robbins, J., Shafazand, S., Walsleben, J., & Weaver, T. (2010). Sleep disturbances, quality of life and ethnicity: The sleep heart health study. *Journal of Clinical Sleep Medicine, 6,* 176–183.

Ballan, A., & Lee, G. (2007). A comparative study of patient perceived quality of life pre and post coronary artery bypass graft surgery. *Australian Journal of Advanced Nursing, 24,* 24–28.

Baker, D. A., & Palmer, R. J. (2006). Examining the effects of perceptions of community and recreation participation on quality of life. *Social Indicators Research, 75*(3), 395–418. doi:10.1007/s11205–004–5298–1

Bayliss, E. A., Ellis, J. L., & Steiner, J. F. (2007). Barriers to self-management and quality-of-life outcomes in seniors with multimorbidities. *Annals of Family Medicine, 5*(5), 395– 402. doi:10.1370/afm.722

Beck, A. T., Ward, C., & Mendelson, M. (1961). Beck Depression Inventory (BDI). *Archives of General Psychiatry, 4,* 561–571.

Bishop, M., Stenhoff, D. M., & Shepard, L. (2007). Psychosocial adaptation and quality of life in multiple sclerosis: Assessment of the disability centrality model. *Journal of Rehabilitation, 73*(1), 3–12.

Borglin, G., Edberg, A. K., & Hallberg, I. R. (2005). The experience of quality of life among older people. *Journal of Aging Studies, 19*(2), 201–220.

Borglin, G., Jakobsson, U., Edberg, A. K., & Hallberg, I. R. (2006). Older people in Sweden with various degrees of present quality of life: Their health, social support, activities, and sense of coherence. *Health & Social Care in the Community, 14*(2), 136–146.

Bounthavong, M., & Law, A. V. (2008). Identifying health-related quality of life (HRQL) domains for multiple chronic conditions (diabetes, hypertension and dyslipidemia: Patient and provider perspectives. *Journal of Evaluation in Clinical Practice, 14,* 1002–1011.

Bowling, A. (1995). *Measuring disease.* Buckingham, England: Open University Press.

Bowling A. (1997). *Measuring health: A review of quality of life measurement scales* (2nd ed.). Buckingham, UK: Open University Press.

Bowling, A., Banister, D., Sutton, S., Evans, O., & Windsor, J. (2002). A multidimensional model of the quality of life in older age. *Aging & Mental Health, 6*(4), 355–371.

Bowling, A., Barber, J., Morris, R., & Ebrahim, S. (2006). Do perceptions of neighbourhood environment influence health? Baseline findings from a British survey on aging. *Journal of Epidemiology and Community Health, 60*(6), 476–483.

Bowling, A., & Gabriel, Z. (2004). An integrational model of quality of life in older age. Results from ESRC/MRC HSRC quality of life survey in Britain. *Social Indicators Research, 69,* 1–36.

Bowling, A., & Gabriel, Z. (2007). Lay theories of quality of life in older age. *Ageing & Society, 27*(6), 827–848.

Bowling, A., Gabriel, Z., Dykes, J., Dowding, L. M., Evans, O., Fleissig, A., et al. (2003). Let's ask them: A national survey of definitions of quality of life and its enhancement among people aged 65 and over. *International Journal of Aging & Human Development, 56,* 269–306.

Bowling, A., & Iliffe, S. (2006). Which model of successful aging should be used? Baseline findings from the British Longitudinal Study on aging. *Age & Ageing, 35*(6), 607–614.

Bowling, A., Seetai, S., Morris, R., & Ebrahim, S. (2007). Quality of life among older people with poor functioning: The influence of perceived control over life. *Age & Ageing, 36*(3), 310–315.

Bramston, P., Chipuer, H., & Pretty, G. (2005). Conceptual principles of quality of life: An empirical exploration. *Journal of Intellectual Disability Research, 49,* 728–733.

Brown, M., & Gordon, W. A. (1994). Quality of life as a construct in health and disability research. *The Mount Sinai Journal of Medicine, 66,* 160–169.

Bukov, A., Maas, I., & Lampert, T. (2002). Social participation in very old age: Cross-sectional and longitudinal findings from BASE. *Journal of Gerontology: Psychological Sciences, 57B*(6), 510–517.

Bullinger, M. (2002). Assessing health related quality of life in medicine. An overview of concepts, methods, and applications in international research. *Restorative Neurology and Neuroscience, 20,* 93–101.

Cooney, A., Murphy, K., & O'Shea, E. (2009). Resident perspectives of the determinants of quality of life in residential care in Ireland. *Journal of Advanced Nursing, 65*(5), 1029–1038. doi:10.111/j.1365–2648.2008.04960.x

Cully, J. A., Phillips, L. L., Kunik, M. E., Stanley, M. A., & Deswal, A. (2010). Predicting quality of life in veterans with heart failure: The role of disease severity, depression and comorbid anxiety. *Behavioral Medicine, 36*(2), 70–76.

Cummins, R. A. (2005). Moving from quality of life concept to a theory. *Journal of Intellectual Disability Research, 49,* 699–706.

Degenholtz, H. B., Kane, R. A., Kane, R. L., Bershadsky, B., & Kling, K. C. (2006). Predicting nursing facility residents' quality of life using external indicators. *Health Services Research, 41*(2), 335–356. doi:10.1111/j.1475–6773.2005.00494.x

Detmar, S. B., Muller, M. J., Schornagel, J. H., Wever, L. D., & Aaronson N. K. (2002). Health-related quality-of-life assessments and patient-physician communication: A randomized controlled trial. *Journal of American Medical Association, 288,* 3027–3034.

Devins, G. M., Bezjak, A., Mah, K., Loblaw, D. A., & Gotowiec, A. P. (2006). Context moderates illness-induced lifestyle disruptions across life domains: A test of the illness-intrusive theoretical framework in six common cancers. *Psycho-Oncology, 15*(3), 221–233.

Drummond, M., O'Brien, B., Stoddart, G., & Torrance, G. (1997). *Methods for the economic evaluation of health care programs.* Oxford, England: Oxford Medical Publications.

Edwards, J. D., Koehoorn, M., Boyd, L. A., & Levy, A. R. (2010). Is health-related quality of life improving after stroke? A comparison of health utilities indicies among Canadians with stroke between 1996 and 2005. *Stroke, 41,* 996–1000.

Erci, B., Sayan, A., Tortumluoglu, G., Kilic, D., Sahin, O., & Gungormus, Z. (2003). The effectiveness of Watson's caring model on the quality of life and blood pressure of patients with hypertension. *Journal of Advanced Nursing, 41*(2), 130–139.

Fagerstrom, C., Holst, G., & Hallberg, I. R. (2007). Feeling hindered by health problems and functional capacity at 60 years and above. *Archives of Gerontology and Geriatrics, 44*(2), 181–200.

Fayers, P. M., & Machin, D. (2000). *Quality of life: Assessment, analysis and interpretation.* New York, NY: Wiley.

Farquhar, M. (1995). Elderly people's definitions of quality of life. *Social Science & Medicine, 41,* 1439–1446.

Ferrans, C. E. (1996). Development of a conceptual model of quality of life. *Scholarly Inquiry for Nursing Practice, 10*(3), 293–304.

Ferriss, A. L. (2006). A theory of social structure and the quality of life. *Applied Research in Quality of Life, 1*(1), 117–123.

Gabriel, Z., & Bowling, A. (2004). Quality of life from the perspectives of older people. *Ageing and Society, 24,* 675–691.

George, J. B. (2002). *Nursing theories: The base for professional nursing practice.* Upper Saddle River, NJ: Prentice Hall.

Gillison, F. B., Skevington, S. M., Sato, A., Standage, M., & Evangelidou, S. (2009). The effects of exercise interventions on quality of life in clinical and healthy populations: A meta-analysis. *Social Science and Medicine, 68,* 1700–1710.

Gurland, B. J., & Gurland, R. V. (2009). The choices, choosing model of quality of life: Description and rationale. *International Journal of Geriatric Psychiatry, 24*(1), 90–95.

Guyatt, G. H., Nogradi, S., Halcrow, S., Singer, J., Sullivan, M. J., & Fallen, E. L. (1989). Development and testing of a new measure of health status for clinical trials in heart failure. *Journal of General Internal Medicine, 4,* 101–107.

Haas, B. K. (1999a). A multidisciplinary concept analysis of quality of life. *Western Journal of Nursing Research, 21*(6), 728–742.

Haas, B. K. (1999b). Clarification and integration of similar quality of life concepts. *Image: Journal of Nursing Scholarship, 31*(3), 215–220.

Hajiran, H. (2006). Toward a quality of life theory: New domestic product of happiness. *Social Indicators Research, 75*(1), 31–43.

Halvorsrud, L., & Kalfoss, M. (2007). The conceptualization and measurement of quality of life in older adults: A review of empirical studies published during 1994–2006. *European Journal on Ageing, 4*(4), 229–246.

Halvorsrud, L., Kirkevold, M., Diseth, A., & Kalfoss, M. (2010). Quality of life model: Predictors of quality of life among sick older adults. *Research and Theory for Nursing Practice: An International Journal, 24*(4), 241–259. doi:10.1891/1541–6577.24.4.241

Harris, K., Chow, E., Zhang, L., Velikova, G., Bezjak, A., Wu, J., . . . Bottomley, A. (2009). Patients' and health care professionals' evaluation of health-related quality of life issues in bone metastases. *European Journal of Cancer, 45,* 2510–2518.

Hee, N. C. (2004). Meaning of the quality of life for persons living with serious mental illness: Human becoming practice with groups. *Nursing Science Quarterly, 17*(3), 220–225.

Hellstrom, Y., Andersson, M., & Hallberg, I. R. (2004). Quality of life among older people in Sweden receiving help from informal and/or formal helpers at home or in special accommodation. *Health & Social Care in the Community, 12,* 504–516.

Hellstrom, Y., & Hallberg, I. R. (2001). Perspectives among elderly people receiving home help on health, care and quality of life. *Health & Social Care in the Community, 9*(2), 61–71.

Ho, T., Wen-Min, L., Lien, C., Ma, T., Kuo, H., Chu, B., . . . Lin, J. (2007). Health-related quality of life in the elderly practicing T'ai Chi Chuan. *Journal of Alternative and Complementary Medicine, 13,* 1077–1084.

Hrisos, S., Eccles, M. P., Francis, J. J., Dickinson, H. O., Kaner, E. F. S., Beyer, F., & Johnston, M. (2009). Are there valid proxy measures of clinical behaviour? A systematic review. *Implementation Science, 4,* 37. doi:10.1186/1748–5908–4-37

Inoguchi, T., & Fujii, S. (2009). The quality of life in Japan. *Social Indicators Research, 92*(2), 227–262. doi:10.1007/s11205–008–9351–3

Irribarren-Diarasarri, S., Aizpuru-Barandiaran, F., Munoz-Martinez, T., Loma-Osorio, A., Hernandez-Lopez, M., Ruiz-Zorilla, J., . . . Vinuesa-Lozano, C. (2009). Health-related quality of life as a prognostic factor of survival in critically ill patients. *Intensive Care Medicine, 35,* 833–839.

Iwasaki, Y. (2007). Leisure and quality of life in an international multicultural context: What are the major pathways linking leisure to quality of life? *Social Indicators Research, 82*(2), 233–264.

Jaeschke, R., Singer, J., & Guyatt, G. (1989). Measurement of health status. Ascertaining the minimally clinically important difference. *Controlled Clinical Trials, 10,* 407–415.

Jenkins, K. R., Pienta, A. M., & Horgas, A. L. (2002). Activity and health-related quality of life in continuing care retirement communities. *Research on Aging, 24*(1), 124–149.

Juniper, E. F., Guyatt, G. H., Epstein, R. S., Ferrie, P. J., Jaeschke, R., & Hiller, T. K. (1992). Evaluation of impairment of health related quality of life in asthma: Development of a questionnaire for use in clinical trials. *Thorax, 47*(2), 76–83.

Karnofsky, D. A., & Burchenal, J. H. (1949). The clinical evaluation of chemotherapeutic agents in cancer (p. 196). In C. M. MacLeod (Ed.), *Evaluation of chemotherapeutic agents.* West Sussex, England: Columbia University Press.

Kershaw, T. S., Mood, D. W., Newth, G., Ronis, D. L., Sanda, M. G., Vaishampayan, U., & Northouse, L. L. (2008). Longitudinal analysis of a model of quality of life in prostate cancer patients and their spouses. *Annals of Behavioral Medicine, 36,* 117–128. doi:10.1007/s12160–008–9058–3

Khemthong, S. (2010). Influence of fatigue on leisure and quality of life in women with chronic conditions. *Annual in Therapeutic Recreation, 18,* 79–86.

King, C. R. (1998). Overview of quality of life and controversial issues. In C. R. King & P. S. Hinds (Eds.), *Quality of life from nursing perspectives* (pp. 23–34). Sudbury, MA: Jones and Bartlett.

King, I. M. (1981). *A theory for nursing: Systems, concepts, process.* New York, NY: Delmar.

King, I. M. (1994). Quality of life and goal attainment. *Nursing Science Quarterly, 7*(1), 29–32.

Kinney, M. R., Burfitt, S. N., Stullenbarger, E., Rees, B., & DeBolt, M. R., (1996). Quality of life in cardiac patient research: A meta-analysis. *Nursing Research, 45*(3), 173–180.

Kloseck, M., Crilly, R. G., & Mannell, R. C. (2006). Involving the community elderly in the planning and provision of health services: Predictors of volunteerism and leadership. *Canadian Journal on Aging, 25*(1), 77–91.

Kostka, T., & Jachimowicz, V. (2010). Relationship of quality of life to dispositional optimism, health locus of control and self-efficacy in older subjects living in different environments. *Quality of Life Research, 19*(3), 351–361. doi:10.1007/s11136–010–9601–0

Krishnan, V., McCormack, M. C., Mathai, S. C., Agarwal, S., Richardson, B., Horton, M. R., . . . Danoff, S. K. (2008). Sleep quality and health-related quality of life in idiopathic pulmonary fibrosis. *Chest, 134,* 693–698.

Kroenke, C. H., Kubzansky, L. D., Adler, N., & Kawachi, I. (2008). Prospective change in health-related quality of life and subsequent mortality among middle-aged and older women. *American Journal of Public Health, 98,* 2085–2091.

Lawton, M. P. (1991). A multidimensional view of quality of life in frail elders. In J. E. Birren, J. E. Lubben, J. C. Cichowlas Rowe, & D. E. Deutchman (Eds.), *The concept and measurement of quality of life in the frail elderly* (pp. 3–27). New York, NY: Academic Press.

Lee, J. J. (2005). An exploratory study on the quality of life of older Chinese people living alone in Hong Kong. *Social Indicators Research, 71*(1–3), 335–361. doi:10.1007/s11205–004-8027-x

Lee, T. W., Ko, I. S., & Lee, K. J. (2006). Health promotion behaviours and quality of life among community-dwelling elderly in Korea: A cross-sectional survey. *International Journal of Nursing Studies, 43*(3), 293–300. doi:10.1016/j.ijnurstu.2005.06.009

Leininger, M. (1978). *Transcultural nursing: Theories, concepts, and practices.* New York, NY: Wiley.

Leininger, M. (1994). Quality of life from a transcultural nursing perspective. *Nursing Science Quarterly, 7*(1), 22–28.

Leksell, J. K., Johansson, I., Wibell, L. B., & Wikblad, K. F. (2001). Power and self-perceived health in blind diabetic and nondiabetic individuals. *Journal of Advanced Nursing, 34*(4), 511–519.

Leventhal, H., & Colman, S. (1997). Quality of life: A process review. *Psychology and Health, 12,* 753–767.

Levasseur, M., Desrosiers, J., & St-Cyr Tribble, D. S. (2008). Subjective quality-of-life predictors for older adults with physical disabilities. *American Journal of Physical Medicine & Rehabilitation, 87*(1), 830–841. doi:10.1097/PHM.0b013e3181861b5bd

Levasseur, M., Desrosiers, J., & Whiteneck, G. (2010). Accomplishment level and satisfaction with social participation of older adults: Association with quality of life and best correlates. *Quality of Life Research, 19*(5), 665–675. doi: 10.1007/s1136–010–9633–5

Lin, P., Yen, M., & Fetzer, S. J. (2007). Quality of life in elders living alone in Taiwan. *Journal of Clinical Nursing, 17*(12), 1610–1617. doi:10.1111/j.1365–2702.2007.02081x

Low, G., & Molzahn, A. E. (2007). Predictors of quality of life in old age: A cross validation study. *Research in Nursing and Health, 30,* 141–150. doi:10.1002/nur.20178

Low, G., Molzahn, A., & Kalfoss, M. (2008). Quality of life of older adults in Canada and Norway: Examining the Iowa Model. *Western Journal of Nursing Research, 30*(4), 458–476.

Lowry, E. G., Curtin, R. B., LePain, N., & Schatell, D. (2003). Medical Outcomes Study Short Form 36: A consistent and powerful predictor of morbidity and mortality in dialysis patients. *American Journal of Kidney Diseases, 41,* 1286–1292.

Lutjens, L. R. J. (1991). *Martha Rogers: The science of unitary human beings.* Newbury Park, CA: Sage.

Mapes, D. L., Lopes, A. A., Satayathum, S., McCullough, K. P., Goodkin, D. A., Locatelli, F., & Port, F. K. (2003). Health-related quality of life as a predictor of mortality and hospitalization: The dialysis outcomes and practice patterns study (DOPPS). *Kidney International, 64,* 339–349.

Masthoff, E. D., Trompenaars, F. J., Van Heck, G. L., Michielsen, H. J., Hodiamont, P. P., & De Vries, J. (2007). Predictors of quality of life: A model based study. *Quality of Life Research, 16,* 309–320. doi: 10.1007/s11136–006–9114-z

McDougall, J., Wright, V., & Rosenbaum, P. (2010). The ICF model of functioning and disability: Incorporating quality of life and human development. *Developmental Neurorehabilitation, 13*(3), 204–211.

McDowell, I., & Newell, C. (1996). *Measuring health: A guide to rating scales and questionnaires* (2nd ed.). New York, NY: Oxford University Press.

Meeburg, G. A. (1993). Quality of life: A concept analysis. *Journal of Advanced Nursing, 18*(1), 32–38.

Michalos, A. C. (1983). Satisfaction and happiness in rural northern resource community. *Social Indicators Research, 13,* 225–252.

Michalos, A. C. (1985). Multiple discrepancies theory (MDT). *Social Indicators Research, 16*(4), 347–413.

Michalos, A. C. (1986). An application of Multiple Discrepancy Theory (MDT) to seniors. *Social Indicators Research, 18*(4), 349–373.

Michalos, A. C. (2004). Social indicators research and health-related quality of life research. *Social Indicators Research, 65*(1), 27–72.

Michalos, A. C., & Kahlke, P. M. (2008). Impacts of arts-related activities on perceived quality of life. *Social Indicators Research, 89*(2), 193–258. doi:10.1007/s11205–007–9236-x

Michalos, A. C., & Kahlke, P. M. (2010). Stability and sensitivity in perceived quality of life measures: Some panel results. *Social Indicators Research, 98,* 403–434. doi:10.1007/s11205–009–9554–2

Mitchell, G. J. (1995). Quality of life: Intimacy in the nurse-person process. *Nursing Science Quarterly, 8*(3), 102–103.

Mo, P. K. H., & Winnie, W. S. M. (2010). The influence of health promoting practices on the quality of life among community adults in Hong Kong. *Social Indicators Research, 95,* 503–517. doi:10.1007/s11205–009–9523–9

Molzahn, A. E. (1991a). Quality of life after organ transplantation. *Journal of Advanced Nursing, 16,* 1042–1047.

Molzahn, A. E. (1991b). The reported quality of life of selected home hemodialysis patients. *American Nephrology Nurses' Association (ANNA) Journal, 18,* 173–181.

Molzahn, A. E., & Kikuchi, J. F. (1998). Children and adolescents with parents receiving home dialysis. *American Nephrology Nurses' Association (ANNA) Journal, 25,* 411–418, 428.

Molzahn, A. E., Northcott, H. C., & Dossetor, J. B. (1997). Perceptions of physicians, nurses and patients regarding quality of life of patients with ESRD. *American Nephrology Nurses' Association (ANNA) Journal, 24,* 325–335.

Molzahn, A. E., Northcott, H. C., & Hayduk, L. (1996). Quality of life of patients with ESRD: A structural equation model. *Quality of Life Research, 5,* 426–432.

Moons, P., Budts, W., & De Geest, S. (2006). Critique on the conceptualization of quality of life: A review and evaluation of different conceptual approaches. *International Journal of Nursing Studies, 43*(7), 891–901.

Netuveli, G., Wiggins, R. D., Hildon, Z., Montgomery, S. M., & Blane, D. (2006). Quality of life at older ages: Evidence from the English longitudinal study of aging (wave 1). *Journal of Epidemiology & Community Health, 60*(4), 357–363.

Ormel, J., Lindenberg, S., Steverink, N., & Vonkorff, M. (1997). Quality of life and social production functions: A framework for understanding health effects. *Social Science & Medicine, 45*(7), 1051–1063.

Parse, R. R. (1981). *Man-living-health: A theory of nursing.* New York, NY: Wiley.

Parse, R. R. (1994). Quality of life: Sciencing and living the art of human becoming. *Nursing Science Quarterly, 7*(1), 16–21.

Parse, R. R. (1996). Quality of life for persons living with Alzheimer's disease: The human becoming perspective. *Nursing Science Quarterly, 9*(3), 126–133.

Paschoal, S. (2005). *Elder quality of life: The construction of an assessment instrument through the clinical method* (Unpublished doctoral dissertation). University of Sao Paulo Faculty of Medicine, Brazil. Retrieved from http://www.teses.usp.br/teses/disponiveis/5/5137/tde-16052005–112538/publico/Sergio_Paschoal_tese.pdf

Paskulin, L. G., & Molzahn, A. E. (2007). Quality of life in older adults in Canada and Brazil. *Western Journal of Nursing Research, 29*(1), 10–26. doi:10.1177/0193945906292550.

Patrick, D. L., & Erickson, J. (1993). *Health status and health policy: Quality of life in health care evaluation and resource allocation.* New York, NY: Oxford University Press.

Peplau, H. E. (1952). *Interpersonal relations in nursing.* New York, NY: Putnam & Sons.

Peplau, H. E. (1994). Quality of life: An interpersonal perspective. *Nursing Science Quarterly, 7*(1), 10–15.

Pilkington, F. B., & Mitchell, G. J. (2004). Quality of life for women living with a gynecologic cancer. *Nursing Science Quarterly, 17*(2), 147–155.

Plummer, M., & Molzahn, A. E. (2009). Quality of life in contemporary nursing theory: A concept analysis. *Nursing Science Quarterly, 22,* 134–40.

Power, M. J., Quinn, K., Schmidt, S., & WHOQOL-OLD Group (2005). Development of the WHOQOL-Old module. *Quality of Life Research, 14,* 2197–2214, 2005.

ProQOLID (n.d.). *Patient reported outcomes and quality of life measurement database.* Retrieved from http://www.proqolid.org/proqolid

Puts, M. T. E., Shekary, N., Widdershoven, G., Helde, J., Lips, P., & Deeg, D. J. H. (2007). What does quality of life mean to older frail and non-frail community-dwelling adults in the Netherlands? *Quality of Life Research, 16*(2), 263–277.

Rapkin, B. D., & Schwartz, C. E. (2004). Toward a theoretical model of quality of life appraisal: Implications of findings from studies of response shift. *Health and Quality of Life Outcomes,* 1–12. Retrieved from http://www.hqlo.com/content/2/1/14

Richard, L., Laforest, S., Dufresne, F., & Sapinski, J. P. (2004). The quality of life of older adults living in an urban environment: Professional and lay perspectives. *Canadian Journal on Aging, 24,* 19–30.

Rogers, M. E. (1970). *An introduction to the theoretical basis of nursing.* Philadelphia, PA: F. A. Davis.

Rogers, M. E. (1990). Nursing: The science of unitary, irreducible, human beings: Update 1990. In E. A. M. Barrett (Ed.), *Visions of Roger's Science-Based Nursing.* New York, NY: National League for Nursing.

Rogers, M. E. (1994). The science of unitary human beings: Current perspectives. *Nursing Science Quarterly, 7*(1), 33–35.

Salek, S. (1999). *Compendium of quality of life instruments.* Chichester, England: Wiley.

Santana, M., & Feeny, D. *The importance of measuring health-related quality of life.* Edmonton, Canada: Institute for Health Economics.

Schok, M. L., & de Vries, J. (2005). Predicting overall quality of life and general health of veterans with and without health problems. *Military Psychology, 17*(2), 89–100.

Schwartz, C. E., & Sprangers, M. A. (1999). Integrating response shift into health-related quality of life research: A theoretical model. *Social Science & Medicine, 48,* 1507–1515.

Scott, L. D., Setter-Kline, K., & Britton, A. S. (2004). The effects of nursing interventions to enhance mental health and quality of life among individuals with heart failure. *Applied Nursing Research, 17*(4), 248–256.

Siegrist, J., & Wahrendorf, M. (2009). Participation in socially productive activities and quality of life in early old age: Findings from SHARE. *Journal of European Social Policy, 19*(4), 317–326. doi:10.1177/1350506809341513

Taillefer, M. C., Dupuis, G., Roberge, M. A., & LeMay, S. (2003). Health-related quality of life models. A systematic literature review. *Social Indicators Research, 64,* 293–323.

Tokuda, Y., Jimba, M., Yanai, H., Fujii, S., & Inoguchi, T. (2008). Interpersonal trust and quality-of-life: A cross-sectional study in Japan. *PloS ONE, 3*(12), e3985. doi:10.1371/journal.pone.0003985

Velikova, G., Booth, L., Smith, A., Brown, P., Lynch, P., Brown, J. M., & Selby, P. (2004). Measuring quality of life in routine oncology practice improves communication and patient well-being: A randomized controlled trial. *Journal of Clinical Oncology, 22,* 714–724.

Ware, J. F., Kosinski, M., & Keller, S. D. (1994). *Physical and mental health summary scales: A user's manual.* Boston, MA: New England Medical Center.

Warner, L. M., Schuez, B., Wurm, S., Ziegelmann, J. P., & Tesch-Roemer, C. (2010). Giving and taking differential effects of providing, receiving and anticipating emotional support on quality of life in adults with multiple illnesses. *Journal of Health Psychology, 15*(5), 660–670. doi:10.1177/1359105310368186

WHOQOL Group. (1998). The development of the World Health Organization WHOQOL-BREF quality of life assessment. *Psychological Medicine, 28,* 551–558.

WHOQOL-HIV Group. (2003). Initial steps to developing the World Health Organisation's Quality of Life Instrument (WHOQOL) module for international assessment of HIV/AIDS. *AIDS Care, 15*(3), 347–357.

WHOQOL-SRPB Group. (2006). A cross-cultural study of spirituality, religion and personal beliefs as components of quality of life. *Social Science and Medicine, 62,* 1486–1497.

Wiggins, R. D., Higgs, P. D. F., Hyde, M., & Blane. D. (2004). Quality of life in the third age: Key predictors of the CASP-19 measure. *Ageing and Society, 24,* 693–708.

Wilhelmson, K., Andersson, C., Waern, M., & Allebeck, P. (2005). Elderly people's perspectives on quality of life. *Ageing and Society, 25*(Part 4), 585–600.

Wilkin, D., Hallam, L., & Doggett, M. (1993). *Measures of need and outcome for primary care* (2nd ed.). Oxford, England: Oxford University Press.

Williams, A., Kitchen, P., Randall, J., & Muhajarine, N. (2008). Changes in quality of life perception in Saskatoon, Saskatchewan: Comparing survey results from 2001 to 2004. *Social Indicators Research, 85*(1), 5–21. doi:10.1007/s11205–007–9129-z

Wilson, I. B., & Cleary, P. D. (1995). Linking clinical variables with health-related quality of life: A conceptual model of patient outcomes. *Journal of the American Medical Association, 273,* 59–65.

World Health Organization (WHO). (2002). *Active ageing—A policy framework.* Retrieved October 17, 2006, from http://www.euro.who.int/ageing

18

HOPE AND HOPELESSNESS

EDITH D. HUNT RALEIGH

ascination with the phenomenon of hope dates back to the Bible. Hope for a better future and salvation is a hallmark of the Scriptures. St. Paul characterized hope as the essence of faith: "But hope that is seen is no hope at all. Who hopes for what he already has? But if we hope for what we do not yet have, we wait for it patiently" (Rom. 8: 24–25, NIV). A 17th century Dutch philosopher and theologian, Baruch de Spinoza, defined hope as a joy that comes from past or future images when something is in doubt (as cited in Bernard, 1977). In the late 20th century, theoretical and scientific interest in the concept of hope developed among investigators and clinicians in psychology, medicine, and nursing.

While the conceptualizations of hope have some variety, there is agreement on the essential characteristics of the concept. Hope, a factor in coping, is future oriented and considered to be multidimensional by most theorists. It enables an individual to cope with a stressful situation by expecting a positive outcome. Because a positive outcome is expected, the individual is motivated to act in the face of uncertainty. Differences in conceptualizations arise as to whether hope has both state and trait components, whether it exists on a continuum with hopelessness, and whether it is an antecedent, a strategy, or an outcome of coping (Raleigh & Boehm, 1994).

Hope is rarely discussed without considering hopelessness and vice versa; however, the relationship between these concepts is not usually explicated. Many authors in the psychology literature link hopelessness with depression. Some, such as Beck (1963, 1967) and Bernard (1977), identify hopelessness as a core characteristic of depression and suicidal ideation behavior (Alloy, Abramson, Metalsky, & Hartlage, 1988; Beck, Kovacs, & Weissman, 1975; Beck, Weissman, Lester, & Trexler, 1974; Grewal & Porter, 2007; Minkoff, Bergman, Beck, & Beck, 1973). In fact, Bernard hypothesized that hope, like depression, may originate from "heredity, physiology and health, environment, and personal and individual orientation—especially the orientation of responsibility" (p. 285). Other authors consider hope and hopelessness to be related, but nonlinear concepts (Farran, Herth, & Popovich, 1995) and to exist simultaneously in the same individual (Dufault & Martocchio, 1985). Still others think hope and hopelessness are on a continuum (McGee, 1984; Stotland, 1969). As the various models of hope are examined, these differences will be presented.

The literature search in preparation for this chapter included books and research and theoretical articles published from 1965 to 2010 by psychologists, physicians, and nurses. Computer and hand searches using MEDLINE and the Cumulative Index to Nursing and Allied Health Literature (CINAHL) were used to identify publications with the word "hope" or "hopelessness" in the title, conceptual framework, or instruments. The focus of the review is nursing models and related research; however, seminal works in psychology were included for background purposes. In the first edition, only research articles that identified the specific hope model were used in the review. Since that time, research on hope has grown exponentially. As a result, research is reviewed that sheds light on models whether or not they were mentioned in the article; grey literature is omitted, however. Just over 100 publications met the review criteria. Since this chapter was initially published, there has been a significant amount of nursing research on hope in different populations including a variety of diagnostic groups and other countries. These will be presented as well. Lastly, additional instruments from the psychology literature have been added to Table 18.1.

Psychologists and physicians presented the earliest explorations of hope in the literature. Later, nurses joined the discussion. The oldest models can be attributed to psychologists, predominately, Lynch (1965) and Stotland (1969). While Lynch and other theorists are frequently mentioned as background for research, Stotland's model is the one that is most often cited as the conceptual framework. In addition, instruments to measure hope have been developed using Stotland's model. Consequently, I have selected it for detailed discussion.

MODELS OF HOPE IN PSYCHOLOGY

With the exception of Stotland (1969), the earliest theorists focused their efforts on developing a definition of hope and offering a few propositions without producing an empirically adequate model. Lynch (1965) considered hope to be "the very heart and center of a human being. It is the best resource of man, always there on the inside, making everything possible when he is in action, or waiting to be illuminated when he is ill" (p. 31). He defined hope as the fundamental knowledge that a difficult situation can be worked out and that goals can be reached. Imagining and wishing are not possible for the hopeless. Hopelessness prevents one from imagining beyond the present.

Melges and Bowlby (1969) proposed that "hope and hopelessness reflect a person's estimate of the probability of his achieving certain goals" (p. 690). The individual determines the probability relative to past successes and failures with similar goals. If there is an expectation of success in meeting goals through one's plans of action, hope exists. If failure is predicted, hopelessness exists. Thus, Melges and Bowlby described hope and hopelessness as opposite expectations and self-efficacy as a fundamental component of self-esteem and a major element in determining whether one feels hopeful or hopeless. Hope encompasses goals that are short-term or long-term and may involve hopefulness about short-term goals simultaneously with hopelessness about long-term goals.

Stotland's Model of Hope

The publication of Ezra Stotland's book, *The Psychology of Hope* (1969), revolutionized the discussions surrounding the concept of hope. Prior to this, many investigators considered hope and hopelessness to be vague and indistinct concepts that prohibited quantification and systematic study. Through a review of the literature, Stotland developed a theory that portrays hope as an expectation of future goal attainment that is mediated by the importance of the goal for the individual and motivates action to achieve the goal. Expectation of goal attainment and importance of the goal are determinants of motivation. The greater the expectation and the greater the importance of the goal to the individual, the greater will be the effort to achieve the goal. If the goal is important and the individual perceives a low probability of attaining it, anxiety will be experienced. Because there is motivation to avoid anxiety, the greater the anxiety, the more the individual will be motivated to escape it. Hope is a component of adaptive action in a difficult situation, and hopelessness is a factor in maladaptive behavior.

Because Stotland's model operationalized hope for the first time, many investigators used it to develop instruments to measure hope and as a framework for their research. What follows is a discussion of studies that used Stotland's model. The discussion will close with an analysis of the model. This pattern will be used through the first section of this chapter. A summary of published instruments (including those not linked to a model discussed in this chapter) is presented in Table 18.1. For in-depth discussion of instruments and relevant research, please refer to *Hope and Hopelessness: Critical Clinical Constructs* (Farran, Herth et al., 1995) and *Hope in Psychiatry: A Review of the Literature* (Schrank, Stanghellini, & Slade, 2008).

Table 18.1 Selected Measures for the Phenomenon of Hope

Name of measure & developer	Variable(s) measured	Brief description	Reliability	Validity	Populations initially studied
Hopelessness Scale (BHS); Beck, Weissman, Lester, & Trexler (1974)	Hopelessness based on Stotland's (1969) conceptualization	20 true/false items scored 0 or 1 and summed. Possible range 0–20.	Internal consistency: Cronbach's alpha = .93	Predictive: Support for hypothesized relationships	Hospitalized suicidal patients (N = 294) (since translated into Turkish)
Hope Scale (HS); Erickson, Post, & Paige (1975)	Hope using Stotland's (1969) conceptualization of expectation of goal attainment	20 goals common in our society rated on importance (I) (7-point scale) and probability of occurrence (P) (100-point scale).	Stability: Test-retest (1 week) (I) r = .79 and (P) r = 78	Predictive: Support for hypothesized relationships	Undergraduate college students (N = 140) Male psychiatric patients (N = 100)
Stoner Hope Scale (SHS); Stoner (1982)	Hope using Stotland's (1969) conceptualization and adapted from the Hope Scale (Erickson, Post, & Paige, 1975)	30 goals, 10 each domain: global, interpersonal, intrapersonal. 4-point scale for importance and 4-point scale for probability of occurrence. Possible total score = 480.	Internal consistency: Cronbach's alpha = .93	Divergent: Hopelessness Scale correlation = –.47	Cancer patients (N = 58)
Hopelessness Scale for Children (HSC); Kazdin, French, Unis, Esveldt-Dawson, & Sherick (1983)	Hopelessness using Stotland's (1969) conceptualization and adapted from the Hopelessness Scale	17 true/false items. Scores range from 0–17.	Internal consistency: Cronbach's alpha = .75	Predictive: Support of hypothesized findings	Psychiatric inpatient children (N = 66)

Name of measure & developer	Variable(s) measured	Brief description	Reliability	Validity	Populations initially studied
Hope Index (HI); Staats (1989)	Hope using Stotland's (1969) and Beck's (1967) conceptualizations	16 goal statements rated 0–5; degree of desire and expectation for goal. Possible scores 0–400. Two subscales: Self, Other.	Internal consistency: Cronbach's alpha = .86 Stability: Test-retest (3½–9 weeks) r = .60	Concurrent criterion-related: Satisfaction with life = .41; optimism = .37 Divergent: Hopelessness Scale –.47 Construct: Factor analysis supported 2 factors (subscales)	Undergraduate students = 234 Healthy adults in community = 303
Snyder Hope Scale (SNHS) (AKA Adult Trait Hope Scale or Dispositional Hope Scale); C. Snyder et al. (1991) & C. R. Snyder (2000)	Trait hope based on Stotland's work	12 items on a 4-point scale. 8 hope items plus 4 fillers. Possible scores 12–48.	Internal consistency: Cronbach's alpha Total = .74–.84; Agency subscale alpha = .71–.76; Pathways subscale alpha = .63–.80 Stability: Test-retest (8-week) r = .73 (3-week) r = .85	Construct: Factor analysis found 2 factors Criterion-related with self-esteem (r = .58), expectancy for success (r = .55), life experience (r = .54), and life orientation (r = .60) Divergent: Hopelessness Scale r = -.51	Healthy adults and adults with psychiatric illnesses (N = 2,753) (since translated into Hebrew)
Multidimensional Hope Scale (MHS); Raleigh & Boehm (1994)	Hope based on Stotland's (1969) work	Adapted from Stoner Hope Scale (Stoner, 1982). 37 items on 4-point scale for importance and 4-point scale for probability of occurrence of hope. Weighted probability score. Possible range: –222 to +222. Six subscales: Civic Interest, Health, Spirituality, Self-Actualization, Resource to Others, Social Support.	Internal consistency: Cronbach's alpha Total scale = .95; Subscales = .77–.92 Stability: (2-week) r = .82	Construct: Factor analysis confirmed 6 factors (subscales) Divergent: Hopelessness Scale r = -.45	Adults with chronic conditions in the community (N = 450)

(Continued)

Table 18.1 (Continued)

Name of measure & developer	Variable(s) measured	Brief description	Reliability	Validity	Populations initially studied
Miller Hope Scale (MHS); Miller & Powers (1988)	Hope using theological, philosophical, psychological, socioanthropological, biological, and nursing literature	40 items on a 5-point scale. Possible scores 40–200. Three subscales: Satisfaction with Self, Others, and Life; Avoidance of Hope Threats; Anticipation of a Future.	Stability: Test-retest (2-week) r = .82 Internal Consistency: Cronbach's alpha = .93, subscales = .82–.91	Divergent: Hopelessness Scale correlation = -.54 Criterion-related : Psychological well-being = .71, Existential well-being = .82 Construct: Factor analysis supported 3 factors (subscales)	College students (N = 522)
Hopefulness Scale for Adolescents (HSA); Hinds & Gattuso (1991)	Hope using Hinds' (1984) conceptualization of hope	24-item visual analogue scale. Possible scores 0–2,400. Consists of two alternate forms.	Internal consistency Cronbach's alpha = .76–.94	Construct: Reported claimed but no findings have been published	Healthy, acutely ill, and chronically ill adolescents (N = 400)
Herth Hope Scale (HHS); K. A. Herth (1991)	Hope using Dufault & Martocchio (1985) model	30 items rated on a 4-point summated scale. Possible scores 0–90. Subscales: Temporality and Future, Positive Readiness and Expectancy, Interconnectedness.	Internal consistency: Cronbach's alpha = .75–.89 Stability: Test-retest (3 weeks) r = .89–.91	Construct: Factor analysis supported 3 hypothesized factors (subscales)	Pretest with adult cancer patients (N = 60) Healthy adults (N = 185), elderly in community (N = 40), elderly widow(er)s (N = 75)
Herth Hope Index (HHI); Herth (1992)	Hope using Dufault & Martocchio (1985) model	Shortened version of the Herth Hope Scale. 12 items on a 4-point scale. 3 subscales of HHS.	Internal consistency: Cronbach's alpha = .94–.98 Stability: (2-week) r = .91	Concurrent: Criterion-related with HHS r = .92 Construct: Factor analysis confirmed 3 factors (subscales)	Acutely ill, chronically ill, and terminally ill adults (N = 172) (since translated into Chinese, Japanese, Norwegian, Swedish)

444

Name of measure & developer	Variable(s) measured	Brief description	Reliability	Validity	Populations initially studied
Gottschalk Hope Scale (GHS); Gottschalk (1974)	Hope = a measure of optimism that a favorable outcome is likely to occur	Content analysis of 5-minute speech samples. The scale has 7 categories weighted +1 or –1.	Interrater Reliability: Cronbach's alpha = .85	Predictive: Studies demonstrated significant differences in mental health crisis group vs. normative adult group	Psychiatric outpatients (N = 68)
Hope Index Scale (HIS); Obayuwana et al. (1982)	Hope using an aggregation of theories and concepts found in literature	60 yes-no items. Scores range 0–500.	Internal consistency: Kuder-Richardson's formula 20 =.61	Divergent: Hopelessness Scale correlation = –.88	Graduate students (N = 150) Psychiatric patients (N = 150)
Geriatric Hopelessness Scale; (GHS) Fry (1984)	Hopelessness derived from interviews with subclinically depressed elderly adults	30 true/false items. Scores range from 0–30.	Internal consistency: Cronbach's alpha = .69–71 Spearman-Brown split-half reliability = .70–73	Construct: Factor analysis supported 4 factors Predictive: Support for hypothesized relationships with depression and self-esteem	Older adults in the community (N = 78)
Nowotny Hope Scale (NHS); Nowotny (1989)	Hope using psychological, theological, psychiatric, and nursing literature	29 items on a 4-point scale (reduced from 47 items). Six subscales: Active Involvement, Confidence, Relates to Others, Spiritual Beliefs, Comes From Within, Future Is Possible.	Internal consistency: Cronbach's alpha Total Scale = .90; subscales = .51–75	Divergent: Hopelessness Scale = –.47 Construct: Factor analysis confirmed 6 factors (subscales)	Healthy adults (N = 156) Cancer patients (N = 150) (since translated into Danish, Italian, Norwegian)
Children's Hope Scale; C. R. Snyder et al. (1997)	Trait hope using Snyder Hope Theory (C. Snyder, 1994)	6 items: 3 agency and 3 pathways.	Internal Consistency: Cronbach's alpha = 0.72–86, M = 77 Temporal Stability: test-retest at 1 month = 0.71	Construct: Factor analysis found 2 factors Convergent: Parent rating r = .37 & .38; .50 & .53. Divergent: Child Depression Inventory r = –.27, –.40, –.48	Children ages 8–16 Arthritis, cancer, or sickle cell anemia DX (B = 48; G = 43) ADHD (B = 170) Cancer survivors (B = 70; G = 73) Public school children (B = 154; G = 168)

(Continued)

Table 18.1 (Continued)

Name of measure & developer	Variable(s) measured	Brief description	Reliability	Validity	Populations initially studied
State Hope Scale; C. R. Snyder et al. (1996)	State Hope based on Snyder Hope Model (C. Snyder, 1994)	6 items: 3 Agency and 3 Pathways. Reworded items from Trait Hope Scale (C. Snyder et al., 1991).	Internal consistency: Cronbach's alpha = .82–.95 (daily analyses) Agency alpha = .83–.95 Pathways alpha = .74–.93 Temporal Variability: correlations = .48–.93	Construct: Factor analysis found 2 factors	College students (N = 444; women = 233, men = 211) Tested each day for 30 days
Hope Differential; Nekolaichuk, Jevne, & Maguire (1999)	Hope using Nekolaichuk Hope model (Nekolaichuk et al., 1999)	24 bipolar adjective pairs rate concepts related to hope; 3 subscales: personal spirit, risk, authentic caring.	Not reported	Construct: Factor analysis found 3 factors	Healthy adults (N = 146), adults with chronic or life-threatening experience (N = 159), and nurses (N = 206)
Hope Differential–Short; Nekolaichuk & Bruera (2004)	Hope using Nekolaichuk Hope model (Nekolaichuk et al., 1999)	Shortened version of Hope Differential with 9 bipolar adjective pairs related to hope (3 from each subscale). Rated on a scale of 1 to 7 anchored "extremely" on each end with 4 as "both or neither."	Internal consistency: Cronbach's alpha: Factor I = 0.83; Factor II = 0.69; Total = 0.83	Construct: Factor analysis confirmed 2 factors: authentic spirit and comfort Concurrent: Moderate positive correlations between Factors I and II and Herth Hope Index (0.64, 0.43), Hope Visual Analog Scale (0.56, 0.40) Divergent: Anxiety (−0.42, −0.39); Depression (−0.40, −0.25)	Advanced cancer patients (N = 35)

Research That Used Stotland's Model

The literature search resulted in several studies that were explicitly based on Stotland's (1969) model. The proposed relationship between hopefulness and mental health has been supported by studies involving hospitalized psychiatric patients and college students (Erickson, Post, & Paige, 1975), where significant relationships were found between lower levels of hope and psychopathology and greater anxiety. Similarly, in community-based older adults (Farran & McCann, 1989; Farran & Popovich, 1990) and geropsychiatric inpatients (Farran, Wiken, & Fidler, 1995) the best predictors of hope were mental health, social support, physical health, and activities of daily living. Additionally, hope has been positively related to social function and morale (Rideout & Montemuro, 1986).

The Stotland model of hope has also been used in studies of populations with physical illnesses. In support of Stotland's proposition that hope is a component of adaptive action, significant positive relationships have been found between level of hope and level of coping (Chapman & Pepler, 1998; Herth, 1989; Popovich, Fox, & Bandagi, 2007) and strong religious convictions (Brandt, 1987; Buckley & Herth, 2004; Davis, 2005; Herth, 1989; Popovich et al., 2007; Raleigh, 1992) in adult patients with cancer and other chronic conditions. Unpredictability or uncertainty has been found to be inversely related to hopefulness and motivation (Mishel, Hostetter, King, & Graham, 1984; Staples & Jeffrey, 1997; Wonghongkul, Moore, Musil, Schneider, & Deimling, 2000); that is, the greater the unpredictability of a situation, the less the expectation of achievement (or hope) and motivation to act. Support for Stotland's proposition that increased anxiety motivates the individual to try to escape it was found in studies of individuals with a variety of chronic conditions including cancer (Buckley & Herth, 2004; Raleigh, 1992; Rustoen, Cooper, & Miaskowski, 2010) and geropsychiatric inpatients (Farran, Wiken et al., 1995). Strategies for improving hopefulness reported by participants in these studies included keeping active, participating in religious activities, thinking about other things, and talking with others—all means of distracting one from the source of anxiety.

In numerous studies, researchers have found no significant differences in level of hope based on phase of illness in adults with cancer (Ballard, Green, McCaa, & Logsdon, 1997; Brandt, 1987; Chen, 2003; Herth, 1991; Heszen-Niejodek, Gottschalk, & Januszek, 1999; Raleigh, 1992; Stoner & Keampfer, 1985; Vellone, Rega, Galletti, & Cohen, 2006). This may suggest no support for the proposition that hope is perceived probability of goal attainment; however, it may be a function of what the patient perceives as the goal. Raleigh (1992) and other investigators (Buckley & Herth, 2004; Ezzy, 2000; Felder, 2004) have found that patients at different stages of illness reported hopes with different time lines. Those who were terminally ill tended to focus on hopes in the short term; nevertheless, they considered themselves very hopeful. On the other hand, this was not the case in one study of Danish patients with cancer who demonstrated a slight deterioration of hope scores over time (Esbensen, Østerlind, & Hallberg, 2006).

Analysis of Stotland's Model of Hope

Stotland's Model of Hope has been widely used and tested by nurse researchers as well as psychologists, leading to significant support for many relationships in the model. According to Walker and Avant (1995), "a theory is an internally consistent group of relational statements that presents a systematic view about a phenomenon and that is useful for description, explanation, prediction, and/or control" (p. 26). Stotland's (1969) Model of Hope provides an understanding of the concept that meets these requirements. The model is logically adequate in that predictions can and have been made from it. Several researchers have tested these predictions, they make sense, and there are no obvious logical fallacies. Stotland's model has proven to be useful. It has been used to develop several measures of hope and hopelessness and has been used by many researchers as a conceptual framework. It is broadly generalizable to various populations and situations as demonstrated by the variety of research it has generated. It also has parsimony in that it can be described using few concepts and relationships, yet it is broad in its application. If the theory is to be empirically testable, the components of the model must have operational definitions (Fawcett, 1984). Stotland initiated the study of hope by being the first to operationalize it. As a result, many studies have been conducted that demonstrate that the model has empirical adequacy as well.

MODELS OF HOPE IN NURSING

The concept of hope has immediate application for nursing practice. In the process of caring for the whole individual, the presence or absence of hopefulness is evident to the nurse. Anecdotally, nurses report instances where hopefulness or hopelessness appeared to impact the client outcome. The North American Nursing Diagnosis Association (NANDA) recognizes the nursing diagnosis of "hopelessness," which is defined as "perception of limited or no alternatives or personal choices available and unable to mobilize energy on own behalf" (Gordon, 2007, p. 265). Conceptualizations of hopefulness and hopelessness began to appear in the nursing literature long before NANDA developed hopelessness as a diagnosis. Two of the earliest nurse authors in this area were Travelbee (1971) and Lange (1978). In the early 1980s, nurses began to use hope models in their research.

Travelbee (1971) addressed hope and hopelessness in discussing the critical care nurse's role. She proposed that "hope is something halfway between knowing and willing" (p. 161) what will happen in the future. It suggests solutions to

problems, imparts security in this knowledge, and generates energy that produces motivation to act. Based on this definition, Travelbee advocated for the nurse's role in fostering hopefulness in patients. Later, Lange (1978) described the concept of hope and differentiated it from similar concepts of wishing, expectation, and optimism. A model of hope was beginning to take form in nursing with Lange's explication of the hope structure as a process for maintaining hope. Soon after this, nurses began to develop and test their models, beginning with Miller (1983). These models are presented in this chapter. Models with supporting subsequent research are detailed in greater depth.

Miller's Model of Hope

Miller (1983, 2000) states that hope is a complex multidimensional construct. It is more than goal attainment; it encompasses a state of being. It involves a confident expectation of an ongoing good state or liberation from a difficult situation. According to Miller, hope exists at three levels complemented by three levels of psychic energy and despair (Figure 18.1).

Figure 18.1 Levels of Hope, Despair, and Psychic Energy

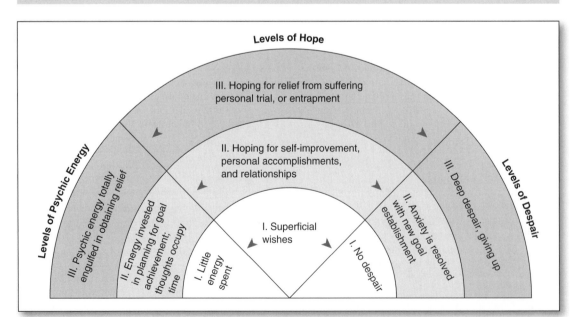

The first level of hope focuses on *superficial wishes,* is characterized by shallow optimism, requires little psychic energy to maintain, and produces no despair when it is not actualized. The second level focuses on hoping for *relationships, self-improvement,* and *personal accomplishments* and involves greater *psychic energy* than the first level. If these hopes are not actualized, *anxiety* is the result. The third level is related to a desire for *relief from suffering, personal trial,* or *entrapment* and involves a total dedication of *psychic energy.* If the individual perceives that relief is not impending, *deep despair* or *giving up* occurs.

Miller and Powers (1988) identified 11 essential elements of hope from interviews of critically ill patients. *Mutuality and affiliation* pertain to interpersonal relationships and the experience of unconditional love. *Sense of the possible* involves a global attitude that there is potential in life. *Avoidance of absolutizing* entails allowing flexibility in one's expectations and avoiding an all-or-nothing attitude. *Anticipation* embraces the confident expectation of some future good combined with acceptance of the need to patiently wait. *Establishing and achieving goals* are the "objects of one dimension of hope" (p. 418). *Psychologic well-being and coping* are factors that empower the individual to have the necessary psychic energy. *Purpose and meaning in life* give the individual something to live for and receive a sense of satisfaction with life. *Freedom* is the ability to recognize that the individual can impact an outcome and maintain a positive attitude. *Reality surveillance* involves cognitive tasks designed to obtain information that confirms the reality of the hope. *Optimism* is essential for hope. *Mental and physical activation* encompasses energy that is used to counteract apathy of despair. Miller (2000) proposes that hope may be inspired by others and presents a model that focuses on nursing strategies designed to inspire hope. These will be discussed later in this chapter.

Research That Used Miller's Hope Model

Many studies have used the Miller Hope Scale (MHS) as the measure of hope, but most of these used a conceptual framework related to other variables, such as uncertainty, and are, therefore, not included in this review (Brackney & Westman, 1992; Fehring, Miller, & Shaw, 1997; Irvin & Acton, 1997; McGill & Paul, 1993; Zorn & Johnson, 1997). In addition, some research used Miller's Hope Model as the conceptual framework but focused the study on the hope-despair model by Miller (1992), a model of hope-inspiring strategies, discussed later.

The findings of lower scores on the MHS for a sample of elderly adults living in a long-term care facility compared to the young, healthy population used by Miller and Powers (1988) in their original psychometric testing (Beckerman & Northrop, 1996) supports the importance of mutuality and affiliation and establishing and achieving goals in hopefulness. These elements of hope are also supported by findings of a significant positive correlation between the MHS factor Avoidance of Hope Threats and social support (Hirth & Stewart, 1994) and the positive correlation between hope and self-care agency in adolescents (Canty-Mitchell, 2001).

The roles of psychological well-being and coping in hope are supported by findings of a significant positive correlation between hope and caregiver well-being (Irvin & Acton, 1997). Additionally, hope was shown to be a mediator of the relationship between stress and well-being. While significant positive correlations were found between hope and education and financial status in one study of elderly (McGill & Paul, 1993), there was no correlation with education in another study (Mishel et al., 1984). Higher education and income would be expected to increase sense of well-being and avoidance of hope threats.

Support for the roles of purpose and meaning in life and mutuality and affiliation can be found in significant positive correlations between religious well-being/intrinsic religiosity and hope (Fehring et al., 1997; Zorn & Johnson, 1997) and self-esteem and social support and hope (Foote, Piazza, Holcomb, Paul, & Daffin, 1990). Furthermore, hope accounted for 31% of the variance in religious well-being, the only significant predictor in this study.

A negative correlation between hope and external locus of control suggests that the perception of chance associated with external locus of control reduces perceptions of ability to attain relief from a personal trial or suffering (Brackney & Westman, 1992). No relationship was found between hope nor hopelessness and the measure of internal locus of control.

Analysis of Miller's Model of Hope

Miller's (1983, 2000) Model of Hope focuses on definitions of concepts related to hope with few statements of relationships among the concepts. This reduces its ability to explain, predict, or control phenomena. The sparseness of relational statements also hinders the model's logical adequacy in that relationships cannot be diagramed (Walker & Avant, 1995). Miller's model has proven to have limited usefulness to researchers who used the MHS but chose to use another conceptual framework. It is broadly generalizable to many populations and situations and has been used with various groups from college students (Miller & Powers, 1988) to elderly (Beckerman & Northrop, 1996; Fehring et al., 1997) and the chronically ill (Hirth & Stewart, 1994; Miller, 2000) to critically ill (Miller, 1989) and their spouses (Patel, 1996). It lacks parsimony in that it uses many concepts and unclear relationships. Miller has developed an operational definition of hope that lends itself to testing. As a result, many studies have been conducted that use the MHS to operationalize hope, but its empirical adequacy has not been demonstrated.

Self-Sustaining Process Model

Hinds and Martin (1988) took the grounded theory approach to develop a definition of hope and the Self-Sustaining Process model. Grounded theory approach is an inductive research technique first described by Glaser and Strauss (1967). A theory evolves from the research process that involves formulation, testing, and redevelopment of propositions.

According to Hinds (1984), hope, for adolescents, is defined as "the degree to which an adolescent believes that a personal tomorrow exists" (p. 360). There are four hierarchical levels of believing in this model: (1) *forced effort,* (2) *personal possibilities,* (3) *expectation of a better tomorrow,* and (4) *anticipation of a personal future.* With *forced effort* the adolescent exhibits a more positive attitude that is artificial. *Personal possibilities* refers to the adolescent's belief that second chances exist for the self. A general positive future orientation is characteristic of *expectation of a better tomorrow* and a specific positive future orientation is evident in *anticipation of a personal future.*

Hinds and Martin (1988) conceptualized the Self-Sustaining Process by which adolescents help themselves achieve hopefulness during their illness experience. This process involves four sequential phases; each phase has specific strategies associated with it (Figure 18.2).

The first phase of the Self-Sustaining Process is *cognitive discomfort,* the degree to which mental uneasiness is experienced related to disheartening or negative thoughts. The second phase is *distraction,* in which the negative thoughts are replaced with neutral or positive thoughts and conditions through cognitive and behavioral activities. The third phase is *cognitive comfort,* which encompasses the experience of solace, lifted spirits, and consideration of future possibilities. The fourth phase is *personal competence,* in which adolescents see themselves as "resilient, resourceful, and adaptable in the face of serious health threats" (p. 339). The researchers concluded that the Self-Sustaining Process is variable in that it can occur in minutes or weeks. Some phases take longer than others and may be bypassed. They also found positive relationships among the concepts (e.g., greater cognitive discomfort relates to more attempts at distraction). Also, behaviors and attitudes of others, including nurses, can influence the adolescent's moving through the process.

Research That Used the
Self-Sustaining Process Model

Four studies were found that used the Self-Sustaining Process Model and the Hopefulness Scale for Adolescents. Connelly (1998) examined the relationship between adolescent pregnancy status and hopefulness and found none; however, hope scores for the sample are not reported. Two of these studies support the importance of the perception that "others have hope for me" as described in the Self-Sustaining Process. A longitudinal, correlational study of 25 adolescents receiving treatment for substance abuse (Hinds, 1988) found a positive correlation between hope and adolescents' perception of degree of caring by the nurses. Another study of 99 high school students found that hopefulness helps to explain the relationship between perceived social support and general well-being (Yarcheski, Scoloveno, & Mahon, 1994). These researchers surmised that greater social support fosters adolescent hopefulness or

Figure 18.2   The Substantive Theory: Categories, Core Concepts, and the Central Organizing Construct

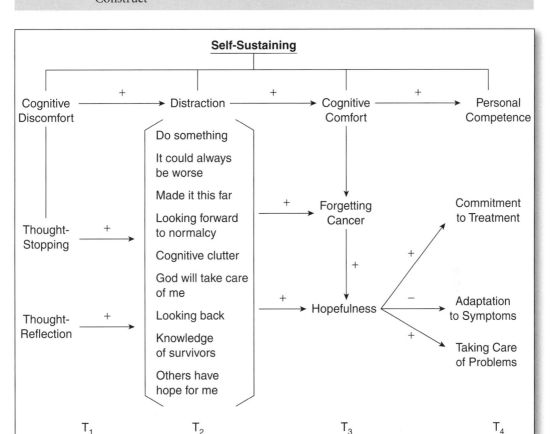

SOURCE: From "Hopefulness and the Self-Sustaining Process in Adolescents With Cancer," by P. S. Hinds and J. Martin, 1988, *Nursing Research*, 37(6), p. 337. Copyright © 1988 by AJN. Reprinted with permission of Lippincott, Williams, & Wilkins.

NOTE: T1–T4 are time frames.

the "comforting life-sustaining belief that a personal and positive future exists" (Hinds, 1984, p. 3) which contributes to general well-being. A case study of seven adolescents followed them during their cancer experience. Five of the adolescents progressed through the process after being told of their diagnosis while two, who were told only indirectly, did not (Ishibashi et al., 2010). Much additional research is needed to support the adequacy of this model.

Analysis of the Self-Sustaining Process Model

The Self-Sustaining Process (Hinds & Martin, 1988) provides a unidimensional understanding of hopefulness in adolescents that shows promise for description, explanation, prediction, and control. The model is logically adequate in that relationships are clear and predictions can be made from it (Walker & Avant, 1995). This model may prove to be useful in a narrow population of adolescents. It has been used to develop a measure of hope, although it has not been used widely as a conceptual framework. It is narrowly generalizable to the adolescent population, and it has parsimony in that it can be described using relatively few concepts and relationships. The Self-Sustaining Process model operationalizes hope for the adolescent and should stimulate more research to test its empirical adequacy.

Dufault and Martocchio's Model of Hope

Dufault and Martocchio (1985) also used the grounded theory approach to arrive at a conceptualization of hope. The researchers described their methodology as "participant observation in multiple settings" (pp. 379–380). Hope is defined as "a multidimensional dynamic life force characterized by a confident yet uncertain expectation of achieving a future good which, to the hoping person, is realistically possible and personally significant" (p. 380). Dufault and Martocchio describe hope as a process, not a trait.

It has two spheres and six common dimensions (Figure 18.3). The spheres are *generalized hope* and *particularized hope*. Generalized hope relates to a sense of an indeterminate future good. "Generalized hope protects against despair when a person is deprived of particular hopes, and preserves or restores the meaningfulness of life—past, present, and future—in circumstances of all kinds" (p. 380). Particularized hope

focuses on a specific hope object which "may be concrete or abstract, explicitly stated or implied" (p. 380) and stimulates coping with obstacles and strategies for attaining the hope object.

The researchers described six dimensions of hope: *affective, cognitive, behavioral, affiliative, temporal,* and *contextual.* "The affective dimension focuses upon sensations and emotions that are part of the hoping process" (p. 382). It involves feelings of confidence, uncertainty, and personal significance about the outcome. "The cognitive dimension focuses upon the processes by which individuals wish, imagine, wonder, perceive, think, remember, learn, generalize, interpret, and judge in relation to hope" (p. 384). "The behavioral dimension focuses upon the action orientation of the hoping person in relation to hope" (p. 385). Actions taken may be those designed to directly achieve a hope or those motivated by, but not directly affecting, the desired outcome, such as praying or following religious customs. "The affiliative dimension focuses upon the hoping person's sense of relatedness or involvement beyond self as it bears upon hope" (p. 386). This dimension pertains to relationships with people and God and may be expressed as a reliance upon or receptivity to help from others. "The temporal dimension focuses upon the hoping person's experience of time (past, present, and future) in relation to hopes and hoping. Hope is directed toward a future good, but past and present are also involved in the hoping process" (p. 387). "The contextual dimension focuses upon those life situations that surround, influence, and are a part of persons' hope. In a sense, the contexts serve as the circumstances that occasion hope, the opportunity for the hoping process to be activated, or as a situation for testing hope" (p. 388).

Dufault and Martocchio do not consider hope and hopelessness to be polar opposites on a continuum. Individuals may be hopeful for one outcome and hopeless in relation to another outcome. The multidimensionality and process orientation of hope ensures that there is always hope for something.

Figure 18.3   Spheres and Dimensions of Hope

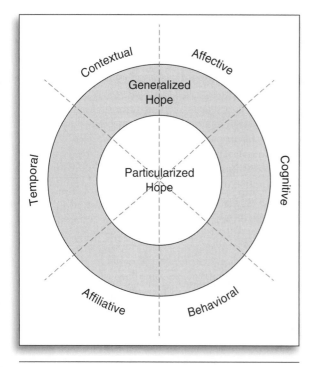

SOURCE: From "Hope: Its Spheres and Dimensions," by K. Dufault and B. C. Martocchio, 1985, *Nursing Clinics of North America, 20*(2), p. 382. Copyright © 1985 by W. B. Saunders Co. Reprinted by permission.

Research That Used Dufault and Martocchio's Model of Hope

Because few relationships are proposed in the Dufault and Martocchio model of hope, research using this model tends to focus on confirming variables that can be related to hope. Thus, researchers are using an inductive method to add to the model. Significant positive relationships have been found between higher levels of hope and level of coping response, strong faith, and no interference with family role responsibilities in a sample of adult cancer patients (Herth, 1991). This offers initial confirmation of the role of these variables in hopefulness. In a sample of elderly widow(er)s, Herth (1990a) has also found a positive relationship between level of hope and the use of positive coping styles identified by Jalowiec (1987) as confrontive, optimistic, palliative, supportant, and self-reliant. A significant negative relationship was found between level of hope and negative coping styles: evasive, emotive, and fatalistic. These findings support the positive role particularized hope plays in coping. The researcher found a significant positive relationship between level of hope and level of grief resolution, which can be a result of effective coping. Hope accounted for 79% of the variance in grief resolution.

Research has resulted in a greater understanding of the temporal dimension as well. A study of caregivers of people with serious mental illness found that hope was "grounded in the present, with a view to a future that enabled a shift from the difficult present to a better future." The researchers also found a "close connection between hope for the future and loss in the present" (Bland & Darlington, 2002, p. 63). Interviews of healthy older adults revealed differences in focus and future orientation of hope "based on age, place of residence, health status, and functional ability" (Herth, 1993, p. 146).

Analysis of Dufault and Martocchio's Model of Hope

Dufault and Martocchio's (1985) Model of Hope defines the elements of hope but presents few relational statements. As with Miller's Model of Hope, this reduces its ability to explain, predict, or control phenomena and hinders the model's logical adequacy (Walker & Avant, 1995). The proposed relationship between hope and coping has proven to have usefulness to researchers who have developed measures of hope and/or used it as a conceptual framework for their studies. It is broadly generalizable to many populations and situations and has been used with various groups from healthy elderly to individuals with cancer. It lacks parsimony in that it uses many concepts and few relationships are clear. Dufault and Martocchio have developed an operational definition of hope that has resulted in instrument development and testing. Due to the limited number of studies using this model, empirical adequacy has not been demonstrated.

Other Nursing Models

Along with producing an increasing amount of research on hope and hopelessness, nurses have continued to develop middle-range and practice theories related to the concept. Various methodologies have been used. Some examples will be presented here. Kylma (2006) conducted a meta-synthesis of her studies to construct a theory of the dynamics of hope in significant others of adults with HIV/AIDS. Johnson, Dahlen, and Roberts (1997) present a practice model for nursing care of patients with congestive heart failure calling it the "Hopeless Model." Cotter (2009) used concept analysis to identify critical attributes of hope in early-stage dementia. Holtslander, Duggleby, Williams, and Wright (2005) used grounded theory method to develop a theory of hope from the point of view of informal caregivers of palliative care patients. Duggleby and Wright (2005) also used grounded theory method to develop their theory related to elderly palliative care patients. There are more examples to be found in the nursing literature. The Coping Process Nursing Model developed by Herth (2000) depicts hope and coping resources as equal components in the coping process that affect the coping response either positively or negatively.

REVIEW OF HOPE RESEARCH WITH VARIOUS POPULATIONS

This section and the following section on variables will provide a review of the literature in specific populations. As we conduct this review, you will notice that the literature, for the most part, does not build upon what has already been done. None of the studies are replications of previous work; however, findings are similar in the various populations. One consistency is that many of these studies use the Herth Hope Index (HHI) (Herth, 1992) to measure hope.

Hope Experience in Diagnostic Groups

Cancer. Studies of individuals with cancer and their families make up the largest number of studies for a particular diagnostic group in relation to their hope experience. Benzein and Berg (2005) found that the level of hope as measured by the HHI was lower among family members than for the patients who were in palliative care. Additionally, they found negative correlations with other variables: the older the family member, the lower their hope score and the greater the reported hopelessness and fatigue. In this sample, the older patients had higher reported levels of hopelessness than the younger patients. Another study found less hope in those living alone, especially in younger people (Rustøen & Wiklund, 2000). In a study of 194 outpatients with a cancer diagnosis, a variety of demographic variables were found to be determinants of hope and coping, and physical and psychosocial functioning were revealed as contributors to hope (Bunston, Mings, Mackie, & Jones, 1995).

Vellone et al. (2006) found an inverse association between hope and anxiety and depression in Italian cancer patients and positive correlations with "self-esteem, coping, adjustment to the illness, well-being, relationship with the family, relationships with healthcare professionals, family's support, healthcare professionals' support, friends' support, satisfaction with information received from healthcare professionals, and comfort in the hospital" (p. 362).

Another study examined hope, uncertainty in illness, and stress appraisal in relation to coping in breast cancer survivors. A regression analysis found uncertainty influenced hope and hope influenced positive reappraisal coping (Wonghongkul et al., 2000). The investigators also found a high level of hope in this sample with the Herth Hope Scale. Palliative care patients reported hopefulness in spite of the advanced stage of their disease (Benzein, Norberg, & Saveman, 2001) as found in studies discussed under the Stotland Model of Hope.

Cardiovascular Conditions. A study of quality of life of 93 women after a cardiac event reported a high level of hope on the HHI, comparable to the levels of hope reported by patients with cancer (Beckie, Beckstead, & Webb, 2001). A study of families of stroke survivors also found a high level of hope on the HHI (Bluvol & Ford-Gilboe, 2004). Both of these studies will be discussed further below. Another study of stroke patients explored their hopes and found patients identified general and specific hopes related to their recovery and future. Similar to cancer patients, they reported hope was inspired by their families and their spiritual beliefs/practices (Popovich et al., 2007). Rustøen, Howie, Eidsmo, and Moum (2005) compared hospitalized patients with heart failure to the general Norwegian population. The patients had significantly higher mean global hope scores than the general population, controlling for demographic variables. They also found significant correlation between hope and comorbid diseases (skin and psychiatric). Consistent with findings in cancer patients, hope was not correlated with stage of the primary illness.

Neurological Conditions. Several studies have examined hope in a variety of neurovascular conditions including amyotrophic lateral sclerosis (ALS), spinal cord injury, brain injury, and multiple sclerosis (MS). Using the HHI–Japanese version in a study of 50 Japanese ALS patients using invasive mechanical ventilator (IMV), the investigators found a moderately high hope level for all groups (grouped according to decision making regarding IMV initiation) (Hirano & Yamazaki, 2010). Those who received sufficient prior information regarding the IMV from physicians and nurses had higher hope levels than those without sufficient information or the opportunity to reflect and prepare. This high level of hope was consistent with findings in another study of ALS patients by Vitale and Genge (2007).

A study of patients with spinal cord injury (SCI) found a positive correlation between hope and greater life satisfaction during the initial acute rehabilitation period (Kortte, Gilbert, Gorman, & Wegener, 2010). This is an important finding since life satisfaction is reported as predictive of better health status overall (Siahpush, Spittal, & Singh, 2008), and increasing evidence suggests hope can be facilitated through intervention (Cook et al., 2009; Manos, Sebastián, Mateos, & Bueno, 2009). Another phenomenological study looked at the hope experience for

Norwegian SCI patients 3 to 4 years following SCI. The author identified three main themes: life-related hopes, body-related hopes, and creative and expanding hopes (Lohne, 2009).

Hope was hypothesized to be a predictor of adherence to pharmacologic therapy in patients with multiple sclerosis (MS). The authors found that hope did not predict adherence to glatiramer acetate therapy in a sample of 199 patients (Fraser, Hadjimichael, & Vollmer, 2003) but it did predict adherence to Copaxone therapy in a sample of 341 MS patients (Fraser, Hadjimichael, & Vollmer, 2001).

Mental Health Conditions. The literature is replete with studies examining the relationship between hopelessness and depression or suicide. Indeed, much of the original research on hope began with such investigations. Holdcroft and Williamson (1991) examined hope levels in hospitalized psychiatric patients and chemically dependent patients. Hope scores were measured on admission and discharge. Those with psychiatric conditions had significantly lower hope scores than those with chemical dependency on admission. Both groups had higher hope scores at discharge. Another study examined adults with obsessive-compulsive disorder and found that the relationship between hope and depressive symptoms was mediated by coping; hope was positively correlated with social support coping strategies (Geffken et al., 2006). In a study of a statewide Illness Management and Recovery Program for adults (*n* = 324) with severe mental illnesses, investigators found an increase in levels of hope and self-management of illness at 6 and 12 months after baseline measurement (Salyers et al., 2009). Finally, a study of chemically dependent adolescents (*n* = 369) found a statistically significant relationship between hope and use of alcohol, tobacco, and marijuana (Wilson, Syme, Boyce, Battistich, & Selvin, 2005).

Hope Experience of Caregivers

Hope has also been studied in caregivers, both nonprofessional and professional. Family members providing palliative home care have been queried in phenomenological studies. The studies found similar themes of concern for things that erode or interfere with hope, the need to "hang on to hope," and hope fostered by relationships with God, the patient, and/or family (Holtslander et al., 2005, p. 290; Borneman, Stahl, Ferrell, & Smith, 2002; Clukey, 2007). Benzein and Berg (2005) compared patients and family members in palliative care. They found that family members had significantly lower levels of hope than the patients.

Duggleby and Wright (2007) studied 113 professional palliative caregivers in Canada using the HHI and survey questions. Nurses reported significantly lower hope subscores (temporality and future) than other health care providers. The investigators identified things that foster hope for these caregivers: (a) making a difference, (b) spirituality, (c) adequate resources, (d) peace, (e) patient comfort, and (f) supportive relationships. Those things that hinder hope were identified as the opposites of these. In another study by Duggleby, Cooper, and Penz (2009), Canadian Continuing Care Assistants reported that "faith, relationships, helping others and positive thinking helped them to have hope" (p. 2376).

Hope Experience in Other Cultures

A significant part of the growth in hope research has been studies of individuals in countries other than the United States. Nursing studies that were found in the database searches included research done with individuals in Australia (1), Denmark (4), England (3), Finland (1), Israel (1), Italy (1), Norway (8), Sweden (3), Taiwan (6), Thailand (1), and Turkey (3). These studies examined the hope experience in relation to specific variables, specific health conditions, and normative data and conducted psychometric testing of translated hope measures.

The reports of the hope experience in these different countries do not differ on the surface from similar studies of the hope experience in people in the United States. One notable exception was related to a Swedish psychometric study of a translation of the Herth Hope Index. The investigators found difficulty translating the items that may be interpreted by many people as linked to religion, suggesting that this may affect construct validity due to the cultural differences related to religion. Additionally the words "value" and "worth" are commonly translated as "värde" in Swedish, leading to difficulty in translating "I feel my life has value and worth" (Benzein & Berg, 2003, p. 413). These findings are similar to studies in Norway where faith items received lower scores (Rustøen et al., 2003).

REVIEW OF HOPE RESEARCH WITH SPECIFIC VARIABLES

Hope and Quality of Life

Several studies have attempted to analyze any relationship between hope and quality of life (QOL). Staples and Jeffrey (1997) found lower quality of life and hope scores associated with uncertainty for patients and spouses before coronary artery bypass surgery. Beckie et al. (2001) attempted to model the relationship between QOL and perceived health status, hope, and optimism in 93 women after a cardiac event. They found a concept they called *outlook* that subsumed hope and dispositional optimism. This concept explained two-thirds of the variance in patient-reported QOL. Another study of 40 moderately to severely impaired stroke survivors and their spouses found positive correlation between hope and quality of life in both partners (Bluvol & Ford-Gilboe, 2004). Evangelista, Doering, Dracup, Vassilakis, and Kobashigawa (2003) studied 50 female heart transplant recipients. They exhibited moderately low hope levels as measured by HHI. The authors found a strong positive correlation between hope, mood states, and the mental component summary of the SF-12 Health Survey (a measure of QOL). The authors concluded that hope was an independent predictor of mood states and QOL.

A study of elderly Norwegians with newly diagnosed cancer found a low level of hope to be significantly related to a low level of quality of life (Esbensen, Østerlind, Roer, & Hallberg, 2004). Similar results were found in 3-month and 6-month follow-up studies of these patients, with decreasing hope scores and decreasing QOL scores (Esbensen et al., 2006; Esbensen, Østerlind, & Hallberg, 2007). Hope was found to be negatively correlated with measures of psychological distress and physical symptoms, and positively correlated with the ability to perform activities of daily living and QOL in 80 Italian cancer patients (Vellone et al., 2006). A study of Norwegian patients with primary antibody deficiency found a moderate level of hope that accounted for 20.6% of the total variance in the QOL scores (Sigstad, Stray-Pedersen & Frøland, 2005).

Hope and Information

A few studies have examined the relationship between provision of information and hope.

One study in the Netherlands examined hope in family members of traumatic coma patients in intensive care. Interviews of 22 family members found information helped families to understand their loved one's care and condition and to develop realistic hope, which the family members defined as based upon information that is correct and complete as possible. This was similar to other findings (Gelling, Fitzgerald, & Blight, 2002; Johnson & Roberts, 1996; Miller 1989, 1991). They also found, in contrast to misinterpretation by professionals, that strong hope expressed by family members was not a denial of reality but a clinging to the small chance of a positive outcome. Another study of 124 Taiwanese cancer patients examined the relationship between diagnostic disclosure and hope. The investigators found higher levels of hope in those who had been informed of their diagnosis as opposed to those who were not informed. Hope decreased over 12 months after diagnosis, but not statistically.

Hope and Coping

Most often hope is described as a coping strategy (Bruhn, 1984; Korner, 1970; Lazarus & Folkman, 1984; Raleigh & Boehm, 1994) but it may also be described as an antecedent to coping (Dufault & Martocchio, 1985; Owen, 1989; Weisman, 1979) or as an outcome of coping (Engel, 1968; Farran & McCann, 1989). In fact, hope may have a role in all three aspects of coping. As an antecedent, hope influences how the individual perceives the situation that may be a challenge or threat to goals. As a coping strategy, hope enables the individual to appraise the situation as a challenge rather than a threat and to muster problem-focused or emotional-focused resources (Farran, Herth et al., 1995). Finally, as an outcome, hope results from the use of coping strategies, such as prayer and interpersonal interaction (Raleigh, 1992). On the other hand, hopelessness occurs when coping becomes ineffective (Farran, Herth et al., 1995; Stotland, 1969).

Some research supports hope as a coping strategy. In a study of adolescents with cancer, Hinds (1988) found that participants reported using two strategies, forgetting cancer and hopefulness, to achieve cognitive comfort, which is part of the larger coping process. Other research suggests that hope is an outcome of using coping mechanisms. In a study of 45 individuals with chronic conditions, Raleigh (1992) found that participants reported using strategies to maintain hope such as physical activity, religious activities, mental distraction, or interaction with others. Herth (1989) found that hope and coping responses were related in a study of 120 cancer patients and suggested that fostering hope in the cancer patient is important for the coping response. Bland and Darlington (2002) found that hope was an important factor in helping family cope with mental illness of a loved one.

Other research has looked at the relationship between hope and specific coping styles. Hope correlated with confrontive coping and emotive coping in a sample of 61 family members of people with terminal cancer (Chapman & Pepler, 1998) confirming similar findings by Herth (1990a). The authors also found inverse relationships between emotive coping and hopefulness, and hope and despair. Wonghongkul et al. (2000) found that hope influenced positive reappraisal coping. They also found a positive relationship between hope and coping style use and coping effectiveness, consistent with other findings (Felder, 2004; Herth, 1989; 1993). A study of HIV-infected African American women found a positive correlation between hope and total coping score and a negative relationship between hope and avoidance coping (Phillips & Sowell, 2000). Consistent with these findings, a positive relationship was found between hope and coping style use (optimistic, confrontive, and evasive) and coping effectiveness in 183 patients with a cancer diagnosis (Felder, 2004). In a study of psychological adjustment to spinal cord injury, hope was a significant predictor of coping (Kennedy, Evans, & Sandhu, 2009). These findings suggest that hope plays a significant role in coping. Further research is essential so that we can understand this role better.

IMPLICATIONS FOR THEORY, PRACTICE, AND RESEARCH

Nursing Theory Implications

Nurse investigators have focused attention on developing models of hope through exploring the "lived experience" of hope in various populations. There has also been a significant effort to conduct concept analysis of hope and relate it to specific populations. For the most part, theorists have focused on the meaning of hope to the individual in their circumstances. Hope, more than most concepts, is nebulous, almost ethereal, and it makes sense that much of the research to date has focused on understanding its meaning and attempting to draw conclusions about it. What has been missing in most models is the lack of relational statements that would lead to research that explains, predicts, and controls the phenomenon. Nursing research needs to move hope theory forward by proposing and testing relationships between hope and outcomes. While significant research has focused on testing relationships between hope and particular variables, what continues to be missing in any significant amount is research that tests these models specifically.

Increasingly, investigators have compared findings across diagnostic groups and within cultures in recent years that has led to understanding of the universality of hope. There is also seminal research that suggests cultural differences, especially related to the spiritual dimension found in most American-developed models. In contrast to the strong spirituality of Americans, populations in other countries may find it less meaningful (Benzein & Berg, 2003). What is missing, however, is replication of studies. The expansion across groups fails to address the critical aspect of good research, which is determining if the findings are consistent when examined in the same population using the same methods. Increasingly, however, researchers have consistently used the Herth Hope Index in studies, which is a step in the right direction for replication.

Nursing Practice Implications

Because much of the research to date has been descriptive and exploratory without providing evidence for expected outcomes of nursing intervention, the various strategies for fostering hope discussed in this section still need to be tested.

An understanding of strategies for fostering hope began with identifying those reportedly used by clients. Several studies (Herth, 1990b, 1993; Miller, 1989; Patel, 1996; Raleigh, 1992) demonstrated fairly consistent findings with regard to strategies individuals report that they use, although the order of use varies according to health status. Subjects include the terminally, critically, and chronically ill, as well as healthy adults. Common categories of reported hope-fostering strategies include (a) cognitive strategies that restructure threatening information to make it less threatening, (b) purposeful activities, (c) conviction that a positive outcome is possible, (d) maintaining a world view that says life has meaning and growth results from struggles, (e) spiritual beliefs and practices that transcend suffering, (f) a relationship with caregivers who convey positive messages and faith in the patient, (g) relationships with loved ones, (h) a sense of being in control, (i) maintaining goals (small or large, short- or long-term), (j) distraction, (k) humor or lightheartedness, and/or (l) uplifting memories (Buckley & Herth, 2004; Herth, 1990a, 1993, 1995; Patel, 1996; Raleigh, 1992, Vitale & Genge, 2007; Wake & Miller, 1992). In addition, some studies (Buckley & Herth, 2004; Herth, 1990a; Miller, 1989, 2000, 2007; Vitale & Genge, 2007) listed threats to hope identified by these patients. Hopes were threatened or hindered when the patient sensed a physical setback, uncontrollable pain and discomfort, abandonment and isolation, negative hospital experiences, or a devaluation of their personhood.

Interventions to foster hope have been proposed by nurses. Common ones include (a) providing comfort and pain relief (Buckley & Herth, 2004; Herth, 1995; Johnson et al., 1997), (b) facilitating relationships with family and health care providers (Buckley & Herth, 2004; Herth, 1995; Kim, 1989; Popovich et al., 2007), (c) assisting to define and redefine hopes and mutual goal setting (Buckley & Herth, 2004; Herth, 1995; Johnson et al., 1997; Popovich et al., 2007; Vitale & Genge, 2007), (d) facilitating an expression of spirituality (Buckley & Herth, 2004; Herth, 1995; Popovich et al., 2007), and (e) encouraging awareness of small positive aspects of a situation (Herth, 1995; Johnson et al., 1997). Herth's (1995) study of 141 hospice and home health care nurses found that nurses rated similar interventions as useful and effective for terminally and chronically ill patients. Providing pain control and comfort was reported by both groups of nurses as most useful and most effective. Both groups also rated connectedness with others very highly. Buckley and Herth (2004, p. 39) conclude that "[a]spects of care that we know intuitively to be good practice, nurture hope. Sustaining hope is an intuitive part of human nature and of nursing practice. Caring practices are the essence of good care."

Miller (1992) developed a Hope–Despair model that summarizes the types of nursing strategies that may be useful to foster hope in patients. These proposed strategies relate to several of the critical elements of hope described in her conceptual model. According to Miller, nurses may foster hope through the affiliative dimension by promoting sustaining relationships and connectedness with others. Nurses may also enhance patients' sense of control or support them, if it is necessary, to temporarily relinquish control. Nurses may use a life-promoting interpersonal framework by maintaining a positive focus that emphasizes the patient's potential for recovery and/or adaptation. Expanding the patient's and family's coping repertoire and supporting the patient's reality surveillance may also foster hopes. Finally, nurses should provide assistance with identifying and/or revising goals and supporting and encouraging the patient's relationship with God or a meaningful higher being.

There have been a few attempts to test hope-promoting interventions. Early on, Mercer and Kane (1979) examined the effects of enabling increased control and choice through caring for a plant and participating on a resident council among eight elderly nursing home residents. Even though the sample size was very small, the investigators found a significant reduction in hopelessness among the experimental group as opposed to the control group. Staats (1991) attempted to increase hope and quality of life through happiness and/or goal-setting training. While the participants in the combination group expected a higher quality of life in five years, there were no significant differences in hope among the groups. Another early study tested visual imagery group therapy and educational discussion groups in relation to cognition, depression, hopelessness, and life satisfaction (Abraham, 1991). Over 36 weeks of behavioral group therapy intervention and repeated data collection, depression and hopelessness did not change over time and no differences were found between groups.

More recent studies have found more positive results. A study of Norwegian cancer patients tested an intervention designed to increase hope against the "Learning to Live with Cancer" program and a control group. All three groups had high initial hope levels, leaving little room for improvement. The hope intervention group had a significant increase in hope in comparison to the other groups at 2 weeks after the intervention, with a return to baseline and no significant differences at 6 months after intervention (Rustøen, Wiklund, Hanestad, Rokne, & Torbjørn, 1998). Herth (2000) conducted a study using three groups: hope intervention group focused on the components of the Hope Process Framework; attention control group received information about cancer, the human body, and cancer treatment; and a control group. Repeated measures of hope and quality of life found significantly higher hope levels in the hope group versus the other two at 2 weeks, and 3, 6, and 9 months after intervention.

In a study of 188 Spanish women with early-stage breast cancer, the investigators compared those who received a multi-componential psychosocial intervention program with a control group. With measures at baseline, post-treatment and 6 months later, the experimental group reported progressively more hopefulness/optimism over time, while the control group reported progressively less (Manos et al., 2009). These few intervention studies highlight the fact that there is little research that has tested theoretical propositions about hope-fostering interventions.

Implications for Research

In examining the level of theory development for the concepts of hope and hopelessness, it is apparent that, while much theorizing has been done, there has not been much empirical testing of the theories/models. Although investigators routinely identify the conceptual framework for their studies, they seldom address whether the study findings support or are related to the aspects of the model. Efforts have focused on determining relationships that exist between hope and other variables without examining how these variables relate to the conceptual framework of the study.

This lack of focus on specific theory testing may be explained by the fact that much of the theory surrounding hope in the nursing literature is still at the concept development stage (Walker & Avant, 1995). In an effort to determine relational statements, nursing research focuses on finding relationships between hope and other concepts. While the interest in hope has geometrically increased in the last two decades, the research has been broad and unfocused. Some of the research has used nursing hope models as conceptual frameworks, but many other studies have used a variety of concepts other than hope as the framework. There is a significant need for nurses to attend to the purposeful building of theory around the concept of hope. In addition, research needs to focus on the testing of strategies used and reported by nurses for fostering hope. Interventions based on theory and suggested by the research literature should be tested for their empirical effectiveness with a variety of patient populations.

Conclusion

Hope is a concept that is extremely important in understanding the coping process. While several models of hope have been proposed, the role of hope in the coping process is not clearly understood. Hope models need further testing and, specifically, the relationship between hope and the coping process needs to be more carefully examined. In addition, interventions need to be related to current theories, be tested for effectiveness, and be replicated. There is still much work to be done in relation to the concept of hope.

References

Abraham, I. (1991). The Geriatric Depression Scale and Hopelessness Index: Longitudinal psychometric data on frail nursing home residents. *Perceptual and Motor Skills, 72,* 875–878.

Alloy, L. B., Abramson, L. Y., Metalsky, G. I., & Hartlage, S. (1988). The hopelessness theory of depression: Attributional aspects. *British Journal of Clinical Psychology, 27,* 5–21.

Ballard, A., Green, A. B., McCaa, A., & Logsdon, M. C. (1997). A comparison of the level of hope in patients with newly diagnosed and recurrent cancer. *Oncology Nursing Forum, 24,* 899–904.

Beck, A. T. (1963). Thinking and depression. *Archives in General Psychiatry, 9,* 324–333.

Beck, A. T. (1967). *Depression: Clinical, experimental, and theoretical aspects.* New York, NY: Harper & Row.

Beck, A. T., Kovacs, M., & Weissman, A. (1975). Hopelessness and suicidal behavior. *Journal of American Medical Association, 234,* 1146–1149.

Beck, A. T., Weissman, A., Lester, D., & Trexler, L. (1974). The measurement of pessimism: The hopelessness scale. *Journal of Consulting and Clinical Psychology, 42,* 861–865.

Beckerman, A., & Northrop, C. (1996). Hope, chronic illness and the elderly. *Journal of Gerontological Nursing, 22*(5), 19–25.

Beckie, T. M., Beckstead, J. W., & Webb, M. S. (2001). Modeling women's quality of life after cardiac events. *Western Journal of Nursing Research, 23*(2), 179–194.

Benzein, E. G., & Berg, A. (2003).The Swedish version of Herth Hope Index—An instrument for palliative care. *Scandinavian Journal of Caring Sciences, 17*(4), 409–415.

Benzein, E. G., & Berg, A. C. (2005). The level of and relation between hope, hopelessness and fatigue in patients and family members in palliative care. *Palliative Medicine, 19*(3), 234–240.

Benzein, E. Norberg, A., & Saveman, B. I. (2001). The meaning of the lived experience of hope in patients with cancer in palliative home care. *Palliative Medicine, 15,* 117–126.

Bernard, H. W. (1977). Hope vs. Hopelessness. *Humanitas, 13,* 283–290.

Bland, R., & Darlington, Y. (2002). The nature and sources of hope: Perspectives of family of stroke survivors. *Journal of Advanced Nursing, 48*(4), 322–332.

Bluvol, A., & Ford-Gilboe, M. (2004). Hope, health work and quality of life in families of stroke survivors. *Journal of Advanced Nursing, 48*(4), 322–332.

Borneman, T., Stahl, C., Ferrell, B. R., & Smith, D. (2002). The concept of hope in family caregivers of cancer patients at home. *Journal of Hospice & Palliative Nursing, 4*(1), 21–33.

Brackney, B., & Westman, A. (1992). Relationships among hope, psychosocial development, and locus of control. *Psychological Reports, 70,* 864–866.

Brandt, B. T. (1987). The relationship between hopelessness and selected variables in women receiving chemotherapy for breast cancer. *Oncology Nursing Forum, 12*(2), 35–39.

Bruhn, J. G. (1984). Therapeutic value of hope. *Southern Medical Journal, 77*(2), 215–219.

Buckley, J., & Herth, K. (2004). Fostering hope in terminally ill patients. *Nursing Standard, 19*(10), 33–41.

Bunston, T., Mings, D., Mackie, A., & Jones, D. (1995). Facilitating hopefulness: The determinants of hope. *Journal of Psychosocial Oncology, 13*(4), 79–103.

Canty-Mitchell, J. (2001). Life change events, hope, and self-care agency in inner-city adolescents. *Journal of Child and Adolescent Psychiatric Nursing, 14*(1), 18–31.

Chapman, K. J., & Pepler, C. (1998). Coping, hope, and anticipatory grief in family members in palliative home care. *Cancer Nursing, 21*(4), 226–234.

Chen, M. L. (2003). Pain and hope in patients with cancer: A role for cognition. *Cancer Nursing, 26*(1), 61–67.

Clukey, L. (2007). "Just be there": Hospice caregivers' anticipatory mourning experience. *Journal of Hospice & Palliative Nursing, 9*(3), 150–158.

Connelly, C. D. (1998). Hopefulness, self-esteem, and perceived social support among pregnant and nonpregnant adolescents. *Western Journal of Nursing Research, 20,* 195–209.

Cook, J. A., Copeland, M. E., Hamilton, M. M., Jonikas, J. A., Razzano, L. A., Floyd, C. B., . . . Grey, D. D. (2009). Initial outcomes of a mental illness self-management program based on wellness recovery action planning. *Psychiatric Services, 60*(2), 246–249.

Cotter, V. T. (2009). Hope in early-stage dementia: A concept analysis. *Holistic Nursing Practice, 23*(5), 297–301.

Davis, B. (2005). Mediators of the relationship between hope and well-being in older adults. *Clinical Nursing Research, 14*(3), 253–272.

Dufault, K., & Martocchio, B. C. (1985). Hope: Its spheres and dimensions. *Nursing Clinics of North America, 20,* 379–391.

Duggleby, W., Cooper, D., & Penz, K. (2009). Hope, self-efficacy, spiritual well-being and job satisfaction. *Journal of Advanced Nursing, 65*(11), 2376–2385.

Duggleby, W., & Wright, K. (2005). Transforming hope: How elderly palliative patients live with hope. *The Canadian Journal of Nursing Research, 37*(2), 70–84.

Duggleby, W., & Wright, K. (2007). The hope of professional caregivers caring for persons at the end of life. *Journal of Hospice and Palliative Nursing. 9*(1), 42–49.

Engel, G. L. (1968). A life setting conducive to illness: The giving up–given up complex. *Annals of Internal Medicine, 69,* 293–300.

Erickson, R. C., Post, R. D., & Paige, A. B. (1975). Hope as a psychiatric variable. *Journal of Clinical Psychology, 31,* 324–330.

Esbensen, B. A., Østerlind, K., & Hallberg, I. R. (2006). Quality of life of elderly persons with cancer: A 3-month follow-up. *Cancer Nursing, 29*(3), 214–224.

Esbensen, B. A., Østerlind, K., & Hallberg, I. R. (2007). Quality of life of elderly persons with cancer: A 6-month follow-up. *Scandinavian Journal of Caring Science, 21,* 178–190.

Esbensen, B. A., Østerlind, K., Roer, O., & Hallberg, I. R. (2004). Quality of life of elderly persons with newly diagnosed cancer. *European Journal of Cancer Care, 13*(5), 443–453.

Evangelista, L. S., Doering, L. V., Dracup, K., Vassilakis, M. E., & Kobashigawa, J. (2003). Hope, mood states and quality of life in female heart transplant recipients. *The Journal of Heart and Lung Transplantation, 22*(6), 681–686.

Ezzy, D. (2000). Illness narratives: Time, hope and HIV. *Social Science and Medicine, 50,* 605–617.

Farran, C. J., Herth, K. A., & Popovich, J. M. (1995). *Hope and hopelessness.* Thousand Oaks, CA: Sage.

Farran, C. J., & McCann, J. (1989). Longitudinal analysis of hope in community-based older adults. *Archives of Psychiatric Nursing, 3*(5), 272–276.

Farran, C. J., & Popovich, J. M. (1990). Hope: A relevant concept for geriatric psychiatry. *Archives of Psychiatric Nursing, 4,* 124–130.

Farran, C. J., Wiken, C. S., & Fidler, R. (1995). A study of hope in geriatric patients. *Journal of Nursing Science, 1*(1–2), 16–26.

Fawcett, J. (1984).The metaparadigm of nursing: Present status and future refinements. *Image, 16,* 84–87.

Fehring, R. J., Miller, J. F., & Shaw, C. (1997). Spiritual well-being, religiosity, hope, depression, and other mood states in elderly people coping with cancer. *Oncology Nursing Forum, 24,* 663–671.

Felder, B. E. (2004). Hope and coping in patients with cancer diagnoses. *Cancer Nursing, 27*(4), 320–324.

Foote, A., Piazza, D., Holcomb, J., Paul, P., & Daffin, P. (1990). Hope, self-esteem, and social support in persons with multiple sclerosis. *Journal of Neuroscience Nursing, 22,* 155–159.

Fraser, C., Hadjimichael, O., & Vollmer, T. (2001). Predictors of adherence to Copaxone therapy in individuals with relapsing-remitting multiple sclerosis. *The Journal of Neuroscience Nursing, 33*(5), 231–239.

Fraser, C., Hadjimichael, O., & Vollmer, T. (2003). Predictors of adherence to glatiramer acetate therapy in individuals with self-reported progressive forms of multiple sclerosis. *The Journal of Neuroscience Nursing, 35*(3), 163–170.

Fry, P. (1984). Development of a geriatric scale of hopelessness: Implications for counseling and intervention with the depressed elderly. *Journal of Counseling Psychology, 31,* 322–331.

Geffken, G. R., Storch, E. A., Duke, D. C., Monaco, L., Lewin, A. B., & Goodman, W. K. (2006). Hope and coping in family members of patients with obsessive-compulsive disorder. *Journal of Anxiety Disorders, 20*(5), 614–629.

Gelling, L., Fitzgerald, M., & Blight, I. (2002). Hope in ICU: A qualitative study exploring nurses' experiences of the concept of hope. *Nursing in Critical Care, 7,* 271–277.

Glaser, B. G., & Strauss, A. (1967). *The discovery of grounded theory: Strategies for qualitative research.* Chicago, IL: Aldine.

Gordon, M. (2007). *Manual of nursing diagnosis* (11th ed.). Sudbury, MA: Jones and Bartlett.

Gottschalk, L. (1974). A hope scale applicable to verbal samples. *Archives of General Psychiatry, 30,* 779–785.

Grewal, P. K., & Porter, J. D. (2007). Hope theory: A framework for understanding suicidal action. *Death Studies, 31,* 131–154.

Herth, K. (2000). Enhancing hope in people with a first recurrence of cancer. *Journal of Advanced Nursing, 32*(6), 1431–41.

Herth, K. A. (1989). The relationship between level of hope and level of coping response and other variables in patients with cancer. *Oncology Nursing Forum, 16,* 67–72.

Herth, K. A. (1990a). Relationship of hope, coping styles, concurrent losses, and setting to grief resolution in the elderly widow(er). *Research in Nursing & Health, 13,* 109–117.

Herth, K. A. (1990b). Fostering hope in terminally-ill people. *Journal of Advanced Nursing, 15,* 1250–1259.

Herth, K. A. (1991). Development and refinement of an instrument to measure hope. *Scholarly Inquiry for Nursing Practice: An International Journal, 5,* 39–56.

Herth, K. A. (1992). Abbreviated instrument to measure hope: Development and psychometric evaluation. *Journal of Advanced Nursing, 17,* 1251–1259.

Herth, K. A. (1993). Hope in older adults in community and institutional settings. *Issues in Mental Health Nursing, 14,* 139–156.

Herth, K. A. (1995). Engendering hope in the chronically and terminally ill: Nursing interventions. *The American Journal of Hospice and Palliative Care, 12*(5), 31–39.

Heszen-Niejodek, I., Gottschalk, L.A., & Januszek, M. (1999). Anxiety and hope during the course of three different medical illnesses: A longitudinal study. *Psychotherapy and Psychosomatics, 68*(6), 304–312.

Hinds, P. S. (1984). Inducing a definition of hope through the use of grounded theory methodology. *Journal of Advanced Nursing, 9,* 357–362.

Hinds, P. S. (1988). The relationship of nurses' caring behaviors with hopefulness and health care outcomes in adolescents. *Archives of Psychiatric Nursing, 2,* 21–29.

Hinds, P. S., & Gattuso, J. (1991). Measuring hopefulness in adolescents. *Journal of Pediatric Oncology Nursing, 8,* 92–94.

Hinds, P. S., & Martin, J. (1988). Hopefulness and the self-sustaining process in adolescents with cancer. *Nursing Research, 37,* 336–340.

Hirano, Y., & Yamazaki, Y. (2010). Ethical issues in invasive mechanical ventilation for amyotrophic lateral sclerosis. *Nursing Ethics 17*(1), 51–63.

Hirth, A. M., & Stewart, M. J. (1994). Hope and social support as coping resources for adults waiting for cardiac transplantation. *Canadian Journal of Nursing Research, 26*(3), 31–48.

Holdcroft, C., & Williamson, C. (1991). Assessment of hope in psychiatric and chemically dependent patients. *Applied Nursing Research, 4*(3), 129–134.

Holtslander, L. F., Duggleby, W., Williams, A. M., & Wright, K. E. (2005). The experience of hope for informal caregivers of palliative patients. *Journal of Palliative Care, 21*(4), 285–291.

Irvin, B. L., & Acton, G. J. (1997). Stress, hope, and well-being of women caring for family members with Alzheimer's disease. *Holistic Nursing Practice, 11*(2), 69–79.

Ishibashi, A., Ueda, R., Kawano, Y., Nakayama, H., Matsuzaki, A., & Matsumura, T. (2010). How to improve resilience in adolescents with cancer in Japan. *Journal of Pediatric Oncology Nursing, 27*(2), 73–93.

Jalowiec, A. (1987). *Jalowiec Coping Scale* (revised) (Unpublished manuscript). University of Illinois, Chicago.

Johnson, L. H., Dahlen, R., & Roberts, S. L. (1997). Supporting hope in congestive heart failure patients. *Dimensions of Critical Care Nursing, 16,* 65–78.

Johnson, L. H., & Roberts, S. (1996). Hope facilitating strategies for the family of the head injury patient. *Journal of Neuroscience Nursing, 28,* 259–266.

Kazdin, A., French, N., Unis, A., Esveldt-Dawson, K., & Sherick, R. (1983). Hopelessness, depression, and suicidal intent among psychiatrically disturbed inpatient children. *Journal of Consulting and Clinical Psychology, 51,* 504–510.

Kennedy, P., Evans, M., & Sandhu, N. (2009). Psychological adjustment to spinal cord injury: The contribution of coping, hope and cognitive appraisals. *Psychology, Health & Medicine, 14*(1), 17–33.

Kim, R. S. (1989). Hope as a mode of coping in amyotrophic lateral sclerosis. *Journal of Neuroscience Nursing, 21,* 342–347.

Korner, I. N. (1970). Hope as a method of coping. *Journal of Consulting and Clinical Psychology, 34,* 134–139.

Kortte, K. B., Gilbert, M., Gorman, P., & Wegener, S. T. (2010). Positive psychological variables in the prediction of life satisfaction after spinal cord injury. *Rehabilitation Psychology, 55*(1), 40–47.

Kylma, J. (2006). Hope, despair and hopeless in significant others of adult persons living with HIV. *The Journal of Theory Construction and Testing, 9*(2), 49–54.

Lange, S. P. (1978). Hope. In C. E. Carlson & B. Blackwell (Eds.), *Behavioral concepts and nursing interventions* (2nd ed., pp. 171–190). Philadelphia, PA: J. B. Lippincott.

Lazarus, R., & Folkman, S. (1984). *Stress, appraisal and coping.* New York, NY: Springer.

Lohne, V. (2009). Back to life again—Patients' experience of hope three to four years after a spinal cord injury—A longitudinal study. *Canadian Journal of Neuroscience Nursing, 31*(2), 20–25.

Lynch, W. F. (1965). *Images of hope: Imagination as the healer of the hopeless.* Notre Dame, IN: University of Notre Dame Press.

Manos, D., Sebastián, J., Mateos, N., & Bueno, M. J. (2009). Results of a multi-componential psychosocial intervention programme for women with early-stage breast cancer in Spain: Quality of life and mental adjustment. *European Journal of Cancer Care, 18*(3), 295–305.

McGee, R. F. (1984). Hope: A factor influencing crisis resolution. *Advances in Nursing Science, 6*(4), 34–44.

McGill, F. S., & Paul, P. B. (1993). Functional status and hope in elderly people with and without cancer. *Oncology Nursing Forum, 20,* 1207–1213.

Melges, F. T., & Bowlby, J. (1969). Types of hopelessness in psychopathological process. *Archives of General Psychiatry, 20,* 690–699.

Mercer, S., & Kane, R. (1979). Helplessness and hopelessness among the institutionalized aged: An experiment. *Health Social Work, 4*(1), 91–116.

Miller, J. F. (1983). *Coping with chronic illness: Overcoming powerlessness.* Philadelphia, PA: F. A. Davis.

Miller, J. F. (1989). Hope-inspiring strategies of the critically ill. *Applied Nursing Research, 2,* 23–29.

Miller, J. F. (1991). Developing and maintaining hope in families of the critically ill. *AACN Clinical Issues in Critical Care Nursing, 2*(2), 307–315.

Miller, J. F. (1992). *Coping with chronic illness: Overcoming powerlessness* (2nd ed.). Philadelphia, PA: F. A. Davis.

Miller, J. F. (2000). *Coping with chronic illness: Overcoming powerlessness* (3rd ed.). Philadelphia, PA: F. A. Davis.

Miller, J. F. (2007). Hope: A construct central to nursing. *Nursing Forum, 42*(1), 12–19.

Miller, J. F., & Powers, M. (1988). Development of an instrument to measure hope. *Nursing Research, 37,* 6–10.

Minkoff, K., Bergman, E., Beck, A. T., & Beck, R. (1973). Hopelessness, depression and attempted suicide. *American Journal of Psychiatry, 130,* 455–459.

Mishel, M., Hostetter, T., King, B., & Graham, V. (1984). Predictors of psychosocial adjustment in patients newly diagnosed with gynecological cancer. *Cancer Nursing, 7,* 291–299.

Nekolaichuk, C. L., & Bruera, E. (2004). Assessing hope at the end of life: Validation of an experience of hope scale in advanced cancer patients. *Palliative & Supportive Care, 2*(3), 243–253.

Nekolaichuk, C. L., Jevne, R. F., & Maguire, T. O. (1999). Structuring the meaning of hope in health and illness. *Social Science & Medicine. 48*(5), 591–605.

Nowotny, M. (1989). Assessment of hope in patients with cancer: Development of an instrument. *Oncology Nursing Forum, 16,* 57–61.

Obayuwana, A., Collins, J., Carter, A., Rao, M., Mathura, C., & Wilson, S. (1982). Hope index scale: An instrument for the objective assessment of hope. *Journal of the National Medical Association, 74,* 761–765.

Owen, D. C. (1989). Nurses' perspectives on the meaning of hope in patients with cancer: A qualitative study. *Oncology Nursing Forum, 16,* 75–79.

Patel, C. T. C. (1996). Hope-inspiring strategies of spouses of critically ill adults. *Journal of Holistic Nursing, 14*(1), 44–65.

Phillips, K. D., & Sowell, R. L. (2000). Hope and coping in HIV-infected African-American women of reproductive age. *Journal of National Black Nurses' Association, 11*(Part 2), 18–24.

Popovich, J. M., Fox, P. G., & Bandagi, R. (2007). Coping with stroke: Psychological and social dimensions in U.S. patients. *International Journal of Psychiatric Nursing Research, 12*(3), 1474–1487.

Raleigh, E. D. (1992). Sources of hope in chronic illness. *Oncology Nursing Forum, 19*(3), 443–448.

Raleigh, E. D., & Boehm, S. B. (1994). Development of the multidimensional hope scale. *Journal of Nursing Measurement, 2,* 155–167.

Rideout, E., & Montemuro, M. (1986). Hope, morale, and adaptation in patients with chronic heart failure. *Journal of Advanced Nursing, 11,* 429–438.

Rustøen, T., Cooper, B. A., & Miaskowski, C. (2010). The importance of hope as a mediator of psychological distress and life satisfaction in a community sample of cancer patients. *Cancer Nursing, 33*(4), 258–267.

Rustøen, T., Howie, J., Eidsmo, I., & Moum, T. (2005). Hope in patients hospitalized with heart failure. *American Journal of Critical Care, 14*(5), 417–425.

Rustøen, T., Wahl, A. K., Hanestad, B. R., Lerdal, A., Miaskowski, C., & Moum, T., (2003). Hope in the general Norwegian population, measured using the Herth Hope Index. *Palliative & Supportive Care, 1*(4), 309–318.

Rustøen T., & Wiklund, I. (2000). Hope in newly diagnosed patients with cancer. *Cancer Nursing, 23*(3), 214–219.

Rustøen, T., Wiklund, I., Hanestad, B. R., & Moum, T. (1998). Nursing intervention to increase hope and quality of life in newly diagnosed cancer patients. *Cancer Nursing, 21*(4), 235–245.

Salyers, M. P., Godfrey, J. L., McGuire, A. B., Gearhart, T., Rollins, A. L., & Boyle, C. (2009). Implementing the illness management and recovery program for consumers with severe mental illness. *Psychiatric Services, 60*(4), 483–490.

Schrank, B., Stanghellini, G., & Slade, M. (2008). Hope in psychiatry: A review of the literature. *Acta Psychiatrica Scandinavica, 118,* 421–433.

Siahpush, M., Spittal, M., & Singh, G. K. (2008). Happiness and life satisfaction prospectively predict self-rated health, physical health, and the presence of limiting, long-term health conditions. *American Journal of Health Promotion, 23*(1), 18–26.

Sigstad, H. M., Stray-Pedersen, A., & Frøland, S. S. (2005). Coping, quality of life, and hope in adults with primary antibody deficiencies. *Health and Quality of Life Outcomes, 3,* 31–44.

Snyder, C. (1994). *The psychology of hope: You can get there from here.* New York, NY: Free Press.

Snyder, C. R. (2000). The past and possible futures of hope. *Journal of Social and Clinical Psychology, 19*(1), 11–28.

Snyder, C. R., Harris, C., Anderson, J., Holleran, S., Irving, L., Sigmon, S., . . . Harney, P. (1991). The will and the ways: Development and validation of an individual-differences measure of hope. *Journal of Personality and Social Psychology, 60*(4), 570–585.

Snyder, C. R., Hoza, B., Pelham, W. E., Rapoff, M., Ware, L., Danovsky, M., . . . Stahl, K. J. (1997). The development and validation of the Children's Hope Scale. *Journal of Pediatric Psychology, 22,* 399–421.

Snyder, C. R., Sympson, S. C., Ybasco, F. C., Borders, T. F., Babyak, M. A., & Higgins, R. L. (1996). Development and validation of the State Hope Scale. *Journal of Personality and Social Psychology, 70*(2), 321–335.

Staats, S. (1989). Hope: A comparison of two self-report measures for adults. *Journal of Personality Assessment, 53,* 366–375.

Staats, S. (1991). Quality of life and affect in older persons' hope, time frames and training effects. *Current Psychological Research Reviews, 10*(1 & 2), 21–30.

Staples, P., & Jeffrey, J. (1997). Quality of life, hope, and uncertainty of cardiac patients and their spouses before coronary artery bypass surgery. *Canadian Journal of Cardiovascular Nursing, 8*(1), 7–16.

Stoner, M. H. (1982). Hope and cancer patients. *Dissertation Abstracts International, 43,* 1983B-2592B. (University Microfilms No. 83–12,243)

Stoner, M. H., & Keampfer, S. H. (1985). Recalled life expectancy information, phase of illness and hope in cancer patients. *Research in Nursing & Health, 8,* 269–274.

Stotland, E. (1969). *The psychology of hope.* San Francisco, CA: Jossey-Bass.

Travelbee, J. (1971). Hopelessness. In J. Travelbee (Ed.), *Interpersonal aspects of nursing* (pp. 159–177). Philadelphia, PA: F. A. Davis.

Vellone, E., Rega, M. L., Galletti, C., & Cohen, M. Z. (2006). Hope and related variables in Italian cancer patients. *Cancer Nursing, 29*(5), 356–366.

Vitale, A., & Genge, A. (2007). Codman Award 2006: The experience of hope in ALS patients. *Axone, 28*(2), 27–35.

Wake, M. M., & Miller, J. F. (1992). Treating hopelessness. *Clinical Nursing Research, 1,* 347–365.

Walker, L. O., & Avant, K. C. (1995). *Strategies for theory construction in nursing* (3rd ed.). Norwalk, CT: Appleton & Lange.

Weisman, A. D. (1979). *Coping with cancer.* New York, NY: McGraw-Hill.

Wilson, N., Syme, S. L., Boyce, W. T., Battistich, V. A., & Selvin, S. (2005). Adolescent alcohol, tobacco, and marijuana use: The influence of neighborhood disorder and hope. *American Journal of Health Promotion, 20*(1), 11–19.

Wonghongkul, T., Moore, S. M., Musil, C., Schneider, S., & Deimling, G. (2000). The influence of uncertainty in illness, stress appraisal, and hope on coping in survivors of breast cancer. *Cancer Nursing, 23*(6), 422–429.

Yarcheski, A., Scoloveno, M. A., & Mahon, N. E. (1994). Social support and well-being in adolescents: The mediating role of hopefulness. *Nursing Research, 43,* 288–292.

Zorn, C. R., & Johnson, M. T. (1997). Religious well-being in noninstitutionalized elderly women. *Health Care for Women International, 18,* 209–219.

19

SELF-REGULATION

The Common-Sense Model of Illness Representation

NANCY R. REYNOLDS, FAITH MARTIN, ROSE C. NANYONGA, AND ANGELO A. ALONZO

Self-regulation is a term used broadly to refer to the voluntary control of a variety of physiological, psychological, and behavioral processes (see Carver & Scheier, 1982, 1996). As applied in cognitive–behavioral models (e.g., Self-Efficacy Theory [SET], Bandura, 1996; Control Theory [CT], Carver & Scheier, 1982; Common-Sense Model of Illness Representation, Leventhal, Meyer, & Nerenz, 1980), self-regulation is an adaptive process whereby self-monitoring and reliance on perceptual appraisal or feedback guide behavior. As such, self-regulation theories have been useful in broadening an understanding of the dynamic factors involved in health and illness behavior (see Baumeister & Heatherton, 1996; Cameron & Leventhal, 1995; Weinstein, 1993).

This chapter provides a review of the Common-Sense Model (CSM) (Diefenbach & Leventhal, 1996; Leventhal, 1986; Leventhal et al., 1997; Leventhal & Cameron, 1987; Leventhal, Diefenbach, & Leventhal, 1992; Leventhal et al., 1980; Leventhal, Nerenz, & Steele, 1984), a self-regulatory model of health and illness behavior that is particularly useful for the research and practice of nurses. Consistent with a focus in nursing, this model places emphasis on patients' lay, "common-sense" perceptions of their illnesses and provides a framework for understanding the role of symptoms and emotions surrounding a variety of health and illness behaviors. Although

the model is known by a variety of names (e.g., Illness Perceptions Model [IPM], Illness Representations Model, Self-Regulatory Model, Parallel Process Model), for the sake of clarity it will be referred to exclusively in this chapter as the Common-Sense Model (CSM).

BACKGROUND AND FEATURES OF THE COMMON-SENSE MODEL

The Common-Sense Model (CSM) is a complex, multi-level information processing model in which health and illness behaviors are seen as being heavily influenced by the patient's own definition or representation of an illness threat (Cameron & Leventhal, 1995; Diefenbach & Leventhal, 1996; Leventhal, 1986; Leventhal et al., 1997; Leventhal, Brissette, & Leventhal, 2003; Leventhal & Cameron, 1987; Leventhal, et al., 1992; Leventhal et al., 1984). Illness representations do not necessarily conform to scientific views, yet are powerful guides of illness coping and self-management activities.

The CSM was originated by Leventhal and colleagues following a series of studies of fear communications conducted in the late 1960s and early 1970s (see Diefenbach & Leventhal, 1996; Leventhal, 1970). In these studies, high fear messages were found to be more effective in changing attitudes toward a recommended health action in comparison with low fear messages. However, changes in attitudes were found to be rather short lived, lasting only 24 to 48 hours following exposure to the fear messages. Further examination showed that actions, such as getting a protective immunization or stopping smoking, occurred only when the participants exposed to the fear messages also received a second message that facilitated the development of an action plan. Neither the fear messages alone nor the action plans alone resulted in action. Because the combination of action plan and fear message (whether high or low) produced action over a period of days and sometimes weeks, and because subjective feelings of fear and fear-induced attitude change faded within 48 hours, the researchers concluded that the action plan was linked not to fear itself, but to some changed way of thinking about or representing the health threat. The realization that the health threat representation in combination with the action plan was the determining factor for subsequent actions led to a series of additional studies designed to define the nature of the representation and adaptations or coping efforts.

Ultimately, a hierarchically organized model of adaptation was proposed featuring three main constructs: (a) representation of the illness, (b) action planning or coping responses and performance of these, and (c) appraisal of the success or failure of the coping efforts. A particularly unique feature of the CSM was delineation of dual cognitive and emotion processing arms (see Diefenbach & Leventhal, 1996; Leventhal et al., 1997) (Figure 19.1).

Several basic assumptions about the self-regulatory processing of health/illness information form the basis upon which the model is premised (Leventhal et al., 1984).

Active Processing

The individual is conceptualized as an active problem solver. It is assumed that behavior and experience are constructed by an underlying information-processing system that integrates current stimulus information with both innate and acquired information. An individual's experience of the world and its objects, emotional reaction to them, and coping reactions are created and organized by this processing system on a moment-by-moment basis (Leventhal et al., 1984).

Parallel Processing

The individual processes and integrates two responses to information about a health threat: the perceived reality of a health threat and the emotional reaction to this threat (Diefenbach & Leventhal, 1996). The processing of information involves two parallel processing pathways. One

Figure 19.1   A Schematic of the Common-Sense Model (CSM) of Illness Representation

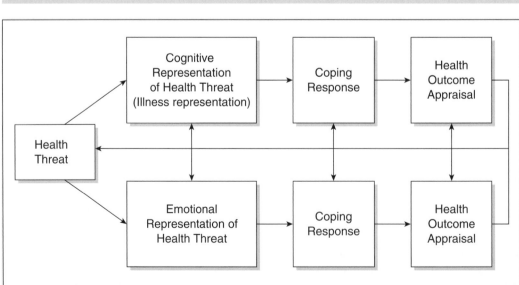

pathway is primarily a conceptual, deliberative system that involves semantic knowledge (derived from culture); controlled, abstract processing; and procedural plans for coping with a health problem. The other is primarily emotional, a concrete, automatic system that involves episodic memories (derived from personal experiences) and perceptual, experiential processing such as somatic sensations, feelings of fear, and impulsive coping responses. The two pathways interact as the individual responds to a health and illness experience. The interaction of the two pathways has important implications for the processing of symptoms and sensations. Emotions are thought, in essence, to create or influence the climate in which symptoms are processed. They can both influence symptom interpretation and generate additional symptoms, which, when incorporated into the person's representation, influence coping and appraisal. Internal and external cues of health threat, therefore, activate conceptual, reasoned efforts to understand and control the health threat. They also elicit concrete, emotional responses and efforts to control these emotions (Leventhal et al., 1997; Leventhal et al., 1984). Motivation to regulate or minimize health-related risks and management strategies selected are consistent with the individual's integrated perceptions of the risk.

Stages in Processing

The processing system operates in three stages: illness representation, coping, and appraisal (Leventhal et al., 1984).

Illness Representation

The first stage creates the definition or the representation of the health threat and the emotion accompanying it. When an individual experiences a health threat, a process of interpretation is brought into play as the individual seeks an understandable explanation. Information is used by the individual to organize, analyze, and interpret the health threat and give it meaning. Individuals are thought to create mental representations of the health threat based on concrete and abstract sources of information available to them. Sources of information include internal, already assimilated general knowledge garnered from sociocultural exposures and past personal

experiences and memories, from the external social environment (e.g., significant others or authoritative sources such as health professionals) and media, or the somatic or symptomatic experience currently being experienced by the individual as well as knowledge of prior illness experiences and effectiveness of management strategies used in those circumstances. Ultimately, it is the perception and interpretation of the different sources of information that lead to the construction of an illness representation. Illness representations have five basic dimensions:

- *Identity:* The label or name given to an illness or condition and the type, location, extent, and feel of the symptoms thought to accompany it.

- *Timeline:* The expected time frame or expected duration of the illness or condition (e.g., whether it is acute, chronic, or cyclic).

- *Cause:* The individual's ideas about the cause of the illness or condition.

- *Controllability:* The individual's perceptions about whether the illness or condition can be controlled or cured and to what extent this is dependent on self or professional intervention.

- *Consequences:* The anticipated ramifications of the illness or condition (e.g., short and long-term outcomes of the illness in terms of personal experiences, economic hardship, or emotional upheaval).

Coping Procedures/Self-Management

How the individual integrates and makes sense of available information about a symptom or health threat, the illness representation, shapes the selection and performance of a coping procedure or management plan. Although an array of options may be available to the individual, one's representation guides how one will act. For example, a symptom interpreted as mild and self-limiting would be acted upon differently than a symptom interpreted as life-threatening and unmanageable without immediate medical intervention.

Appraisal

In the third stage, appraisal, the patient evaluates the efficacy of the coping or management procedure. Once executed, the individual appraises the outcome. Of primary concern is whether or not coping or management procedures have moved the individual closer or farther from desired outcomes formed in response to a health threat. Information from the appraisal stage feeds back into the prior stages. If the patient appraises a particular coping procedure as being ineffective, then this might result in selection of an alternative coping strategy and/or modification of the illness representation.

Thus, the processing system is dynamic, with continuous, recursive feedback among the stages. As individuals obtain new information and evaluate their attempts to manage or cope with an illness, the underlying memory structures are reconstructed and new representations are formed. Illness representations are in effect cumulative and the patient's treatment preferences and coping and management strategies as well as appraisal emerge over time.

Hierarchical Processing

The information processing system is hierarchical, operating at multiple levels ranging from a very simple concrete, experiential level of processing to a highly abstract level (Diefenbach & Leventhal, 1996). The simplest level of processing includes automatic mechanisms that make use of concrete stimulus features, while the most abstract levels make use of conceptual processes such as language, judgment, and synthesis of information.

Inconsistencies can occur between concrete and abstract aspects of an illness experience. For example, a patient may be told that a treatment such as antiretroviral therapy is killing the virus and improving chances for survival, but the patient may actually feel worse because of medication side effects. The abstract information that the patient's condition is improving is inconsistent with the concrete experience the patient is having connected with the therapeutic side effects. Depending on his or her interpretation of this discrepancy, the patient may then alter his or her coping strategies accordingly to achieve greater consistency (e.g., skip doses or stop taking the medication) (Leventhal et al., 1984). This would thus account, in part, for differences in the weightings or priorities of patients in contrast to health professionals.

Use and Testing of the CSM

A considerable amount of research conducted over the past two decades has been guided by precepts of the CSM. The research has enhanced our understanding of the structure of illness representations, factors that influence differences within and across different populations, and the role of illness perceptions in illness coping and self-management behaviors and health outcomes. The model and supporting evidence base is also being used increasingly to guide the development of interventions to improve health outcomes.

Illness Representation

Early work of Leventhal and colleagues suggested a consistent pattern to the way individuals' perceptions of illness are structured (Leventhal & Nerenz, 1982; Leventhal et al., 1984). The five common dimensions (*identity, timeline, cause, controllability*, and *consequences*) were identified through this and subsequent research examining individuals' descriptions of how they think about their illness (see Hagger & Orbell, 2003; Lau & Hartman, 1983; Scharloo & Kaptein, 1997; Skelton & Croyle, 1991). In the years since, researchers have explored the dimensional structure of illness representation across a range of diagnoses and population groups. This has included, for example, representations of HIV (Reynolds et al., 2009; Sacajiu et al., 2007), schizophrenia (Watson et al., 2006), myocardial infarction (Petrie & Weinman, 1997), genetic risk for cardiovascular disease (Meulenkamp et al., 2008), heart failure (Molloy et al., 2009), diabetes (Hamera et al., 1988; Hampson, 1997; Harvey & Lawson, 2009; Nouwen, Law, Hussain, McGovern, & Napier, 2009), dementia (Hamilton-West, Milne, Chenery, & Tilbrook, 2010), trauma (Chaboyer, Lee, Wallis, Gillespie, & Jones, 2010), chronic fatigue syndrome (Moss-Morris, 1997), cancer and pain (Jenson & Karoly, 1991a, 1991b; Morley & Wilkinson, 1995; Orbell et al., 2008; Rozema, Völlink, & Lechner, 2009; S. E. Ward, Wang, Serlin, Peterson, & Murray, 2009), and among persons representing different cultural and socioeconomic circumstances and age groups (e.g., Chen, Tsai, & Lee, 2009; Lam et al., 2008; Meulenkamp et al., 2008; Reynolds et al., 2009; Sacajiu et al., 2007; E. C. Ward, Clark, & Heidrich, 2009).

While studies exploring the illness representations of various population groups vary in emphasis, methodology, and terminology, it has been repeatedly shown that people do hold cognitive representations of their illnesses. There is also substantial support for the five basic cognitive dimensions of illness representation as proposed by Leventhal and colleagues (see Hagger & Orbell, 2003; Lau & Hartman, 1983; Scharloo & Kaptein, 1997; Skelton & Croyle, 1991). Research has shown a pattern of correlations between the dimensions that support the construct and discriminant validity of the dimensions and are indicative of a logical pattern of relationships. For example, persons who perceive an illness as being highly symptomatic (strong illness identity) are more apt to view the illness as uncontrollable, chronic, and having serious consequences for their life (Hagger & Orbell, 2003; Weinman, Petrie, Moss-Morris, & Horne, 1996). Advances in the measurement of illness representation, notably those provided by the development of the Illness Perception Questionnaire (IPQ) (Weinman et al., 1996) (described in detail in *Measurement* section), have been instrumental in furthering the exploration and understanding of the relationship between dimensions of illness representation, as well as how differences in illness representation may vary within and across different types of illnesses and population groups (Petrie, Jago, & Devich, 2007).

The IPQ has also accelerated research informing areas for refinement and additional study. This has included, for example, further differentiation of the illness representation dimensions and relevant processes (Leventhal et al., 1997; Weinman & Petrie, 1997) and informed a revision of the IPQ. The revised instrument, the IPQ–R, (Moss-Morris et al., 2002) broadened the scope of the original IPQ to include an assessment of *illness coherence* and *emotional representations*. The reciprocal influences of emotions and cognitions in the context of an illness threat are an integral feature of the CSM. Consistent with the CSM research in general, the emotional regulation arm was not taken into account in the original version of the IPQ. However, advances in emotion regulation research over the past decade have highlighted the importance of emotional processing and underscored advantages offered by the CSM for furthering an understanding of emotional regulation in the context of illness (see Cameron & Jago, 2008).

In other work, researchers are exploring how past experiences, personal attributes, and the social context may influence an individual's illness perceptions. In keeping with precepts of the CSM, it has been shown that illness representations vary widely among individuals. Even persons living with the same illness may have very disparate views (e.g., perceptions regarding severity of consequences). Emerging research demonstrates how the differences in illness representation may be a function of a variety of factors as illustrated in the following examples.

Age, especially older age, may account for differences in illness representations, especially attribution of symptoms to aging (Gump et al., 2001; Prohaska, Keller, Leventhal, & Leventhal, 1987). Gump and colleagues (2001) found that older adults were more likely to identify "old age" as the primary reason surgical intervention was needed as compared to other factors such as lifestyle or physiologic changes, and the older participants were significantly more likely to believe they had no control over the disease in contrast to younger participants.

Other research has highlighted the influence of experience with an illness. In a study exploring "lay" perceptions regarding depression, schizophrenia, cancer, hypertension, and influenza, Godoy-Izquierdo, López-Chicheri, López-Torrecillas, Vétez, & Godoy (2007) found that persons who had experience with an illness (had suffered from it or lived with an ill relative) had significantly different representations than those who had not. Further, in keeping with the understanding that CSM processes are dynamic and recursive (Diefenbach & Leventhal, 1996), research indicates that representations will vary in accordance with an individual's experience living with a health condition over time. For example, a longitudinal study of patients hospitalized for traumatic injury (Lee, Chaboyer, & Wallis, 2010) showed that perceptions regarding the consequences of the injury were more severe several months following hospitalization as patients continued to experience significant ill health and became aware of the enduring nature of their acquired condition. Similarly, Fischer and colleagues (2010) observed changes over time among patients with a diagnosis of COPD; longer time since diagnosis was associated with perceptions corresponding with a chronic illness model. However, perceptions were also influenced by positive experiences with a treatment program. After completing a rehabilitation program, patients who were more confident that their participation in the program led to achievement of desired outcomes were less concerned about adverse consequences of the illness and had stronger perceptions of personal controllability. Other research indicates that representations of a chronic illness can remain fairly constant over time during periods of relative stability (e.g., Rutter & Rutter, 2007).

Researchers have also demonstrated how specific aspects of the social context may account for variations in illness representations, such as the illness representations of family members and health care providers. Studies comparing spousal representations have shown that both the degree of congruence and the extent to which the perceptions are positively or negatively valenced are influential. Sterba and colleagues (2008) compared the representations of women living with rheumatoid arthritis with those of their partner and found that similar, optimistic spousal representations were associated with the better psychological adjustment and functioning outcomes. When spousal representations differed, better outcomes were observed among women whose husbands overestimated, rather than underestimated, the consequences of living with arthritis. Likewise, positive spousal perceptions were associated with better outcomes following myocardial infarction (Figueiras & Weinman, 2003).

Studies examining the illness representations of children show that they tend to be highly correlated with their parents' representations. The relationship is upheld regardless of their degree of correspondence to medical recommendations (Diefenbach & Leventhal, 1996; Yoos, Kitzman, McMullen, & Sidora, 2003), which has implications for both the shorter- and longer-term welfare of the child. A substantial body of research demonstrates the significance of illness perceptions with respect to health behavior choices and use of health care services; however, the perceptions are often not commensurate with pertinent, evidence-based knowledge and optimal health outcomes (Godoy-Izquierdo et al., 2007; Royer & Zahner, 2009; Yoos et al., 2007). The illness perceptions of the general population were examined in relation to primary health care professionals in a study focusing on arterial hypertension

(van-der Hofstadt, Rodríguez-Marín, Quiles, Mira, & Sitges, 2003). In contrast to the representations of health professionals (nurses and physicians), the lay representations reflected a generally poor understanding of scientifically based medical knowledge. On the other hand, the representations of the health professional reflected a generally poor understanding of knowledge pertaining to the subjective aspects of illness experiences (e.g., symptoms, quality of life, uncertainty), with the exception of nurses who held perceptions that were similar to the general public in this regard.

The influence of the broader sociocultural context and corresponding social norms, roles, and demands have also been examined. Research has shown that representations differ by gender. Grace and colleagues (2005) found that women were more likely to attribute cardiovascular disease to personally controllable causes than men and to perceive the disease as chronic, serious, and difficult to treat. Further, gender-based differences in illness representation may be associated with variations observed in coping response. In a study of depression (Kelly, Sereika, Battista, & Brown, 2007), women were more likely to use emotionally focused coping while men engaged in more avoidance coping. Further, while greater perceived control was associated with adaptive coping and fewer or less serious perceived consequences were associated with greater problem solving among women, this relationship was not seen among men.

Other research has shown that representations may vary by country of origin. For example, in one U.S. sample, the European American participants identified "unknown factors" as the primary cause of depression and "impact on paid work" as the main consequence, while the South Asian immigrant participants identified "stressors" as the primary cause and "domestic role failure" as the main consequence (Karasz, 2005). Another large, multisite study showed differences in illness representations of HIV by country which were associated with frequency and perceived effectiveness of self-care (Reynolds et al., 2009). Sociocultural influences are also evident in research of illness-related stigma. For example, illnesses with high levels of social stigma, such as HIV, are associated with more negative illness representations of HIV, especially consequences which are viewed as more serious and causes which suggest culpability of the individual (Mak et al., 2006). These and findings discussed above have important implications for health outcomes.

Illness Representation and Health Outcomes

In addition to the considerable body of research investigating the content, structure, and determinants of illness representations, a number of studies have focused on the relationship between illness representations and health outcomes. In keeping with precepts of the CSM, illness representations have been linked with important adaptive psychological and behavioral processes and outcomes in a range of acute and chronic illnesses and conditions. The work has been instrumental in furthering an understanding of how individuals self-regulate illness, particularly how illness cognitions affect health behaviors that individuals employ in response to an illness threat ("coping responses" or "coping procedures"). Indeed, the considerable body of research that has amassed provides compelling evidence supporting a relationship between illness representations, coping behaviors, and importantly, illness outcomes.

Early research found the propensity to seek care was more likely for people who held strong representations of "identity" and "cure/control" (Lau, Bernard, & Hartman, 1989). Studies conducted since have further established the prominence of perceptions about the identity of an illness and accompanying symptoms in relation to care-seeking behavior (Burgess et al., 2006; Hunter, Grunfeld, & Ramirez, 2003). For example, Burgess and collegaues (2006) found symptoms commonly and clearly associated with breast cancer, such as a breast lump, were predictive of quicker care seeking. The precision or accuracy of one's interpretation of their symptoms, the illness identity, may be particularly influential, and it should be noted, are potentially highly significant, if successful care-seeking outcomes are time-dependent. This was seen in a study of care-seeking behavior during the acute phase of myocardial infarction (MI) (Petrie & Weinman, 1997); more expeditious care seeking (less delay) was associated with greater family history and correspondence between the symptoms experienced and classic symptoms regarded as critical (e.g., breathlessness, pain). On the other hand, ambiguous symptoms or an inaccurate illness identity may delay appropriate care seeking. In another MI care-seeking study, delay among the sample of lower-income urban women who delayed seeking care was related to misattribution of symptoms experienced to general poor health or minor complaints such as chest cold (Harralson, 2007).

Care seeking has also been associated with other dimensions of illness representation. Just as the individual's correct labeling of symptoms is important, so too are severity, duration, and perceptions about the value and necessity of the available care (Prohaska et al., 1987). A study of young adults with mental health problems showed that greater care seeking was associated with perceptions that treatment could help, help is necessary, cause is internal, and that one cannot manage it oneself, while perceptions that the timeline is cyclic and the mental health difficulties are under personal control were associated with less health care-seeking (Vanheusden et al., 2009). Likewise, Y. J. Wong, Tran, Kim, Van Horne Kerne & Calfa (2010) found that care seeking for depression was more likely when the cause was perceived as outside of one's personal control, due to biological and situational factors. In other research of persons across the lifespan, changes in patterns of care seeking are observed as people age (Leventhal & Crouch, 1997; Prohaska et al., 1987). These changes may be a reflection of age-related modifications in the way that symptoms are perceived and evaluated as people age. While modifications in perceptions may tend toward more benign attributions and possible delays in care seeking, an increased sense of vulnerability combined with the need to reduce health risks and conserve personal resources tends to move older adults toward higher levels of preventative behavior and better adherence to treatment (Leventhal & Crouch, 1997; Prohaska et al., 1987).

Illness representations have also been associated with a number of self-management behaviors, especially adherence to treatment. Early research established symptom perceptions as powerful determinants of adherence behaviors (Baumann & Leventhal, 1985; Hamera et al., 1988) and showed that patients' interpretation of symptoms, or in some cases the absence of symptoms, may influence adherence in several ways. For example, a patient may stop taking medication if she erroneously interprets the absence of symptoms as an indication that her condition or illness is getting better, or she may rely on the presence of certain symptoms to gauge whether or not to take a prescribed medication (e.g., antihypertensive), even if from a medical perspective the symptom fluctuation has little relationship to the illness for which the medication has been ordered. The side effects of medication can also influence adherence if they are interpreted by the patient as making his condition worse or are regarded by the patient as more problematic than the symptoms of the condition when untreated (Reynolds, 2003; W. K. T. Wong & Ussher, 2008). A prominent line of research conducted by Horne and others (Gonzalez et al., 2007; Horne, 1997; Horne & Weinman, 2002; Horne et al., 2004; Horne, Cooper, Gellaitry, Date, & Fisher, 2007) has also shown that patients' beliefs about the necessity and efficacy of medications may be tempered by their concerns about the potential for harm. High perceived necessity and low concern for adverse effects is associated with better adherence, while greater concern for harm is related to nonadherence.

Much of the research conducted to date has focused on the illness representation of persons living with the condition in relation to health behavior outcomes. However, attention has also been directed to how people perceive a condition they do not have, with the implicit aim of establishing the applicability of the CSM in primary prevention. For example, adolescents' illness representations of sexually transmitted infections (STIs) were explored (Royer, 2008; Royer & Zahner, 2009) and several misconceptions identified: many adolescents did not seem to know of the severe consequences of chlamydia, and many believed that no STI could be transmitted via oral sex. Whilst this research did not attempt to connect these beliefs to risk or testing behaviors, the authors concluded the framework is of potential use in this area. In another study, Sullivan et al. (2010) found that representations were associated with preventive health behaviors including screening for colon cancer, nonsmoking for lung cancer, and sunscreen use in relation to skin cancer. Likewise, Cameron (2008) found that beliefs about identity and timeline of skin cancer risk were linked to worry, and a more vivid and emotionally charged type of representation was associated with greater intentions and subsequent protective behaviors, such as skin self-examination.

Application of the CSM with respect to risk reduction or secondary prevention has also been explored among persons who are already living with an illness diagnosis. Research has demonstrated the salience of illness representations in relation to risk reduction in some studies, such as motivation to quit smoking while living with a chronic illness such as cervical cancer (Hall, Weinman, & Marteau, 2004) or HIV (Reynolds, Neidig, & Wewers, 2004), but less so in others. For example, illness representations only weakly predicted smoking, exercise, diet, alcohol use, and medication adherence in a study of patients with chronic heart disease (Byrne, Walsh, & Murphy, 2005).

Researchers have also sought to extend understanding of the CSM processes by examining illness representations, not only in relation to coping response, but to health-related outcomes as well. Illness representations have, for example, been studied in relation to physical function and disability, depression, anxiety, quality of life, and well-being (Evans & Norman, 2009; Kaptein et al., 2006, 2008). The mechanism by which illness representations influence outcomes appears to be only partly explained by their influence on coping response. Findings indicate that outcomes may be influenced directly by illness representations as well. Rozema, Völlink, and Lechner (2009) found that patients who viewed their illness as chronic, uncontrollable, and having serious symptoms and consequences reported worse physical and mental health than those who believed the opposite. Regression analysis showed that, after controlling for external variables, identity and consequences explained 57% of variance in physical health, whereas emotional illness representation and treatment control explained 47% of variance in mental health. In another study, researchers examined "illness helplessness," a cluster of illness representations of serious consequences with poor treatment and personal control, in relationship to health outcomes in patients with cardiac problems. Illness helplessness was associated with emotional well-being and physical functioning outcomes, and shown to have an indirect negative effect through the coping response of wishful thinking (Karademas & Hondronikola, 2010).

Taken together, a substantial body of work demonstrates that illness representations influence coping mechanisms. Systematic examination of findings across studies has identified representations salient in moving an individual toward particular coping action. A review of 101 studies published between 1985 and 1995 by Scharloo and Kaptein (1997) showed that favorable outcomes were associated with: (1) higher scores on "internal control," (2) higher accuracy ratings on "identity" and "causes," (3) a belief that the illness will be intermittent or discontinuous, and (4) a low level of perceived disability or seriousness of the illness. Similarly, a meta-analysis of 45 studies conducted by Hagger and Orbell (2003) showed better coping and health outcomes were associated with higher perceived control, while unfavorable coping and health outcomes were related to perceptions of the illness as highly symptomatic, a chronic timeline, and serious consequences. Recent analyses conducted by Skinner and colleagues (2010) highlight cluster analysis of illness representations as a potentially powerful approach for furthering an understanding of patterns of coping response and health outcomes. This, and other evidence demonstrating predictable relationships between different illness perceptions or clusters of illness perceptions and coping and health outcomes, advances knowledge of self-regulatory processes and provides direction for CSM-based interventions.

CSM-Based Interventions

The strength of findings from research examining illness representations in relation to health behaviors and outcomes suggests the CSM may provide a fertile guide for development of interventions to enhance appropriate health and illness management and reduce the impact of disease. Indeed, a growing number of interventions based on the model are being developed including interventions designed to enhance management of pain and anxiety, medication adherence, cardiac rehabilitation attendance, and diabetes self-management among others.

Ward, Donovan, and colleagues have developed an intervention based on the CSM to address cancer pain, which is often unnecessarily undertreated and distressing to patients because of their unwarranted beliefs about pain as uncontrollable and analgesics becoming addictive (Donovan & Ward, 2001). The face-to-face intervention is delivered by advanced practice nurses who first assess the patients' representations, explore inaccurate representations, and discuss the concerns and misrepresentations with the goal of modifying

these and pain medication use behaviors. Findings to date demonstrate that the intervention is feasible, acceptable, and improves self-reported use of pain medication and confidence to discuss pain and pain management. Ongoing research seeks to establish the intervention's effect on perceived pain, functional status, and objective indicators of appropriate pain medication use.

Other CSM-based interventions have been designed to improve health outcomes following a cardiac event. Petrie and colleagues (2002) conducted a randomized controlled trial to examine whether a brief hospital intervention designed to alter patients' perceptions about their myocardial infarction (MI) would result in a better recovery and reduced disability in comparison to usual care. Patients' illness perceptions were significantly altered by the intervention. Although attendance at cardiac rehabilitation did not improve significantly, patients in the intervention group reported they were better prepared for leaving hospital, returned to work faster, and reported a significantly lower rate of angina symptoms at the 3-month follow-up.

Broadbent, Ellis, Thomas, Gamble, and Petrie (2009) later tested a brief in-hospital illness perception intervention for MI patients delivered in three half-hour patient sessions and one half-hour patient-and-spouse session. Guided discussion regarding patient and spouse perceptions about the MI, patient education to correct misconceptions, and information and planning for appropriate rehabilitation activities were included. Findings were similar to the earlier study. At discharge, there were significant changes in the illness perceptions in intervention group and higher perceived understanding of their condition, a better understanding of the information given in hospital, higher intentions to attend cardiac rehabilitation classes, lower anxiety about returning to work, greater increases in exercise, and fewer phone calls were made to their general practitioner about their heart condition at follow-up. The intervention group also returned to work faster than the control group.

Several self-management interventions have also been based on the CSM. In one trial, patients with diabetes benefitted from a group education program addressing beliefs, including illness representations, about health and condition management (Davies et al., 2008). Findings showed improvements in health behaviors (weight loss and smoking cessation) and health beliefs, particularly the patient's own role in causing and controlling their diabetes. A CSM-based self-management intervention designed to improve HIV medication adherence has also shown improvements in both adherence behavior and health outcomes (HIV-1 RNA) in two separate clinical trials (Reynolds, Alonzo, & Nagaraja, 2008; Reynolds et al., 2010). In another study described above (Skinner et al., 2010), the cluster analysis of data from an intervention trial showed that patients' patterns of responding to illness could be predicted by illness representations, suggesting a potentially useful way of identifying groups of patients in need of similar intervention.

Taken together, CSM-based interventions tested to date show promise. Findings suggest that illness representations may be modified to effect positive, albeit modest, improvements in health behaviors and outcomes. An important element to note when considering CSM-informed interventions is that many address illness representations (the cognitive pathway) without consideration of emotional representations. Further, some of the interventions include multiple components, including goal setting and action planning, which are specific coping behaviors themselves, making it difficult to identify the active ingredient of the intervention. Further intervention work is warranted that integrates more features of the model and uses methods that allow for elucidation of the mechanism of action. Pertinent to these objectives, Leventhal and colleagues have recently outlined important theoretical and methodological considerations when using the CSM to design interventions for prevention and management of chronic illness which are being examined in their ongoing work (see McAndrew et al., 2008).

MEASUREMENT

Different measurement approaches have been used to assess illness representation. Much of the early research used semi-structured or open-ended interviews to elicit patients' illness representations. Several different instruments were used as well, many specific to a particular illness and dimension of illness representation (Leventhal & Nerenz, 1985; Scharloo & Kaptein, 1997; Weinman et al., 1996). While this work was productive, it was often time consuming and produced large variations in the quantity and quality of response (Weinman et al., 1996). Further, several of the measures were not theoretically derived and, in some cases, inconsistent with the CSM. Nevertheless, the major theoretical and empiric contributions and potential demonstrated by this body of work stimulated Weinman and colleagues (1996) to develop the Illness Perception Questionnaire (IPQ). The explicit aim was to produce a questionnaire that was theoretically based and conceptually congruent with the CSM, psychometrically sound, but also flexible enough to be used to assess representations of different population groups and illnesses.

In keeping with these objectives, the Illness Perception Questionnaire (IPQ) (Weinman et al., 1996) enables researchers to assess each of the five cognitive representations of illness as described by Leventhal et al. (Diefenbach & Leventhal, 1996; Leventhal, 1986; Leventhal & Cameron, 1987; Leventhal et al., 1984, 1992, 1997) across population groups and lends itself to the study of interactions among the variables. The instrument consists of five subscales, one for each of the attributes (identity, timeline, cause, cure-control, and consequences). Identity is measured using a list of 15 symptoms. Timeline, cause, cure-control, and consequences are measured using a 34-item, Likert-type scale.

Derivatives of the IPQ include a revised version of the IPQ, the IPQ–R (Moss-Morris et al., 2002), and the Brief-IPQ (Broadbent et al., 2006). The IPQ has also recently been adapted to assess spouses' illness perceptions (Sterba & DeVellis, 2009). The IPQ–R was developed to improve the measurement properties of the IPQ as the timeline dimension was found to have less than desirable internal consistency and the cure-control scale loads on two factors. In the IPQ–R, the control dimension is split into personal control and treatment control. It also incorporates a cyclical time dimension, emotional representation, and overall comprehension of illness (Moss-Morris et al., 2002). The measure is long, however, making it difficult to use in some settings (see Table 19.1). The brief IPQ (Broadbent et al., 2006) was developed to provide a rapid assessment of illness perceptions. It provides a more appropriate tool for very ill patients or when there is limited time for assessment. Studies and reviews comparing the reliability and validity of this measure and others show favorable psychometric properties (Coutu et al., 2008; Hagger & Orbell, 2005).

Table 19.1 Selected CSM-Based Measures

Measure	Aim	CSM dimensions	Items	IC*	IR**	Languages
Illness Perception Questionnaire (IPQ) Weinman et al., 1996	First CSM-based, psychometrically sound measure of the five illness representation dimensions	Identity, Causes, Consequences, Cure-Control, Timeline	38	.73–.82		English, French, Italian, Norwegian, Romanian, Sinhalese (Sri Lankan), Samoan, Tongan
Illness Perception Questionnaire–Revised (IPQ–R) Moss-Morris et al., 2002	Modification of two of the original IPQ subscales and inclusion of new subscales	Identity, Causes, Consequences, Personal Control, Treatment Control, Timeline—acute/chronic, Timeline—cyclical, Illness Coherence, Emotional Representation	70	.79–.89	.46–.88	Chinese, Dutch, English, French, German, Greek, Hebrew, Hungarian, Italian, Icelandic, Norwegian, Persian, Portuguese, Slovenian, Spanish, Swedish, Turkish
Brief Illness Perception Questionnaire (B-IPQ) Broadbent, Petrie, Main, & Weinman, 2006	Rapid assessment of the cognitive and emotional representations of illness	Identity, Causes, Consequences, Personal Control, Treatment Control, Timeline, Coherence, Emotional Representation, Illness Concern	9		.42–.75	Chinese, Danish, Dutch, English, French, German, Greek, Gujarati, Hebrew, Hindi, Italian, Japanese, Norwegian, Persian, Portuguese, Polish, Samoan, Russian, Slovenian, Spanish, Thai, Tongan, Turkish
Barts Explanatory Model Inventory (BEMI) Rüdell, Bhui, & Priebe, 2009	Designed to capture culturally variable beliefs	Identity, Causes, Consequences, Cure-Control, Timeline, Treatment Distress	12 open-ended questions		< .81	Language used in interview
Survey of Illness Beliefs in Heart Failure (HF) Albert and Zeller, 2007	Designed to measure accuracy and certainty of beliefs about HF	Accuracy-Inaccuracy of HF Representations of Identity, Timeline, Consequences, Control	14	.73		English

(Continued)

Table 19.1 (Continued)

Measure	Aim	CSM dimensions	Items	IC*	IR**	Languages
Beliefs about Medicines Questionnaire (BMQ) Horne, Weinman, & Hankins, 1999	Measure of treatment representations	General Overuse, General Harm, Specific Necessity, Specific Concerns	14	.60–.86		English, Spanish
Asthma Illness Representation Scale (AIRS) Sidora-Arcoleo, Feldman, Serebrisky, & Spray, 2010	Measure of parental illness representations of their children's asthma	Nature of Asthma Symptoms, Facts About Asthma, Attitudes Toward Medication Use, Treatment Expectations, Emotional Aspects of Medication Use	37	.82		English, Spanish
Illness Cognition Questionnaire (ICQ) Evers et al., 2001	Assesses three ways of cognitively evaluating the stressful and aversive character of a chronic illness	Helplessness, Acceptance, Disease Benefits	18	.84–.91	r > .67	English, Spanish
Menopause Representations Questionnaire (MRQ) M. Hunter & O'Dea, 2001	Measures cognitive representations of menopause	Identity, Cause, Consequence, Cure-Control, Timeline	37	.60–.79	.54–.92	

* Internal Consistency

**Interrater Reliability

The IPQ instruments have been translated to several different languages and used to assess the illness representations of a variety of chronic illnesses and found to be internally consistent and reliable. The IPQ is now considered by most researchers as the measure of choice in CSM studies, and its widespread use in CSM research is credited with substantial advancement in the field (Hagger & Orbell, 2005).

Several other instruments with sound psychometric properties are also used in CSM research. Some have been developed to elicit illness representations of a particular diagnostic group. For example, the Personal Models of Diabetes Interview (Hampson, Glasgow, & Toobert, 1990) was designed to determine a wide range of beliefs of diabetic patients, including five components of illness representations. The Illness in Heart Failure Tool was developed by Albert and Zeller (2007) to measure the accuracy and certainty of illness beliefs with respect to heart failure. The Asthma Illness Representation Scale (AIRS) (Sidora-Arcoleo, Feldman, Serebrisky, & Spray, 2010) provides a structured assessment of the key components of asthma illness representations among pediatric and adolescent patients, while the Menopause Representation Questionnaire (MRQ) (M. Hunter & O'Dea, 2001) is a short questionnaire designed to assess women's cognitive representations of menopause.

The Beliefs about Medicines Questionnaire developed by Horne, Weinman, and Hankins (1999) extends the assessment of illness representations to representations of illness treatments that have been found important in relation to self-management behavior, namely medication adherence behavior. Another recently developed instrument, the Barts Explanatory Model Inventory (Rüdell, Bhui, & Priebe, 2009), was designed to provide a more culturally sensitive assessment of illness representations that captures culturally variable beliefs.

Other instruments are conceptually consistent with the CSM but not guided by the precepts in the model. For example, the Illness Cognition Questionnaire (ICQ) assesses illness cognitions across different chronic illnesses and shows both unfavorable and favorable ways to adjust to a chronic illness (Evers et al., 2001).

IMPLICATIONS FOR THEORY, PRACTICE, AND RESEARCH

Consistent with the emphasis of nursing, the focal point of the CSM is the patient. The model suggests that an understanding of patients' responses to health threats is obtained by understanding their perceptions or implicit models of the threats they face. Particular emphasis is placed on the significance of the patient's interpretation of symptoms, as well as on the individual as an active participant in the health care process.

The CSM provides a strong paradigm for integrating findings from diverse lines of research, and it can guide new research in nursing. The model has been used by nurses to guide exploration of a broad range of health and illness experiences such as self-care processes (Keller, Ward, & Baumann, 1989; Reynolds et al., 2008), cardiac delay (The Acute Myocardial Infarction Coping Model; Alonzo & Reynolds, 1998), recovery from illness episodes (Massey & Pesut, 1991), diabetic adherence (Hamera et al., 1988; O'Connell et al., 1984; O'Connell, Hamera, Schorfheide, & Guthrie, 1990), responses to diabetes (Newbern, 1990), functioning in schizophrenia (Hamera, Peterson, Handley, Plumlee, & Frank-Ragan, 1991), cancer and cancer therapies

(J. E. Johnson, 1996; Johnson, Fieler, Wlasowicz, Mitchell, & Jones, 1997; S. E. Ward, Leventhal, Easterling, Luchterhand, & Love, 1991; S. E. Ward et al., 2009), pressure ulcers (Sebern, 1996), genital herpes (Keller, Jadack, & Mims, 1991), and recovery from surgery (J. E. Johnson, Fuller, Endress, & Rice, 1978; Johnson, Rice, Fuller, & Endress 1978).

Although considerable support has been rendered for some of the major precepts of the model, this review of the literature raises some issues and limitations. First, there is support for the five cognitive dimensions of representation. However, there is growing awareness that other processes need to be incorporated and/or the current dimensions need further delineation (Horne, 1997; Leventhal et al., 1997; Weinman & Petrie, 1997). For example, in addition to assessing illness perceptions, there is a need to understand people's views about the treatment or advice they have received. Further, research shows that certain patterns of illness representations may be associated with better psychological and physical outcomes. A growing body of research identifies combinations of illness representations associated with coping behaviors and outcomes. While there is support for links between illness representations and coping behaviors, little data is available about how particular coping strategies are selected. The importance and role of emotional representations and types of appraisal processes that inform coping behaviors and their interaction with illness cognitions remain poorly understood. This knowledge is important to guide development of effective intervention strategies that need to consider the role of emotions.

The CSM has not been widely used to guide nursing practice explicitly, but several aspects appear to be used implicitly (e.g., Garvin, Huston, & Baker, 1992). Research by Johnson and colleagues (J. A. Johnson & King, 1985; J. E. Johnson, 1996; J. E. Johnson et al., 1997; J. E. Johnson, Lauver, & Nail, 1989; Johnson, Nail, Lauver, King, & Keys, 1988; Johnson, Rice, Fuller, & Endress, 1978; Leventhal & Johnson, 1983) provides a foundation for the development of preparatory information interventions in nursing. It has also been suggested that patients' implicit models should routinely be explored as part of providing information to patients and families (Keller et al., 1989; S. E. Ward, 1993; Yoos et al., 2007). This would enable delivery of information to patients that is congruent with, rather than antithetical to, the patients' own representations. Implicit belief systems may, however, be difficult to uncover because patients may not realize that they hold these beliefs or, if they are recognized, patients may hide them because they do not conform to medical knowledge (Lowery, 1993). Instruments designed to assess illness representations for research purposes may have clinical applicability.

Clearly, there is considerable complexity in illness representations that needs to be addressed further. Indeed, research testing the complete theory, including emotional representations and appraisals processes, is needed. Questions remain about the cognitive and emotional processes involved in people's representations of health and illness. Leventhal et al. (1997) has stressed the importance of enhancing an understanding of self-regulatory processes within the social and cultural contexts in which they occur. While a considerable number of studies conducted over the past decade have advanced an understanding, additional work is needed to elaborate the influence of social system variables.

Summary

The Common-Sense Model of illness representation provides a useful framework for broadening our understanding of the dynamic factors involved in the perceptions of health and illness behaviors. It has stimulated research and intervention design, with increasingly robust findings across different patient types, conditions, and cultures. Many features of the model as initially conceptualized have been supported empirically. The model is particularly useful for knowledge development in nursing, as it places emphasis on the role of symptoms and emotions surrounding a variety of health behaviors, and places emphasis on patients' perceptions of their illnesses. Findings from this exciting body of work offer direction for research and practice.

References

Albert, N. M., & Zeller, R. A. (2007). Development and testing of the Survey of Illness Beliefs in Heart Failure tool. *Progress in Cardiovascular Nursing, 22*(2), 63–71.

Alonzo, A. A. & Reynolds, N. R. (1998). The structure of emotions during acute myocardial infarction: A model of coping. *Social Science and Medicine, 46*, 1099–1110.

Bandura, A. (1996). Failures in self-regulation: Energy depletion or selective disengagement? *Psychological Inquiry, 7*(1), 20–24.

Baumann, L., & Leventhal, H. (1985). I can tell when my blood pressure is up: Can't I? *Health Psychology, 4*, 203–218.

Baumeister, R. F., & Heatherton, T. F. (1996). Self-regulation failure: An overview. *Psychological Inquiry, 7*(1), 1–15.

Broadbent, E., Ellis, C. J., Thomas, J., Gamble, G., & Petrie, K. J. (2009). Can an illness perception intervention reduce illness anxiety in spouses of myocardial infarction patients? A randomized controlled trial. *Journal of Psychosomatic Research, 67*(1), 11–15.

Broadbent, E., Petrie, K. J., Main, J., & Weinman, J. (2006). The brief illness perception questionnaire. *Journal of Psychosomatic Research, 60*(6), 631–637.

Burgess, C. C., Potts, H. W. W., Hamed, H., Bish, A. M., Hunter, M. S., Richards, M. A., et al. (2006). Why do older women delay presentation with breast cancer symptoms? *Psycho-Oncology, 15*(11), 962–968.

Byrne, M., Walsh, J., & Murphy, A. W. (2005). Secondary prevention of coronary heart disease: Patient beliefs and health-related behaviour. *Journal of Psychosomatic Research, 58*(5), 403–415.

Cameron, L. D. (2008). Illness risk representations and motivations to engage in protective behavior: The case of skin cancer risk. *Psychology and Health, 23*(1), 91–112.

Cameron, L. D., & Jago, L. (2008). Emotion regulation interventions: A common-sense model approach. *British Journal of Health Psychology, 13*, 215–231.

Cameron, L. D., & Leventhal, H. (1995). Vulnerability beliefs, symptom experiences, and the processing of health threat information: A self-regulatory perspective. *Journal of Applied Social Psychology, 25*, 1859–1883.

Carver, C. S., & Scheier, M. F. (1982). Control theory: A useful conceptual framework for personality, social, clinical, and health psychology. *Psychological Bulletin, 92*(1), 111–135.

Carver, C. S., & Scheier, M. F. (1996). Self-regulation and its failures. *Psychological Inquiry, 7*(1), 32–40.

Chaboyer, W., Lee, B. O., Wallis, M., Gillespie, B., & Jones, C. (2010). Illness representations predict health-related quality of life 6 months after hospital discharge in individuals with injury: A predictive survey. *Journal of Advanced Nursing, 66*, 2743–2750.

Chen, S., Tsai, J., & Lee, W. (2009). The impact of illness perception on adherence to therapeutic regimens of patients with hypertension in

Taiwan. *Journal of Clinical Nursing, 18*(15), 2234–2244.

Coutu, M. F., Durand, M. J., Baril, R., Labrecque, M. E., Ngomo, S., Côté, D., & Rouleau, A. (2008). A review of assessment tools of illness representations: Are these adapted for a work disability prevention context? *Journal of Occupational Rehabilitation, 18,* 347–361.

Davies, M. J., Heller, S., Skinner, T. C., Campbell, M. J., Carey, M. E., Cradock, S., et al. (2008). Effectiveness of the diabetes education and self management for ongoing and newly diagnosed (DESMOND) programme for people with newly diagnosed type 2 diabetes: Cluster randomised controlled trial. *British Medical Journal, 336*(7642), 491–495.

Diefenbach, M. A., & Leventhal, H. (1996). The common-sense model of illness representation: Theoretical and practical considerations. *Journal of Social Distress and the Homeless, 5,* 11–38.

Donovan, H. S., & Ward, S. (2001). A representational approach to patient education. *Journal of Nursing Scholarship: An Official Publication of Sigma Theta Tau International Honor Society of Nursing/Sigma Theta Tau, 33*(3), 211–216.

Evans, D., & Norman, P. (2009). Illness representations, coping and psychological adjustment to Parkinson's disease. *Psychology and Health, 24*(10), 1181–1196.

Evers, A., Kraaimaat, F., van Lankveld, W., Jongen, P., Jacobs, J. W., Bijlsma, J. W., et al. (2001). Beyond unfavorable thinking: The illness cognition questionnaire for chronic diseases. *Journal of Consulting and Clinical Psychology, 69,* 1026–1036.

Figueiras, M. J., & Weinman, J. (2003). Do similar patient and spouse perceptions of myocardial infarction predict recovery? *Psychology and Health, 18*(2), 201–216.

Fischer, M., Scharloo, M., Abbink, J., van 't Hul, A., van Ranst, D., Rudolphus, A., Weinman, J., Rabe, K., & Kaptein, A. A. (2010). The dynamics of illness perceptions: Testing assumptions of Leventhal's Common-Sense Model in a pulmonary rehabilitation setting. *British Journal of Health Psychology, 15,* 887–903.

Garvin, B. J., Huston, G. P., & Baker, C. F. (1992). Information used by nurses to prepare patients for a stressful event. *Applied Nursing Research, 5,* 158–163.

Godoy-Izquierdo, D., López-Chicheri, I., López-Torrecillas, F., Vélez, M., & Godoy, J. F. (2007). Contents of lay illness models dimensions for physical and mental diseases and implications for health professionals. *Patient Education and Counseling, 67*(1–2), 196–213.

Gonzalez, J. S., Penedo, F. J., Llabre, M. M., Durán, R. E., Antoni, M., Schneiderman, N., et al. (2007). Physical symptoms, beliefs about medications, negative mood, and long-term HIV Medication adherence. *Annals of Behavioral Medicine, 34*(1), 46–55.

Grace, S. L., Krepostman, S., Brooks, D., Arthur, H., Scholey, P., Suskin, N., et al. (2005). Illness perceptions among cardiac patients: Relation to depressive symptomatology and sex. *Journal of Psychosomatic Research, 59*(3), 153–160.

Gump, B. B., Matthews, K. A., Scheier, M. F., Schulz, R., Bridges, M. W., & Magovern, G. J. (2001). Illness representations according to age and effects on health behaviors following coronary artery bypass graft surgery. *Journal of the American Geriatrics Society, 49*(3), 284–289.

Hagger, M. S., & Orbell, S. (2003). A meta-analytic review of the Common-Sense Model of Illness Representations. *Psychology and Health, 18*(2), 141–184.

Hagger, M. S., & Orbell, S. (2005). A confirmatory factor analysis of the revised illness perception questionnaire (IPQ-R) in a cervical screening context. *Psychology and Health, 20*(2), 161–173.

Hall, S., Weinman, J., & Marteau, T. M. (2004). The motivating impact of informing women smokers of a link between smoking and cervical cancer: The role of coherence. *Health Psychology 23*(4), 419–424.

Hamera, E., Cassmeyer, V. O, Connell, K. A., Weldon, G. T., Knapp. T. M., & Kyner, J. L. (1988). Self-regulation in individuals with type II diabetes. *Nursing Research, 37*(6), 363–367.

Hamera, E. K., Peterson, K. A., Handley, S. M., Plumlee, A. A., & Frank-Ragan, E. (1991). Patient self-regulation and functioning in schizophrenia. *Hospital & Community Psychiatry, 42*(6), 630–631.

Hamilton-West, K. E., Milne, A. J., Chenery, A., & Tilbrook, C. (2010). Help-seeking in relation to signs of dementia: A pilot study to evaluate the utility of the Common-Sense Model of Illness Representations. *Psychology, Health & Medicine, 15,* 540–549.

Hampson, S. E. (1997). Illness representations and the self-management of diabetes. In K. J. Petrie & J. A. Weinman (Eds.), *Perceptions of health & illness* (pp. 323–349). Amsterdam, Netherlands: Harwood Academic Publishers.

Hampson, S. E., Glasgow, R. E., & Toobert, D. J. (1990). Personal models of diabetes and their relations to self-care activities. *Health Psychology, 9,* 632–646.

Harvey, J. N., & Lawson, V. L. (2009). The importance of health belief models in determining self-care behaviour in diabetes. *Diabetic Medicine, 26,* 5–13.

Harralson, T. L. (2007). Factors influencing delay in seeking treatment for acute ischemic symptoms among lower income, urban women. *Heart Lung, 36*(2), 96–104.

Horne, R. (1997). Representations of medication and treatment: Advances in theory and measurement. In K. J. Petrie and J. A. Weinman (Eds.) *Perceptions of health & illness.* Amsterdam, Netherlands: Harwood Academic Publishers.

Horne, R., Buick, D., Fisher, M., Leake, H., Cooper, V., & Weinman, J. (2004). Doubts about necessity and concerns about adverse effects: Identifying the types of beliefs that are associated with non-adherence to HAART. *International Journal of STD & AIDS, 15,* 38–44.

Horne, R., Cooper, V., Gellaitry, G., Date, H. L., & Fisher, M. (2007). Patients' perceptions of highly active antiretroviral therapy in relation to treatment uptake and adherence. *Journal of Acquired Immune Deficiency Syndromes, 45*(3), 337–341.

Horne, R., & Weinman, J. (2002). Self-regulation and self-management in asthma: Exploring the role of illness perceptions and treatment beliefs in explaining non-adherence to preventer medication. *Psychology and Health, 17*(1), 17–32.

Horne, R., Weinman, J., & Hankins, M. (1999). The Beliefs about Medicines Questionnaire: The development and evaluation of a new method for assessing the cognitive representation of medication. *Psychology and Health, 14,* 1–24.

Hunter, M. S., Grunfeld, E. A., & Ramirez, A. J. (2003). Help-seeking intentions for breast-cancer symptoms: A comparison of the self-regulation model and the theory of planned behaviour. *British Journal of Health Psychology, 8*(3), 319–333.

Hunter, M., & O'Dea, I. (2001). Cognitive appraisal of the menopause: The Menopause Representations Questionnaire (MRQ) *Psychology, Health & Medicine, 6,* 65–76.

Jensen, M. P., & Karoly, P. (1991a). Pain-specific beliefs, perceived symptom severity, and adjustment to chronic pain. *Clinical Journal of Pain, 8,* 123–130.

Jensen, M. P., & Karoly, P. (1991b). Control beliefs, coping efforts, and adjustment to chronic pain. *Journal of Consulting and Clinical Psychology, 59,* 431–438.

Johnson, J. A., & King, K. B. (1985). Influence of expectations about symptoms on delay in seeking treatment during myocardial infarction. *American Journal of Critical Care, 4*(1), 29–35.

Johnson, J. E. (1996). Coping with radiation therapy: Optimism and the effect of preparatory interventions. *Research in Nursing and Health, 19,* 2–12.

Johnson, J. E., Fieler, V. K., Wlasowicz, G. S., Mitchell, M. L., & Jones, L. S. (1997). The effects of nursing care guided by self-regulation theory on coping with radiation therapy. *Oncology Nursing Forum, 24*(6), 1041–1050.

Johnson, J. E., Fuller, S. S., Endress, M. P., & Rice, V. H. (1978). Altering patient's responses to surgery: An extension and replication. *Research in Nursing and Health, 1,* 111–121.

Johnson, J. E., Lauver, D. R., & Nail, L. M. (1989). Process of coping with radiation therapy. *Journal of Consulting and Clinical Psychology, 57,* 358–364.

Johnson, J. E., Nail, L. M., Lauver, D., King, K. B., & Keys, H. (1988). Reducing the negative impact of radiation therapy on functional status. *Cancer, 6*(1), 46–51.

Johnson, J. E., Rice, V. H., Fuller, S. S., & Endress, M. P. (1978). Sensory information, instruction in coping strategy, and recovery from surgery. *Research in Nursing & Health, 1,* 4–7.

Kaptein, A. A., Helder, D. I., Scharloo, M., Van Kempen, G. M. J., Weinman, J., Van Houwelingen, H. J. C., et al. (2006). Illness perceptions and coping explain well-being in patients with Huntington's disease. *Psychology and Health, 21*(4), 431–446.

Kaptein, A. A., Scharloo, M., Fischer, M. J., Snoei, L., Cameron, L. D., Sont, J. B., et al. (2008). Illness perceptions and COPD: An emerging field for COPD patient management. *Journal of Asthma, 45,* 625–629.

Karademas, E. C., & Hondronikola, I. (2010). The impact of illness acceptance and helplessness to subjective health, and their stability over time: A prospective study in a sample of cardiac patients. *Psychology and Health, 15*(3), 336–346.

Karasz, A. (2005). Cultural differences in conceptual models of depression. *Social Science & Medicine, 60,* 1625–1635.

Keller, M., Jadack, R., & Mims, F. (1991). Perceived stressors and coping responses in persons with recurrent genital herpes. *Research in Nursing and Health, 14,* 421–430.

Keller, M. L., Ward, S., & Baumann, L. J. (1989). Processes of self-care: Monitoring sensations and symptoms. *Advances in Nursing Science, 12,* 54–66.

Kelly, M. A. R., Sereika, S. M., Battista, D. R., & Brown, C. (2007). The relationship between beliefs about depression and coping strategies: gender differences. *British Journal of Clinical Psychology, 46*(Part 3), 315–332.

Lam, W. W. T., Tsuchiya, M., Chan, M., Chan, S. W. W., Or, A., & Fielding, R. (2008). Help-seeking patterns in Chinese women with symptoms of breast disease: a qualitative study. *Journal of Public Health, 31*(1), 59–68.

Lau, R. R., & Hartman, K. A. (1983). Common-sense representations of common illnesses. *Health Psychology, 2,* 167–185.

Lau, R., Bernard, T., & Hartman, K. (1989). Further exploration of common-sense representations of common illnesses. *Health Psychology, 2,* 195–219.

Lee, B.-O., Chaboyer, W., & Wallis, M. (2010). Illness representations in patients with traumatic injury: A longitudinal study. *Journal of Clinical Nursing, 19,* 556–563.

Leventhal, H. (1970). Findings and theory in the study of fear communications. In L. Berkowitz (Ed.), *Advances in experimental social psychology, Vol. V* (pp. 120–186). New York, NY: Academic Press.

Leventhal, H. (1986). Symptom reporting: A focus on process. In S. McHugh & T. M. Vallis (Eds.), *Illness behavior: A multidisciplinary model* (pp. 219–237). New York, NY: Plenum Press.

Leventhal, H., Benyamini, Y., Brownlee, S., Diefenbach, M., Leventhal, E. A., PatrickMiller, L., & Robitaille, C. (1997). Illness representations: Theoretical foundations. In K. J. Petrie & J. A. Weinman (Eds.), *Perceptions of health and illness: Current research and applications* (pp. 1945). Singapore: Harwood Academic Publishers.

Leventhal, H., Brissette, I., & Leventhal, E. A. (2003). The common-sense model of self-regulation of health and illness. In L. D. Cameron & H. Leventhal (Eds.), *The self-regulation of health and illness behaviour* (pp. 42–65). London, England: Routledge.

Leventhal, H., & Cameron, L. (1987). Behavioral theories and the problem of compliance. *Patient Education and Counseling, 10,* 117–138.

Leventhal, H., Diefenbach, M., & Leventhal, E. A. (1992). Illness cognition: Using common sense to understand treatment adherence and affect cognition interactions. *Cognitive Therapy and Research, 16,* 143–163.

Leventhal, E. A., & Crouch, M. (1997). Are there differences in perceptions of illness across the lifespan? In K. J. Petrie & J. A. Weinman (Eds.), *Perceptions of health & illness.* Netherlands: Harwood Academic Publishers.

Leventhal, H., & Johnson, J. E. (1983). Laboratory and field experimentation: Development of a theory of self-regulation. In P. J. Wooldridge, M. H. Schmitt, J. K. Skipper, et al. (Eds.), *Behavioral science and nursing theory.* St. Louis, MO: Mosby.

Leventhal, H., Meyer, D., & Nerenz, D. (1980). The common sense representation of illness danger. In S. Rachman (Ed.), *Medical psychology* (Vol. II, pp. 7–30), New York, NY: Pergamon Press.

Leventhal, H., & Nerenz, D. (1982). Representations on threat and the control of stress. In D. Meichenbaum & M. Jaremko (Eds.), *Stress prevention and management: A cognitive behavioral approach.* New York, NY: Plenum.

Leventhal, H., & Nerenz, D. (1985). The assessment of illness cognition. In P. Karoly (Ed.), *Measurement strategies in health psychology* (pp. 517–555). New York, NY: Wiley.

Leventhal, H. L., Nerenz, D. R., & Steele, D. J. (1984). Illness representations and coping with health threats. In A. Baum, S. E. Taylor, & J. E. Singer (Eds.), *Handbook of psychology and health* (pp. 219–252). Hillsdale, NJ: Lawrence Erlbaum.

Lowery, B. J. (1993). Response to "The Common Sense Model: An organizing framework for knowledge development in nursing." *Scholarly Inquiry for Nursing Practice: An International Journal, 7,* 91–94.

Mak, W. W. S., Mo, P. K. H., Cheung, R. Y. M., Woo, J., Cheung, F. M., & Lee, D. (2006). Comparative stigma of HIV/AIDS, SARS, and tuberculosis in Hong Kong. *Social Science & Medicine, 63*(7), 1912–1922.

Massey, J. A., & Pesut, D. J. (1991). Self-regulation strategies of adults. *Western Journal of Nursing Research, 13*(5), 627–634.

McAndrew, L. M., Musumeci-Szabó, T. J., Mora, P. A., Vileikyte, L., Burns, E., Halm, E. A., Leventhal, E. A., & Leventhal, H. (2008). Using the common sense model to design interventions for the prevention and management of chronic illness threats: From description to process. *British Journal of Health Psychology, 13,* 195–204.

Meulenkamp, T. M., Tibben, A., Mollema, E. D., van Langen, I. M., Wiegman, A., de Wert, G. M., et al. (2008). Predictive genetic testing for cardiovascular diseases: impact on carrier children. *American Journal of Medical Genetics. Part A, 146A*(24), 3136–3146.

Molloy, G. J., Gao, C., Johnston, D. W., Johnston, M., Witham, M. D., Struthers, A. D., & MMcMurdo, M. E. T. (2009). Adherence to angiotensin-converting-enzyme inhibitors and illness beliefs in older heart failure patients. *European Journal of Heart Failure: Journal of the Working Group on Heart Failure of the European Society of Cardiology, 11*(7), 715–720.

Morley, S., & Wilkinson, L. (1995). The pain beliefs and perceptions inventory: A British replication. *Pain, 61,* 427–433.

Moss-Morris, R. (1997). The role of illness cognitions and coping in the aetiology and maintenance of the chronic fatigue syndrome. In K. J. Petrie & J. Weinman (Eds.), *Perceptions of health and illness: Current research and applications* (pp. 411–439). London, England: Harwood Academic Publishers.

Moss-Morris, R., Weinman, J., Petrie, K. J., Horne, R., Cameron, L. D., & Buick, D. (2002). The

Revised Illness Perception Questionnaire (IPQ-R). *Psychology and Health, 17*(1), 1–16.

Newbern, V. B. (1990). Application of self-regulation theory to the year of denouement for an insulin dependent diabetic. *Holistic Nursing Practice, 5*(1), 36–44.

Nouwen, A., Law, G. U., Hussain, S., McGovern, S., & Napier, H. (2009). Comparison of the role of self-efficacy and illness representations in relation to dietary self-care and diabetes distress in adolescents with type 1 diabetes. *Psychology & Health, 24*(9), 1071–1084.

O'Connell, K. A., Hamera, E. K., Knapp, T. M., Cassmeyer, V. L., Eaks, G. A., & Fox, M. A. (1984). Symptom use and self-regulation in type II diabetes. *Advances in Nursing Science, 6*(3), 19–28.

O'Connell, K., Hamera, E., Schorfheide, A., & Guthrie, D. (1990). Symptom beliefs and actual blood glucose in type II diabetes. *Research in Nursing and Health, 13,* 145–151.

Orbell, S., O'Sullivan, I., Parker, R., Steele, B., Campbell, C., & Weller, D. (2008). Illness representations and coping following an abnormal colorectal cancer screening result. *Social Science & Medicine, 67*(9), 1465–1474.

Petrie, K. J., Cameron, L. D., Ellis, C. J., Buick, D., & Weinman, J. (2002). Changing illness perceptions after myocardial infarction: An early intervention randomized controlled trial. *Psychosomatic Medicine, 64,* 580–586.

Petrie, K. J., Jago, L. A., & Devich, D. A. (2007). The role of illness perceptions in patients with medical conditions. *Current Opinion in Psychiatry, 20,* 163–167.

Petrie, K. J., & Weinman, J. A. (1997). Illness representations and recovery from myocardial infarction. In K. J. Petrie & J. A. Weinman (Eds.), *Perceptions of health & illness* (pp. 441–463). Netherlands: Harwood Academic Publishers.

Prohaska, T. R., Keller, M. L., Leventhal, E. A., & Leventhal, H. (1987). Impact of symptoms and aging attribution on emotions and coping. *Health Psychology, 6,* 495–514.

Reynolds, N. R. (2003). The problem of antiretroviral adherence: A self-regulatory model for intervention. *AIDS Care, 15*(1), 117–124.

Reynolds, N. R., Alonzo, A.A., & Nagaraja, H.N. (2008). A telephone-delivered adherence intervention improves clinical outcomes. *AIDS 2008—XVII International AIDS Conference.* Abstract no. CDB0506.

Reynolds, N. R., Neidig, J. L., & Wewers, M. E. (2004). Illness representation and smoking behavior: a focus group study of HIV-positive men. *Journal of the Association of Nurses in AIDS Care, 15,* 37–47.

Reynolds, N. R., Eller, L. S., Nicholas, P. K., Corless, I. B., Kirksey, K., Heamilton, M. J., et al. (2009). HIV illness representation as a predictor of self-care management and health outcomes: A multi-site, cross-cultural study. *AIDS Behavior, 13*(2), 258–267.

Reynolds, N. R., Testa, M. A., Su, M., Chesney, M. A., Neidig, J. L., Frank, I., Smith, S., Ickovics, J., & Robbins, G. K. AIDS Clinical Trials Group 731 and 384 Teams (2008). Telephone support to improve antiretroviral medication adherence: A multisite, randomized controlled trial. *Journal of Acquired Immune Deficiency Syndromes, 47,* 62–68.

Royer, H. R. (2008). *Young women's representations of sexually transmitted infections and sexually transmitted infection testing* (Doctoral dissertation). University of Wisconsin–Madison. Available from ProQuest Dissertations and Theses database. (AAT 3314299)

Royer, H. R., & Zahner, S. J. (2009). Providers' experiences with young people's cognitive representations and emotions related to the prevention and treatment of sexually transmitted infections. *Public Health Nursing, 26*(2), 161–172.

Rozema, H., Völlink, T., & Lechner, L. (2009). The role of illness representations in coping and health of patients treated for breast cancer. *Psycho-Oncology, 18*(8), 849–857.

Rüdell, K., Bhui, K., & Priebe, S. (2009). Concept, development and application of a new mixed method assessment of cultural variations in illness perceptions: Barts Explanatory Model Inventory. *Journal of Health Psychology, 14,* 336–347.

Rutter, C. L., & Rutter, D. R. (2007). Longitudinal analysis of the illness representation model in patients with irritable bowel syndrome (IBS). *Journal of Health Psychology, 12*(1), 141–148.

Sacajiu, G., Fox, A., Ramos, M., Sohler, N., Heller, D., & Cunningham, C. (2007). The evolution of HIV illness representation among marginally housed persons. *AIDS Care, 19*(4), 539–545.

Scharloo, M., & Kaptein, A. (1997). Measurement of illness perceptions in patients with chronic somatic illnesses: A review. In K. J. Petrie & J. A. Weinman (Eds.), *Perceptions of health & illness.* Netherlands: Harwood Academic Publishers.

Sebern, M. D. (1996). Explication of the construct of shared care and the prevention of pressure ulcers in home health care. *Research in Nursing & Health, 19,* 183–192.

Sidora-Arcoleo, K., Feldman, J., Serebrisky, D., & Spray, A. (2010). Validation of the Asthma Illness Representation Scale (AIRS). *Journal of Asthma, 47,* 33–40.

Skelton, J. A., & Croyle, R. T. (Eds.). (1991). *Mental representation in health and illness.* New York, NY: Springer-Verlag.

Skinner, T. C., Carey, M. E., Cradock, S., Dallosso, H. M., Daly, H., Davies, M. J., et al. (2010). Comparison of illness representations dimensions and illness representation clusters in predicting outcomes in the first year following diagnosis of type 2 diabetes: Results from the DESMOND trial. *Psychology & Health, 26*(3), 321–335.

Sterba, K. R., & DeVellis, R. F. (2009). Developing a spouse version of the Illness Perception Questionnaire–Revised (IPQ–R) for husbands of women with rheumatoid arthritis. *Psychology & Health, 24*(4), 473–487.

Sterba, K. R., DeVellis, R. F., Lewis, M. A., DeVellis, B. M., Jordan, J. M., & Baucom, D. H. (2008). Effect of couple illness perception congruence on psychological adjustment in women with rheumatoid arthritis. *Health Psychology, 27*(2), 221–229.

Sullivan, H. W., Rutten, L. J. F., Hesse, B. W., Moser, R. P., Rothman, A. J., & McCaul, K. D. (2010). Lay representations of cancer prevention and early detection: Associations with prevention behaviors. *Preventing Chronic Disease, 7*(1), A14.

van-der Hofstadt, C. J., Rodríguez-Marín, J., Quiles, M. J., Mira, J. J., & Sitges, E. (2003). Illness representation of arterial hypertension in a sample of health professionals and the general public. *Psychology, Health & Medicine, 8*(1), 81–87.

Vanheusden, K., van der Ende, J., Mulder, C. L., van Lenthe, F. J., Verhulst, F. C., & Mackenbach, J. P. (2009). Beliefs about mental health problems and help-seeking behavior in Dutch young adults. *Social Psychiatry & Psychiatric Epidemiology, 44*(3), 239–246.

Ward, S. E. (1993). The common sense model: An organizing framework for knowledge development in nursing. *Scholarly Inquiry for Nursing Practice, 7*(2), 79–90.

Ward, E. C., Clark, L., & Heidrich, S. (2009). African American women's beliefs, coping behaviors, and barriers to seeking mental health services. *Qualitative Health Research, 19*(11), 1589–1601.

Ward, S., Leventhal, H., Easterling, D., Luchterhand, C., & Love, R. (1991). Social support, self-esteem, and communication in patients receiving chemotherapy. *Journal of Psychosocial Oncology, 9,* 95–116.

Ward, S. E., Wang, K. K., Serlin, R. C., Peterson, S. L., & Murray, M. E. (2009). A randomized trial of a tailored barriers intervention for Cancer Information Service (CIS) callers in pain. *Pain, 144,* 49–56.

Watson, P. W. B., Garety, P. A., Weinman, J., Dunn, G., Bebbington, P. E., Fowler, D., et al. (2006). Emotional dysfunction in schizophrenia spectrum psychosis: The role of illness perceptions. *Psychological Medicine, 36*(6), 761–770.

Weinman, J. A., & Petrie, K. J. (Eds). (1997). Perceptions of health and illness. *Perceptions of health & illness* (pp. 1–19). Netherlands: Harwood Academic Publishers.

Weinman, J., Petrie, K. J., Moss-Morris, R., & Horne, R. (1996). The Illness Perception Questionnaire: A new method for assessing illness perceptions. *Psychology and Health, 11,* 431–446.

Weinstein, N. D. (1993). Testing four competing theories of health-protective behavior. *Health Psychology, 12,* 324–333.

Wong, W. K. T., & Ussher, J. (2008). How do subjectively-constructed meanings ascribed to anti-HIV treatments affect treatment-adherent practice? *Qualitative Health Research, 18,* 458–468.

Wong, Y. J., Tran, K. K., Kim, S.-H., Van Horn Kerne, V., & Calfa, N. A. (2010). Asian Americans' lay beliefs about depression and professional help seeking. *Journal of Clinical Psychology, 66*(3), 317–332.

Yoos, H. L., Kitzman, H., McMullen, A., & Sidora, K. (2003). Symptom perception in childhood asthma: How accurate are children and their parents? *Journal of Asthma, 40*(1), 27–39.

Yoos, H. L., Kitzmann, H., Henderson, C., McMullen, A., Sidora-Arcoleo, K., Halterman, J. S., et al. (2007). The impact of the parental illness representation on disease management in childhood asthma. *Nursing Research, 56*(3), 167–174.

20

STRESS, SELF-EFFICACY, AND HEALTH

DEBRA SIELA AND ANN W. WIESEKE

With the rapidly evolving health care system and the growing emphasis on self-care, professional nurses are seeking theories that explain and predict initiation and maintenance of health behaviors that can be used to guide nursing practice. One construct that addresses the factors involved in initiation and maintenance of self-care behavior is self-efficacy (SE), derived from Bandura's broader social cognitive theory (SCT) (Bandura, 1977, 1986, 1989, 1997). SE is becoming widely recognized by nurses as a construct that has theoretical and practical application related to the initiation and maintenance of self-care health behaviors, including those related to stress and coping.

Searches in several electronic databases show that self-efficacy was first referenced in the nursing research literature in 1977. Since that time there have been almost 6,000 publications referenced. In the past 5 years, more than 1,400 publications or about 25% of the total cited self-efficacy as a keyword; most were research reports. Nurse researchers, in particular, have used self-efficacy, as defined by Bandura, more frequently in the past decade as evidenced by more than 500 studies. The Health Promotion Model, rooted in Bandura's SCT, recognizes the importance of cognitive-perceptual factors such as self-efficacy and modifying factors such personal characteristics that influence the occurrence of health-promoting behaviors. Both frameworks recognize the individual as self-determining in relation to health behaviors.

The first section of this chapter provides an overview of the SCT. The second contains a review of self-efficacy research literature. Research from both nursing and nonnursing disciplines is discussed. The third section describes the development of self-efficacy measures, and the last section discusses the implications of SE for nursing research and practice. The research is limited to that related to health behavior published in the past three decades (1980–2010). The majority of the studies reviewed have used descriptive and/or correlational designs rather than predictive or clinical trial designs.

SOCIAL COGNITIVE THEORY

Bandura refined social learning theory (SLT) to formulate a middle-range theory known as the social cognitive theory (SCT) as a framework for examining human motivations, thoughts, and actions. Social learning theory posits that people learn from one another via observation, imitation, and modeling. This theory has often been called a bridge between behaviorist and cognitive learning theories because it encompasses attention, memory, and motivation (Bandura, 1977).

Social cognitive theory is based on the premise that people learn by observing others. It involves understanding how human cognitions, actions, motivations, and emotions affect one another reciprocally. SCT asserts that people are self-reflective and self-regulative and can mold their environment because of these attributes. Through symbolic interactions, individuals create models of experience in their mental processes. The created models are then used to test hypothetical courses of action, to predict outcomes, and as a framework to communicate these experiences to others. People perform behaviors that are purposive or goal directed because they have a previous model based on their symbolizing capacity. People develop standards for behavior and evaluate behaviors against these standards. According to the SCT, individuals are able to analyze their own thoughts, experiences, and behaviors. When they use self-reflection, they create the cognitive base for self-regulation or control of subsequent behaviors (Bandura, 1986).

Self-Efficacy and Triadic Reciprocality

In 1989, Bandura broadened the principle of *reciprocal determinism* to that of *triadic* reciprocality. Triadic reciprocality added the interaction of inner personal factors to the previously conceptualized interaction of environmental and behavioral factors. Inner personal factors include cognition, emotion, and biological events. On the basis of triadic determinism, the original definition of *self-efficacy—one's belief in one's ability to perform a specific behavior or set of behaviors required to produce an outcome—was changed to include beliefs about the individual's capability to exercise control over their destinies* (Bandura, 1997, p. 8). Self-efficacy then referred to perceptions that initially evolved from the interactions of inner personal factors (particularly cognitive factors) with behavior, environmental events, and other inner personal factors. The three factors of environmental events, inner personal events, and behavior may not directly interact, and they may not affect each other simultaneously or with equal strength. People respond cognitively, behaviorally, and emotionally to environmental events. Through cognition, people exert control over (self-regulate) their behavior or emotions in response to events. Self-regulation involves self-appraisal of one's abilities. The process of self-appraisal leads to the development of efficacy expectations and outcome expectations that are synthesized into perceptions of self-efficacy that help to determine

whether an individual ultimately initiates or maintains a specific behavior or both. Self-efficacy, as noted previously, is determined by efficacy expectations and outcome expectations. *Efficacy expectations* are beliefs about one's ability to perform a given behavior that will produce an expected outcome. *Outcome expectations* are the beliefs that engaging in a certain behavior or behaviors will result in a specific outcome. See Figure 20.1 for a schematic of these relationships.

Dimensions of Efficacy Expectations

Efficacy expectations can be assessed on three dimensions: (a) magnitude, (b) strength, and (c) generality. Magnitude of efficacy expectations refers to the ordering of tasks by difficulty. People may have high efficacy expectations at lower levels of difficulty and lower efficacy expectations at higher levels of difficulty. Strength of efficacy expectations refers to a judgment of the certainty one has of the ability to perform a certain behavior. Most of the early research has measured only the strength dimension when assessing efficacy expectations (Holden, 1991; O'Leary, 1985; Strecher, DeVillis, Becker, & Rosenstock, 1986).

Generality of efficacy expectations refers to the extent to which efficacy expectations about a specific behavior and its related outcome generalize to other situations. Bandura (1986) initially proposed that self-efficacy beliefs were situation specific and were not generalizable. In 1991, however, Bandura broadened the beliefs, stating that generalization can occur if

Figure 20.1   Self-Efficacy

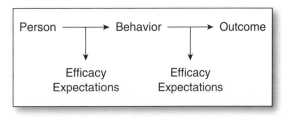

SOURCE: From A. Bandura, "Self-Efficacy: Toward a Unifying Theory of Behavioral Change." *Psychological Review, 84,* 191–215. Copyright © 1977 by the American Psychological Association. Reprinted with permission.

other situations are similar in social structure so that the development of skills and behaviors covary (Bandura, 1991).

Sources of Efficacy Information

Not only does the nursing profession need to recognize the dimensions of efficacy expectations but also the sources of efficacy information that must be acquired to support use of the theory for nursing practice. Efficacy expectations evolve from (a) cognitive appraisal of previous performance accomplishments, (b) vicarious experience, (c) verbal persuasion, and (d) autonomic arousal found within the personal, behavioral, and environmental factors of a situation (Bandura, 1982). High levels of efficacy expectations will not result in the performance of a desired behavior if deficits are present in an individual's perceived capabilities as identified through cognitive appraisal of information available. Given perceptions of adequate skills, resources, and incentives, efficacy expectations are a major determinant of behavior choice, amount of effort, and persistence with a behavior (Bandura, 1986).

Mastery, one source of efficacy information, also called "enactive attainment," originates from an individual's personal experiences. Mastery is attained after performing given behavior successfully numerous times. Many believe that this is the most persuasive of all sources of efficacy information in determining positive perceptions for performing a behavior.

Vicarious learning or modeling is another source of efficacy information. When people see others with similar attributes and situations performing a behavior successfully, they have a sense that they too may be able to perform the behavior successfully.

A third source of efficacy information is verbal persuasion. Verbal persuasion is the act of talking someone into believing that they can successfully perform a desired behavior. The effectiveness of this source depends on the perceived expertness, trustworthiness, and attractiveness of the source (Petty & Cacioppo, 1981). This source of efficacy information is not as effective for increasing efficacy expectations as mastery or vicarious experiences.

The physiological state of the individual (i.e., degree of autonomic arousal) is the fourth source of efficacy information. This information

about physiologic state includes that of somatic arousal in stressful situations, such as fear, fatigue, shortness of breath, and pain. People with high somatic arousal tend to have lower self-efficacy for performing certain behaviors (Bandura, 1986).

Summary of Social Cognitive Theory

SCT proposes that the influences of environmental events, behavior, and inner personal factors interact with each other in a reciprocal fashion. Inner personal factors include cognition, emotion, and biologic events. Through cognition, people are able to self-reflect, and appraise thoughts, experiences, and behaviors. When people self-reflect, they create the cognitive base for self-regulation or control of subsequent behaviors. Self-reflection leads to perceptions of self-efficacy (Bandura, 1989).

In summary, perceived self-efficacy refers to beliefs in one's capabilities to organize and execute the courses of actions required to produce given actions (Bandura, 1997, p. 3). For the individual to judge capability to perform a behavior, he or she must examine the information from all sources of efficacy information, including enactive attainment, vicarious experience, verbal persuasion, and autonomic arousal. Bandura (1986) wrote that behavior initiation and maintenance is determined by perceptions of self-efficacy that evolve from efficacy and outcome expectations. Efficacy expectations are beliefs about one's ability to engage or execute a given behavior that will result in an expected outcome. Outcome expectations are the beliefs that engaging in a certain behavior or behaviors will result in a specific result (see Figure 20.1). Efficacy expectations vary on the three dimensions of magnitude, strength, and generality.

Critical Examination of Social Cognitive Theory

The SCT, formulated through a process of deduction for the purpose of explaining behavior initiation, change, and maintenance, is useful in nursing practice. The theory emphasizes variables thought to influence health behaviors. Understanding how the health care consumer can be motivated to initiate and sustain positive behaviors that will promote and/or maintain health is a priority for nursing. The SCT is logical and easy to comprehend, with reciprocal relationships among the variables clearly identified and linked with performance of purposive, goal-directed behavior. The content of the theory provides insights and adds useful information to the body of nursing knowledge. The theory is parsimonious, although it deals with complex phenomena related to human behavior. The process of reciprocal determinism is easy to understand and is generalizable across diverse populations (e.g., Dzewaltowski, Noble, & Shaw, 1990; K. Waller & Bates, 1992; Wieseke, 1991), although the original research involved only adult phobics as subjects (Bandura, 1977). The theory can be applied to nursing practice and health education because teaching and learning involve behavioral initiation, change, and maintenance. The SCT provides a framework for nursing research that critically analyzes and manipulates variables embedded within the theory, providing a basis for nursing interventions and further research. The theory is testable and has been supported through research both within and outside the nursing domain.

Measurement of the variables in SCT, however, is complicated by the interchangeable use of terms such as self-inducements and self-incentives for motivation. Efficacy expectations are also referred to as self-efficacy, perceived self-efficacy, and perceived competence, despite Bandura's (1986) definitions. Outcome expectations are referred to as anticipated consequences. Semantic consistency and clarity would enhance communication, understanding, and application of the theory. A related problem concerns the lack of operational definitions for some concepts found within SCT. Bandura (1986) stated that efficacy expectations vary across the dimensions of magnitude, generality, and strength; no clear guidelines are provided to facilitate consistent measurement of these dimensions across studies, however. As a result, studies have used a variety of methods for measuring efficacy expectations. For example, efficacy expectations have been measured by the means of Likert-type items (Desharnais, Bouillon, & Godin, 1986) and by identifying the percentage of confidence (0–100%) for performing increasingly difficult levels of a behavior (Hilgenkamp, 1987). Variations in scales even occur within methodological types. For example, a one-item Likert-type response format was applied to measuring self-efficacy in

one study (Gortner et al., 1988), whereas another employed a tool with 17 Likert-type items (P. Waller, Crow, Sands, & Becker, 1988).

Clearing-Sky (1986) and Hilgenkamp (1987) measured the dimensions of magnitude and strength in relation to exercise behavior. Subjects were asked to identify the percentage of confidence they had about whether they could successfully perform a specific exercise task (measured by distance arranged in increasing values) and the percentage of confidence they had that they could continue to do the exercise program after the course in which they were enrolled had ended. Generality of efficacy expectations was not assessed.

Dzewaltowski et al. (1990) used a different approach by asking participants to report their exact percentage of confidence in performing an exercise activity three times per week during four different time frames despite any disconfirming experiences. The only dimension of efficacy expectations assessed was that of strength. P. Waller et al. (1988) assessed efficacy expectations using a Likert-type format. Generalization of efficacy expectations was measured in relation to a variety of health promotion behaviors; magnitude and strength dimensions, however, were not measured.

The studies mentioned above illustrate the different methodologies and interpretations employed to investigate efficacy expectations. Consistent measures are needed to enable valid comparisons across studies and the generalization of results to other populations.

RELATIONSHIP OF SELF-EFFICACY TO STRESS AND COPING

Although no research directly compares Bandura's self-efficacy construct to the concepts of stress and coping as proposed by Lazarus and Folkman (1984), both theorists report a relationship between them. Bandura (1997) states that according to the SCT, stress reactions in people occur because of a low sense of self-efficacy to exercise control over unpleasant threats and disturbing environmental demands. If people believe they can control (high self-efficacy) a threat or stressor, they are not as negatively emotionally aroused and they are able to use coping strategies effectively. If people believe they cannot control their environment, they experience stress and cannot function adequately. Bandura agreed with Lazarus and Folkman (1984) that the most important stressors that humans have to cope with involve psychological threats. However, Bandura (1997) believes the intensity of reactions to stress are directly related to levels of self-efficacy for coping rather than the actual threat and environmental factors.

Similar to Bandura's propositions, Lazarus and Folkman (1984) state that part of secondary appraisal of a threat is the probability that a given coping option will accomplish what it is supposed to accomplish and the probability that one can apply a particular coping strategy or set of strategies effectively. Lazarus and Folkman noted that there was a parallel between the concept of situational appraisals and control and self-efficacy. They indicate that efficacy expectations, as identified by Bandura (1982), affect the extent to which a person feels threatened and, thus, direct their coping efforts. Lazarus and Folkman (1984) propose that efficacy expectations are part of secondary appraisal, which includes a total evaluation of alternative coping options that affect emotions and coping.

Bandura (1995) discussed the relationship of threat and self-efficacy, stating that people's beliefs in their coping capabilities affect how much stress and depression they experience in threatening or difficult situations as well as their level of motivation to perform a specific behavior. Efficacy beliefs affect vigilance toward potential threats and how they are perceived and cognitively processed. People who believe, due to low self-efficacy, that potential threats are unmanageable may perceive many aspects of their environment and life as perilous, perpetuating coping deficiencies. Severity of possible threats is exaggerated, and they worry about things that rarely happen. Bandura and Lazarus and Folkman (1984) agree that low self-efficacy for managing threat produces greater stress and impairs level of functioning.

Bandura and Lazarus and Folkman concur that when people perceive outcomes are difficult they use cognitive coping strategies and restructure the cognitive meaning of the outcomes. If recurring difficult situations are uncontrollable, people resort to cognitive coping strategies designed to lessen their stress. Lazarus (1991) identified two concepts that overlap with self-efficacy and are involved in the appraisal process: coping potential and future expectations.

Coping potential and future expectations incorporate appraisal of potential environmental response to a coping action. These appraisals help determine the coping strategies chosen to decrease stress and negative emotional arousal.

Bandura (1997) suggests using coping strategies to meet the challenge of maintaining the quality of life with chronic disease or the aftermath of serious illness by the exercise of control over emotional distress associated with such conditions. Active involvement in purposeful activities is a good coping strategy when appraising and managing distress, feelings of despair, and emptiness in chronic disease states. The theorists agree that these strategies include more positive reappraisals of one's life situation, reordering one's lifestyle priorities, controlling perturbing ideation, alleviating stress by cognitive means, and seeking social support.

Lazarus and Folkman (1991) noted that the main component in coping effectiveness is whether or not the choice of coping strategy is appropriate to the stressful situation. They agree with Bandura that the major criterion for coping effectiveness is the extent to which an outcome is within the person's control. If the outcome is within the person's control, problem-focused forms of coping that are intended to achieve the desired outcome are appropriate, and emotion-focused forms of coping may inhibit coping effectiveness. If the outcome is not perceived to be within the person's control, emotion-focused forms of coping that promote reduction of stress are appropriate.

In conclusion, self-efficacy and stress and coping are strongly related. Secondary appraisal, situational appraisal, coping potential, and future expectations as discussed by Lazarus are intimately intertwined with efficacy expectations and outcome expectations as discussed by Bandura. Research focused on stress and coping and self-efficacy has addressed health behaviors. The theorists noted that health behaviors can be effective coping strategies for managing stressful situations.

SELF-EFFICACY AND HEALTH BEHAVIOR RESEARCH

The following sections summarize information reported in meta-analyses of self-efficacy research and provide examples of studies that addressed the relationships of both efficacy expectations and outcome expectations in relation to self-efficacy, health behavior, and stress and coping. Next, a discussion of research related to specific health concerns from the perspectives of both nursing and nonnursing disciplines is provided.

Self-efficacy has been studied extensively for its role in initiation, change, and maintenance of health behaviors in both well and ill populations. Holden (1991), O'Leary, (1985), and Strecher et al. (1986) reviewed self-efficacy research studies grouped by health concerns. Health concerns addressed included cardiac rehabilitation, chronic lung disease, cigarette smoking, weight control, eating disorders, alcohol abuse, adherence to medical regimens, pain, depression, stress management, and contraceptive behavior.

O'Leary (1985) examined several studies on self-efficacy and health outcomes such as smoking cessation. He found that high levels of self-efficacy were associated with increased adherence to medical regimens, especially when the individual recognized the perceived health threat and the desired outcomes of related health behaviors. Strecher et al. (1986) reviewed studies that had examined self-efficacy in relation to cigarette smoking, weight control, contraceptive behavior, alcohol abuse, and exercise. All studies indicated that the level of self-efficacy consistently predicted short- and long-term success in initiating and maintaining health behavior. Most important, as proposed by Bandura (1986), in studies that measured both efficacy and outcome expectations self-efficacy was an even stronger predictor of health behavior.

Holden (1991) performed a meta-analysis on 56 studies examining the relationship between self-efficacy and health behaviors and found self-efficacy consistently predicted health-related behavioral outcomes. His analysis revealed a statistically significant negative correlation between observed effect sizes and the length of time from the individual's self-efficacy appraisal to actual performance of the behavior. Holden also concluded that self-efficacy was not merely a component of other general constructs regarding the self, such as self-esteem or locus of control, but also a uniquely predictive construct. In addition, Holden found that self-efficacy predicted a variety of behavioral outcomes, including those related to cigarette smoking, pain, weight loss, exercise, and dental care. Interestingly, the

relationship was much weaker for weight loss and pain-related behavioral outcomes—a phenomenon that needs additional investigation.

Hofstetter et al. (1990) examined self-efficacy and the relationship between efficacy and outcome expectations. The sample for the study consisted of 2,053 male and female residents selected from the population of San Diego, California. Variables measured included self-efficacy, modeling, social support, benefits, knowledge about exercise, normative beliefs, medical history, exercise history, heart-healthy diet habits, smoking, body mass index, education, and sex—all variables identified as pertinent in the SCT. Results of the study revealed that self-efficacy was not unidimensional but rather multidimensional as well as highly domain specific. The researchers found that outcome expectations were distinct from efficacy expectations. As indicated by Bandura (1986), if the individual does not desire the outcome, measuring efficacy expectations is of little relevance.

Grembowski et al. (1993) investigated self-efficacy and health behavior among older adults who were enrollees ($N = 2,524$) in a Medicare program. They found that adults with higher self-efficacy for health behaviors based on efficacy expectations, including those related to exercise, dietary fat intake, weight control, alcohol intake, and smoking, had better functional, mental, and self-rated health than those with lower self-efficacy. Outcome expectations were correlated negatively with perceived health risks, suggesting that outcome expectations may have some influence on the initiation and achievement of behavior change in older adults. Outcome expectations, however, were not related significantly to health status, providing support for the SCT assumption that outcome expectations may be dependent only partially on self-efficacy. The study provided support for the assumptions, including triadic reciprocity of the SCT.

If only efficacy expectations are measured, results may not be as valid, reliable, and applicable as results from studies that measure both efficacy and outcome expectations. Findings will also be more accurate if researchers first determine whether the individual desires the specified outcome and then measure efficacy expectations for being able to perform the necessary behaviors to achieve that outcome. If the outcome is not desired, efficacy expectations for performing the pertinent behaviors to achieve the outcome will be low.

Cardiovascular Disease

Since nurses began to conduct studies on the effect of self-efficacy on adults with disease or illness, much of that research has been with clients/patients diagnosed with cardiovascular disease. Several of those research studies were completed during the 1990s (Allen, Becker, & Swank, 1990; Burns, Camaione, Froman, & Clark, 1998; Carroll, 1995; Clark & Dodge, 1999; Gillis et al., 1993; Gulanick, 1991; Shuster & Waldron, 1991; Schuster, Wright, & Tomich, 1995; Sullivan, LaCroix, Russo, & Kathon, 1998; Thomas, 1993; Vidmar & Robinson, 1994). Results of those studies showed that high levels of self-efficacy were related to and predictive of exercise activity, adherence to cardiac rehabilitation regimens, improved social and physical function, and increased exercise tolerance.

Schuster and Waldron (1991) conducted a longitudinal exploratory study to investigate gender differences in anxiety, self-efficacy, activity tolerance, and adherence in cardiac rehabilitation patients with diagnosed coronary artery disease ($N = 101$). Results of the study indicated that on enrollment in a cardiac rehabilitation program, women were significantly less self-efficacious, more anxious, and less able to tolerate physical activity than men. Although not statistically significant, the data revealed that women attended the cardiac rehabilitation sessions less regularly than did men. These findings are congruent with those of Verbrugge (1985), who found that females showed higher morbidity for both acute and chronic diseases, restricted activities more because of health problems, and spent more days in bed than men. The researchers recommended that before entry to cardiac rehabilitation, assessments should be made of self-efficacy, anxiety, activity tolerance, and adherence to individualize rehabilitation strategies, facilitate attainment of rehabilitation goals, and promote adherence to the program. Schuster and Waldron also suggested that results related to adherence may reflect a phenomenon identified by Bandura (1986) in that both too much and too little self-efficacy may be related to the absence or decreased performance of physical activity. High self-efficacy of men and low self-efficacy of women may both have hindered adherence to the program. No other studies in the reviewed literature were found to support this assumption, however. A question can be asked as to why males and females respond in different ways to cardiac experiences. Also, why do their responses, although opposite, sometimes result in the same behavioral outcomes?

Schuster et al. (1995) conducted a subsequent study to explore gender differences in the behavioral outcomes of postoperative coronary artery bypass graft (CABG) surgery patients ($N = 73$) in home programs compared to those in structured cardiac rehabilitation programs. No significant differences were found over time between home and structured programs for males and females on self-efficacy, length of time before return to work, diet adherence, smoking cessation, and medication adherence. Self-efficacy for physical activity and knowledge did significantly increase over time, regardless of the type of program or gender. The researchers concluded that self-efficacy related to the ability to endure exercise and complete activities of daily living improved over time as physical status improved. Additional research needs to be conducted to examine the relationships between and predictability of study variables in relation to physical activity, especially self-efficacy.

In another study of clients in cardiac rehabilitation, Vidmar and Robinson (1994) examined the relationship between self-efficacy and exercise compliance. Significant positive relationships were found between total self-efficacy and exercise compliance, exercise barriers, and exercise behavior. Individuals who perceived many barriers to exercise tended to exercise at a higher level to overcome barriers. Exercise barriers efficacy was found to be the most significant predictor of exercise behavior. Research must be performed to determine if subjects who respond in this way interpret overcoming barriers as a challenge rather than a threat. On the basis of the findings, the researchers recommended that to increase self-efficacy and exercise compliance strategies related to the sources of self-efficacy information should be implemented, such as (a) offering a variety of exercise modalities, (b) educating about use of equipment and physiologic responses to exercise, (c) allowing individuals to take part in structured activities when desired as a means to increase motivation by observing others exercising, (d) providing verbal encouragement, (e) suggesting alterations in exercise regimens, and (f) recommending counseling regarding setting and attaining goals. They also suggested that self-efficacy be reinforced regularly during long-term treatment regimens, such as dietary changes, smoking cessation, and stress management.

Carroll (1995) evaluated self-efficacy, self-care agency, and self-care and recovery behaviors at four points in time in elderly people after CABG surgery. Results revealed that self-efficacy increased during the recovery period, as did self-care agency and the ability to perform self-care and recovery behaviors. Women were found to be less self-efficacious before surgery, at discharge, and at 6 weeks after surgery than men. By 12 weeks after surgery, however, men and women reported equal self-efficacy. Women obviously increased their self-efficacy more than men during the 12 weeks after surgery. In addition, self-efficacy was found to be a mediator between self-care agency and self-care and recovery behaviors of walking, climbing stairs, and general activities. No explanation for gender differences was offered, and additionally research must be conducted to explore this issue. Carroll suggested that reported increased self-efficacy, increased self-care agency, and improved activity performance might be influenced by the physiologic recovery because recovery provides physiologic arousal efficacy information. In addition, Carroll suggested that nurses provide coaching and guidance to the patients. Coaching should include encouraging performance of self-care behaviors in a supportive environment before discharge, assisting with setting and supporting realistic daily goals of performance, and mandatory attendance at an educational offering before discharge. These coaching strategies lead to increased self-efficacy because they use all sources of efficacy information.

Allen et al. (1990) investigated self-efficacy and functional status after CABG surgery. The longitudinal study involved 125 male patients. Women were purposely excluded from the study because they constituted only 19% of all CABG surgeries and because potential gender differences might confound results. Self-efficacy was found to be a significant and independent predictor of 6-month postoperative physical activity and social and leisure activity. Men with higher self-efficacy performed more physical, social, and leisure activities. Self-efficacy was a better predictor of functional status than disease severity, functional capacity, comorbidity, or preoperative functioning. On the basis of study results, attempts should be made to increase self-efficacy in cardiac rehabilitation programs.

Between 2000 and 2010, there have been 78 studies related to cardiovascular disease or illness using self-efficacy as a variable conducted by health care professionals. When searching for more research articles of self-efficacy and specific cardiovascular diseases or illnesses for the same decade, you will be able to locate many articles for hypertension, heart failure, coronary artery disease, myocardial infarction, cardiac surgery, and cardiac rehabilitation. Research studies that examine self-efficacy and how it relates to heart failure and hypertension lead the list of cardiovascular diseases and disorders. Several of the past decade's self-efficacy related to cardiovascular disorders studies are cited here (Al-Duhoun, 2005; Arnold, Ranchor, DeJonste, & Gerard, 2005; Cheng & Boey, 2002; English, 2001; Garry, 2006; Hitunen, Winder, Rait, & Buselli, 2005; J. Jones, 2004; Mason, 2002; Perry, 2000; Sarikonda-Woitas, 2001; Sharp, 2008). See Table 20.1 for numbers of research studies related to cardiovascular disease, illness, and disorders.

In summary, self-efficacy has been shown to be a strong predictor of functional outcomes and physical activity in people with cardiac illness or who have had cardiac surgery. Clearly, more research is needed involving women because the results predominantly reflect the reportings of men. Additional research must examine self-efficacy over time, across cultures, and across interventions.

Pulmonary Disease

Self-efficacy in patients with pulmonary disease is another area of health behavior research. A few studies appeared in the literature back in the 1990s (Atkins, Kaplan, Timms, Reinsch, & Lofback, 1984; Devins & Edwards, 1988; Gormley, Carrieri-Kohlman, Douglas, & Stulbarg, 1993; Kaplan, Ries, Prewitt, & Eakin, 1994; Scherer & Schmieder, 1997; Toshima, Kaplan, & Ries, 1990, 1992). High levels of self-efficacy were shown to be associated with enhanced symptom management, decreased perceptions of dyspnea, improved functional status, and increased exercise and increased exercise tolerance.

Table 20.1 Number of Research Studies Examining Self-Efficacy as a Factor in the Initiation, Change, and/or Maintenance of Health Behaviors in Well and Ill Populations

Health problem	2000–2010 number of studies
Exercise	592
Physical activity	480
Depression	350
HIV	341
Older adults	325
Diabetes	239
Cancer	235
AIDS	227
Diet	210
Pain	203
Nutrition	197
Smoking cessation	129
Caregivers	125
Alcohol	119
Symptom management	99
Arthritis	82
Falls	79
Cardiovascular	78
Breast cancer	72
Substance abuse	66
STD	60
Asthma	47
Stroke	47
Hypertension	41
Dementia	38
Multiple sclerosis	33
Heart failure	30
Glucose control	29
Prostate cancer	29
Childbirth	28
Cardiac rehabilitation	25
Pulmonary disease	25
Coronary artery disease	20
Dyspnea	20
Spinal cord injury	20
Breastfeeding	19
Eating disorders	19
Cardiac surgery	18
Dialysis	17
COPD	15
Menopause	11
Myocardial infarction	11
Alzheimer's disease	10
Joint replacement	10
Renal failure	10
Pulmonary rehabilitation	9
Lung cancer	6
Brain injury	4

Based on a ProQuest Search. Note an overlap of publications can occur between populations and areas of study.

Atkins et al. (1984) examined efficacy expectations of patients with chronic obstructive pulmonary disease (COPD) in a walking program. The researchers also investigated the relationship between locus of control and self-efficacy. The sample included 22 men and 38 women with moderate to severe COPD, as determined by forced expiratory volume in 1 second (FEV_1) percent predicted. Researchers measured efficacy expectations after the exercise prescription was given and 3 months later. Statistically significant differences were found in distance walked and exercise tolerance in participants who were in the experimental treatment groups compared to those in the control group at the end of 3 months. Those in treatment groups walked farther and tolerated the activity better. Results suggested that interventions based on sources of efficacy information, particularly mastery and verbal persuasion, improved self-efficacy in walking in adults with COPD, as proposed in the SCT. In addition, Atkins et al. reported that health locus of control had a weaker relationship with walking and behavior change during the 3 months. These findings support Bandura's assumption that self-efficacy, because it is behavior specific, is more predictive of a health behavior than the more general concept of health locus of control.

Another study examined self-efficacy in 119 patients (32 women and 87 men) with stable COPD who were undergoing pulmonary rehabilitation. Researchers measured exercise endurance, quality of well-being, depression, and self-efficacy (Toshima et al., 1990, 1992). Participants were assigned either to an education control group that received exercise training or to an education control group that did not receive exercise training. After 6 months, the exercise training group had a significant increase in exercise tolerance. Although self-efficacy in walking did improve from baseline, in contrast to findings of Schuster et al. (1995), it was not a significant change. Members of the exercise training group, who initially had higher self-efficacy scores for treadmill walking, demonstrated the greatest endurance on the treadmill. Toshima et al. asserted that physiological feedback was a strong source of efficacy information for people with COPD because they experience discomfort, such as dyspnea and fatigue, with activity and sometimes even at rest, creating a negative autonomic feedback. When people with COPD perceive aversive autonomic feedback while attempting behaviors such as exercise, this autonomic source of efficacy information may limit efficacy expectations and subsequently self-efficacy. Thus, if people with COPD are helped to experience a more positive autonomic state or are able to avoid focusing on negative autonomic feedback, they may perceive a greater degree of self-efficacy. Another consideration is that women and men may experience not only their disease symptoms but also exercise treatment differently.

Devins and Edwards (1988) conducted a study of self-efficacy and smoking reduction in COPD patients. Participants (27 men and 21 women) had smoked for at least 15 years and were currently smoking at least 10 cigarettes a day. Through an educational process, study participants were exposed to the various behavioral techniques used to reduce smoking. Participants were then asked to rate the perceived effectiveness of each technique, thus measuring their outcome expectations. The strength of efficacy expectations was measured by rating their confidence in being able to perform each of the smoking-cessation techniques. The researchers

also measured motivation to stop smoking using a motivational index and a smoking index. At 1 month and 3 months post–original testing and educational sessions, self-efficacy was the only significant predictor of reduced smoking. Measuring both efficacy and outcome expectations specific to a behavior, as Bandura (1986) did, yielded information about the multidimensional concept of self-efficacy, thus enhancing the generalizability of study findings.

In 1993, Gormley et al. examined treadmill self-efficacy and walking performance in 52 patients with COPD. FEV_1, percentage predicted was lower in men than women before interventions started. Subjects were randomly assigned to a monitored exercise group or a coached exercise group. Self-efficacy was defined as the level that corresponded to the highest treadmill speed and grade for which participants had the greatest confidence. Results showed that both self-efficacy and walking performance increased significantly over time for both groups; there were no significant differences between the two groups, however.

Gormley et al. (1993) suggested that through the efficacy information of mastery by exercise, the dyspnea-inactivity-dyspnea cycle for the COPD patients was interrupted. In addition, participants were probably inactive because aversive autonomic feedback, such as dyspnea and fatigue, decreased confidence in the ability to perform exercise activity. Interestingly, this supposition was supported because most of the participants consistently underestimated their ability to exercise. Gormley et al. stated that the reason there were no differences between the groups in self-efficacy is that both groups exercised in a safe, monitored setting with a nurse present. The presence of the nurse was enough to increase self-efficacy and security even in participants who were only monitored and received no coaching. Both groups were provided mastery experiences for their exercise, the strongest source of efficacy information.

Another important finding was that women increased their self-efficacy significantly more than did men, as also occurred in the Carroll (1995) study. In the beginning, women reported lower self-efficacy than men, even when they reported better walking performance. The researchers suggested that women focused more on their uncomfortable autonomic state than did men during the initial exercise test—thus the initial low level of self-efficacy. In addition, past experiences and socialization may have influenced the women's perceptions. Many of the women were of the generation in which women were taught that they were not capable of great physical tasks—thus the lower self-efficacy for physical tasks. The researchers recommended that clinicians assess self-efficacy related to exercise in all COPD patients, especially women, attending pulmonary rehabilitation programs. By recognizing patients with lower self-efficacy, strategies could then be used to improve both self-efficacy and walking performance.

Kaplan et al. (1994) investigated the relationships of self-efficacy to FEV_1, diffusing capacity for carbon monoxide (DL_{CO}; measures how well the lung transfers gas from inspired air to blood), VO_2 max (standard measure of exercise tolerance, maximum oxygen uptake), and arterial oxygen level as predictors of mortality among 119 patients (32 women and 87 men) with COPD. Self-efficacy was measured with an instrument that asked subjects to rate their expectations for walking progressively longer distances for longer periods of time. Results indicated that self-efficacy for walking was a significant predictor of survival, as were FEV_1, VO_2 max, and DL_{CO}. The pO_2 (partial pressure of oxygen) was not a significant predictor of survival. Statistical analysis, however, revealed that FEV_1 accounted for the greatest amount of variance in the prediction of survival. The researchers noted that self-reports of self-efficacy could compete favorably with physiologic measures to predict mortality in COPD patients. They proposed that efficacy expectations in COPD patients were affected by the seriousness of the underlying illness producing an aversive autonomic state.

Scherer and Schmieder (1997) investigated the effect of a pulmonary rehabilitation program on self-efficacy and the ability to manage or avoid breathing difficulty in certain situations. Results indicated that self-efficacy increased significantly over time from pretest to posttest at 1 month but decreased slightly at 6 months postoutpatient pulmonary rehabilitation (OPR) in relation to managing or avoiding breathing difficulty associated with physical exertion. Higher scores on the COPD Self-Efficacy Scale (CSES) indicated greater confidence in the ability to manage or avoid breathing difficulty and were correlated with lower scores of perceived dyspnea.

Self-efficacy was still greater at 6 months post-OPR than before OPR; therefore, periodic reinforcement or review sessions are recommended to maintain high levels of self-efficacy. Interestingly, in contrast to the findings of Gormley et al. (1993), the researchers reported no significant differences between men and women on pre- and postprogram scores on the CSES, Dyspnea Scale, and 12-minute distance.

Between 2000 and 2010, 25 research studies were conducted using self-efficacy as a variable related to health behaviors in patients with pulmonary disease or illness. These studies included specific self-efficacy research related to people with COPD and asthma, and those who attended pulmonary rehabilitation programs (Arnold et al., 2005; Kaul, 2007; Mackin, 2007; Ries, Kaplan, Myers, & Prewitt, 2003; Siela, 2003; Srof, 2004). See Table 20.1 for numbers of abstracts and research articles.

In summary, multiple studies involving subjects with COPD have provided support for predictive relationships between self-efficacy and symptom management, exercise tolerance, and endurance. Additional studies must be conducted across a wider section of participants and situations to develop reliable, valid instruments for measuring self-efficacy in COPD patients.

Physical Activity and Exercise

The relationship between physical activity and self-efficacy is an area of research that has been investigated only to a limited extent by nurses but to a much greater extent by other professionals (Bosscher & Van Der, 1995; Courneya & McAuley, 1994; Godin & Shephard, 1985; Kingery & Glasglow, 1989; McAuley, 1994; McAuley, Courneya, & Lettunich, 1991; Parkatti, Deeg, Bosscher, & Launer, 1998). The following discussion provides a sample of the self-efficacy research that has been completed and that provided support for a positive relationship, even a predictive relationship, between self-efficacy and physical activity.

Godin and Shephard (1985) conducted a study on gender differences in perceived physical self-efficacy among older individuals. Data analysis revealed significant differences between men and women in total physical self-efficacy and perceived physical ability, with women having lower scores. No significant differences were found based on age. Godin and Shephard suggested that gender differences in self-efficacy, and therefore actual physical activity, were due to sociocultural influences of a particular era rather than biological differences. The differences in self-efficacy levels need to be identified and incorporated into design and implementation of programs to enhance physical activity of older adults.

McAuley et al. (1991) examined the effects of acute (single-graded exercise test) and long-term (structured exercise program) exercise on perceptions of personal efficacy with respect to physical capabilities. Results revealed that men had significantly higher sit-up self-efficacy than women at both times. The researchers suggested that the difference in sit-up self-efficacy was a physiologic advantage that men had over women because men were leaner and took longer to reach the targeted heart rate. Both men and women increased bicycle and walk and jog self-efficacy during the 20-week time period, with the levels of self-efficacy equal across genders at 20 weeks. Women, however, actually had greater increases in self-efficacy levels because their levels were lower initially for the three physical activities than those of the men. Interestingly, men had more bicycle self-efficacy than women at baseline and Time 2. McAuley et al. suggested that gender differences at baseline in sit-up, bicycle, and walk and jog self-efficacy were related to beliefs about physical abilities based on past physical experiences and different sociocultural upbringing of men and women.

Additional research related to self-efficacy and physical activity and exercise has been conducted during 2000 to 2010. As expected, the findings suggest that high self-efficacy for behaviors related to increasing physical activity and/or exercise facilitate the desired outcomes (Allison, 2000; D'Alonzo, 2002; Dutton et al., 2009; Ferrier, Dunlop, & Blanchard, 2010; Gleeson-Kreig, 2004; Haas, 2001; Lee, Laffrey, & Cloutier, 2008; Kohlbry, 2006; Marquez & McCauley, 2006; McCauley, Konopack, Morris, & Moti, 2006; Morris, McAuley, & Moti, 2008; Netz & Raviv, 2004; Paxton, Moti, Aylward, & Nigg, 2010; Perkins, Multhalp, Perkins, & Barton, 2008; Rogers, Shah, Dunnington, & Greive, 2005). Refer to Table 20.1 to view numbers of these studies.

Diabetes Management

A limited number of studies in the 1990s explored the relationship between self-efficacy and diabetes management (J. Davis, 1997; Holcomb et al., 1998; Hurley & Shea, 1992; Kingery & Glasglow, 1989; Leonard, Skay, & Rheinberger, 1998; Skelly, Marshall, Haughey, Davis, & Dunford, 1995; Wang, Wang, & Lin, 1998). Examples of research that provides evidence of a positive relationship between levels of self-efficacy and health-promotive behaviors in diabetes management are presented here.

Skelly et al. (1995) assessed the influence of perceptions of self-efficacy and confidence in outcomes related to diabetes self-care regimens in a sample of 118 middle-aged, inner-city African American women. At the time of the initial interview, subjects reported high levels of self-efficacy about self-care related to medications and glucose monitoring but not diet or exercise. At Time 2, self-efficacy levels had increased for all the behaviors; they were still lower for diet and exercise, however, as evidenced by less adherence for these behaviors. Additional research needs to be conducted on this phenomenon.

The Insulin Management Diabetes Self-Efficacy Scale and the Diabetes Self-Care Scale were used by Hurley and Shea (1992) in a study examining diabetes management behaviors in a sample of 142 adults who self-administered insulin. Subjects had high levels of self-efficacy at both times, and strong positive correlations were found between self-efficacy and self-care behaviors of general diabetes management and diet control. There was also a strong positive correlation between insulin self-efficacy beliefs and self-care. Higher levels of self-efficacy enabled individuals to optimize self-care skills. The provided personal mastery experiences, vicarious experiences available, verbal persuasion, and emotional support provided by the nurses in the safe hospital environment enhanced self-efficacy and improved the likelihood of self-care behavior for diabetes management.

Kingery and Glasgow (1989) examined self-efficacy and outcome expectations in the self-regulation of non-insulin-dependent diabetes mellitus. The sample consisted of 127 diabetic outpatients (85 women and 42 men). The researchers found that exercise self-efficacy was a more significant predictor of exercise levels in women than in men. They found, however, that outcome expectations were a more significant predictor of exercise levels for men than for women. Kingery and Glasgow suggested that different educational strategies need to be used for men and women to increase self-efficacy with subsequent improved exercise levels for diabetes management. Women may need assistance in increasing self-efficacy related to exercise skills, whereas men may need increased self-efficacy to increase understanding of the importance of exercise for diabetes management.

From 2000 to 2010, a ProQuest literature search revealed approximately 239 research studies of self-efficacy in adults with diabetes and 29 for glucose control (see Table 20.1). Perception of self-efficacy was used to predict its effect on the attainment of successful outcomes of disease self-management, exercise, and glucose control. It should be noted that high levels of self-efficacy predicted attainment of desired outcomes related to diabetes care and glucose control (Mann, Ponieman, Leventhal, & Haim, 2009; Nichols, 2009; Sander, Odell, & Hood, 2010; Serrano, Leiferman, & Dauber, 2007; Temple, 2003; Trief, Teresi, Eimicke, Shea, & Weinstock, 2009).

Arthritis

A few studies in the 1990s supported self-efficacy as a mediator of health outcomes for individuals diagnosed with rheumatoid arthritis (Barlow, 1998; Lorig, Chastain, Ung, Shoor, & Holman, 1989; Riemsma et al., 1998). Lorig et al. (1989) explored this relationship in an experimental study involving 144 adults measured by the Beck Depression Scale. Self-efficacy was measured using the Arthritis Self-Efficacy Scale developed by the researchers that contained three subscales related to pain, function, and other symptoms (fatigue, activity regulation, and depression). Subjects who received the intervention significantly increased self-efficacy levels and decreased levels of depression and pain. Function improved, possibly because of the increase in self-efficacy.

In the period between 2000 and 2010, approximately 82 studies were conducted regarding self-efficacy and arthritis and were published as reports or abstracts in journals according to a ProQuest search. Most of these studies examined the relationship of self-efficacy to successful self-management, pain control, and physical activity/mobility (Arthur et al., 2009; Pariser, O'Hanlon, & Espinoza, 2005). See Table 20.1 for numbers over the decade.

Other Disorders

Several other studies have examined levels of self-efficacy as a factor in the initiation, change, and maintenance of health behaviors in other ill populations or disorders. Following are citations of research report articles that use self-efficacy as a variable to examine how it affects health behavior adoption for people with various disorders. Access these research articles and dissertations for additional information.

Joint Replacement: Akhavan, 2008; Moon & Backer, 2000.

Cancer, Breast Cancer and Prostate Cancer: Blacklock, Rhodes, Blanchard, & Gaul, 2010; Champion, Skinner, & Menon, 2005; Crowley, 2003; Fisher & Howell, 2010; Haas, 2001; McGhan, 2007; Rogers et al., 2005; Rogers, McAuley, Courneya, & Verhuist, 2008; Weber et al., 2007.

Stroke, Multiple Sclerosis, and Spinal Cord Injury: Airlie, Baker, Smith, & Young, 2001; Ferrier et al., 2010; Fraser & Polito, 2007; Hampton, 2004; Hampton & Marshall, 2000; F. Jones, Mandy, & Partridge, 2009; Morris et al., 2008; Pang, Eng, & Miller, 2007.

Pain: Menzies, 2004; Rahman et al., 2008; Reneman, Geetzen, Groothoff, & Brouwer, 2008; Rokke, Fleming-Ficek, Sieman, & Hegstad; Vong, Cheing, Chan, Chan, & Leung, 2009.

Psychosocial Concerns

The 1990s produced studies related to psychosocial concerns and self-efficacy. Self-efficacy was shown to be related to adjustment in cancer patients (Beckham, Burker, Lytle, Feldman, & Costakis, 1997), maternal depression and child temperament (Gross, Conrad, Fogg, & Wothke, 1994), psychological distress and problem-focused coping (Sharts-Hopko, Regan-Kubinski, Lincoln, & Heverly, 1996), adaptation in battered women (Varvaro & Palmer, 1993), stress and coping in early psychosis (MacDonald, Pica, McDonald, Hayes, & Baglioni, 1998), coping with labor (Lowe, 1991), decreasing mental frailty in at-risk elders (McDougall & Balver, 1998), functional ability and depression after elective total hip replacement surgery (Kurlowicz, 1998), and distress and adjustment in Mexican American college students (Solberg & Villarreal, 1997). Overall, high levels of self-efficacy were negatively correlated with depression, mental frailty, and stress and positively correlated with enhanced coping and adaptation as well as health outcomes (less fatigue and pain).

Many of the studies used instruments designed by the researchers to be behavior specific, as did Varvaro and Palmer (1993). Varvaro and Palmer developed the Self-Efficacy Scale for Battered Women to assess self-efficacy needs of and develop treatment plans for abused women ($N = 43$) who presented to the emergency room. The women were found to have low levels of self-efficacy for asking for help, shrugging off self-doubts, saying what they think, and feeling without fear. Subjects were found to have a need for information on abuse, safety, and self-empowerment to decrease fear and promote adaptive psychosocial functioning. Individualized treatment plans were developed with components that addressed the sources of efficacy information. These components included providing the women with abuse information and information on where and how to get help, helping them create a plan for safety, and helping them identify, create, and practice coping skills. When assessing eight of the subjects after they attended an educational support group for battered women for 12 weeks in which the intervention plan was implemented, the researchers found a significant increase in self-efficacy. The increase in self-efficacy was translated into better control over patients' lives.

See Table 20.1 for the numbers of studies related to psychosocial concerns conducted between 2000 and 2010. There are many more studies compared to those in the 1990s. The research of the relationship between self-efficacy and depression included a few studies (Bray, Kehle, Lawless, & Theodore, 2003; Perraud, Fogg, Kopytko, & Gross, 2006). One area of research that has increased by using self-efficacy as a variable is how it affects the role of caregivers (Penacoba, Losada, Lopez, & Marquez-Gonzalez, 2008; Reich, Bickman, & Heflinger, 2004; Sardi, 2003).

Preventive Behaviors

Self-efficacy has been investigated in two areas of behavior that are considered preventive and promotive in nature. It has been found to be predictive of behavior related to obtaining regular mammograms (Allen, Sorensen, Stoddard, Colditz, & Peterson, 1998) and breast self-examination (Gonzalez, 1990). In addition, self-efficacy has been found to be related to condom use by college students (Brafford & Beck, 1991) and Black adolescent women (Jemmott & Jemmott, 1992); safe sex behaviors (Cecil & Pinkerton, 1998; Goldman & Harlow, 1993; Kalichman, Roffman, Picciano, & Bolan, 1998); and AIDS preventive behaviors among 10th-grade students (Kasen, Vaughan, & Walter, 1992) and female drug users (Brown, 1998). Researchers have developed behavior-specific self-efficacy scales, with most measuring only the strength dimension.

For example, high levels of self-efficacy were found to be positively correlated with performance of breast self-examination when Mexican American subjects who attended a local health clinic were given guidance and training that were sensitive to cultural needs (Gonzalez, 1990). High levels of self-efficacy were positively associated with frequency of breast self-examination, supporting the proposition that self-examination was central to the behavior. Gonzalez suggested that to increase self-efficacy in relation to a specific behavior, the nurse must carefully assess cultural and language variables and use gathered data to help individualize care plans and optimize health outcomes.

See Table 20.1 for numbers of publications about self-efficacy related to exercise, physical activity, nutrition, and diet during 2000 to 2010. There was a negative patient outcome for preventive behaviors speculated to reduce its numbers. This is the number of patient falls. In the decade of 2000 to 2010, several studies regarding the relationship of self-efficacy for performing preventive behaviors for falls have been conducted (Anderson, Wolinsky, Miller, & Wilson, 2006; Hauer et al., 2010; Hellstrom, Vahlberg, Urell, & Emtner, 2009; Li et al., 2005; Liu-Ambrose, Khan, Donaldson, & Eng, 2006; Michael, Allen, & Macko, 2006; Pang & Eng, 2008; Whitehead, Miller, & Crotty, 2003).

Smoking Cessation, Eating Disorders, and Substance Abuse

Studies have demonstrated a predictive relationship between self-efficacy and successful smoking cessation (De Vries, Mudde, Dijkstra, & Willemsen, 1998; Kowalski, 1997; Pohl, Martinelli, & Antonakos, 1998). Kowalski, for example, explored self-efficacy in relation to smoking cessation behaviors and adherence in 75 adult subjects at the beginning of a smoking cessation program and 3 months after completion of the program. Self-efficacy scores at the beginning of the program significantly predicted whether or not subjects would be smoking 3 months after completion of the program. Subjects with higher self-efficacy scores at the beginning were more likely to stop smoking and maintain the status of nonsmoker 3 months after completion of the program. Kowalski suggested that believing that one could stop smoking forever influences the level of motivation, energy, and commitment necessary to break the habit.

Refer to Table 20.1 for numbers of smoking cessation, eating disorders, and alcohol use abstracts and research articles during 2000 to 2010. These are areas in which high levels of self-efficacy plays a key role in changing bad behaviors to healthy ones. Examples of self-efficacy research in these areas are few (Badr & Moody, 2005; Boardman, Catley, Mayo, & Ahiuwalia, 2005; Garg, Serwint, Hiugman, & Kanof, 2007; Gregory, 2001; Kranz, 2003; Warnecke et al., 2001).

In summary, research has provided ongoing support for the assumptions of the SCT in the areas of health behavior. Additional research must be conducted to assess the impact of additional environmental, behavioral, and inner personal factors on self-efficacy and subsequently on health behavior. In addition, research that would be beneficial should be that which examines the relationships between self-efficacy, stress and coping, and health behaviors, with the end result being the design of effective interventions.

SELF-EFFICACY SCALE/TOOL/ INSTRUMENT DEVELOPMENT

Many scales, tools, and instruments have been developed to measure self-efficacy in relation to health behaviors. Some of the instruments measure only the strength dimension of efficacy expectations. Conner and Norman (1995) suggested that to truly be able to measure self-efficacy a scale must assess risk perception, outcome expectancy, and all dimensions of efficacy expectations. The researchers suggested that outcome expectancy statements should be worded as "if-then" statements, whereas efficacy expectations statements should be worded as confidence statements. They also suggested that

self-efficacy scales should include positive and negative outcomes. Self-efficacy instruments, some of which apply the guidelines suggested by Conner and Norman, include the Cardiac Diet Self-Efficacy and Cardiac Exercise Self-Efficacy instruments (Hickey, Owen, & Froman, 1992); Knowledge, Attitude, and Self-Efficacy Asthma Questionnaire (Wigal et al., 1993); COPD Self-Efficacy Scale (Wigal, Creer, & Kotses, 1991); Self-Efficacy Scale (Sherer et al., 1982); Self-Efficacy Scale for Battered Women (Varvaro & Palmer, 1993); Maternal Self-Efficacy Scale (Gross et al., 1994); Cancer Self-Efficacy Scale (Beckham et al., 1997); Long-Term Medication Behaviour Self-Efficacy Scale (De Geest, Abraham, Gemoets, & Evers, 1994); Epilepsy Self-Efficacy Scale (Dilorio, Faherty, & Manteuffel, 1992); Headache Self-Efficacy Scale (Martin, Holroyd, & Rokicki, 1993); Preoperative Self-Efficacy Scale (Oetker & Taunton, 1994); General Perceived Self-Efficacy Scale (Schwarzer & Jerusalem, 1995); Osteoporosis Self-Efficacy Scale (Horan, Kim, Gendler, Froman, & Patel, 1998); Hormone Replacement Therapy Self-Efficacy Scale (Ali, 1998); and the Insulin Management Diabetes Self-Efficacy Scale (Hurley, 1990). Examination of the instruments reveals a variety of approaches to measuring self-efficacy; most, however, use a Likert-type format. Even within this structure different descriptors are used, including very confident to not at all confident, strongly agree to strongly disagree, and very likely to very unlikely. In addition, all the scales do not measure both outcome and efficacy expectations, or all three dimensions of efficacy expectations.

Hurley (1990) provides a good example of self-efficacy instrument development. The Insulin Management Diabetes Self-Efficacy Scale was designed to assess and identify individuals who would benefit from individualized care in addition to traditional diabetes health education. The 28-item instrument also could be used as an outcome measure of post-diabetes education. Items on the instrument were borrowed from other instruments and created by the researcher to reflect self-efficacy in relation to diabetes activities of daily living. Items contained action words that were not outcomes, contained only one behavior, used positive or negative wording related to ability, used the word "diabetic" as an adjective and not a noun, contained descriptors of varied situational variables, and used the term "insulin" rather than "medication." Strength and magnitude of efficacy expectations were measured in different items. Generalizability does not appear to be addressed by the scale. Behaviors measured included general, diet, exercise, foot care, monitoring, insulin administration, and detecting, preventing, or treating high and low blood glucose reactions. Ten items were negatively phrased. Subjects were asked to respond to each behavioral item using a Likert-type scale, with a possible score of strongly agree (1) to strongly disagree (6).

Validity and reliability have been tested in more than eight studies with inpatients or outpatients or both. Sample sizes have ranged from 5 to more than 127. Expert review, exploratory factor analysis, and convergent validity have provided support for construct and content validity of the instrument. Reliability was confirmed by Cronbach's alpha statistic, test-retest stability,

and interrater reliability assessment. The majority of the self-efficacy instruments have not been tested as extensively as the Insulin Management Self-Efficacy Scale, and such testing needs to be completed to be able to use findings when designing, implementing, and evaluating interventions to enhance self-efficacy and health behavior.

In the decade of 2000 to 2010, numerous self-efficacy scales and tools were developed and tested for psychometric validity and reliability. A literature search provided over 90 new self-efficacy scales and instruments. These scales included measurement of self-efficacy in people with diabetes, heart failure, COPD, rheumatoid arthritis, multiple sclerosis, medication adherence, depression, and exercise. See Table 20.2 for examples of new self-efficacy scales and tools.

Table 20.2   Self-Efficacy Measurement Tools (2000–2010)

Medication adherence

- Medication Adherence Self-Efficacy Scale in hypertensive African Americans (Fernandez, Chaplin, Schoenthaler, & Ogedegba, 2008)
- Osteoporosis Medication Adherence Scale (Resnick, Wehren, & Orwig, 2004)
- Pictographic Medication Adherence Self-Efficacy Scale for low literacy patients (Kalichman, Cain, Fuhrel, Eaton, & Di Fonzo, 2005)
- HIV Medication Taking Self-Efficacy Scale (Erlen, Cha, Kim, Caruthers, & Serika, 2010)
- HIV Treatment Adherence Self-Efficacy Scale (Johnson, Neilands, Dilworth, Morin, & Remien, 2007)

Sickle cell disease

- Sickle Cell Self-Efficacy Scale (Adegbola, 2007)

Multiple sclerosis

- Multiple Sclerosis Self-Efficacy Scale (Airlie, Baker, Smith, & Young, 2001)

Rheumatoid arthritis

- Rheumatoid Arthritis Self-Efficacy Scale (Hewlett et al., 2001)

COPD

- Exercise Self-Regulatory Efficacy Scale for individuals with chronic obstructive pulmonary disease (A. Davis, Aurelio, Fahy, & Rawiworrakul, 2007)

Heart failure

- Heart Failure Self-Efficacy Scale (Perry, 2000)

Diabetes

- Confidence in Diabetes Self-Care Scale (Van der Ven et al., 2003)
- Perceived Diabetes Self-Management Scale (Wallston, Rothman, & Cherrington, 2007)
- Self-Efficacy for Adults with Diabetes Scale (Hall, 2000)

(Continued)

Table 20.2 (Continued)

Older adults

- Task Self-Efficacy Scale for everyday activities in older adults (Roberts, Dolansky, & Weber, 2010)
- Self-Efficacy to Walk for Health Scale for use with midlife and older, low-income, African Americans women (Rowe, 2004)
- Multidimensional Outcome Expectations for Exercise Scale for older adults (Wojcicki, White, & McAuley, 2009)

Physical activity and exercise

- Stage-Specific Self-Efficacy Scale for physical activity (Masse, Heesch, Eason, & Wilson, 2006)
- Multidimensional Self-Efficacy for Exercise Scale (Rodgers, Wilson, Hall, Fraser, & Murray, 2008)
- Outcome Expectations for Exercise Scale: Utility and Psychometrics (Resnick, Zimmerman, Orwig, Furstenburg, & Magaziner, 2000)

Adolescent parenting

- Parenting Self-Efficacy Scale for parents of young adolescents (James, 2008)

Breast-feeding and care of infants

- Breastfeeding Self-Efficacy Scale (Dennis, 2003)
- Prenatal Breast-feeding Self-Efficacy Scale (Wells, Thompson, & Kloeblen-Tarver, 2006)
- Self-Efficacy in Infant Care Scale (Prasopkittikun, Tilokskulchai, Sinsuksai, & Sitthimongkol, 2006)

Pap smear

- Self-Efficacy Scale for Pap Smear Screening Participation in Sheltered Women (Hogenmiller et al., 2007)

Incontinence

- Broome Pelvic Muscle Self-Efficacy Scale for African American women with incontinence (Broome, 2001)

Abused women

- Self-Efficacy Scale for Abused Women (May & Limandri, 2004)

Mammography

- Mammography Self-Efficacy Scale (Champion, Skinner, & Menon, 2005)

Smoking

- Smoking Self-Efficacy Scale (Etter, Bergman, Humair, & Perneger, 2000)

Pain

- Pain Self-Efficacy Scale (Vong, Cheing, Chan, Chan, & Leung, 2009)

Falls

- Falls Efficacy Scale (Hauer et al., 2010)

Depression

- Depression Coping Self-Efficacy Scale (Perraud, Fogg, Kopytko, & Gross, 2006)

Mental disorders

- Mental Health Confidence Scale (Carpinello, Knight, Markowitz, & Pease, 2000)

Dementia caregivers

- Revised Scale for Caregiving Self-Efficacy for dementia caregivers (Penacoba, Losada, Lopez, & Marquez-Gonzalez, 2008)

Relocation

- Relocation Self-Efficacy Scale (Rossen & Gruber, 2007)

IMPLICATIONS OF SELF-EFFICACY

Bandura (1986) stated that behavior is influenced by self-efficacy as based on perceived efficacy expectations and outcome expectations. These evolve from cognitive appraisal of the sources of information found within the inner personal, behavioral, and environmental components of a situation as also reported by Lazarus. Self-efficacy has been associated with and has predicted behavioral choice, behavioral change, initiation of behavior, behavioral elimination, the amount of effort expended to perform a behavior, and persistence of a variety of health behaviors. High levels of self-efficacy were revealed to (a) enhance smoking cessation behaviors, increasing length of abstinence and decreasing risk of relapse; (b) enhance weight management; (c) increase control of eating disorders and decrease risk of relapse; (d) increase pain tolerance and enhance pain management behaviors; (e) increase adherence to medical regimens; (f) be instrumental in the control of addictive behaviors; (g) increase exercise activity during and after cardiac and pulmonary rehabilitation; (h) enhance the effects of health education; (i) improve stress management; and (j) increase performance of health-promotion behaviors in general. Support has been found for generalization of self-efficacy to similar situations and behaviors.

Interventions designed to produce behavioral change have been found to be more effective if the assumptions of the SCT are incorporated in their design and implementation. Interventions evolving from the mastery source of information, such as participatory exercise classes with individuals with similar characteristics and experiences grouped together, are the most potent in influencing self-efficacy and related behavior. Mastery is achieved more quickly if behaviors are broken down into components and each component is addressed in a logical manner separately, possibly mastering from simple to complex. Verbal persuasion and emotional arousal appear to be the most common methods of intervention to increase self-efficacy and improve health behaviors. Health education and public advertisements, although not as effective sources of information as mastery, are appropriate for helping identify barriers, benefits, and consequences of a behavior while identifying desired outcomes. In addition, research has shown that to maintain a behavioral change, reinforcement must be provided intermittently as appropriate for the behavior being addressed. Verbal persuasion and emotional arousal are excellent sources of information for reinforcement.

Additional research using conceptual and operational definitions consistent with the SCT must be conducted to support the reliability, validity, and applicability of the theory to nursing practice and research in the areas of health behavior and stress and coping. More research needs to be completed that addresses outcome expectations and all three dimensions of efficacy expectations to evaluate the multidimensional character of self-efficacy. Most studies have not addressed all four sources of efficacy information involved in cognitive appraisal and subsequent behavior. Research also must be conducted to develop reliable, valid instruments that can be used, or modified for use, across behavioral categories and populations. Items on a self-efficacy instrument need to reflect the four sources of efficacy information and three dimensions of efficacy expectations as well as outcome expectations. Specific positive and negative consequences of a behavior need to be identified within the instrument. Ideally, the individual would identify expected outcomes because these must be relevant to the individual in a specific situation to be cognitively appraised in relation to efficacy expectations and actual behavioral performance.

REFERENCES

Adegbola, M. (2007). *The relationship among spirituality, self-efficacy, and quality of life in adults with sickle cell disease* (Unpublished doctoral dissertation). The University of Texas at Arlington.

Airlie, J., Baker, G. A., Smith, S. J., & Young, C. A. (2001). Measuring the impact of multiple sclerosis on psychosocial functioning: The development of a new self-efficacy scale. *Clinical Rehabilitation, 15*(3), 259–265.

Akhavan, J. (2008). *The effect of a dyadic intervention on self-efficacy, physical functioning, and anxiety/depression in older adults post joint replacement surgery* (Unpublished doctoral dissertation). University of California, Los Angeles.

Al-Duhoun, A. (2005). *Effect of cardiac rehabilitation attendance on social support for exercise, motivation, and self-efficacy after cardiac surgery* (Unpublished doctoral dissertation). Case Western Reserve University (Health Sciences), Cleveland, OH.

Ali, N. (1998). The hormone replacement therapy self-efficacy scale. *Journal of Advanced Nursing, 28*(5), 1115–1119.

Allen, J., Becker, D., & Swank, R. (1990). Factors related to functional status after coronary artery bypass surgery. *Heart & Lung, 19*(4), 337–343.

Allen, J., Sorensen, G., Stoddard, A., Colditz, G., & Peterson, K. (1998). Intention to have a mammogram in the future among women who have underused mammography in the past. *Health Education Behavior, 25*(4), 474–488.

Allison, M. (2000). *The effect of a social cognitive theory-based intervention of self-efficacy and physical activity in older adults post coronary event* (Unpublished doctoral dissertation). The University of Texas Health Science Center at San Antonio.

Anderson, E., Wolinsky, F., Miller, J., & Wilson, M. (2006). Cross-sectional and longitudinal risk factors for falls, fear of falling, and falls efficacy in a cohort of middle-aged African Americans. *The Gerontologist, 46*(2), 249–257.

Arnold, R., Ranchor, A., DeJongste, M., & Gerard, K. (2005). The relationship between self-efficacy and self-reported physical functioning in chronic obstructive pulmonary disease and chronic heart failure. *Behavioral Medicine, 31*(3), 107–115.

Arthur, B., Kopec, J., Kinkhoff, A., Adam, P., Carr, S., et al. (2009). Readiness to manage arthritis: A pilot study using stages-of-change measures for arthritis rehabilitation. *Rehabilitation Nursing, 34*(2), 64–73.

Atkins, C., Kaplan, R., Timms, R., Reinsch, S., & Lofback, K. (1984). Behavioral exercise programs in the management of chronic obstructive pulmonary disease. *Journal of Counseling and Clinical Psychology, 52*(4), 591–603.

Badr, H., & Moody, P. (2005). Self-efficacy: A predictor for smoking cessation contemplators in Kuwaiti adults. *International Journal of Behavioral Medicine, 12*(4), 273–277.

Bandura, A. (1977). Self-efficacy: Toward a unifying theory of behavioral change. *Psychological Review, 84*, 191–215.

Bandura, A. (1982). Self-efficacy mechanism in a human agency. *American Psychologist, 37*, 122–147.

Bandura, A. (1986). Social foundations of thought and action: A social cognitive theory. Englewood Cliffs, NJ: Prentice Hall.

Bandura, A. (1989). Human agency in social cognitive theory. *American Psychologist, 44*(9), 1175–1184.

Bandura, A. (1991). Self-efficacy mechanism in physiological activation and health-promoting behavior. In J. Madden (Ed.), *Neurobiology of learning, emotion and affect* (pp. 229–270). New York, NY: Raven Press.

Bandura, A. (1995). Exercise of personal and collective efficacy in changing societies. In A. Bandura (Ed.), *Self-efficacy in changing societies* (pp. 1–45). New York, NY: Cambridge University Press.

Bandura, A. (1997). *Self-efficacy: The exercise of control*. New York, NY: Freeman.

Barlow, J. (1998). Understanding exercise in the context of chronic disease: An exploratory investigation of self-efficacy. *Perception and Motor Skills, 87*(2), 439–446.

Beckham, J., Burker, E., Lytle, B., Feldman, M., & Costakis, M. (1997). Self-efficacy and adjustment in cancer patients: A preliminary report. *Behavioral Medicine, 23*(3), 138–142.

Blacklock, R., Rhodes, R., Blanchard, C., & Gaul, C. (2010). Effects of exercise intensity and self-efficacy on state anxiety with breast cancer survivors. *Oncology Nursing Forum, 37*(2), 206–212.

Boardman, T., Catley, D., Mayo, M., & Ahiuwalia, J. (2005). Self-efficacy and motivation to quit during participation in a smoking cessation program. *International Journal of Behavioral Medicine, 12*(4), 266–272.

Bosscher, R., & Van Der, H. (1995). Physical performance and physical self-efficacy in the elderly. *Journal of Aging & Health, 7*(4), 459–475.

Brafford, L., & Beck, K. (1991). Development and validation of a condom self-efficacy scale for college students. *College Health, 39*, 219–225.

Bray, M., Kehle, T., Lawless, K., & Theodore, L. (2003). The relationship of self-efficacy and depression to stuttering. *American Journal of Speech-Language Pathology, 12*(4), 425–431.

Broome, B. (2001). Psychometric analysis of the Broome pelvic muscle self-efficacy scale in African American women with incontinence. *Urologic Nursing, 21*(4), 289–297.

Brown, E. (1998). Female injecting drug users: Human immunodeficiency virus risk behavior and intervention needs. *Journal of Professional Nursing, 14*(6), 361–369.

Burns, K., Camaione, D., Froman, R., & Clark, B. (1998). Predictors of referral to cardiac rehabilitation. *Clinical Nursing Research, 7*(2), 1054–1077.

Carpinello, S., Knight, E., Markowitz, F., & Pease, E. (2000). The development of the mental health confidence scale: A measure of self-efficacy in individuals diagnosed with mental disorders. *Psychiatric Rehabilitation Journal, 23*(3), 236–243.

Carroll, D. (1995). The importance of self-efficacy expectations in elderly patients recovering from coronary artery bypass surgery. *Heart & Lung, 24*, 50–59.

Cecil, H., & Pinkerton, S. (1998). Reliability and validity of a self-efficacy instrument for protective sexual behaviors. *Journal of American College Health, 47*(3), 113–121.

Champion, V., Skinner, C., & Menon, U. (2005). Development of a self-efficacy scale for mammography. *Research in Nursing & Health, 28*(4), 329–336.

Cheng, T. & Boey, K. (2002). The effectiveness of a cardiac rehabilitation program on self-efficacy and exercise tolerance. *Clinical Nursing Research, 11*(1), 10–21.

Clark, N., & Dodge, J. (1999). Exploring self-efficacy as a predictor of disease management. *Health Education & Behavior, 26,* 1090–1981.

Clearing-Sky, M. (1986). *A path analysis of the biopsychosocial variables related to exercise performance and adherence* (Unpublished doctoral dissertation). Michigan State University, East Lansing.

Conner, M., & Norman, P. (1995). *Predicting health behaviour: Research and practice with social cognition models* (pp. 163–196). Buckingham, UK: Open University Press.

Courneya, K., & McAuley, E. (1994). Are there different determinants of the frequency, intensity, and duration of physical activity? *Behavioral Medicine, 20*(2), 84–90.

Crowley, S. (2003). *The effect of a structured exercise program on fatigue, strength, endurance, physical self-efficacy, and functional wellness in women with early stage breast cancer* (Unpublished doctoral dissertation). University of Michigan, Ann Arbor, MI.

D'Alonzo, K. (2002). *Effects of an intervention to enhance exercise self-efficacy among Black and Hispanic college-age women* (Unpublished doctoral dissertation). The State University of New Jersey.

Davis, A., Aurelio, J., Fahy, B., & Rawiworrakul, T. (2007). Reliability and validity of the exercise self-regulatory efficacy scale for individuals with chronic obstructive pulmonary disease. *Heart & Lung, 36*(3), 205.

Davis, J. (1997). *The relationship between self-efficacy of diabetes management and health-promoting behaviors* (Unpublished manuscript).

De Geest, S., Abraham, I., Gemoets, H., & Evers, G. (1994). Development of the Long Term Behaviour Self-Efficacy Scale: Qualitative study for item development. *Journal of Advanced Nursing, 19,* 233–238.

Dennis, C. (2003). The Breastfeeding Self-Efficacy Scale: Psychometric assessment of the short form. *Journal of Obstetric, Gynecologic, and Neonatal Nursing, 32*(6), 734–744.

Desharnais, R., Bouillon, J., & Godin, G. (1986). Self-efficacy and outcome expectations as

determinants of exercise adherence. *Psychological Reports, 59,* 1155–1159.

Devins, G., & Edwards, P. (1988). Self-efficacy and smoking reduction in chronic obstructive pulmonary disease. *Behavior Research Therapy, 26*(2), 127–135.

De Vries, H., Mudde, A., Dijkstra, A., & Willemsen, M. (1998). Differential beliefs, perceived social influences, and self-efficacy expectations among smokers in various motivational phases. *Previews in Medicine, 27*(5), 681–689.

Dilorio, C., Faherty, B., & Manteuffel, B. (1992). The development and testing of an instrument to measure self-efficacy in individuals with epilepsy. *Journal of Neuroscience Nursing, 24,* 9–13.

Dutton, G., Tan, F., Provost, B., Sorenson, J., Allen, B., et al. (2009). Relationship between self-efficacy and physical activity among patients with type 2 diabetes. *Journal of Behavioral Medicine, 32*(3), 270–277.

Dzewaltowski, D., Noble, J., & Shaw, J. (1990). Physical activity participation: Social cognitive theory versus the theories of reasoned action and planned behavior. *Journal of Sport & Exercise Psychology, 12,* 388–405.

English, L. (2001). *Relationship of perceived self-efficacy of disease management and hospital utilization among patients with heart failure* (Unpublished doctoral dissertation). Grand Valley State University, Allendale, MI.

Erlen, J., Cha, E., Kim., K., Caruthers, D., & Sereika, S. (2010). The HIV Medication Taking Self-Efficacy Scale: psychometric evaluation. *Journal of Advanced Nursing, 66*(11), 2560.

Etter, J., Bergman, M., Humair, J., & Perneger, T. (2000). Development and validation of a scale measuring self-efficacy of current and former smokers. *Addiction, 95*(6), 901–913.

Fernandez, S., Chaplin, W., Schoenthaler, A. M., & Ogedegbe, G. (2008). Revision and validation of the Medication Adherence Self-Efficacy Scale (MASES) in hypertensive African Americans. *Journal of Behavioral Medicine, 31*(6), 453–462.

Ferrier, S., Dunlop, N., & Blanchard, C. (2010). The role of outcome expectations and self-efficacy in explaining physical activity behaviors of individuals with multiple sclerosis. *Behavioral Medicine, 36*(1), 7–11.

Fisher, M., & Howell, D. (2010). The power of empowerment: An ICF-based model to improve self-efficacy and upper extremity function of survivors of breast cancer. *Rehabilitation Oncology, 28*(3), 19–25.

Fraser, C., & Polito, S. (2007). A comparative study of self-efficacy in men and women with multiple sclerosis. *Journal of Neuroscience Nursing, 39*(2), 102–106.

Garg, A., Serwint, J., Hiugman, S., & Kanof, A. (2007). Self-efficacy for smoking cessation counseling patients in primary care: An office-based intervention for pediatricians and family physicians. *Clinical Pediatrics, 46*(3), 252–257.

Garry, R. (2006). Exercise self-efficacy in older women with diastolic heart failure: Results of a walking program and education intervention. *Journal of Gerontological Nursing, 32*(7), 31–39.

Gillis, C., Gortner, S., Hauck, W., Shinn, J., Sparacino, P., & Tompkins, C. (1993). A randomized clinical trial of nursing care for recovery from cardiac surgery. *Heart & Lung, 22*(2), 125–133.

Gleeson-Kreig, J. (2004). *Daily activity records: Effects on physical activity self-efficacy and behavior in people with type 2 diabetes* (Unpublished doctoral dissertation). The University of Connecticut, Storrs, CT.

Godin, G., & Shephard, R. (1985). Gender differences in perceived self-efficacy among older individuals. *Perceptual and Motor Skills, 60*, 599–602.

Goldman, J., & Harlow, L. (1993). Self-perception variables that mediate AIDS preventive behavior in college students. *Health Psychology, 12*(6), 489–498.

Gonzalez, J. (1990). Factors relating to frequency of breast self-examination among low-income Mexican-American Women. *Cancer Nursing, 13*(3), 134–142.

Gormley, J., Carrieri-Kohlman, V., Douglas, M., & Stulbarg, M. (1993). Treadmill self-efficacy and walking performance in patients with COPD. *Journal of Cardiopulmonary Rehabilitation, 13*, 424–431.

Gortner, S., Gilliss, C., Shinn, J., Sparacino, P., Rankin, S., Leavitt, M., . . . Hudes, M. (1988). Improving recovery following cardiac surgery: A randomized clinical trial. *Journal of Advanced Nursing, 13*, 649–661.

Gregory, V. (2001). *Stage of change, level of self-efficacy (confidence), and level of temptation after participating in a smoking cessation program* (Unpublished doctoral dissertation). Texas Tech University, Lubbock, TX.

Grembowski, D., Patrick, D., Diehr, P., Durham, M., Beresford, S., Kay, E., & Hecht, J. (1993). Self-efficacy and health behavior among older adults. *Journal of Health and Social Behavior, 34*, 89–104.

Gross, D., Conrad, B., Fogg, L., & Wothke, W. (1994). A longitudinal model of maternal self-efficacy, depression, and difficult temperament during toddlerhood. *Research in Nursing and Health, 17*, 207–215.

Gulanick, M. (1991). Is phase 2 cardiac rehabilitation necessary for early recovery of patients with

cardiac disease? A randomized, control study. *Heart & Lung, 20*, 9–15.

Haas, B. (2001). *Fatigue, self-efficacy for physical activity and quality of life in women with breast cancer* (Unpublished doctoral dissertation). The University of Texas at Austin.

Hall, A. (2000). *Psychometric analysis of the self-efficacy for adults with diabetes scale* (Unpublished doctoral dissertation). Saint Louis University, St. Louis, MO.

Hampton, N. (2004). Subjective well-being among people with spinal cord injuries: The role of self-efficacy, perceived social support, and perceived health. *Rehabilitation Counseling Bulletin, 48*(1), 31–37.

Hampton, N., & Marshall, A. (2000). Culture, gender, self-efficacy, and life satisfaction: A comparison between Americans and Chinese people with spinal cord injuries. *Journal of Rehabilitation, 66*(3), 21–28.

Hauer, K., Yardley, L., Beyer, N., Kempen, G., Dias, N., et al. (2010). Validation of the Falls Efficacy Scale and Falls Efficacy Scale International in Geriatric Patients with and without cognitive impairment: Results of self-report and interview-based questionnaires. *Gerontology, 56*(2), 190–199.

Hellstrom, K., Vahlberg, B., Urell, C., & Emtner, M. (2009). Fear of falling, fall-related self-efficacy, anxiety and depression in individuals with chronic obstructive pulmonary disease. *Clinical Rehabilitation, 23*(2), 1136–1144.

Hewlett, S., Cockshott, Z., Kirwan, J., Barrett, J., Stamp, J., et al. (2001). Development of a self-efficacy scale for use in British patients with rheumatoid arthritis (RASE). *Rheumatology, 40*(11), 1221.

Hickey, M., Owen, S., & Froman, R. (1992). Instrument development: Cardiac diet and exercise self-efficacy. *Nursing Research, 41*(6), 347–351.

Hilgenkamp, K. (1987). *The role of self-efficacy in various stages of exercise involvement among novice female runners* (Unpublished doctoral dissertation). University of Nebraska, Lincoln.

Hiltunen, E., Winder, P., Rait, M., & Buselli, E. (2005). Implementation of efficacy enhancement nursing interventions with cardiac elders. *Rehabilitation Nursing, 30*(6), 221–229.

Hofstetter, C., Sallis, J., Hovell, M., Byron, M., Jones, S., Rummani, S., . . . Weiss, D. (1990). Some health dimensions of self-efficacy: Analysis of theoretical specificity. *Social Medicine, 31*(9), 1051–1056.

Hogenmiller, J., Atwood, J., Lindsey, A., Johnson, D., Hertzog, M., et al. (2007). Self-efficacy scale for pap smear screening participation in sheltered women. *Nursing Research, 56*(6), 369.

Holcomb, J., Lira, J., Kingery, P., Smith, D., Lane, D., & Goodway, J. (1998). Evaluation of Jump into Action: A program to reduce the risk of non-insulin dependent diabetes mellitus in school children on the Texas-Mexico border. *Journal of School Health, 68*(7), 282–288.

Holden, G. (1991). The relationship of self-efficacy appraisals to subsequent health-related outcomes: A meta-analysis. *Social Work in Health Care, 16,* 53–93.

Horan, M., Kim, K., Gendler, P., Froman, R., & Patel, M. (1998). Development and evaluation of the Osteoporosis Self-Efficacy Scale. *Research in Nursing and Health, 21*(5), 395–403.

Hurley, A. (1990). Measuring self care ability in patients with diabetes: The Insulin Management Diabetes Self-Efficacy Scale. In O. Strickland & C. Waltz (Eds.), *Measurement of nursing outcomes* (pp. 28–44). New York, NY: Springer.

Hurley, A., & Shea, C. (1992). Self-efficacy: Strategy for enhancing diabetes self-care. *The Diabetes Educator, 18*(2), 146–150.

James, S. (2008). *I think I can: Parenting self-efficacy in parents of young adolescents* (Unpublished doctoral dissertation). University of Massachusetts, Amherst, MA.

Jemmott, L., & Jemmott, J. (1992). Increasing condom-use intentions among sexually active black adolescent women. *Nursing Research, 41*(5), 273–279.

Johnson, M., Neilands, T., Dilworth, S., Morin, S., & Remien, R. (2007). The role of self-efficacy in HIV treatment adherence: Validation of the HIV Treatment Adherence Self-Efficacy Scale (HIV-ASES). *Journal of Behavioral Medicine, 30*(5), 359–370.

Jones, F., Mandy, A., & Partridge, C. (2009). Changing self-efficacy in individuals following a first time stroke: preliminary study of a novel self-management intervention. *Clinical Rehabilitation, 23*(6), 522–533.

Jones, J. (2004). *Effect of a health promotion program on self-efficacy, health behaviors, and blood pressure within an adult hypertensive population* (Unpublished doctoral dissertation). Louisiana State University Health Sciences Center School of Nursing, New Orleans, LA.

Kalichman, S., Cain, D., Fuhrel, A., Eaton, L., Di Fonzo, K., et al. (2005). Assessing medication adherence self-efficacy among low-literacy patients: Development of a pictographic visual analogue scale. *Health Education Research, 20*(1), 24–35.

Kalichman, S., Roffman, R., Picciano, J., & Bolan, M. (1998). Risk for HIV infection among bisexual men seeking HIV-prevention services and risks posed to their female partners. *Health Psychology, 17*(4), 320–327.

Kaplan, R., Ries, A., Prewitt, L., & Eakin, E. (1994). Self-efficacy expectations predict survival for patients with chronic obstructive pulmonary disease. *Health Psychology, 13*(4), 366–368.

Kasen, S., Vaughan, R., & Walter, H. (1992). Self-efficacy and AIDS preventive behaviors among tenth grade students. *Health Education Quarterly, 19*(2), 187–202.

Kaul, T. (2007). *The relationship between self-efficacy beliefs toward self-management of asthma and asthma self-management behaviors in urban African American children* (Unpublished doctoral dissertation). Marquette University, Milwaukee, WI.

Kingery, P., & Glasglow, R. (1989). Self-efficacy and outcome expectations in the self regulation of non-insulin dependent diabetes mellitus. *Health Education, 20*(7), 13–19.

Kohlbry, P. (2006). *Exercise self-efficacy, stages of exercise change, health promotion behaviors, and physical activity in postmenopausal Hispanic women* (Unpublished doctoral dissertation). University of San Diego, San Diego, CA.

Kowalski, S. (1997). Self-esteem and self-efficacy as predictors of success in smoking cessation. *Journal of Holistic Nursing, 15*(2), 128–142.

Kranz, K. (2003). Development of the alcohol and other drug self-efficacy scale. *Research on Social Work Practice, 13*(6), 724–741.

Kurlowicz, L. (1998). Perceived self-efficacy, functional ability, and depressive symptoms in older elective surgery patients. *Nursing Research, 47*(4), 219–226.

Lazarus, R. (1991). *Emotion & adaptation.* New York, NY: Oxford University Press.

Lazarus, R., & Folkman, S. (1984). *Stress, appraisal, and coping.* New York, NY: Springer.

Lazarus, R., & Folkman, S. (1991). The concept of coping. In A. Monet & R. Lazarus (Eds.), *Stress and coping: An anthology* (pp. 189–227). New York, NY: Columbia University Press.

Lee, Y., Laffrey, S., & Cloutier, S. (2008). Exercise and self-efficacy among employed Hispanic men and women. *Hispanic Health Care International, 6*(1), 21–26.

Leonard, B., Skay, C., & Rheinberger, N. (1998). Self-management development in children and adolescents with the role of maternal self-efficacy and conflict. *Journal of Pediatric Nursing, 13*(4), 224–233.

Li, F., Fisher, K., Harmer, P., & McAuley, E. (2005). Falls Self-Efficacy as a mediator of fear of falling in an exercise intervention for older adults. *The Journal of Gerontology, 60B*(1), P34–40.

Liu-Ambrose, T., Khan, K., Donaldson, M., & Eng, J. (2006). Falls-related self-efficacy is independently associated with balance and mobility in older women with low bone mass. *The Journal of Gerontology, 61A*(8), 832–838.

Lorig, K., Chastain, R., Ung, E., Shoor, S., & Holman, H. (1989). Development and evaluation of a scale to measure perceived self-efficacy in people with arthritis. *Arthritis and Rheumatism, 32,* 37–44.

Lowe, N. (1991). Maternal confidence in coping with labor. *Journal of Obstetrics, Gynecology, & Neonatal Nursing, 20*(6), 457–463.

MacDonald, E., Pica, S., McDonald, S., Hayes, R., & Baglioni, A. (1998). Stress and coping in early psychosis: Role of symptoms, self-efficacy, and social support in coping with stress. *British Journal of Psychiatry, 172*(Suppl. 33), 122–127.

Mackin, L. (2007). *A beginning look at the effect of age on dyspnea, physical functioning and self-efficacy for home walking and managing shortness of breath in adults with chronic obstructive pulmonary disease* (Unpublished doctoral dissertation). University of California, San Francisco.

Mann, D. Ponieman, D., Leventhal, H., & Haim, E. (2009). Predictors of adherence to diabetes medications: the role of disease and medication beliefs. *Journal of Behavioral Medicine, 32*(3), 278–284.

Marquez, D., & McAuley, E. (2006). Social cognitive correlates of leisure time physical activity among Latinos. *Journal of Behavioral Medicine, 29*(3), 281–289.

Martin, N., Holroyd, K., & Rokicki, M. (1993). The Headache Self-Efficacy Scale: Adaptation to recurrent headaches. *Headache, 33,* 244–248.

Mason, V. (2002). *Cardiac rehabilitation, home-walking, health status, and self-efficacy* (Unpublished doctoral dissertation). University of Massachusetts, Amherst.

Masse, L., Heesch, K., Eason, K., & Wilson, M. (2006). Evaluating the properties of a stage-specific self-efficacy scale for physical activity using classical test theory, confirmatory factor analysis and item response modeling. *Health Education Research, 21 S1,* 133–146.

May, B., & Limandri, B. (2004). Instrument development of the self-efficacy scale for abused women. *Research in Nursing & Health, 27*(3), 208–214.

McAuley, E. (1994). Self-efficacy and intrinsic motivation in exercising middle-aged adults. *Journal of Applied Gerontology, 13*(4), 355–370.

McAuley, E., Courneya, K., & Lettunich, J. (1991). Effects of acute and long-term exercise on self-efficacy responses in sedentary, middle-aged males and females. *The Gerontologist, 31*(4), 534–542.

McAuley, E., Konopack, J., Morris, K., & Moti, R. (2006). Physical activity and functional limitations in older women: Influence of self-efficacy. *The Journals of Gerontology, 618*(S), P270–277.

McDougall, G., & Balver, J. (1998). Decreasing mental frailty in at-risk elders. *Geriatric Nursing, 19*(4), 222–224.

McGhan, G. (2007). *Enhancing self-efficacy: Will it improve quality of life and lymphedema management for patients with breast cancer related lymphedema?* (Unpublished doctoral dissertation). University of Manitoba (Canada).

Menzies, V. (2004). *Effects of guided imagery on outcomes of pain, functional status, and self-efficacy in persons diagnosed with fibromyalgia* (Unpublished doctoral dissertation). University of Virginia.

Michael, K., Allen, J., & Macko, R. (2006). Fatigue after stroke: Relationship to mobility, fitness, ambulatory activity, social support, and falls efficacy. *Rehabilitation Nursing, 31*(5), 210–217.

Moon, L., & Backer, J. (2000). Relationships among self-efficacy, outcome expectancy, and postoperative behaviors in total joint replacement patients. *Orthopaedic Nursing, 19*(2), 77–85.

Morris, K., McAuley, E., & Moti, R. (2008). Self-efficacy and environmental correlates of physical activity among older women and women with multiple sclerosis. *Health Education Research, 23*(4), 744–752.

Netz, Y., & Raviv, S. (2004). Age differences in motivational orientation toward physical activity: An application of social-cognitive theory. *The Journal of Psychology, 138*(1), 35–48.

Nichols, J. (2009, April). The impact of a self-efficacy intervention on short-term breast-feeding outcomes. *Health Education & Behavior, 36*(3), 250–258.

Oetker, S., & Taunton, R. (1994). Evaluation of a Self-Efficacy Scale for Preoperative Patients. *American Operating Room Nurse Journal, 60,* 43–50.

O'Leary, A. (1985). Self-efficacy and health. *Behavioral Research and Therapy, 23*(4), 437–451.

Pang, M., & Eng, C. (2008). Fall-related self-efficacy, not balance and mobility performance, is related to accidental falls in chronic stroke survivors with low bone mineral density. *Osteoporosis International, 19*(7), 919–927.

Pang, M., Eng, J, & Miller, W. (2007). Determinants of satisfaction with community reintegration in older adults with chronic stroke: Role of balance self-efficacy. *Physical Therapy, 87*(3), 282–291

Pariser, D., O'Hanlon, A., & Espinoza, L. (2005). Effects of telephone intervention on arthritis self-efficacy, depression, pain, and fatigue in older adults with arthritis. *Journal of Geriatric Physical Therapy, 28*(3), 67–73.

Parkatti, T., Deeg, D., Bosscher, R., & Launer, L. (1998). Physical activity and self-rated health among 55 to 89 year old Dutch people. *Journal of Aging & Health, 10*(3), 311–326.

Paxton, R., Moti, R., Aylward, A., & Nigg, C. (2010). Physical activity and quality of life: The complementary influence of self-efficacy for physical activity and mental health difficulties. *International Journal of Behavioral Medicine, 17*(4), 255–263.

Penacoba, C., Losada, A., Lopez, J., & Marquez-Gonzalez, M. (2008). Confirmatory factor analysis of the Revised Scale for Caregiving Self-Efficacy in a sample of dementia caregivers. *International Psychogeriatrics, 20*(6), 1291–1293.

Perkins, J., Multhalp, K., Perkins, W., & Barton, C. (2008). Self-efficacy and participation in physical and social activity among older adults in Spain and the United States. *The Gerontologist, 48*(1), 51–58.

Perraud, S., Fogg, L., Kopytko, E., & Gross, D. (2006). Predictive validity of the Depression Coping Self-Efficacy Scale (DCSES). *Research in Nursing & Health, 29*(2), 147–160.

Perry, K. (2000). *Psychometric assessment of the Heart Failure Self-Efficacy Scale-34.* Unpublished doctoral dissertation. University of Illinois at Chicago Health Sciences Center.

Petty, R., & Cacioppo, J. (1981). *Attitudes and persuasion: Classic and contemporary approaches.* Dubuque, IA: William C. Brown.

Pohl, J., Martinelli, A., & Antonakos, C. (1998). Predictors of participation in a smoking cessation intervention group among low-income women. *Addictive Behaviors, 23*(5), 699–704.

Prasopkittikun, T., Tilokskulchai, F., Sinsuksai, N., & Sitthimongkol, Y. (2006). Self-efficacy in Infant Care Scale: Development and psychometric testing. *Nursing and Health Sciences, 8*(1), 44–50.

Rahman, A., Reed, E., Underwood, M., Shipley, M. E., & Omar, R. Z. (2008). Factors affecting self-efficacy and pain intensity in patients with chronic musculoskeletal pain seen in a specialist rheumatology pain clinic. *Rheumatology 47*(12), 1803–1808.

Reich, S., Bickman, L., & Heflinger, C. (2004). Covariates of self-efficacy: Caregiver characteristics related to mental health services self-efficacy. *Journal of Emotional and Behavioral Disorders, 12*(2), 99–106.

Reneman, M., Geetzen, J., Groothoff, J., & Brouwer, S. (2008). General and specific self-efficacy reports of patients with chronic low back pain: Are they related to performances in a functional capacity evaluation? *Journal of Occupational Rehabilitation, 18*(2), 183–189.

Resnick, B., Wehren, L., & Orwig, D. (2004). Reliability and validity of the Self-Efficacy and Outcome Expectations for Osteoporosis Medication Adherence Scales. *Orthopaedic Nursing, 22*(2), 139–147.

Resnick, B., Zimmerman, S., Orwig, D., Furstenburg, A., & Magaziner, J. (2000). Outcome expectations for exercise scale: Utility and psychometrics. *The Journal of Gerontology, 558*(6), S352–356.

Riemsma, R., Rasker, J., Taal, E., Griep, E., Wouters, J., & Wiegman, O. (1998). Fatigue in rheumatoid arthritis: The role of self-efficacy and problematic social support. *British Journal of Rheumatology, 37*(10), 1042–1046.

Ries, A., Kaplan, R., Myers, R., & Prewitt, L. (2003). Maintenance after pulmonary rehabilitation in chronic lung disease: A randomized trial. *American Journal of Respiratory and Critical Care Medicine, 167*(6), 880–888.

Roberts, B., Dolansky, M., & Weber, B. (2010). Psychometric properties of the task self-efficacy scale for everyday activities in older adults. *Research and Theory for Nursing Practice, 24*(2), 113–127.

Rodgers, W. M., Wilson, P. M., Hall, C. R., Fraser, S. N., & Murray, T. C. (2008). Evidence for a multidimensional self-efficacy for exercise scale. *Research Quarterly for Exercise and Sport, 79*(2), 222–234.

Rogers, L., McAuley, E., Courneya, K., & Verhuist, S. (2008). Correlates of physical activity self-efficacy among breast cancer survivors. *American Journal of Health Behavior, 32*(6), 594–603.

Rogers, L., Shah, P., Dunnington, G., & Greive, A. (2005). Social Cognitive Theory and physical activity during breast cancer treatment. *Oncology Nursing Forum, 32*(4), 807–815.

Rokke, P., Fleming-Ficek, S., Sieman, N., & Hegstad, H. (2004). Self-efficacy and choice of coping strategies for tolerating acute pain. *Journal of Behavioral Medicine, 27*(4), 343–360.

Rossen, E., & Gruber, K. (2007). Development and psychometric testing of the relocation self-efficacy scale. *Nursing Research, 56*(4), 244.

Rowe, K. (2004). *Development and psychometric properties of a self-efficacy to walk for health scale for use with midlife and older, low-income, African American women* (Unpublished doctoral dissertation). The University of Texas at Austin.

Sander, E. P., Odell, S., & Hood, K. K. (2010). Diabetes-specific family conflict and blood glucose monitoring in adolescents with type 1 diabetes: Mediational role of diabetes self-efficacy. *Diabetes Spectrum, 23*(2), 89–94.

Sardi, V. (2003). *The relationship among the use and non-use of eldercare services, self-efficacy, and job satisfaction on the perceived stress of employed* caregivers of older adults (Unpublished doctoral dissertation). The George Washington University, Washington, DC.

Sarikonda-Woitas, C. M. (2001). *The relationship between self-efficacy, exercise barriers efficacy, and exercise adherence in a cardiac rehabilitation population* (Dissertation). Medical College of Toledo, OH.

Scherer, Y., & Schmieder, L. (1997). The effect of a pulmonary rehabilitation program on self-efficacy, perception of dyspnea, and physical endurance. *Heart & Lung, 26,* 15–22.

Schuster, P., & Waldron, J. (1991). Gender differences in cardiac rehabilitation patients. *Rehabilitation Nursing, 16*(5), 248–253.

Schuster, P., Wright, C., & Tomich, P. (1995). Gender differences in the outcomes of participants in home programs compared to those in structured cardiac rehabilitation programs. *Rehabilitation Nursing, 20*(2), 93–101.

Schwarzer, R., & Jerusalem, M. (1995). Generalized Self-Efficacy Scale. In J. Weinman, S. Wright, & M. Johnstone (Eds.), *Measures in health psychology: A user's portfolio. Causal and control beliefs* (pp. 35–37). Windsor, UK: NFER-NELSON.

Serrano, E., Leiferman, J., & Dauber, S. (2007). Self-efficacy and health behaviors toward the prevention of diabetes among high risk individuals living in Appalachia. *Journal of Community Health, 32*(2), 121–133.

Sharp, P. (2008). *Self-efficacy and barriers to health-promoting behavior in cardiac rehabilitation participants and nonparticipants* (Unpublished doctoral dissertation). Virginia Commonwealth University, Richmond.

Sharts-Hopko, N., Regan-Kubinski, M., Lincoln, P., & Heverly, M. (1996). Problem focused coping in HIV infected mothers in relation to self-efficacy, uncertainty, social support, and psychological distress. *Image: Journal of Nursing Scholarship, 28*(2), 107–111.

Sherer, M., Maddux, J., Mercandate, B., Prentice-Dunn, S., Jacobs, B., & Rogers, R. (1982). The Self-Efficacy Scale: Construction and validation. *Psychological Reports, 51,* 663–671.

Siela, D. (2003). Use of self-efficacy and dyspnea perceptions to predict functional performance in people with COPD. *Rehabilitation Nursing, 28*(6), 197–204.

Skelly, A. H., Marshall, J. R., Haughey, B. P., Davis, P. J., & Dunford, R. G. (1995). Self-efficacy and confidence in outcomes as determinants of self-care practices in inner city, African-American women with insulin-dependent diabetes. *The Diabetic Educator, 21,* 38–46.

Solberg, V., & Villarreal, P. (1997). Examination of self-efficacy, social support, and stress. *Hispanic Journal of Behavioral Sciences, 19*(2), 182–193.

Srof, B. (2004). *A study of the effects of asthma related coping skills training on asthma self-efficacy, asthma related quality of life, social support, and asthma diary parameters among teens with asthma* (Unpublished doctoral dissertation). Loyola University of Chicago, IL.

Strecher, V., DeVillis, B., Becker, M., & Rosenstock, I. (1986). The role of self-efficacy in achieving health behavior change. *Health Education Quarterly, 13,* 72–91.

Sullivan, M., LaCroix, A., Russo, J., & Kathon, W. (1998). Self-efficacy and self reported functional status in coronary heart disease: A six month prospective study. *Psychosomatic Medicine, 60*(4), 473–478.

Temple, A. (2003). *The effects of diabetes self-management education on diabetes self-care, diabetes self-efficacy, and psychological adjustment to diabetes* (Unpublished doctoral dissertation). Louisiana State University Health Sciences Center School of Nursing, New Orleans, LA.

Thomas, J. (1993). Cardiac inpatient education: The impact of educational methodology on self-efficacy. *Journal of Cardiopulmonary Rehabilitation, 13,* 398–405.

Toshima, M., Kaplan, R., & Ries, A. (1990). Experimental evaluation of rehabilitation in chronic obstructive pulmonary disease: Short-term effects on exercise endurance and health status. *Health Psychology, 9*(3), 237–252.

Toshima, M., Kaplan, R., & Ries, A. (1992). Self-efficacy expectancies in chronic obstructive pulmonary disease rehabilitation. In R. Schwarzer (Ed.), *Self-efficacy: Thought control of action* (pp. 325–354). Washington, DC: Hemisphere.

Trief, P., Teresi, J., Eimicke, J., Shea, S., & Weinstock, R. (2009). Improvement in diabetes self-efficacy and glycemic control using telemedicine in a sample of older, ethnically diverse individuals who have diabetes: The IDEATel project. *Age and Ageing, 38*(2), 219–225.

Van der Ven, N. C. W., Ader, H., Weinger, K., Vand der Ploeg, H. M., Yi, J., Snoek, F. J. & Pouwer, F. (2003). The confidence in diabetes self-care scale: Psychometric properties of a new measure of diabetes-specific self-efficacy in Dutch and U.S. patients with type 1 diabetes. *Diabetes Care, 26*(3), 713–718.

Varvaro, F., & Palmer, M. (1993). Promotion of adaptation in battered women: A self-efficacy approach. *Journal of the American Academy of Nurse Practitioners, 5*(6), 264–270.

Verbrugge, L. (1985). Gender and health: An update on hypotheses and evidence. *Journal of Health and Social Behavior, 26,* 156–182.

Vidmar, P., & Robinson, L. (1994). The relationship between self-efficacy and exercise compliance in a cardiac population. *Journal of Cardiopulmonary Rehabilitation, 14,* 246–254.

Vong, S. K. S., Cheing, G. L. Y., Chan, C. C. H., Chan, F., & Leung, A. S. L. (2009). Measurement of structure of the Pain Self-Efficacy Questionnaire in a sample of Chinese patients with chronic pain. *Clinical Rehabilitation, 23*(11), 1034–1043.

Waller, K., & Bates, R. (1992). Health locus of control and self-efficacy beliefs in a health elderly sample. *American Journal of Health Promotion, 6*(4), 302–309.

Waller, P., Crow, C., Sands, D., & Becker, H. (1988). Health related attitudes and health promoting behaviors: Differences between health fair attenders and a community comparison group. *American Journal of Health Promotion, 3,* 17–24.

Wallston, K., Rothman, R., & Cherrington, A. (2007). Psychometric properties of the perceived diabetes self-management scale (PDSMS). *Journal of Behavioral Medicine, 30*(5), 395–401.

Wang, J., Wang, R., & Lin, C. (1998). Self-care behaviors, self-efficacy, and social support effect on the glycemic control of patients newly diagnosed with non-insulin dependent diabetes mellitus. *Kao Hsuing I Hsueh Ko Hseuh Tsa Chih, 14*(12), 807–815.

Warnecke, R., Morera, O., Turner, L., Mermeistein, R., et al. (2001). Changes in self-efficacy and readiness for smoking cessation among women with high school or less education. *Journal of Health and Social Behavior, 42*(1), 97–110.

Weber, B., Roberts, B., Yarandi, H., Mills, T., Chambler, N., & Wajsman, Z. (2007). The impact of dyadic social support on self-efficacy and depression after radical prostatectomy. *The Journal of Aging and Health, 19*(4), 630–645.

Wells, K., Thompson, N., & Kloeblen-Tarver, A. (2006). Development and psychometric testing of the prenatal breast-feeding self-efficacy scale. *American Journal of Health Behavior, 30*(2), 177–187.

Whitehead, C., Miller, M., & Crotty, M. (2003). Falls in community-dwelling older persons following hip fracture: Impact on self-efficacy, balance, and handicap. *Clinical Rehabilitation, 17*(8), 899–906.

Wieseke, A. (1991). *Self-care attributes and correlates identified by individuals with chronic disease* (Unpublished manuscript).

Wigal, J., Creer, T., & Kotses, H. (1991). The COPD Self-Efficacy Scale. *Chest, 99*(5), 1193–1196.

Wigal, J., Stout, C., Brandon, M., Winder, J., McConnaughy, K., Creer, T., & Kotses, H. (1993). The Knowledge, Attitude, and Self-Efficacy Asthma Questionnaire. *Chest, 104,* 1144–1148.

Wojcicki, T., White, S., & McAuley, E. (2009). Assessing outcome expectations in older adults: The multidimensional outcome expectations for exercise scale. *The Journals of Gerontology, 64B1,* 33–40.

21

STRESS, UNCERTAINTY, AND HEALTH

MERLE H. MISHEL AND CECILIA R. BARRON

Uncertainty is a part of life and inherent in the stress, coping, and illness experience (Babrow, Kasch, & Ford, 1998; Fjelland, Barron, & Foxall, 2008) when persons lack an adequate explanatory framework for understanding their situations and predicting outcomes (Yoshida, 1997). The link between uncertainty and stress has been repeatedly confirmed over the years (e.g., Barron, 2000; Clayton, Mishel, & Belyea, 2006; L. M. Johnson, Zautra, & Davis, 2006; Mast, 1998; Mishel, 1988; Santacroce & Lee, 2006). Uncertainty is recognized as the greatest source of psychosocial stress for persons with acute and chronic illnesses (Barron, 2000; Koocher, 1985; Mishel, 1988; Mishel, 1990; Reich, Johnson, Zautra, & Davis, 2006) and that is why it is important for nursing.

A search of the Cumulative Index for Nursing and Allied Health Literature (CINAHL) database using the word "uncertainty" for the time period 1983 through December 2010 yielded 1,123 records. A similar search for the last decade (2000–2010) revealed 785 "Uncertainty" and 245 "Uncertainty in Illness" research studies. More than one-third (96) of the latter studies had used one of Mishel's theoretical models (1981, 1988, 1990). The majority used one of Mishel's measures for assessing uncertainty, or they have interpreted qualitative findings with reference to Mishel's writings (Mishel 1983a, 1983b; Mishel & Epstein, 1990; Mishel et al., 2005).

In general, the studies show that uncertainty can reduce coping and hopefulness. It can increase anxiety, negative mood, fear, and the characteristic post-trauma symptoms—intrusive thoughts, hyper-arousal such as sleep difficulties, and hyper-vigilance to symptoms (Reich et al., 2006). Also, research has shown that high levels of uncertainty were most often associated with stress-related events, less hope, more illness intrusiveness, and greater emotional distress. Mullins et al. (1995) found illness uncertainty to be the strongest predictor of psychological distress in a post-polio syndrome population.

In a recent study of young breast cancer survivors, uncertainty at baseline was associated with higher levels of fatigue and menopausal-type symptoms (Germino et al., 2011). Chronic fear of recurrence and uncertainty about the meaning of symptoms may account for the relationship between uncertainty and negative moods (Porter et al., 2006). Stress resulting from continual uncertainty may stimulate inflammatory pathways (Antoni et al., 2006), and enduring uncertainty may be like other conditions of chronic stress. Cognitive impairment, fearful memories, depression, and disordered sleep can heighten uncertainty and undermine constructive uncertainty management (Mishel, 1988, 1990).

The concept of uncertainty is central to understanding various aspects of the stress, coping, and illness experience, including diagnosis (Fillion, Lemyre, Mandeville, & Piché, 1996) and treatment phases (Barron, 2000; Christman, 1990; Mishel & Sorenson, 1991) as well as living with chronic illness (Hilton, 1988; L. M. Johnson et al., 2006; Mishel, 1990). Also, the literature on uncertainty is not limited to the patient, but it also includes friends and family members

(Dickerson, 1998; Theobald, 1997; Wright, Afari, & Zautra, 2009). Moreover, uncertainty is the central concept in the Theory of Uncertainty in Illness related to acute (Mishel, 1981, 1988) and chronic (Mishel, 1990) illness and is implicit in self-regulation models of coping with the illness experience (J. E. Johnson, Fieler, Jones, Wlasowicz, & Mitchell, 1997; Leventhal, Diefenbach, & Leventhal, 1992). Because of the prominence of Mishel's conceptualizations in the nursing literature, the evolution and description of the theory of uncertainty in illness related to acute (Mishel, 1981, 1988) and chronic (Mishel, 1990) illness is presented here, followed by a review of uncertainty research.

UNCERTAINTY IN ILLNESS

Mishel's Theory of Uncertainty in Acute Illness

Acute Illness

According to Mishel (1984, 1988), uncertainty is the inability to determine the meaning of illness-related events and occurs when insufficient cues prevent the person from adequately structuring or categorizing an event, thus inhibiting the person's ability to predict outcomes adequately. The first pictorial representation, the Model of Perceived Uncertainty in Illness, focused on uncertainty related to acute illness (Mishel, 1981) (see Figure 21.1).

This theory was based on a cognitive appraisal model and incorporated many conceptual ideas from the writings of Lazarus (Lazarus, 1974; Lazarus & Folkman, 1984) and other theorists, such as Moos and Tsu (1977), Norton (1975), and Wyler (1974). In the model, factors within the person and characteristics of the stimuli influence the person's perception of illness-related events. When stimuli are perceived as uncertain or ambiguous, the person is unable to subjectively evaluate the illness, treatment, and hospitalization events. Lack of a cognitive structure of the illness and related events hinders the person from adequately appraising the situation, thus influencing subsequent decision making. Events perceived as uncertain are appraised as threatening and necessitate coping. Stress occurs when the person is unable to resolve the uncertainty, therefore, Mishel's (1981) original model conceptualized uncertainty as negative.

Development of the Mishel Uncertainty in Illness Scale (MUIS) (Mishel, 1981) facilitated research on this concept, which in turn contributed to revision of the model (Mishel, 1988). The focus of the revised model remained on uncertainty during acute illness or downward illness trajectory (Mishel, 1988) in patients undergoing active medical treatment (Mishel, 1988, 1995). Key concepts of the model include *stimuli frame, cognitive capacity,* and *structure providers* as antecedents to uncertainty; *inference* and *illusion* as part of the *appraisal process; coping;* and *adaptation.* A diagram of Mishel's (1988) modified model is shown in Figure 21.2.

The major changes in the model included (a) the use of the word "uncertainty" within the pictorial representation, (b) adaptation as the major outcome of coping with uncertainty, (c) uncertainty appraised as an opportunity or a "danger" (as either positive or negative), (d) greater elaboration of stimuli characteristics, and (e) the addition of resources (structure providers).

According to the revised model, *stimuli frame* refers to characteristics of the stimulus as perceived by the individual and consists of three components: symptom pattern, event familiarity, and event congruency. Uncertainty is likely to be present when the person perceives: (a) inconsistency in symptoms to form a pattern (symptom pattern), (b) the environment as sufficiently novel (event familiarity), and (c) little or no congruency between expectations and experiences in the illness-treatment situation (event congruency).

Cognitive capacity refers to the ability to process information. This capacity includes the ability to attend to information. Pain, medication, nutrition, and perceptions that the environment is dangerous may influence the person's ability to attend to information. Moreover, information overload, as well as the disease process such as dementia, also may influence attention, encoding, and recall.

Structure providers are the available resources for assistance with interpretation of the stimuli frame and include credible authority (trust and confidence in the health care provider), social support (availability of individuals for assistance), and education. Education contributes to the knowledge base from which relevant cognitive maps are developed and used for comparison with current illness-treatment stimuli. It provides the person with the ability to modulate the uncertainty. Structure providers directly

Figure 21.1   Original Model of Perceived Uncertainty in Illness

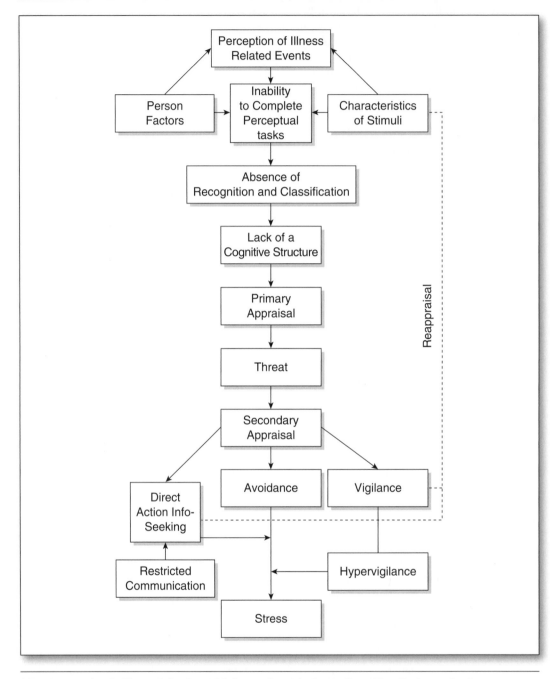

SOURCE: Reproduced with permission from Mishel, 1988. Copyright © 1988 Sigma Theta Tau International.

reduce uncertainty and indirectly reduce it through the stimuli frame components.

Appraisal in uncertainty involves the processes of inference and illusion. *Inferences* refer to general beliefs about the self and one's interaction with the environment and to the evaluation of uncertainty based on related situations from the past. Personality dispositions, such as learned

Figure 21.2   Model of Perceived Uncertainty in Illness

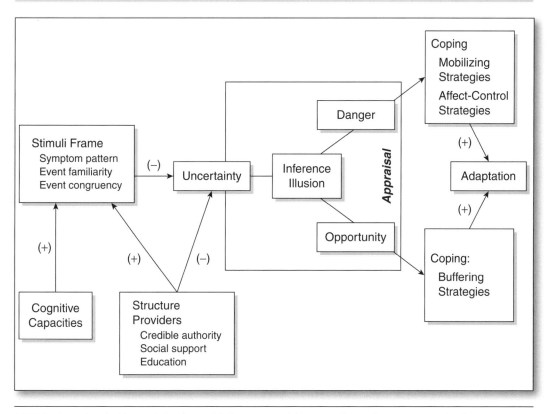

resourcefulness, sense of mastery, and locus of control, may affect the development of inferences by influencing perceptions and interpretations of current stimuli that are then encoded into memory. *Illusions* refer to beliefs arising from uncertainty and generally reflect a positive outlook. Significant others and health care providers may help the person maintain hope by fostering illusions. Inferences and illusions result in appraisals of danger or opportunity. Mishel emphasizes the experience of uncertainty as neutral until it is appraised.

When uncertainty is appraised as a danger, *Coping* is initiated to reduce the uncertainty and to manage the emotions through mobilizing and affect-management strategies. When uncertainty is appraised as an opportunity, coping is initiated to maintain uncertainty so as to sustain the belief in a positive outcome. Buffering methods are used to block the input of new stimuli that could alter the person's appraisal of uncertainty as an

opportunity. *Buffering strategies* include *avoidance, selective inattention to information, minimization of threatening information,* and the *reordering of priorities.* Effective coping via buffering, mobilizing, affect-control strategies, or all three, promotes adaptation. *Adaptation* serves as the outcome for effective coping with uncertainty.

Theory of Uncertainty and Chronic Illness

The original theory of uncertainty in illness (Mishel, 1981) and the modification (Mishel, 1988) were developed and tested primarily within the context of acute illness or downward illness trajectory and did not address (a) the experience of living with uncertainty within the context of chronic illness or a treatable acute phase with probable recurrence, (b) the nonlinear impact of antecedent variables on the appraisal of uncertainty across time, and (c) the possibility that growth or increased complexity, as opposed to adaptation, may be the desired outcome state (Mishel, 1990). Moreover, contrary to the original theory that postulates opportunity appraisals only in situations characterized by a high probability of negative consequences (i.e., downward trajectory), uncertainty was viewed as an opportunity in long-term chronic illness without a downward trajectory (Mishel & Murdaugh, 1987). In response to these problems, Mishel (1990) reconceptualized the theory for use in chronic illness. The "new view" assumes those with chronic illness are receiving maintenance treatments for their conditions (Mishel, 1990, 1995).

The theory of uncertainty in chronic illness (Mishel, 1990) incorporates the following characteristics: (a) As an open system, the person interchanges energy with the environment; (b) the person can change over time; (c) the person's appraisal of uncertainty is not static but evolves over time; and (d) the desired state may not be equilibrium but rather increased complexity. On the basis of insights obtained from chaos theory (Pool, 1989), uncertainty in illness was viewed as beginning in one part of the human system and having the potential to spread to the entire system. The more uncertainty spreads, the greater the likelihood that it will invade significant aspects of the person's life and threaten the stability of the personal system. Continual and pervasive uncertainty can destroy the cognitive structures that give life meaning, which in turn promotes disorganization.

When instability in the personal system reaches a critical threshold, the person is propelled toward a new state characterized by a higher-order, more complex orientation toward life. Structure providers, previous life experiences, and the person's physiological status influence the formation of a new life orientation. The new worldview being constructed is characterized by probabilistic and conditional thinking and necessitates the person's acceptance of uncertainty as inherent in life. The person gradually moves from an uncertainty appraisal of danger to an appraisal of opportunity.

Because the new orientation toward life is fragile, the person needs assistance from the environment to support the necessary cognitive restructuring. The process of reevaluation of uncertainty can be blocked or prolonged when (a) the person does not interact with potential social resources, (b) structure providers do not

support the person's probabilistic or conditional view of life, (c) the provider's approach to the provision of health care communicates an overt or covert devaluation of the probabilistic view, and (d) the person's role responsibilities compete with the psychological work necessary for structuring of the new value system.

In response to a critical review (Mast, 1995) of the research on adult uncertainty in illness, Mishel (1995) emphasized that the two conceptualizations (Mishel, 1988, 1990) are not interchangeable. Whereas the first conceptualization (Mishel, 1988) addresses persons receiving active medical treatment for the acute phase of an illness, the second conceptualization (Mishel, 1990) addresses persons receiving maintenance treatment for stabilization of a long-term illness. Therefore, studies addressing one conceptualization cannot be interpreted in terms of the other. Mishel cautioned, however, that the theory was re-conceptualized *"not to disregard the existing theoretical statements and linkages but to expand them to account for a perspective of growth and self-organization"* as an outcome of coping with uncertainty in chronic illness (p. 258).

Uncertainty and Stress

The most stressful experiences of uncertainty can occur in chronic conditions such as breast cancer where the fear of recurrence is common. Beyond the diagnosis and treatment phase, many breast cancer survivors experience the stressor of continual uncertainty about the possibility of recurrence and the enduring effects from cancer and treatment–induced functional limitations (Mishel et al., 2005). Among long-term survivors, uncertainty reduces one's sense of control over life, and increases emotional distress (Dirkson, 2000). It may be this uncertainty about what lies ahead that accounts for the perception among cancer survivors that the world is less controllable and more random (Tomich & Helgeson, 2002).

Furthermore, studies with fibromyalgia patients support that over time illness uncertainty interacted with interpersonally stressful daily events and predicted reduced positive affect. Illness uncertainty was a risk factor during stressful times (Reich et al., 2006). Levels of distress have been reported to increase the further patients move away from the end of active treatment. Uncertainty accounted for nearly

70% of the change over time. The experience of having cancer can be a traumatic stressor that influences the transition from cancer patient to survivor. Traumatic stress is usually intense and can intensify into full-blown cognitive crises accompanied by emotional distress (Garofalo, Choppala, Haman, Heidi, & Gjerde, 2009).

In studies of younger adult survivors of childhood cancer who are at risk for late effects from treatment, this can lead to the development of post-traumatic stress symptoms. Uncertainty has been found to function as a mediator of the relationship between post-traumatic stress syndrome and health-promotion behaviors (Santacroce & Lee, 2006).

Although there is evidence for a link between stressful events and uncertainty, there is also evidence to support decreasing uncertainty. Studies on uncertainty and stress include research conducted with patients living with implantable cardioverter defibrillators for 7 years. Uncertainty at long-term follow-up was negatively related to quality of life. Uncertainty did decline over time from a score of 63.41 at baseline to 60.81 at year 1 and 52.56 at long-term follow-up. It seems that in some conditions, such as the one tested here, uncertainty becomes less of a problem the longer the chronically ill patient lives with continuous uncertainty (Flemme et al., 2005). In a study of patients with atrial fibrillation, those with higher education and/or greater social support perceived less uncertainty and persons with greater social support perceived less uncertainty (Kang, Daly, & Kim, 2004). Furthermore, there is evidence that as cancer survivors age, they experience less symptom bother resulting in less uncertainty and distress and improved well-being during survivorship (Clayton, Mishel, & Belyea, 2006). Although age is not a factor in uncertainty theory, inclusion of this finding provides information on how the theory functions under various conditions. This raises questions about the subjective interpretation of illness and the extent to which it determines perceptions of stress and uncertainty. According to the uncertainty in illness theory, uncertainty is inherently neutral but can be appraised as an opportunity or a threat.

Uncertainty and Management Interventions

In her work, Mishel conducted a number of uncertainty management interventions that have been effective in promoting uncertainty management and in decreasing uncertainty, thus decreasing stress (Germino et al., 2011; Mishel, Germino, Lin, Pruthi, & Wallen, 2009). As an example, two of the studies are summarized here. One (Mishel, Germino, Belyea et al., 2003) was conducted with men with localized prostate cancer. This was a telephone-delivered intervention providing the men with skills in cognitive reframing, problem solving patient–provider communication, and cancer information. A key finding was that the men in the intervention gained significant improvement in two uncertainty management skills, cognitive reframing and problem solving, 4 months following treatment. These early months after treatment were the most distressful in terms of worsening of incontinence and severe distress about impotence. This intervention study provided these men with new skills for coping with the disruption in their lives and for managing extreme treatment side effects during the time of highest distress.

The second study (Mishel, Germino, Gil et al., 2005) was of 509 older recurrence-free breast cancer survivors (360 Caucasian and 149 African American women) with a mean age of 64; they were 5 to 9 years post-treatment. Women were randomly assigned to either intervention or usual care control. The intervention was delivered during four weekly telephone sessions in which nurse interveners guided the cancer survivors in the use of audio-taped cognitive behavioral strategies to manage uncertainty about recurrence, and a self-help manual designed to help women understand and manage long-term treatment side effects and other symptoms. Treatment outcome data on uncertainty management were gathered at pre-intervention baseline, at 10 months later, and again at 20 months post-baseline.

At 10 months post-baseline, training in uncertainty management resulted in improvements in cognitive reframing, cancer knowledge, patient–health care provider communication, and gains in obtaining symptom and lymphedema information/resources. With no contact between 10 and 20 months, the women post–20 months in the intervention group maintained their improvements in cognitive reframing, cancer knowledge, coping skills, and maintenance of the gain in symptom and lymphedema information that was given between baseline and 10 months. More important, the women in the intervention at 20 months declined in illness uncertainty and had increased personal growth over time. These results suggest that the intervention is important in helping women derive positive benefits from the cancer experience, including developing a new view of life and finding meaning or purpose in the experience.

In conclusion, uncertainty can threaten one's sense of coherence and has the potential to produce stress and physiological consequences over time. However, there is some recent evidence that uncertainty can be managed and, in some situations, it can be reduced. Further work is needed to identify and capitalize on such situations so that uncertainty becomes manageable across the continuum of chronic illness.

MEASURES OF UNCERTAINTY

Uncertainty in Illness Scales

Uncertainty in illness scales are the primary paper-and-pencil tools used to assess the uncertainty phenomenon (Mishel, 1981, 1983a, 1983b, 1984; Mishel & Epstein, 1990). The original work on instrument development began with the Mishel Uncertainty in Illness Scale (MUIS) in 1981. The 30-item scale was constructed to examine uncertainty in adults undergoing treatment for an active disease process. The MUIS uses a 5-point, Likert-type format and has undergone several revisions as a result of multiple psychometric evaluations. Versions range from 28 to 34 items and yield 2 to 4 factors: (a) ambiguity of illness cues, (b) complexity related to cues about the treatment and the system of care, (c) inconsistency related to information received, and (d) unpredictability of illness outcomes from illness and treatment cues. Factor reliabilities range from .71 to .91 and are strongest for ambiguity and complexity (Mishel & Epstein, 1990).

Diagnostic-specific versions of the uncertainty scale have been developed over the years to enhance clinical application of the questionnaires to specific diagnostic groups (Mishel, 1983a). Persons with various health problems, such as cardiovascular and lupus patients, completed the MUIS, and cluster analyses were used to develop the diagnostic-specific versions. The specific diagnostic version is administered together with the MUIS to allow for comparison across diagnostic entities.

Whereas the MUIS was designed for use with hospitalized adults, a 28-item community version (MUIS-C) is being used for non-hospitalized adults. The community version can be used by family members of the non-hospitalized chronically ill (Mishel & Epstein, 1990). A 34-item Parents' Perception of Uncertainty Scale (PPUS) (Mishel, 1983b) was used to evaluate the degree of uncertainty perceived by parents of an ill child and can be modified for use by a spouse or relative of an ill family member.

The MUIS has been translated into Swedish, German, Chinese, Egyptian, Thai, Korean, and Hebrew (Mishel & Epstein, 1990). Initial work on a Swedish version of the MUIS provides support for the cultural equivalence of the uncertainty concept (Hallberg & Erlandsson, 1991; Mishel, 1991), although questions remain regarding the consistency of the definition of uncertainty in the Swedish language and culture (Mishel, 1991, 1997).

Hilton (1994) developed the Uncertainty Stress Scale (USS), which is intended to measure uncertainty, the stress occurring from that uncertainty, and the degree to which uncertainty is perceived as threatening or positive or both. The first part of the measure (60 items) asks respondents to rate their degree of uncertainty about their health condition and their coping with that uncertainty using a 5-point scale. Respondents are given the option of indicating whether the item is applicable or not applicable. The second part of the questionnaire asks respondents to rate their degree of stress related to each of the uncertainty items on a 3-point scale. The third part uses visual analog scales to measure global uncertainty, global stress, global threat, and perceptions of positive feelings arising from the uncertain state. A subscale score for each section can be obtained by summing the responses for each section.

The USS has undergone several revisions, and the author expects additional reduction of items to create a more streamlined version (Hilton, 1994). Factor analysis yielded two factors: (a) indefiniteness and lack of clarity about the present and future state of the disorder and (b) being unsettled or having doubts about coping. Internal consistency reliabilities for the factors are .96 and .94, respectively. Construct validity of the USS has been reported (Hilton, 1994). Clauson (1996) adapted the USS to create a high-risk pregnancy version.

The Appraisal of Uncertainty Scale is a 15-item questionnaire derived from a scale designed to assess coping responses (Folkman,

1982; Lazarus & Folkman, 1984). Each item represents an emotional state, such as sad, fearful, and hopeful. Respondents rate the degree to which they feel each emotion in response to the uncertainty perceived using a 6-point Likert scale ranging from "not at all" (1) to "a great deal" (6). Eight items comprise the Danger Appraisal subscale, and seven items comprise the Opportunity Appraisal subscale. Coefficient alphas range from .76 (opportunity) to .87 (danger) (Mishel & Sorenson, 1991). See Table 21.1 for psychometric properties of uncertainty measures.

Table 21.1   Selected Measures for the Phenomenon of Uncertainty

Measure	Reference and population	Reliability and validity[1,2]
Appraisal of Uncertainty Scale	Mishel, Padilla, Grant, & Sorenson (1991); Adults: 100 women receiving treatment for gynecological cancer	.82 (danger), .76 (opportunity); CV-HT
	Mishel & Sorenson (1991); Adults: 131 women receiving treatment for gynecological cancer	.87 (danger), .82 (opportunity); CV-HT
	Padilla, Mishel, & Grant (1992); Adults: 100 women receiving treatment for newly diagnosed gynecological cancer	.82 (danger), .76 (opportunity); CV-HT
	Wineman, Durand, & Steiner (1994); Adults: 433 (multiple sclerosis [MS]) and 257 (spinal cord injury [SCI])	.88 for danger (MS), .86 for danger (SCI); .80 for opportunity (MS), .83 for opportunity (SCI); CV-HT
Mishel Uncertainty in Illness (MUIS)	Ellett & Young (1997); Adolescents: 105 (68 with inflammatory bowel disease, 20 with irritable bowel syndrome, and 17 healthy)	.84–.89; CV-HT
	Galloway & Graydon (1996); Adults: 40 cancer patients following surgical resection of colon cancer	.80 (total scale), .53 (complexity); alpha for ambiguity factor not reported; CV-HT
	Germino et al. (1998); Adults: 403 (201 men with prostate cancer and their family caregivers)	Coefficient alphas > .70 (specific Cronbach's alpha coefficients not reported); CV-HT
	Mast (1998); Adults: 109 women with breast cancer (58 Stage I, 50 Stage II, and 1 Stage III)	.90 (total score); CV-HT
	McCain, Zeller, Cella, Urbanski, & Novak (1996); Adults: 45 men with HIV disease	.83 (total score); CV-HT
	Mishel (1981); Adults: 134 medical, 51 rule-out, and 68 surgical patients	.91 (total scale); construct validity (known groups)
	Mishel (1984); Adults: 100 hospitalized medical patients from a Veterans Administration hospital	.89 (multiattributed ambiguity), .72 (unpredictability); CV-HT
	Mishel et al. (1991); Adults: 100 women receiving treatment for gynecological cancer	.91 (total scale); CV-HT
	Mishel & Sorenson (1991); Adults: 131 women receiving treatment for gynecological cancer	.90 (total scale); CV-HT
	Moser, Clements, Brecht, & Weiner (1993); Adults: 94 systemic sclerosis patients	.84 (total scale); CV-HT

(Continued)

Table 21.1   (Continued)

Measure	Reference and population	Reliability and validity[1,2]
	Northouse, Dorris, & Charron-Moore (1995); Adults: 155 (81 women with a first recurrence of breast cancer and 74 husbands)	.90 (patients); CV-HT
	Northouse, Jeffs, Cracchiolo-Caraway, Lampman, & Dorris (1995); Adults: 300 women awaiting a breast biopsy and their spouses (265)	.80 (patients); CV-HT
	Padilla et al. (1992); Adults: 100 women receiving treatment for newly diagnosed gynecological cancer	.91 (total scale); data from current study support a three-factor structure: ambiguity about illness-wellness state ($\alpha = .88$), lack of information/complexity of events information ($\alpha = .83$), unpredictability of illness/treatment outcomes ($\alpha = .72$); CV-HT
	Redeker (1992); Adults: 129 nonemergency first-time coronary artery bypass surgery (CABS) patients	One-week post-CABS $\alpha = .84$ (ambiguity) and .75 (complexity); 6-week post-CABS $\alpha = .89$ (ambiguity) and.78 (complexity); CV-HT
	Sheer & Cline (1995); Adults: 56 clinic cardiac patients	.80 and .89 for clinic pre- and post-visits, respectively; CV-HT
	Steele, Tripp, Kotchick, Summers, & Forehand (1997); Adults and children: 65 families (father, mother, and one child at least 7 years of age) in which the father had hemophilia	Alphas for father and mother data not reported; $\alpha = .83$ for child sample; CV-HT
	White & Frasure-Smith (1995); Adults: male angioplasty (22) and bypass (25) patients at 1 and 3 months after treatment	.82; CV-HT
	Wineman (1990); Adults: 38 men and 80 women with MS	.82; CV-HT
	Wineman et al. (1994); Adults: 433 (MS) and 257 (SCI)	.84 (MS) and.89 (SCI); CV-HT
	Wineman, Schwetz, Goodkin, & Rudick (1996); Adults: 59 patients with progressive MS	.74; CV-HT
	Wong & Bramwell (1992); Adults: 25 mastectomy patients	Predischarge $\alpha = .91$ (total scale), .87 (ambiguity), .82 (complexity); post-discharge $\alpha = .86$ (total scale), .71 (ambiguity), .77 (complexity); CV-HT

1. Reliability coefficients refer to internal consistency alphas.

2. CV-HT indicates that study results support the construct validity of the measure through hypothesis testing. The hypothesis is either directly posed in the study or can be inferred based on the literature review or the framework that guided the study or both.

RESEARCH RELATED TO UNCERTAINTY IN ILLNESS

Mishel's uncertainty in illness theory related to acute (Mishel, 1981, 1988) and chronic (Mishel, 1990) illness remains the sole mid-range nursing theory specifically addressing uncertainty in illness. Linkages among concepts can be supported through direct testing of the linkages or by explaining study findings in light of existing conceptualizations (Mishel, 1997). The direct testing of linkages provides for the greatest precision because the researcher can ensure, at the outset of the study, that concepts are operationalized and other parameters are established in accordance with the theory to be tested. When the theory has not driven the proposal development decisions, the "fit" between the findings and the existing conceptualization referenced is likely to be less adequate. Selected measures and studies for the phenomenon of uncertainty are in Table 21.1.

On the basis of a review of the literature, 61 articles were found that used the MUIS, an adaptation (e.g., PPUS), or parts of the instrument. The majority of studies using the MUIS, however, were not based on any of Mishel's (1981, 1988, 1990) conceptualizations. Some studies tested an investigator-developed framework, and others were atheoretical with linkages to Mishel's (1981, 1988, 1990) conceptualizations made in light of the findings. Studies of illness uncertainty can be divided into eight categories by type of illness (acute, chronic), person experiencing uncertainty (patient or family member), and developmental age of person (child or adult). Because Mishel's (1981, 1988) original conceptualizations were related to the acutely ill adult, most of the research is in this area. Studies to evaluate uncertainty in the chronically ill adult and in family members were stimulated when the MUIS was adapted for these populations. The evaluation of uncertainty in children and adolescents (Ellett & Young, 1997; Steele, Tripp, Kotchick, Summers, & Forehand, 1997), either as the patients or as family members has been limited but is growing (Sammarco, 2001; Santacroce & Lee, 2006). In keeping with the original model (Mishel, 1981, 1988), this review of the literature on uncertainty in illness focuses on acute illness in adults and uses the major concepts of the model (Mishel, 1988) as the organizing force. Next, research on uncertainty related to chronic illness in adults, children and adolescents, and family members is discussed.

Acute Illness in Adults

Mast (1995) evaluated the literature on adult uncertainty in both acute and chronic illness, whereas Mishel (1997) focused on uncertainty in acute illness, including the adult patient and the family member of an acutely ill adult or child. The purpose of this discussion is to highlight the consistencies and inconsistencies related to findings on uncertainty in acute illness and Mishel's model (1988). (See Figure 21.2.)

Stimuli Frame

Stimuli frame (characteristics of the stimulus as perceived by the individual) is proposed to be an antecedent of uncertainty, but interpretation of findings is difficult because the majority of studies in illness uncertainty did not directly test the linkage between stimuli frame and uncertainty. Mishel and Braden (1988) tested the linkage directly in women with gynecological cancer and found that symptom pattern predicted ambiguity but not complexity, whereas event familiarity predicted complexity but not ambiguity.

Diagnostic specificity may be considered an aspect of stimuli frame. Uncertainty is expected to be higher prior to diagnostic specificity when symptoms are present but a diagnosis is absent or before all diagnostic information is complete (Mishel, 1988). Overall, studies supported a linkage between diagnostic specificity and uncertainty (Fillion et al., 1996; Mishel, 1981; Northouse, Jeffs, Cracchiolo-Caraway, Lampman, & Dorris, 1995).

Cognitive Capacity

Cognitive capacity (the ability to process information) is proposed to influence uncertainty indirectly through stimuli frame. No studies in the illness uncertainty literature were found that directly tested this linkage. Severity of illness may be considered an indirect measure of cognitive capacity because severity of illness and its intensive treatment, such as the experience of pain and the use of pain medication, may influence an individual's capacity to perceive and interpret stimuli.

The majority of studies indicate a positive relationship between illness severity and uncertainty, but the findings are not conclusive (Mishel, 1997). The approaches used to assess severity of illness are varied and range from recurrence of illness (Hilton, 1994) and objective pathological indices (Staples & Jeffrey, 1997) to self-report measures of symptom distress (Christman, 1990) and functional status (Christman et al., 1988; Staples & Jeffrey, 1997). Some consistency of measuring illness severity is sorely needed. Moreover, clarification of relationships among the concepts of cognitive capacity, stimuli frame, and uncertainty requires studies that directly measure cognitive capacity.

Structure Providers

Structure providers (available resources) are proposed to influence uncertainty directly and indirectly by providing assistance in interpretation of the stimuli frame (Mishel, 1988). The literature provides greater support for the structure providers of credible authority and social support and less support for education (Mishel, 1997).

Several studies (Bennett, 1993; Davis, 1990; Mishel & Braden, 1987, 1988; White & Frasure-Smith, 1995) support an inverse relationship between social support and uncertainty across diverse populations, such as cardiac (Bennett, 1993; Davis, 1990; White & Frasure-Smith, 1995), gynecological cancer (Mishel & Braden, 1987, 1988), and trauma and postsurgical (Davis, 1990) patients. Although increased social support has been linked to less uncertainty, Mast (1995) notes that little is known about how social support ameliorates uncertainty and how unsupportive relationships may heighten the patient's uncertainty.

Credible authority was also associated with decreased uncertainty (Mishel & Braden, 1988; Molleman, Pruyn, & van Knippenberg, 1986), but the indirect path through symptom pattern was not supported in a sample of gynecological cancer patients (Mishel & Braden, 1988). In a study of 56 cardiac patients, illness uncertainty was lower in patients who perceived they had received adequate information from a credible health care provider (Sheer & Cline, 1995). Uncertainty was not decreased, however, in newly diagnosed diabetic patients when a provider-centered style of communication discouraged patients from seeking answers to their questions (Mason, 1985).

Findings related to education are inconsistent. Some studies found an inverse relationship between education and uncertainty (Christman et al., 1988; Hilton, 1994; Mishel, Hostetter, King, & Graham, 1984), whereas other studies found the opposite (Galloway & Graydon 1996; Mishel, 1984; Wong & Bramwell, 1992). There is evidence that the influence of education and social support on uncertainty may change over time (Christman et al., 1988; Mishel & Braden, 1987). Therefore, research is needed to determine the influence of structure providers across the illness process. Through the process of cognitive appraisal, the person judges the event to be a threat or an opportunity, and this in turn influences the type of coping to be used (Mishel, 1988). Although Mishel's (1988) model highlights the importance of cognitive appraisal to coping and adaptation, few model-based studies were found that sought to investigate variables influencing the cognitive appraisals of danger and opportunity. The majority of studies focused on the relationships between uncertainty or mastery and cognitive appraisals.

Appraisal

High levels of uncertainty were associated with threat of cancer recurrence in acute and chronic breast cancer survivors (Hilton, 1989), danger in women receiving treatment for gynecological cancer (Mishel, Padilla, Grant, & Sorenson, 1991; Mishel & Sorenson, 1991), and less hope in cancer patients receiving radiotherapy (Christman, 1990). There is evidence, however, that the relationship between uncertainty and cognitive appraisal is mediated by mastery (Mishel et al., 1991; Mishel & Sorenson, 1991)—that is, the person's perception of personal resources to manage potential stressors.

Mishel (1995) identified several concepts, such as optimism (Mishel et al., 1984), sense of personal control (Braden, 1990a), and learned resourcefulness (Braden, 1990a), that may serve as other potential mediators related to inference in cognitive appraisal. Research is needed to identify other variables that may mediate between uncertainty and cognitive appraisal and to test interventions that incorporate strategies related to cognitive appraisals for promotion of healthy adaptation. In Mishel's (1988) model, cognitive appraisal mediates uncertainty and coping. Several studies (Mishel et al., 1991;

Mishel & Sorenson, 1991) of uncertainty in gynecological oncology patients support this relationship, with uncertainty appraised as a danger-predicting, emotion-focused coping and uncertainty appraised as an opportunity-predicting, problem-focused coping.

Coping

Most investigations of uncertainty and coping have examined this linkage directly rather than indirectly through appraisals of danger and opportunity. Testing of direct relationships indicated that uncertainty was associated with coping that is focused on controlling emotional distress (Mast, 1995; Mishel, 1997). Inconsistencies in the testing of direct relationships were noted, however, when subjects were studied over time (Christman et al., 1988; Mishel, 1997; Redeker, 1992).

Few studies have examined uncertainty and coping during the course of an acute illness using a repeated measures design. Also, it remains unclear how the type of acute illness, such as myocardial infarction, and previous illness experiences influence the relationship among uncertainty, coping, and adaptation. Moreover, the conceptualization and measurement of the coping variable may influence results. New measures of coping are needed that incorporate strategies relevant to reducing the stress of uncertainty (Mishel, 1997). Qualitative studies that investigate coping with uncertainty across types of illness and over time are needed to generate items for inclusion in coping scales and to determine if there is sufficient variation in responses to warrant the tailoring of coping scales to specific clinical populations similar to Mishel's (1983a) tailoring of uncertainty scales.

Mishel (1988) proposed that coping mediates the relationship between appraisal and adaptation. In a study of 131 women receiving treatment for gynecological cancer, Mishel and Sorenson (1991) found little support for coping strategies as mediators between emotional distress and appraisals of danger or opportunity. Only two coping strategies, wishful thinking and focus on the positive, were found to mediate between danger or opportunity appraisals and emotional distress, and the mediation effect for each was small. A replication testing of the mediation effect of coping in a more heterogeneous sample of women also found limited support (Mishel et al., 1991).

Adaptation

Most studies have not tested coping as a mediator between uncertainty and adaptation but rather the direct relationship between uncertainty and adaptation. Moreover, adaptation has been operationalized in various ways, such as anxiety, emotional distress, quality of life, health, recovery, and adjustment (Mast, 1995; Mishel, 1988, 1997). In general, research has demonstrated a relationship between uncertainty and poorer psychosocial outcomes. Uncertainty has been linked to anxiety, depression, and emotional distress as well as to poorer psychosocial adjustment and quality of life in a variety of populations, such as in breast biopsy (Northouse, Jeffs et al., 1995), breast cancer (Wong & Bramwell, 1992), cardiac (Bennett, 1993; Christman et al., 1988; Webster & Christman, 1988), gynecological cancer (Mishel & Braden, 1987; Mishel & Sorenson, 1991; Mishel et al., 1984; Padilla, Mishel, & Grant, 1992), and hysterectomy patients (Warrington & Gottlieb, 1987). Similar results were found in studies of adults with chronic illness, such as patients with arthritis (Braden, 1990b), diabetes (Landis, 1996), and spinal cord injury and multiple sclerosis (Wineman, Durand, & Steiner, 1994; Wineman, Schwetz, Goodkin, & Rudick, 1996).

In her review article, Mast (1995) posed the question of whether uncertainty inevitably produces negative patient outcomes and concluded that studies of adaptation to long-term uncertainty, such as in chronic illness, may demonstrate the phenomenon of positive reappraisal that Mishel (1990) hypothesized in her theory reconceptualization. There is evidence in the research literature that the degree and type of uncertainty may change over time, leading to the phenomenon of positive reappraisal (Hilton, 1988; Nyhlin, 1990).

Chronic Illness in Adults

There is a growing body of research related to uncertainty in chronic illness across a wide variety of populations, ranging from patients with abdominal aortic aneurysm (C. Patterson & Faux, 1993), atrial fibrillation (Kang et al., 2004), and AIDS and HIV (Barroso, 1997; Gaskins & Brown, 1992; McCain & Cella, 1995; Regan-Kubinski & Sharts-Hopko, 1995; Sharts-Hopko, Regan-Kubinski, Lincoln, & Heverly, 1996; Weitz, 1989) to patients with stroke (Häggström, Axelsson, & Norberg, 1994), breast cancer survival (Mishel et al., 2005; Porter et al., 2006), and ulcerative colitis (Dudley-Brown, 1996). Approximately half of the studies reviewed used a qualitative approach, with phenomenological or grounded theory designs predominating.

Antecedents to Uncertainty

Several studies examined severity of illness as an antecedent to uncertainty. Uncertainty was positively correlated with severity of illness as measured by repeated surgeries in peripheral vascular disease (Ronayne, 1989) and perceptions of illness severity in rheumatoid arthritic (Braden, 1990a, 1990b) and asthmatic patients (Janson-Bjerklie, Ferketich, & Benner, 1993). Mast (1998), however, found no relationship between uncertainty and disease state in breast cancer survivors. Hawthorne and Hixon (1994) found that diminished functional status was associated with uncertainty in heart failure patients and noted that patients grouped by functional status had different illness trajectories, supporting the importance of assessing severity of illness in chronicity.

Other studies have investigated the structure provider variables of education and social support as antecedents to uncertainty in chronic illness. Studies reviewed generally found an inverse relationship between education and uncertainty in persons who had been diagnosed with breast cancer (Mast, 1998), multiple sclerosis (Wineman et al., 1996), and abdominal aortic aneurysm (C. Patterson & Faux, 1993), extending the linkage proposed by Mishel (1988) to chronic illness. Although there was no significant difference in uncertainty between multiple sclerosis patients who agreed to participate in a clinical trial and those who refused, acceptors reported a higher educational mean (Armer, McDermott, & Schiffer, 1996).

Social Support

Uncertainty was positively correlated with perceptions of unsupportiveness or dissatisfaction with social support in 118 adults diagnosed with multiple sclerosis (Wineman, 1990). Moreover, unsupportiveness was related to purpose in life through the variable of uncertainty. Although there was a dearth of quantitative studies investigating social support and uncertainty in chronicity, social support was an important theme in many qualitative studies (Lugton, 1997; Nelson, 1996; Regan-Kublinski & Sharts-Hopko, 1995; Thibodeau & MacRae, 1997).

Similar to Mishel's (1990) description of environmental supports needed to promote a person's new and fragile life, breast cancer survivors used supportive persons to nourish their changing identities (Lugton, 1997), as did long-term survivors of AIDS, who renegotiated interpersonal relationships to maintain their reconstructed lives within the context of HIV (Barroso, 1997). For diabetic patients, searching for support, advice, and information was important in coming to terms with the uncertainty caused by the disease and the inadequacy of the health care system (Nyhlin, 1990). The "doctor-centered" style of communication used by health professionals, however, was not helpful to diabetics as they attempted to resolve their uncertainty (Mason, 1985).

Appraisal

Uncertainty was positively correlated with the appraisal of danger in persons with asthma (Janson-Bjerklie et al., 1993) and rheumatoid arthritis (Bailey & Nielsen, 1993). Ambiguity was moderately correlated with an appraisal of danger in persons with abdominal aortic aneurysm, although there was no relationship between total uncertainty scores and appraisals of danger or opportunity (C. Patterson & Faux, 1993). The sample size was small ($N = 27$), however, and subjects experienced many other chronic illnesses, such as arthritis, in addition to the chronic aneurysm. For both multiple sclerosis and spinal cord injury patients, danger appraisals yielded more emotion-focused coping, whereas opportunity appraisals yielded more problem-focused coping (Wineman et al., 1994). Choice of coping strategies did not explain emotional well-being once selected demographic and disability-related variables were controlled, possibly due to the coping instrument's deficiency in defining the coping dimensions important to that clinical population (Wineman et al., 1994).

Outcomes of Coping With Uncertainty

Uncertainty was associated with poorer psychosocial adjustment (Moser, Clements, Brecht, & Weiner, 1993; Mullins et al., 1995), more depression (Wineman, 1990) and psychological distress (Landis, 1996; McCain & Cella, 1995; Wineman et al., 1996), poorer quality of life (Hawthorne & Hixon, 1994), and a lower sense of purpose in life (Wineman, 1990). Mishel's (1990) reformulation, however, allowed for growth rather than merely stability and equilibrium. The concept of growth is more clearly reflected in the qualitative studies in chronicity.

Selder (1989) proposed a life transition theory that describes how people who experience a disruption of their reality reorganize or reconstruct the existing one to create new meaning and resolve uncertainty. The idea of the process of transition was found in several qualitative studies that were reviewed. For example, breast cancer survivors learned new ways of being in the world and of putting uncertainty into life's perspective (Nelson, 1996). Cancer survivors spoke of the preciousness of life (Hilton, 1988) and changes in beliefs, values, goals, and roles that may serve as a positive experience (Halldórsdóttir & Hamrin, 1996; Hilton, 1988).

Confronting a life-threatening illness caused breast cancer survivors to think about metaphysical issues, such as the nature and meaning of life and the universe (Thibodeau & MacRae, 1997). Reappraising life and creating positive meanings were reflected in the interviews of diabetic patients facing long-term complications (Nyhlin, 1990). Women who survived a cardiac event redefined their priorities and focused on those activities that provided them with meaning and purpose (Fleury, Kimbrell, & Kruszewski, 1995).

Some studies have sought to understand uncertainty in chronicity by sampling subjects with a wide range of time since diagnosis—as much as a 53-year time span (Landis, 1996)—by collecting data cross-sectionally at only one point in time or at several points within a brief time period. Type and characteristics of uncertainty, however, may change over time. To develop an understanding of how uncertainty, appraisal, coping, and well-being can change over time and to determine what factors facilitate or deter such changes, longitudinal studies are needed to track persons from their initial diagnosis. Mixed designs, employing both quantitative and qualitative strategies, can be used to test hypothesized linkages while exploring factors less understood, such as identification of coping strategies relevant to the clinical population at each phase of the chronicity process. Finally, studies are needed to clarify how illnesses reflecting different levels of threat to life, such as arthritis versus AIDS, influence uncertainty and the process of transition in chronic illness.

Children and Adolescents

Most studies of ill children and adolescents have focused on uncertainty in the parent and not the child. Few studies were found that focused on uncertainty from the ill child's perspective. Haase and Rostad (1994) used a phenomenological approach to explore the children's perspective of experiencing the completion of cancer treatment in seven children ages 5 to 18 years. Whereas parents' fear of recurrence focused on the child's diminished chance of survival, children's fear of recurrence focused more on having to re-experience the side effects of chemotherapy. For children, talking about their fear of recurrence was associated with a belief that their cancer would return. This study indicates the influence of the developmental stage on perceptions of and coping with uncertainty.

The MUIS was used to assess uncertainty in adolescents with cystic fibrosis, whereas the PPUS was used to assess uncertainty in parents (Yarcheski, 1988). On the basis of the results, Yarcheski postulated that some of the items on the total MUIS and PPUS may be extraneous to the concerns of adolescents with cystic fibrosis and their parents. It is also possible, however, that the MUIS and PPUS did not adequately capture the uncertainty concerns of the adolescents and their parents. Collectively, the two studies indicate the need for tailoring the measurement of uncertainty to the developmental stage and illness-related concerns of the respondent.

Family Members

Thirty-seven articles were reviewed related to studies of uncertainty in family members; the majority (20) described qualitative studies. Almost half (16) reported on studies of parents of ill children (Cohen, 1993, 1995; Cohen & Martinson, 1988; Sparacino et al., 1997), whereas 10 articles reported on spouses of ill adults (Dickerson, 1998; O'Brien, Wineman, & Nealon, 1995; Stetz, 1989). The remaining articles reported on studies of multiple family members or did not clarify whether other family members in addition to spouses were investigated (Brown & Powell-Cope, 1991; Jamerson et al., 1996; Malone, 1997).

Parents

Miles, Funk, and Kasper (1992) used the PPUS to study uncertainty in parents of pre-term infants. Results indicated that the highest level of uncertainty was in the area of unpredictability, with mothers reporting higher levels of unpredictability than fathers. Uncertainty about the effects of prematurity on their child's development was also found in a qualitative study of parents attending a neonatal intensive care unit follow-up clinic, indicating a need for the provision of more developmental and parenting information (Hussey-Gardner, Wachtel, & Viscardi, 1998). Grounded theory was used to explore the dimensions of uncertainty of parents whose children were hospitalized in an intensive care unit (Turner, Tomlinson, & Harbaugh, 1990). The results were similar to those found in the PPUS; uncertainty related to the family system and the parent-child role, however, extended Mishel's work (Turner et al., 1990).

Uncertainty or mastering uncertainty was a central theme of several qualitative studies related to parents of chronically ill children (MacDonald, 1995, 1996; Sparacino et al., 1997). The use of hope or optimism (Siegl & Morse, 1994; Sterken, 1996) and creating meaning and purpose (Siegl & Morse, 1994) as coping strategies reflects Selder's (1989) proposal of a life transition that disrupts reality and requires creation of a new meaning and resolution of uncertainty.

Spouses

A major theme of spouses whose partners had suffered a myocardial infarction was "crushing uncertainty" (Theobald, 1997). Spouses had greater uncertainty about the illness than did cardiac (Staples & Jeffrey, 1997) and recurrent breast cancer patients (Northouse, Laten, & Reddy, 1995). Uncertainty predicted emotional distress in women experiencing recurrent breast cancer and their spouses (Northouse, Dorris, & Charron-Moore, 1995), in individuals with multiple sclerosis (MS) and their spouses (Wineman, O'Brien, Nealon, & Kaskel, 1993), and in women awaiting a breast biopsy but not

in their respective spouses (Northouse, Jeffs et al., 1995). Although illness uncertainty was an essential factor in determining family satisfaction for the MS spouse, the congruence between each partner's perception of uncertainty was the crucial factor in determining family satisfaction for the well spouse (Wineman et al., 1993). Collectively, research in this area demonstrates the importance of investigating uncertainty in the spouse and the need to expand and test Mishel's acute (1988) and chronic (1990) illness models to incorporate the spouse and the influence of each partner's uncertainty on the well-being and growth of the other.

Other Family Members

The remaining research either studied multiple family members or did not clarify whether other family members in addition to spouses were investigated. In general, when studies investigated multiple family members results were reported as family findings rather than by specific relationship. The relative's illness and negotiating the health care system served as sources of uncertainty (Jamerson et al., 1996). Adult siblings often felt left out of the decision-making process and perceived that they had not received enough basic information about their relative's illness, suggesting information may not be uniformly communicated throughout the family. Family members of patients with heart transplantation (Mishel & Murdaugh, 1987), childhood cancer (Clarke-Steffen, 1997), and AIDS experienced "transitions through uncertainty" (Brown & Powell-Cope, 1991). Collectively, these studies indicate the importance of extending and testing life transition theory (Selder, 1989) in family members of those with chronic illness. Moreover, these findings indicate the importance of studying uncertainty in the family to determine how uncertainty in each of its members influences the well-being of the others.

Uncertainty and Biomarkers

Over the past 10 years, there have been a growing number of studies examining associations between biomarkers and uncertainty about symptoms such as fatigue and sexual dysfunction, as well as studies examining biomarkers as outcomes of psychosocial interventions. Recent work has addressed whether uncertainty of the diagnosis adversely affects biochemical stress levels. According to Lang, Berbaum, & Lutgendorf (2009), four salivary cortisol samples per day for 5 days were collected after large-core breast biopsy from 150 women. T tests were used to compare diurnal cortisol slopes among three groups: patients who did not have a final diagnosis (uncertain group), patients who knew they had cancer (known malignant group), and patients who knew they have benign disease (known benign group). The mean cortisol slope for the women with uncertain disease was significantly flatter (less desirable) than that for women who learned they had benign disease but was not significantly different from women who learned they had malignant disease. The uncertainty about the final diagnosis after breast biopsy was associated with substantial biochemical distress that can have negative effects on immune defenses and wound healing.

Others have reported that prolonged and recurrent stress associated with uncertainty and fear of recurrence can be detrimental to survivors' adjustment and health (Lebel, Rosberger, Edgar, & Devins, 2007). Enduring uncertainty may be comparable to other conditions of chronic stress when physiological systems are negatively affected by prolonged exposure to steroids such as cortisol and DHEA and to the biomarkers of inflammation. In a pilot study, intrusive thoughts were correlated with the inflammatory cytokines IL-1β, IL-1ra, and IL-8, which have been related to depression and poorer quality of life among younger breast cancer survivors (Cordova, Cunningham, Carlson, & Andrykowski, 2001; Sammarco, 2001; Stanton, Danoff-Burg, & Huggins, 2002).

HEALTH-RELATED UNCERTAINTY

Although Mishel's (1981, 1988, 1990) conceptualizations have spawned a large body of research on uncertainty in illness, some investigators have extended the study of uncertainty beyond acute and chronic illness. An in-depth discussion of the theoretical and research literature in this area is beyond the scope of this chapter. Literature in this domain, however, bears mentioning to appreciate the breadth of and opportunities for research related to uncertainty.

Life Transitions and Events

Uncertainty has been studied in relation to normal life transitions, such as in pregnancy (E. T. Patterson, Freese, & Goldenberg, 1986), menopause (Lemaire & Lenz, 1995), infant adoption (Lobar & Phillips, 1996), and after natural disasters (Coffman, 1996). The majority of the studies reviewed used a qualitative design in which uncertainty emerged as a key concept. Models related to uncertainty in normal life transitions and following natural (or manmade) disasters are needed so that systematic research in these areas can be conducted.

Genetic Testing

As the revolution in molecular biology and genetics continues, genetic testing for various diseases is likely to become more available. Healthy persons with a family history of a potentially inheritable disease may experience substantial stress because of uncertainty about their risk for developing the disease. For diseases caused by inherited defects, such as Huntington's disease, testing is likely to produce different benefits and costs than those for diseases with multiple causes, such as breast cancer (Baum, Friedman, & Zakowski, 1997). Whereas genetic testing for Huntington's disease may decrease risk uncertainty, a positive result for the gene is likely to cause emotional distress. Cast in stress theory, Baum and associates (1997) presented a model that predicts long-term stress in genetic testing when risk uncertainty is minimally reduced, when testing results suggest a high risk or are at odds with preventive actions already taken, and when people lack the resources for coping with a high-risk result. As the use of genetic testing continues to increase, testing of this model and development of other models related to anticipation and consequences of genetic testing should prove to be fruitful areas for nursing research.

Dispositional Intolerance of Uncertainty

Whereas Mishel focuses on uncertainty in illness, several researchers, primarily from the discipline of psychology, have focused on various personality traits related to an individual's intolerance of uncertain situations (Freeston,

Rhéaume, Letarte, Dugas, & Ladouceur, 1994; Krohne, 1993; Sorrentino & Short, 1986). Those who are habitually intolerant of uncertainty are likely to employ consistent vigilant behaviors by directing attention to threat-relevant information so as to avoid surprises and decrease uncertainty (Krohne, 1993). If individuals are simultaneously intolerant of emotional arousal (anxiety), however, vigilance will serve to heighten their anxiety. The end result is less effective coping characterized by fluctuations between vigilance to decrease uncertainty and avoidance to decrease anxiety. Research is needed to determine how intolerance of uncertainty and emotional arousal influences cognitive appraisal of uncertainty in illness and subsequent coping.

Implications of Uncertainty for Theory, Research, and Practice

Theory and Research

A review of the nursing literature indicates high interest in the concept of uncertainty in illness. The majority of quantitative studies have been atheoretical with reference to one of Mishel's (1981, 1988, 1990) conceptualizations made in "hindsight." An understanding of the strengths and needed revisions of the current conceptualizations (Mishel, 1988, 1990) is unlikely to occur until more research is conducted in which the relevant conceptualization (acute and chronic) drives proposal development decisions.

Most studies referencing one of Mishel's (1981, 1988, 1990) conceptualizations have investigated uncertainty in ill adults. Few studies (Yarcheski, 1988) have investigated uncertainty in illness in acutely and chronically ill children and adolescents, even though developmental stage may influence perceptions of and coping with uncertainty (Haase & Rostad, 1994). Research is needed in this area and is likely to necessitate the development of different methods and measures for the assessment of uncertainty relevant to acute and chronic illness in youth. Moreover, most quantitative studies on uncertainty have used a cross-sectional design. Longitudinal studies are needed to determine how uncertainty, appraisal, coping, and adaptation and growth are

related; how these relationships change over the course of acute and chronic illnesses; and what facilitates or deters healthy movement.

In addition to the need for the development of methods and measures for assessment of uncertainty in youth, Mast (1995) questioned whether the MUIS adequately measures the concept of uncertainty experienced in chronic illness because it was originally developed to assess uncertainty in acute illness. Moreover, Mishel (1997) recommended that new measures of coping are needed to incorporate strategies specific to stress reduction in uncertainty.

Most of the studies reviewed that examined illness uncertainty in family members used qualitative methods. Quantitative studies were primarily atheoretical, with results interpreted using Mishel's (1981, 1988, 1990) conceptualizations. There is evidence that uncertainty in the ill person and in the family member are interrelated (Steele et al., 1997), with issues and problems related to the family system being a source of concern for parents of ill children (Turner et al., 1990). Collectively, research in this area points to the need for determining the unique dimensions of and relationships between uncertainty in the ill person and family member, given the specific characteristics of and demands made by the illness. As research in this area progresses, it is likely that the current uncertainty conceptualizations (Mishel, 1988, 1990), which were developed with respect to ill adults, will be modified to incorporate antecedents to and consequences of uncertainty in family members.

Mishel (1997) noted that the role of personality dispositions as predictors of uncertainty or mediators between uncertainty and cognitive appraisal is limited, with some support for the mediating role of mastery. No research was found, however, that examined the relationship between uncertainty and the personality variable of intolerance for uncertainty. It is likely that dispositional intolerance for uncertainty will influence perceptions of illness uncertainty and cognitive appraisals, and this bears investigation. In addition, research (Germino et al., 1998) indicates that ethnicity influenced the relationship between uncertainty and coping. Therefore, Mast's (1995) observation that the majority of studies have examined uncertainty in Caucasian, middle-class samples indicates the need for research on uncertainty in diverse cultural populations.

Practice

Although few studies were found that investigated interventions related to illness uncertainty, most found uncertainty decreased following intervention (Braden, 1991, 1992; Hawthorne & Hixon, 1994). For example, the Self-Help Intervention Project (SHIP) for women receiving breast cancer treatment uses interventions for uncertainty management based on five goals: (a) reinforcement of opportunity appraisals; (b) promotion of elements related to cognitive structure, such as provision of information; (c) reduction of inappropriate or incorrect certainty associated with negative outcomes; (d) regulation of emotional response; and (e) promotion of personal control and probabilistic thinking (Braden, Mishel, & Longman, 1998). Although the extent to which weekly telephone interventions from the nurse contributed to a decrease in uncertainty is unclear, the study serves as a good beginning for determining the effectiveness of uncertainty interventions. Mishel (1997) concluded that the most effective interventions were educational in nature, providing information and skill building related to management of uncertainty.

Uncertainty is not necessarily detrimental (Mishel, 1988, 1990). On the basis of a literature review related to uncertainty, Wurzbach (1992) developed a guide to assess the client's degree of uncertainty and proposed interventions for use when certainty and uncertainty are deemed to be detrimental. Strategies for certainty and uncertainty are similar to strategies found in the SHIP (Braden et al., 1998) and include (a) cognitive reappraisal, (b) information provision, and (c) personal control strategies (Wurzbach, 1992). As descriptive studies further delineate the type, degree, and health consequences of uncertainty experienced throughout the illness experience, interventions can be developed and tested to target effective resolution of detrimental uncertainty (or certainty).

Conclusion

Although the focus of this chapter was on acute and chronic illness-related uncertainty in ill persons and their families, it should be noted that some research has focused on uncertainty in nursing (Thompson & Dowding, 2001; Vaismoradi, Salsali, & Ahmadi, 2011). In addition, studies have investigated decision making (Baumann, Deber, & Thompson, 1991), moral uncertainty about withholding or withdrawing artificial nutrition and hydration (Wurzbach, 1995, 1996), and risk uncertainty in working with AIDS patients (Reutter & Northcott, 1993). The most systematic research found, however, was in the area of perceived environmental uncertainty.

Attempts to control increasing health care costs have led to changes in the delivery of care, the availability of health care resources, and the acuity level of the patient population (Salyer, 1995; Salyer & Hamric, 2004). To determine how these changes influence nursing's job performance, Salyer (1995, 1996) proposed and tested a four-stage model that identified characteristics of the environment and of the nurse predicted to influence nursing performance. A key concept of the model was perceived environmental uncertainty, which was operationalized by the 11-item Perceived Environmental Uncertainty in Hospitals Scale and defined as the perception of uncertainty resulting from the need for information and the complexity, dynamism, and environmental dominance of the organization (Salyer, 1995, 1996). Research on the model is limited, and support is mixed, ranging from partial (Salyer, 1995, 1996; Salyer & Hamric, 2004) to minimal (Callahan, Young-Cureton, Zalar, & Wahl, 1997).

Allred and associates (Allred, Hoffman, Fox, & Michel, 1994; Allred, Michel et al., 1994) also investigated perceived environmental uncertainty through their Perceived Environmental Uncertainty Questionnaire (PEUQ), designed to measure the "degree of complexity, change, unpredictability, and uncertainty associated with the information, resources, or relationship factors identified as most important to providing patient care" (Allred et al., 1995, pp. 130–131). For a complete description of the four-part questionnaire with results of psychometric testing, consult articles by Allred and associates (Allred, Hoffman et al., 1994; Allred, Michel et al., 1994). The PEUQ identified three distinct nursing practice environments characterized by increasing levels of complexity, change, unpredictability, and uncertainty (Allred, Michel et al., 1994). With the capacity to differentiate nursing practice environments, this questionnaire provides an opportunity for designing and testing practice models to facilitate effective and efficient nursing practice outcomes.

In conclusion, the nursing literature is replete with references to uncertainty. Based on the Cumulated Index for Nursing and Allied Health Literature (CINAHL), there have been 908 citations for uncertainty in illness since 1981. In the last decade (2000–2010), there have been 661 research citations for uncertainty in illness, 40 of which are international studies, 60 are dissertation studies, and 61 specify Mishel's mid-range Uncertainty in Illness Theory. There is also a systematic and growing body of research related to perceived environmental uncertainty and efficient quality of care. Opportunities for research on uncertainty abound, whether the researcher is interested in focusing on the patient, the family, or the nursing practice environment.

REFERENCES

Allred, C. A., Arford, P. H., Michel, Y., Veitch, J. S., Dring, R., & Carter, V. (1995). Case management: The relationship between structure & environment. *Nursing Economics, 13,* 32–51.

Allred, C. A., Hoffman, S. E., Fox, D. H., & Michel, Y. (1994). A measure of perceived environmental uncertainty in hospitals. *Western Journal of Nursing Research, 16*(2), 169–182.

Allred, C. A., Michel, Y., Arford, P. H., Carter, V., Veitch, J. S., Dring, R., . . . Finch, N. J. (1994). Environmental uncertainty: Implications for practice model design. *Nursing Economics, 12*(6), 318–326.

Antoni, M. H., Lutgendorf, S. K., Cole, S. W., Dhabhar, F. S., Sephton, S. E., McDonald, P. G., et al. (2006). The influence of bio-behavioural factors on tumour biology: Pathways and mechanisms. *National Review of Cancer, 6*(3), 240–248.

Armer, J. M., McDermott, M. P., & Schiffer, R. B. (1996). Psychological characteristics of MS patients: Determining differences based upon participation in a therapy regimen. *Rehabilitation Nursing Research, 5*(3), 102–112.

Babrow, A. S., Kasch, C. R., & Ford, L. A. (1998). The many meanings of uncertainty in illness: Toward a systematic accounting. *Health Communication, 10,* 1–23.

Bailey, J. M., & Nielsen, B. I. (1993). Uncertainty and appraisal of uncertainty in women with rheumatoid arthritis. *Orthopaedic Nursing, 12*(3), 63–67.

Barron, C. R. (2000). Stress, uncertainty, and health. In V. H. Rice (Ed.), *Handbook of stress, coping, and health: Implications for nursing research, theory, and practice* (pp. 517–539). Thousand Oaks, CA: Sage.

Barroso, J. (1997). Social support and long-term survivors of AIDS. *Western Journal of Nursing Research, 19,* 554–582.

Baum, A., Friedman, A. L., & Zakowski, S. G. (1997). Stress and genetic testing for disease risk. *Health Psychology, 16,* 8–19.

Baumann, A. O., Deber, R. B., & Thompson, G. G. (1991). Overconfidence among physicians and nurses: The "micro-certainty, macro-uncertainty" phenomenon. *Social Science and Medicine, 12,* 167–174.

Bennett, S. J. (1993). Relationships among selected antecedent variables and coping effectiveness in postmyocardial infarction patients. *Research in Nursing & Health, 16,* 131–139.

Braden, C. J. (1990a). Learned self-help response to chronic illness experience: A test of three alternative learning theories. *Scholarly Inquiry for Nursing Practice, 4,* 23–41.

Braden, C. J. (1990b). A test of the self-help model: Learned response to chronic illness experience. *Nursing Research, 39,* 42–47.

Braden, C. J. (1991). Patterns of change over time in learned response to chronic illness among participants in a systemic lupus erythematosus self-help course. *Arthritis Care and Research, 4,* 158–167.

Braden, C. J. (1992). Description of learned response to chronic illness: Depressed versus nondepressed self-help class participants. *Public Health Nursing, 9,* 103–108.

Braden, C. J., Mishel, M. H., & Longman, A. J. (1998). Self-help intervention project: Women receiving breast cancer treatment. *Cancer Practice, 6*(2), 87–98.

Brown, M. A., & Powell-Cope, G. M. (1991). AIDS family caregiving: Transitions through uncertainty. *Nursing Research, 40,* 338–345.

Callahan, P., Young-Cureton, G., Zalar, M., & Wahl, S. (1997). Relationship between tolerance/intolerance of ambiguity and perceived environmental uncertainty in hospitals. *Journal of Psychosocial Nursing & Mental Health Services, 35*(11), 39–44.

Christman, N. J. (1990). Uncertainty and adjustment during radiotherapy. *Nursing Research, 39,* 17–20, 47.

Christman, N. J., McConnell, E. A., Pfeiffer, C., Webster, K. K., Schmitt, M., & Ries, J. (1988). Uncertainty, coping, and distress following myocardial infarction: Transition from hospital to home. *Research in Nursing & Health, 11,* 71–82.

Clarke-Steffen, L. (1997). Reconstructing reality: Family strategies for managing childhood cancer. *Journal of Pediatric Nursing, 12*(5), 278–287.

Clauson, M. I. (1996). Uncertainty and stress in women hospitalized with high-risk pregnancy. *Clinical Nursing Research, 5*(3), 309–325.

Clayton, M. F., Mishel, M., & Belyea, M. (2006). Testing a model of symptoms, communication, uncertainty, and well-being in older breast cancer survivors. *Research in Nursing and Health, 29*(1), 18–39.

Coffman, S. (1996). Parents' struggles to rebuild family life after hurricane Andrew. *Issues in Mental Health Nursing, 17,* 353–367.

Cohen, M. H. (1993). The unknown and the unknowable—Managing sustained uncertainty. *Western Journal of Nursing Research, 15,* 77–96.

Cohen, M. H. (1995). The stages of the prediagnostic period in chronic, life-threatening childhood illness: A process analysis. *Research in Nursing & Health, 18,* 39–48.

Cohen, M. H., & Martinson, I. M. (1988). Chronic uncertainty: Its effect on parental appraisal of a child's health. *Journal of Pediatric Nursing, 3*(2), 89–96.

Cordova, M. J., Cunningham, L. L., Carlson, C. R., & Andrykowski, M. A. (2001). Social constraints, cognitive processing, and adjustment to breast cancer. *Journal of Consulting and Clinical Psychology, 69*(4), 706–711.

Davis, L. L. (1990). Illness uncertainty, social support, and stress in recovering individuals and family care givers. *Applied Nursing Research, 3*(2), 69–71.

Dickerson, S. S. (1998). Cardiac spouses' help-seeking experiences. *Clinical Nursing Research, 7,* 6–28.

Dirkson, S. R. (2000). Predicting well being among breast cancer survivors, *Journal of Advanced Nursing, 32*(4), 932–943.

Dudley-Brown, S. (1996). Living with ulcerative colitis. *Gastroenterology Nursing, 19*(2), 60–64.

Ellett, M. L., & Young, R. J. (1997). Development of the Vulnerability Scale. *Gastroenterology Nursing, 20*(3), 82–86.

Fillion, L., Lemyre, L., Mandeville, R., & Piché, R. (1996). Cognitive appraisal, stress state, and cellular immunity responses before and after diagnosis of breast tumor. *International Journal of Rehabilitation and Health, 2*(3), 169–187.

Fjelland, J. E., Barron, C. R., & Foxall, M. (2008). A review of instruments measuring two aspects of meaning: Search for meaning and meaning in illness. *Journal of Advanced Nursing, 62*(4), 394–406.

Flemme, I., Edvardsson, N., Hinic, H., Jinhage, B. M., Dalman, M., Fridlund, B., & Linkoping, H. (2005). Long-term quality of life and uncertainty in patients living with an implantable cardioverter defibrillator. *Heart and Lung, 34,* 386–392.

Fleury, J., Kimbrell, C., & Kruszewski, M. A. (1995). Life after a cardiac event: Women's experience in healing. *Heart & Lung, 24*(6), 474–482.

Folkman, S. (1982). An approach to the measurement of coping. *Journal of Occupational Behavior, 3,* 56–107.

Freeston, M. H., Rhéaume, J., Letarte, H., Dugas, M. J., & Ladouceur, R. (1994). Why do people worry? *Personality and Individual Differences, 17,* 791–802.

Galloway, S. C., & Graydon, J. E. (1996). Uncertainty, symptom distress, and information needs after surgery for cancer of the colon. *Cancer Nursing, 19,* 112–117.

Garofalo, J.P., Choppala, S., Haman, Heidi, A., Gjerde, J. (2009). Uncertainty during transition from cancer patient to survivor, *Cancer Nursing, 32(4),* 8–14.

Gaskins, S., & Brown, K. (1992). Responses among individuals with human immunodeficiency virus infection. *Applied Nursing Research, 5,* 111–121.

Germino, B. B., Mishel, M. H., Alexander, G. R., Jenerette, C., Blyler, D., Baker, C . . . Long, D. G. (2011). Engaging African American breast cancer survivors in an intervention trial: Culture, responsiveness and community. *Journal of Cancer Survival, 5*(1), 82–91.

Germino, B. B., Mishel, M. H., Belyea, M., Harris, L., Ware, A., & Mohler, J. (1998). Uncertainty in prostate cancer: Ethnic and family patterns. *Cancer Practice, 6*(2), 107–113.

Haase, J. E., & Rostad, M. (1994). Experiences of completing cancer therapy: Children's perspectives. *Oncology Nursing Forum, 21*(9), 1483–1494.

Häggström, T., Axelsson, K., & Norberg, A. (1994). The experience of living with stroke sequelae illuminated by means of stories and metaphors. *Qualitative Health Research, 4*(3), 321–337.

Hallberg, L. R.-M., & Erlandsson, S. I.-M. (1991). Validation of the Swedish version of the Mishel Uncertainty in Illness Scale. *Scholarly Inquiry for Nursing Practice: An International Journal, 5,* 57–67.

Halldórsdóttir, S., & Hamrin, E. (1996). Experiencing existential changes: The lived experience of having cancer. *Cancer Nursing, 19,* 29–36.

Hawthorne, M. H., & Hixon, M. E. (1994). Functional status, mood disturbance and quality of life in patients with heart failure. *Progress in Cardiovascular Nursing, 9,* 22–32.

Hilton, B. A. (1988). The phenomenon of uncertainty in women with breast cancer. *Issues in Mental Health Nursing, 9,* 217–238.

Hilton, B. A. (1989). The relationship of uncertainty, control, commitment, and threat of recurrence to coping strategies used by women diagnosed with breast cancer. *Journal of Behavioral Medicine, 12,* 39–54.

Hilton, B. A. (1994). The Uncertainty Stress Scale: Its development and psychometric properties. *Canadian Journal of Nursing Research, 26*(3), 15–30.

Hussey-Gardner, B. T., Wachtel, R. C., & Viscardi, R. M. (1998). Parent perceptions of an NICU follow-up clinic. *Neonatal Network, 17,* 33–39.

Jamerson, P. A., Scheibmeier, M., Bott, M. J., Crighton, F., Hinton, R. H., & Cobb, A. K. (1996). The experiences of families with a relative in the intensive care unit. *Heart & Lung, 25,* 467–474.

Janson-Bjerklie, S., Ferketich, S., & Benner, P. (1993). Predicting the outcomes of living with asthma. *Research in Nursing & Health, 16,* 241–250.

Johnson, J. E., Fieler, V. K., Jones, L. S., Wlasowicz, G. S., & Mitchell, M. L. (1997). *Self-regulation theory: Applying theory to your practice.* Pittsburgh, PA: Oncology Nursing Press.

Johnson, L. M., Zautra, A. J., & Davis, M. C. (2006). The role of illness uncertainty on coping with fibromyalgia symptoms. *Health Psychology, 25*(6), 696–703.

Kang, Y., Daly, B. J., & Kim, J. S (2004) Uncertainty and its antecedents in patients with atrial fibrillation. *Western J. of Nursing Research, 26*(7), 770–783.

Koocher, G. P. (1985). Psychosocial care of the child cured of cancer. *Pediatric Nursing, 11*(2), 91–93

Krohne, H. W. (1993). Vigilance and cognitive avoidance as concepts in coping research. In H. W. Krohne (Ed.), *Attention and avoidance: Strategies in coping with aversiveness* (pp. 19–50). Seattle, WA: Hogrefe & Huber.

Landis, B. J. (1996). Uncertainty, spiritual well-being, and psychosocial adjustment to chronic illness. *Issues in Mental Health Nursing, 17,* 217–231.

Lang, E. V., Berbaum, K. S., & Lutgendorf, S. K. (2009). Large-core breast biopsy: Abnormal salivary cortisol profiles associated with uncertainty of diagnosis. *Radiology, 250*(3), 631–637.

Lazarus, R. S. (1974). Psychological stress and coping in adaptation and illness. *International Journal of Psychiatry in Medicine, 5,* 321–333.

Lazarus, R. S., & Folkman, S. (1984). *Stress, appraisal, and coping.* New York, NY: Springer.

Lebel, S., Rosberger, Z., Edgar, L., & Devins, G. M. (2007). Comparison of four common stressors across the breast cancer trajectory. *Journal of Psychosomatic Research, 63*(3), 225–232.

Lemaire, G. S., & Lenz, E. R. (1995). Perceived uncertainty about menopause in women attending an educational program. *International Journal of Nursing Studies, 32,* 39–48.

Leventhal, H., Diefenbach, M., & Leventhal, E. A. (1992). Illness cognition: Using common sense to understand treatment adherence and affect cognition interactions. *Cognitive Therapy and Research, 16,* 143–163.

Lobar, S. L., & Phillips, S. (1996). Parents who utilize private infant adoption: An ethnographic analysis. *Issues in Comprehensive Pediatric Nursing, 19,* 65–76.

Lugton, J. (1997). The nature of social support as experienced by women treated for breast cancer. *Journal of Advanced Nursing, 25,* 1184–1191.

MacDonald, H. (1995). Chronic renal disease: The mother's experience. *Pediatric Nursing, 21*(6), 503–507, 574.

MacDonald, H. (1996). Mastering uncertainty: Mothering the child with asthma. *Pediatric Nursing, 22,* 55–59.

Malone, J. A. (1997). Family adaptation: Adult sons with long-term physical or mental illnesses. *Issues in Mental Health Nursing, 18,* 351–363.

Mason, C. (1985). The production and effects of uncertainty with special reference to diabetes mellitus. *Social Science and Medicine, 21,* 1329–1334.

Mast, M. E. (1995). Adult uncertainty in illness: A critical review of research. *Scholarly Inquiry for Nursing Practice: An International Journal, 9,* 3–24.

Mast, M. E. (1998). Survivors of breast cancer: Illness uncertainty, positive reappraisal, and emotional distress. *Oncology Nursing Forum, 25*(3), 555–562.

McCain, N. L., & Cella, D. F. (1995). Correlates of stress in HIV disease. *Western Journal of Nursing Research, 17*(2), 141–155.

McCain, N. L., Zeller, J. M., Cella, D. F., Urbanski, P. A., & Novak, R. M. (1996). The influence of stress management training in HIV disease. *Nursing Research, 45*(4), 246–253.

Miles, M. S., Funk, S. G., & Kasper, M. A. (1992). The stress response of mothers and fathers of preterm infants. *Research in Nursing & Health, 15,* 261–269.

Mishel, M. H. (1981). The measurement of uncertainty in illness. *Nursing Research, 30,* 258–263.

Mishel, M. H. (1983a). Adjusting the fit: Development of uncertainty scales for specific clinical populations. *Western Journal of Nursing Research, 5*(4), 355–370.

Mishel, M. H. (1983b). Parents' perception of uncertainty concerning their hospitalized child. *Nursing Research, 32,* 324–330.

Mishel, M. H. (1984). Perceived uncertainty and stress in illness. *Research in Nursing and Health, 7,* 163–171.

Mishel, M. H. (1988). Uncertainty in illness. *Image: Journal of Nursing Scholarship, 20*(4), 225–232.

Mishel, M. H. (1990). Reconceptualization of the Uncertainty in Illness theory. *Image: Journal of Nursing Scholarship, 22*(4), 256–262.

Mishel, M. H. (1991). Response to "Validation of the Swedish version of the Mishel Uncertainty in Illness Scale." *Scholarly Inquiry for Nursing Practice: An International Journal, 5,* 67–70.

Mishel, M. H. (1995). Response to "Adult uncertainty in illness: A critical review of research." *Scholarly Inquiry for Nursing Practice: An International Journal, 9,* 25–29.

Mishel, M. H. (1997). Uncertainty in acute illness. *Annual Review of Nursing Research, 15,* 57–80.

Mishel, M. H., Belyea, M., Germino, B. B., Stewart, J. L., Bailey, D. E., Robertson, C. N., & Mohler, J. (2002). Helping patients with localized prostate carcinoma manage uncertainty and treatment side effects. *Cancer, 94*(6), 1854–1866.

Mishel, M. H., & Braden, C. J. (1987). Uncertainty: A mediator between support and adjustment. *Western Journal of Nursing Research, 9,* 43–57.

Mishel, M. H., & Braden, C. J. (1988). Finding meaning: Antecedents of uncertainty in illness. *Nursing Research, 37*(2), 98–103, 127.

Mishel, M. H., & Epstein, D. (1990). *Uncertainty in Illness Scales manual.* Available from M. H. Mishel, University of North Carolina at Chapel Hill, School of Nursing, CB #7140 Carrington Hall, Chapel Hill, NC 27599–7140.

Mishel, M. H., Germino, B. B., Belyea, M., Stewart, J. L., Bailey, D. E., Jr., Mohler, J., & Robertson, C. (2003). Moderators of an uncertainty management intervention: For men with localized prostate cancer. *Nursing Research, 52*(2), 89–97.

Mishel, M. H., Germino, B. B., Gil, K. M., Belyea, M., LaNey, I. C., Stewart, J., . . . Clayton, M. (2005). Benefits from an uncertainty management intervention for African-American and Caucasian older long-term breast cancer survivors. *Psycho-Oncology, 14,* 962–978.

Mishel, M. H., Germino, B. B., Lin, L., Pruthi, R. S., & Wallen, E. M. (2009). Efficacy of a decision making uncertainty management intervention in early stage prostate cancer. *Patient Education and Counseling, 77*(3), 349–359.

Mishel, M. H., Hostetter, T., King, B., & Graham, V. (1984). Predictors of psychosocial adjustment in patients newly diagnosed with gynecological cancer. *Cancer Nursing, 7,* 291–299.

Mishel, M. H., & Murdaugh, C. L. (1987). Family experiences with heart transplantation: Redesigning the dream. *Nursing Research, 36,* 332–338.

Mishel, M. H., Padilla, G., Grant, M., & Sorenson, D. S. (1991). Uncertainty in Illness theory: A replication of the mediating effects of mastery and coping. *Nursing Research, 40,* 236–240.

Mishel, M. H., & Sorenson, D. S. (1991). Uncertainty in gynecological cancer: A test of the mediating functions of mastery and coping. *Nursing Research, 40,* 167–171.

Molleman, E., Pruyn, J., & van Knippenberg, A. (1986). Social comparison processes among cancer patients. *British Journal of Social Psychology, 25,* 1–13.

Moos, R. H., & Tsu, V. D. (1977). The crisis of physical illness: An overview. In R. H. Moos (Ed.), *Coping with physical illness.* New York, NY: Plenum.

Moser, D. K., Clements, P. J., Brecht, M. L., & Weiner, S. R. (1993). Predictors of psychosocial adjustment in systemic sclerosis: The influence of formal education level, functional ability, hardiness, uncertainty, and social support. *Arthritis & Rheumatism, 10,* 1398–1405.

Mullins, L. L., Chaney, J. M., Hartman, V. L., Albin, K., Miles, B., & Roberson, S. (1995). Cognitive and affective features of postpolio syndrome: Illness uncertainty, attributional style, and adaptation. *International Journal of Rehabilitation and Health, 1*(4), 211–222.

Nelson, J. P. (1996). Struggling to gain meaning: Living with the uncertainty of breast cancer. *Advances in Nursing Science, 18*(3), 59–76.

Northouse, L. L., Dorris, G., & Charron-Moore, C. (1995). Factors affecting couples' adjustment to recurrent breast cancer. *Social Science and Medicine, 41,* 69–76.

Northouse, L. L., Jeffs, M., Cracchiolo-Caraway, A., Lampman, L., & Dorris, G. (1995). Emotional distress reported by women and husbands prior to a breast biopsy. *Nursing Research, 44*(4), 196–201.

Northouse, L. L., Laten, D., & Reddy, P. (1995). Adjustment of women and their husbands to recurrent breast cancer. *Research in Nursing & Health, 18,* 515–524.

Norton, R. W. (1975). Measurement of ambiguity tolerance. *Journal of Personality Assessment, 39,* 607–619.

Nyhlin, K. T. (1990). Diabetic patients facing long-term complications: Coping with uncertainty. *Journal of Advanced Nursing, 15,* 1021–1029.

O'Brien, R. A., Wineman, N. M., & Nealon, N. R. (1995). Correlates of the caregiving process in multiple sclerosis. *Scholarly Inquiry for Nursing Practice: An International Journal, 9*(4), 323–338.

Padilla, G. V., Mishel, M. H., & Grant, M. M. (1992). Uncertainty, appraisal and quality of life. *Quality of Life Research, 1,* 155–165.

Patterson, C., & Faux, S. A. (1993). Uncertainty, and appraisal in patients diagnosed with abdominal aortic aneurysms. *Canadian Journal of Cardiovascular Nursing, 4,* 4–10.

Patterson, E. T., Freese, M. P., & Goldenberg, R. L. (1986). Reducing uncertainty: Self-diagnosis of pregnancy. *Image, 18*(3), 105–109.

Pool, R. (1989). Chaos theory: How big an advance? *Science, 245,* 26–28.

Porter, L., Clayton, M. F., Belyea, M., Mishel, M., Gill, K. M., & Germino, B. (2006). Predicting negative mood state and personal growth in African American and White long-term breast cancer survivors. *Annals of Behavioral Medicine, 31*(3), 195–204.

Redeker, N. S. (1992). The relationship between uncertainty and coping after coronary bypass surgery. *Western Journal of Nursing Research, 14,* 48–61.

Regan-Kubinski, M. J., & Sharts-Hopko, N. (1995). Illness cognition of HIV-infected mothers. *Issues in Mental Health Nursing, 16,* 327–344.

Reich, J. W., Johnson, L., Zautra, A., & Davis M. (2006). Uncertainty of illness relationships with mental health and coping processes in fibromyalgia patients. *Journal of Behavioral Medicine, 29*(4), 307–316.

Reutter, L. I., & Northcott, H. C. (1993). Making risk meaningful: Developing caring relationships with AIDS patients. *Journal of Advanced Nursing, 18,* 1377–1385.

Ronayne, R. (1989). Uncertainty in peripheral vascular disease. *Canadian Journal of Cardiovascular Nursing, 1*(2), 26–30.

Salyer, J. (1995). Environmental turbulence: Impact on nurse practitioner. *Journal of Nursing Administration, 25*(4), 12–20.

Salyer, J. (1996). Development and psychometric evaluation of an instrument to measure staff nurses' perception of uncertainty in the hospital environment. *Journal of Nursing Management, 4,* 33–48.

Salyer, J., & Hamric, A. (2004). Evolving specialties and innovative opportunities for advanced practice nursing. In A. Hamric, J. Spross, & C. Hansen (Eds.), *Advanced nursing practice: An integrated approach* (3rd ed., pp. 677–702). Philadelphia, PA: W. B. Saunders.

Sammarco, A. (2001). Perceived social support, uncertainty, and quality of life of younger breast cancer survivors. *Cancer Nursing, 24*(3), 212–219.

Santacroce, S. J., & Lee, Y.-L. (2006). Uncertainty, posttraumatic stress, and health behavior in young adult childhood cancer survivors. *Nursing Research, 55*(4), 259–266.

Selder, F. (1989). Life transition theory: The resolution of uncertainty. *Nursing & Health Care, 10,* 437–451.

Sharts-Hopko, N. C., Regan-Kubinski, M. J., Lincoln, P. S., & Heverly, M. A. (1996). Problem-focused coping in HIV-infected mothers in relation to self-efficacy, uncertainty, social support, and psychological distress. *Image, 28*(2), 107–111.

Sheer, V. C., & Cline, R. J. (1995). Testing a model of perceived information adequacy and uncertainty reduction in physician-patient interactions. *Journal of Applied Communication Research, 23,* 44–59.

Siegl, D., & Morse, J. M. (1994). Tolerating reality: The experience of parents of HIV positive sons. *Social Science Medicine, 38*(7), 959–971.

Sorrentino, R. M., & Short, J. C. (1986). Uncertainty, motivation, and cognition. In R. M. Sorrentino & E. T. Higgins (Eds.), *The handbook of motivation and cognition: Foundations of social behavior* (pp. 379–403). New York, NY: Guilford.

Sparacino, P. S. A., Tong, E. M., Messias, D. K. H., Foote, D., Chesla, C. A., & Gillis, C. L. (1997). The dilemmas of parents of adolescents and young adults with congenital heart disease. *Heart & Lung, 26*(3), 187–194.

Stanton, A. L., Danoff-Burg, S., & Huggins, M. E. (2002). The first year after breast cancer diagnosis: Hope and coping strategies as predictors of adjustment. *Psycho-Oncology, 11*(2), 93–102.

Staples, P., & Jeffrey, J. (1997). Quality of life, hope, and uncertainty of cardiac patients and their spouses before coronary artery bypass surgery. *Canadian Journal of Cardiovascular Nursing, 8,* 7–16.

Steele, R. G., Tripp, G., Kotchick, B. A., Summers, P., & Forehand, R. (1997). Family members' uncertainty about parental chronic illness: The relationship of hemophilia and HIV infection to child functioning. *Journal of Pediatric Psychology, 22,* 577–591.

Sterken, D. J. (1996). Uncertainty and coping in fathers of children with children. *Journal of Pediatric Oncology Nursing, 13*(2), 81–88.

Stetz, K. M. (1989). The relationship among background characteristics, purpose in life, and caregiving demands on perceived health of spouse caregivers. *Scholarly Inquiry for Nursing Practice: An International Journal, 3*(2), 133–153.

Theobald, K. (1997). The experience of spouses whose partners have suffered a myocardial infarction: A phenomenological study. *Journal of Advanced Nursing, 26,* 595–601.

Thibodeau, J., & MacRae, J. (1997). Breast cancer survival: A phenomenological inquiry. *Advances in Nursing Science, 19*(4), 65–74.

Thompson, C., & Dowding, D. (2001). Responding to uncertainty in nursing practice. *International Journal of Nursing Studies, 38*(5), 609–615.

Tomich, P. L., Helgeson, V. S. (2002). Five years later: A cross-sectional comparison of breast cancer survivors with healthy women. *Psycho-Oncology, 11,* 154–169.

Turner, M. A., Tomlinson, P. S., & Harbaugh, B. L. (1990). Parental uncertainty in critical care hospitalization of children. *Maternal/Child Nursing Journal, 19,* 45–62.

Vaismoradi, M., Salsali, M., & Ahmadi, F. (2011). Nurses' experiences of uncertainty in clinical practice: A descriptive study. *Journal of Advanced Nursing, 67*(5), 991–999.

Warrington, K., & Gottlieb, L. (1987). Uncertainty and anxiety of hysterectomy patients during hospitalization. *Nursing Papers/Perspectives in Nursing, 19,* 59–73.

Webster, K. K., & Christman, N. J. (1988). Perceived uncertainty and coping post myocardial infarction. *Western Journal of Nursing Research, 10*(4), 384–400.

Weitz, R. (1989). Uncertainty and the lives of persons with AIDS. *Journal of Health and Social Behavior, 30,* 270–281.

White, R. E., & Frasure-Smith, N. (1995). Uncertainty and psychologic stress after coronary angioplasty and coronary bypass surgery. *Heart & Lung, 24,* 19–27.

Wineman, N. M. (1990). Adaptation to multiple sclerosis: The role of social support, functional disability, and perceived uncertainty. *Nursing Research, 39*(5), 294–299.

Wineman, N. M., Durand, E. J., & Steiner, R. P. (1994). A comparative analysis of coping behaviors in persons with multiple sclerosis or a spinal cord injury. *Research in Nursing & Health, 17,* 185–194.

Wineman, N. M., O'Brien, R. A., Nealon, N. R., & Kaskel, B. (1993). Congruence of uncertainty between individuals with multiple sclerosis and their spouses. *Journal of Neuroscience Nursing, 25*(6), 356–361.

Wineman, N. M., Schwetz, K. M., Goodkin, D. E., & Rudick, R. A. (1996). Relationships among illness uncertainty, stress, coping, and emotional well-being at entry into a clinical drug trial. *Applied Nursing Research, 9*(2), 53–60.

Wong, C. A., & Bramwell, L. (1992). Uncertainty and anxiety after mastectomy for breast cancer. *Cancer Nursing, 15,* 363–371.

Wright, L. J, Afari, N., & Zautra, A. (2009). The illness uncertainty concept: A review. *Current Pain and Headache Reports, 13,* 133–138.

Wurzbach, M. E. (1992). Assessment and intervention for certainty and uncertainty. *Nursing Forum, 27*(2), 29–35.

Wurzbach, M. E. (1995). Long-term care nurses' moral convictions. *Journal of Advanced Nursing, 21,* 1059–1064.

Wurzbach, M. E. (1996). Long-term care nurses' ethical convictions about tube feeding. *Western Journal of Nursing Research, 18,* 63–76.

Wyler, R. S. (1974). *Cognitive organization and change: An information processing approach.* Hillsdale, NJ: Lawrence Erlbaum.

Yarcheski, A. (1988). Uncertainty in illness and the future. *Western Journal of Nursing Research, 10*(4), 401–413.

Yoshida, K. (1997). Uncertainty in the lives of people with spinal cord injury and rheumatoid arthritis. *Canadian Journal of Rehabilitation, 10,* 5–14.

22

Stress, Coping, Health, and Nursing

The Future

Virginia Hill Rice and Brenda L. Lyon

It is widely accepted that stress is a common experience in life that can affect a person's health positively and negatively. The question is: What is it that we do not understand about the relationships among stress, coping, and health and why is this understanding important to nursing? The purpose of this final chapter is to propose a conceptual model that is a holistic representation of what we currently understand about the relationships among stress, coping, and health and to identify future directions for nursing research, theory, and practice. The task of grasping the knowledge of this wide area of science as a whole is a challenge as studies of the stress, coping, and health relationships have grown exponentially over the past century in nursing as well as other disciplines. As is clear from the preceding chapters, there is still much work to be done in the development of conceptual, measurement, and methodological guidelines to help us to consistently evaluate these phenomena from a nursing perspective. Not only has "stress" been defined and operationalized differently (see Chapters 1 and 2), but our conceptualizations and measurements have varied greatly. Nonetheless, there are some repeatedly supported dynamics among these constructs that can be summarized here.

First, it is clear that there are stress-related factors that are genetic, psychological, physiological, and/or environmental that effect how a person is feeling and doing as well as the body's ability to avoid or overcome disease. The theoretical framework proposed by Lazarus and his colleagues holds considerable promise in explaining on a grand and, with some relationships, a midrange level the dynamics among stress, coping, and health. Figure 22.1 is a visual representation of the stress-related variables and health outcome relationships presented in the chapters of this text. It incorporates major components of Lazarus's (1966) and Lazarus and Folkman's (1984) models of stress and coping along with many of the factors that science has shown affects their relationship.

Our portrayal is not meant to be linear but rather nonrecursive in nature, with some simultaneous occurrences and multiple feedback loops. In addition, solid lines among the variables represent "midrange" relationships that have been empirically supported. Those that rely heavily on theoretical propositions with some, but not necessarily adequate, empirical support are depicted with dashed lines. It is interesting to note that many of the dashed lines are the result of the fact that it is infrequent for

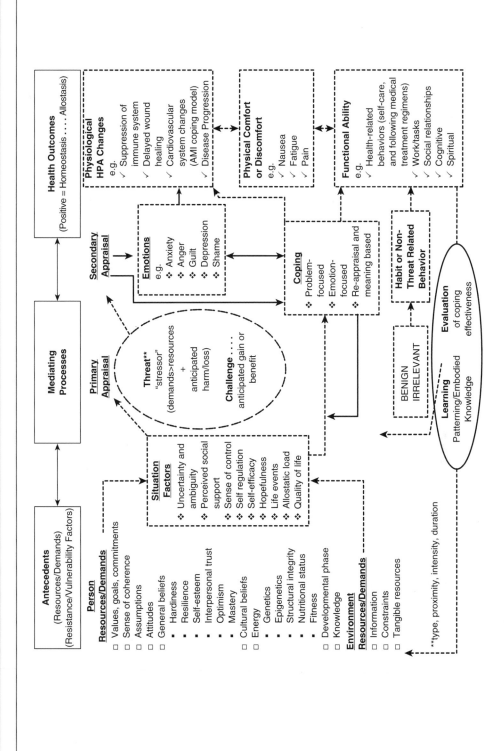

SOURCE: Based on the theoretical structures of Lazarus (1966) and Lazarus and Folkman (1984).

"appraisals" to be measured in stress, coping, and health research.

Antecedent variables in the model include person, environment, and situational resources and demands. The importance of these lies in the possibility that they play a role in making a person resistant or vulnerable to stress experiences. Personal factors include a sense of coherence and individual goals, values, assumptions, and general beliefs that are in turn affected by personality, hardiness, resilience, self-esteem, interpersonal trust, optimism, and mastery. These factors are discussed in detail in Chapters 8, 13, and 19. Other elements include cultural beliefs, and the energy elements of genetics, epigenetics, structural integrity, nutritional status, and physiological and psychological fitness (Chapters 3, 4 and 5). In addition, knowledge and developmental phase (i.e., childhood, adolescence, and early and late adulthood) affects one's personal resources and demands as well. See Chapters 10 and 11, respectively, on childhood and adolescent stress and coping.

Environmental factors include available information (e.g., technological in Chapter 7) and the nature of the information along with tangible resources (e.g., money, housing, and transportation) (Chapter 14). Situational factors arise from the transactions between a person and his or her home or work environment (Chapter 12) and include, but are not limited to, uncertainty and ambiguity (Chapter 21), perceived social support (Chapter 14), sense of control and self-regulation (Chapter 19), self-efficacy (Chapter 20), hopefulness (Chapter 18), the volume of demands in terms of life events (Chapter 6), allostatic load (Chapters 2 and 15), and quality of life (Chapter 17).

There is significant evidence that antecedent variables influence how a person appraises the meaning of a situation to begin with and, therefore, the resultant judgment of whether the situation presents a threat or challenge or is benign/positive or irrelevant (Chapter 9). As discussed in Chapter 13, personality constructs, values, beliefs (general and cultural), and attitudes affect the meaning that a person derives from a given situation. Chapter 19 presents evidence that having information (i.e., reducing uncertainty) in the form of sensory information increases one's sense of personal control, thereby influencing appraisals of health care events. This in turn influences the emotions experienced. Specifically, if a patient who desires information about what

to anticipate during a medical procedure receives that information, then the patient evaluates the situation as less threatening and experiences less anxiety than those who receive no information or information that only describes the medical "mechanics" of the procedure.

The important role that social support plays in affecting health-related outcomes is highlighted in Chapter 14. How social support influences health outcomes, however, is unclear. Although there is research that purports to demonstrate a direct effect of social support on health outcomes, this relationship may be spurious because "threat" tends not to be measured. It is not clear whether social support acts as a coping resource, a mediator, or a moderator of stress. It is possible that the experience of desired and satisfying social support influences the individual's primary and secondary appraisals a priori, thereby acting as a resistance resource (Chapter 8) that reduces threat appraisals and enhances coping potential.

As discussed in Chapter 20, self-efficacy is a factor that influences the initiation and maintenance of behavior, including coping efforts. Behavior is proposed to be a function of the subjective value of an outcome, the subjective probability that a particular behavior or coping effort will achieve the valued outcome in a specific situation, and the individual's efficacy expectations in relation to performance. Efficacy expectations can be assessed on three dimensions (magnitude, strength, and generality) and influenced by four sources of efficacy information (mastery, vicarious experience, verbal persuasion, and physiological arousal). Many systematic reviews have supported the relationship between level of personal self-efficacy and performance of given health behaviors. These are important findings to guide nursing practice as it seeks to enhance the health performance and coping of its patients and clients.

As is clear in Chapter 21, uncertainty, as a situational factor, can either increase or decrease the intensity of perceived threat depending on how a person views a situation. There is evidence that uncertainty is positively correlated with the appraisal of danger, but it is not known what factors lead a person to appraise a similar situation as nonthreatening or as a challenge. This is a classic example of viewing the glass as "half full" instead of "half empty." There is evidence that the relationship between uncertainty and cognitive appraisal of a situation is mediated by mastery, although it is not clear what variables may either moderate uncertainty or mediate between uncertainty and appraisal. Research has demonstrated a positive relationship between high uncertainty and poor psychosocial outcomes, such as anxiety, depression, psychosocial adjustment, and quality of life. It is not clear, however, what pathway or what variables may either moderate or mediate the relationship between uncertainty and psychosocial outcomes. It is also pointed out in Chapter 21 that situational factors interact with one another. For example, the presence of social support decreases perceived uncertainty in some situations.

The burden of many and competing stressors has been examined in terms of allostatic load (Chapter 2), life events and hassles and uplifts (Chapter 6), and quality of life (Chapter 17). All of these situational factors need more extensive nursing research. As Lazarus (1966) and others have noted, in many circumstances it may be more important and "easier" to change the situation than it is to modify one's resources.

In terms of the Mediating Processes (see Figure 22.1) as described by Lazarus in Chapter 9, the appraisal of threat triggers a secondary appraisal that not only influences which emotions are experienced but also influences what determines coping responses. The effect of appraised threat on emotions and coping seemingly occurs simultaneously through the secondary appraisal process. There is considerable evidence that this proposition is valid given that researchers, as discussed in Chapters 9, often find it difficult to determine which comes first, the emotion(s) or the coping effort. Lazarus also proposed that secondary appraisal contributes to the meaning of the situation through three basic judgments: blame or credit, coping potential, and future expectations. He emphasized the role that values, goals, belief systems, and personal resources play, not only in influencing the primary appraisal but also in determining the particular emotion experienced through secondary appraisal that connects the relational meaning of the situation to how the person feels and acts.

As discussed in Chapters 4 and 5, stress emotions and coping responses both influence physiological changes primarily thought to occur through the hypothalamic-pituitary-adrenal (HPA) axis. In addition, there is substantial evidence, as summarized in Chapter 4, that chronic elevations in cortisol, glucocorticoids, catecholamines, and the neuromediators of norepinephrine and epinephrine have been linked to the development of disease, including coronary artery disease, hypertension, cancer, and various infectious diseases. Also, there is significant support for the proposition that elevations in these hormones and the neuromediators depress the immune system, a factor most likely involved in the development of many illnesses (Chapter 3).

The health outcome variables of most of the research have been delimited by a focus on disease or proposed physiological correlates (Chapter 1). Despite the absence of focus on the effects of stress-related variables on symptoms, a body of theoretical work proposes relationships among physiological correlates and selected symptoms, such as sympathetic-mediated contraction of muscles contributing to the experience of tension and migraine headaches. As noted in Chapters 1 and 6 and throughout the book, numerous intervention studies have demonstrated the beneficial effects of relaxation therapy, cognitive interventions, therapeutic touch, sensory stimulation, back rubs and massage, guided imagery, meditation, and behavior modification on the experience of irritable bowel syndrome, temporal-mandibular joint pain, tension and migraine headaches, anxiety, pain, sleep, nausea, and heart rate. It is interesting to note that, except for sleep, there has been little research on how stress affects functional ability, including self-care decisions and self-care behaviors.

As indicated by the authors of Chapter 15, the relationship between psychosocial stress, risk for cardiovascular disease (CVD), and patient outcomes has been extensively studied. However, the relationships among stress, physiological responses, and the mechanisms leading to heart disease development continue to mystify researchers. Explaining these relationships is imperative for several reasons. Firstly, CVD remains the number one killer of American women and men despite advances in technology and science that have significantly reduced mortality and morbidity (see Roger et al., 2011). Second, the traditional risk factors of CVD, including smoking, obesity, and diabetes, only account for 58% to 75% of the incidence of heart disease, consequently, a significant portion of disease causation remains unexplained. Thirdly, some of the causal mechanisms of heart disease, including inflammation and coagulation, have been well established, but mediating and moderating factors have not. Fourthly, advances in acute care and primary prevention strategies have led to improved survival rates and resulted in a significant number of patients with chronic disease. Finally, the identification of mechanisms and determinants of CVD need to open an extensive line of inquiry focused on the design and testing of interventions.

The Acute Myocardial Infarction (AMI) Coping Model described in Chapter 16 begins to explain the relationship between awareness of cardiac symptoms and the decision to seek care, but there is still very little consideration of what role emotions and situational or social constraints play in symptom interpretation and care-seeking behavior. Symptoms are conceptualized in the AMI model as "demands" that tax a person's resources and trigger coping responses proposed to occur in four phases: (a) symptom recognition, which includes formulation of a hypothesis about the meaning of the symptom and possible coping strategies; (b) covert construction of an action plan with the intent of restoring equilibrium; (c) overt behavior that implements the action plan (if the overt behavior does not restore equilibrium, then the process is recursive); and (d) assessment and consummation.

Many of the linkages among the variables demonstrate that how we think affects how we feel and function and vice versa (see Figure 22.1). Stress-related variables help us to consider how our perceptions can trigger negative or positive emotions and how emotions affect autonomic and endocrine influences throughout the body. How a person is feeling and doing is not separate from his or her thoughts or emotions (Chapters 9). Appraisal of threat appears to involve a simultaneous activation of biological and psychological system changes. It is accompanied by a systemic arousal produced by the sympathetic nervous system and the hypothalamic-pituitary-adrenocortical axis (HPA) (Chapters 2 and 5). At the same time, depending on the meaning of the situation, stress emotions are triggered along with coping efforts that may in turn alter the physiological and psychological responses (Chapter 9).

It is striking that despite all the research conducted to date, very little has examined the relationship between stress-related variables and subjective health outcomes, including somatic discomfort (e.g., nausea, fatigue, and pain) and functional ability. In particular, because of nursing's concern about comfort and physical performance, it is surprising that nurse researchers have not focused more on the effects of appraised threat, stress emotions, and coping responses on somatic symptoms or functional problems. It is even more surprising when one considers the increasing evidence of a high incidence of chronic stress-related illnesses (including but not limited to somatoform disorders) as noted in Chapters 1, 15, and 21.

Nursing can make a major contribution toward enhancing the experience of wellness and well-being, even in the presence of disease and illness, and therefore increase patients' quality of life and decrease their health care costs. The development of nursing interventions to help patients alter stress-related responses to enhance somatic comfort (psychological, physical, and emotional) and functional ability is essential and should be a priority for the nursing research agenda.

FUTURE DIRECTIONS FOR NURSING THEORY, RESEARCH, AND PRACTICE

Nursing's concern centers on the human experience of "illness" and "wellness." As noted in Chapter 1 and discussed in many other chapters, human beings can experience wellness or illness in the presence or absence of disease. More important, there is sufficient reason, both research-based and anecdotal-based, to propose that middle-range stress-related phenomena, such as stress appraisals, stress emotions, and coping, influence the subjective experience of illness—in other words, how one is feeling and doing. Therefore, it is proposed here that a scientific goal for nursing is the identification of transaction patterns between stress-related variables that predict susceptibility or vulnerability to illness experiences and that predict resilience to stress and enhanced wellness experiences. Specifically, what patterns predict the experience of somatic discomforts, including stress emotions and physical discomforts and declines in functional ability below capability level, or what patterns predict somatic comfort and functional ability at or near capability level? To achieve this goal, we must (1) focus on the development of midrange theories regarding the linkages or patterns among variables (there are many midrange and situation-specific relationships embedded but not explicated in Figure 22.1); (2) develop clear and consistent conceptual and operational definitions of the constructs; (3) develop new or use existing methodologies that allow us to capture recursive, and sometimes simultaneous, changes in variables; (4) use analysis techniques that adequately capture the nature of the relationships or influences that we are proposing; and (5) replicate and extend our nursing research studies to validate our nursing knowledge. Also, it is important that researchers develop programs of research from a nursing perspective (using nursing theories and/or concepts) that will help explicate the patterns of variables that contribute to the experiences of illness, wellness, and QOL (Chapter 17) over the lifespan.

Midrange theories of stress-related variables could include addressing the following questions: What factors contribute to a person being stress resistant or stress vulnerable? For example, does low self-esteem, lack of hardiness, and a pessimistic outlook place a person "at risk" for a stress-related illness in situations in which demands chronically exceed resources? Furthermore, do self-originated demands, such as expecting oneself to measure up to an "ideal" or holding onto unrealistic expectations of others, contribute to stress appraisals and, concomitantly, the stress emotions of guilt and anger? What pattern of variables predicts a threat appraisal over a challenge appraisal? Is the "hardy" person who has high self-esteem with a high degree of personal control, commitment, mastery, social support, and an optimistic disposition more likely to experience demanding or taxing situations as positively toned challenges? How are coping strategies learned? That is, are coping efforts learned through modeling, information, trial and error, or some other method? How do people determine if their coping responses are effective? Are the primary questions considered in determining coping effectiveness the following: (a) was the purpose accomplished and (b) did it not cost too much? Are there other factors? How are self-care behaviors and coping responses similar or different? Which personal and environment factors, in addition to stress emotions and coping, are most likely to lead to specific physical discomforts or functional disability problems?

It is clear that our understanding of how stress-related variables affect health is evolving. However, there is tremendous promise for nursing research, theory, and practice in the area of stress, coping, and health. As we enter the second millennium, the role that nursing can play in helping people experience high-level wellness, even in the presence of disease, or to not experience illness in the absence of disease, will become increasingly important to policymakers and payers of health care services. It is imperative that nursing research efforts not only clearly document the factors or relationships among stress, coping, and health across the life span that are affected by health outcome interventions, but also document the cost–benefit ratio of the outcomes achieved through effective nursing interventions.

In summary, the importance of nursing research in the area of stress, coping, and health continues to grow in this era of managed care and capitated payment for health care services. It is widely recognized that as many as 65% of visits to physician offices are for illnesses that have no discernible medical cause, and many of these illnesses are thought to be stress-related. Furthermore, productivity in the workplace for nurses and other health professionals is greatly affected by the deleterious effects of stress (Chapter 12). Future directions for nursing research will need to focus on (1) the effects of psychological and physiological stress on the somatic sense of self, functional ability, the experience of illness, and aberrant behaviors such as abuse and use of alcohol and drugs; (2) the identification of patterns that predict vulnerability or at-risk status for stress-related illness experiences and aberrant behaviors; (3) intervention studies designed to alter factors that make a person vulnerable to stress-related illnesses across the life span; and (4) intervention studies to evaluate the effects of various stress management strategies, including cognitive restructuring, on stress-related threats and illnesses.

REFERENCES

Lazarus, R. S. (1966). *Psychological stress and the coping process.* New York, NY: McGraw-Hill.

Lazarus, R. S., & Folkman, S. (1984). *Stress, appraisal, and coping.* New York, NY: Springer.

Roger, V. L., Go, G. S., Lloyd-Jones, D. M., Adams, R. J., Berry, J. D., Brown, T. M., . . . Wylie-Rosett, J. (2011). Heart disease and stroke statistics—2011 update: A report from the American Heart Association. *Circulation, 123,* e18–e209.

NAME INDEX

NOTE: Page numbers referring to tables are followed by (table).

SUBJECT INDEX

NOTE: Page numbers referring to tables and figures are followed by (table) and (fig.).

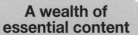
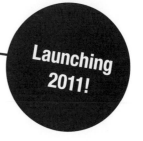
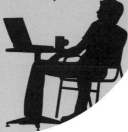
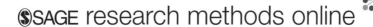